Age-Related Macular Degeneration

Age-Related Macular Degeneration

edited by

Jennifer I. Lim

Doheny Eye Institute
University of Southern California Keck School of Medicine
Los Angeles, California

MARCEL DEKKER, INC.

NEW YORK · BASEL

ISBN: 0-8247-0682-X

This book is printed on acid-free paper.

Headquarters
Marcel Dekker, Inc.
270 Madison Avenue, New York, NY 10016
tel: 212-696-9000; fax: 212-685-4540

Eastern Hemisphere Distribution
Marcel Dekker AG
Hutgasse 4, Postfach 812, CH-4001 Basel, Switzerland
tel: 41-61-260-6300; fax: 41-61-260-6333

World Wide Web
http://www.dekker.com

The publisher offers discounts on this book when ordered in bulk quantities. For more information, write to Special Sales/Professional Marketing at the headquarters address above.

Current printing (last digit)
10 9 8 7 6 5 4 3 2 1

PRINTED IN THE UNITED STATES OF AMERICA

Foreword

Age-related macular degeneration (AMD) has become a scourge of modern, developed societies. In such groups, where improved living conditions and medical care extend human longevity, degeneration of bodily tissues slowly but relentlessly occurs as the life span increases. Sooner or later, the "warranty" on such tissues expires, and so do critically important cells that, in the case of the macula, would have allowed normal visual function if they had survived. Those cells occupy a tiny area having a diameter of only about 2 to 3 mm in human eyes. When the cells lose their function or die and disappear, sharp central visual acuity fails, and lifestyle is compromised—often severely. The ability to read, drive, recognize faces, or watch television can be impaired or lost. This group of diseases—AMD—has become the leading cause of visual impairment in those countries where increasingly large numbers of individuals live to a so-called "ripe old age." Most of these senior citizens had anticipated, with pleasure, the opportunity to enjoy their mature and less frenetic years, but too many of these individuals, ravaged physically and emotionally with AMD, frequently and understandably complain that the golden years are not quite so golden. This is the human and emotional side of AMD, a group of disorders now under intense scientific and clinical scrutiny, as ably summarized herein by Dr. Jennifer Lim and her expert group of coauthors.

The chapters in this book are devoted to pathophysiology, clinical features, diagnostic tests, current and experimental therapies, rehabilitation, and research. They represent what we know today. They also tell us explicitly or by inference what we need to know tomorrow. In effect, they are cross-sectional analyses of the present state of knowledge, analogous to photos in an album, for example. Here, in this book, we have comprehensive, definitive, analytic reviews of the current state of macular affairs. Such albums and books are often informative and beautiful, but they best realize their inherent potential, as does this book, by whetting our appetite for more information, both for today as well as for tomorrow. For example, what are the precise etiology and pathophysiology of AMD? Will they change? What are the best diagnostic tests for different forms of AMD? (Parenthetically, it is historically noteworthy to realize that fluorescein angiography remains the definitive test for diagnosing the presence of choroidal neovascularization and related phenomena in AMD, despite having been developed almost half a century ago.) What are the best therapies of today and how might we improve them in the future? At present, we think primarily of thermal laser photocoagulation and photodynamic therapy.

How can they be enhanced? What roles, if any, will other techniques play? Will they include low-power transpupillary thermal or x-irradiation, antiangiogenic drugs, genetic manipulation, or surgery? Will combinations of these or even newer modalities be demonstrated to be both safe and effective? Will wide-scale population-based preventive measures, including antioxidants, for example, be more important than therapeutic intervention ex post facto?

Clairvoyance is an imperfect attribute, but the largely palliative and incompletely successful treatments of today are quite frustrating. There is a compelling mandate for intense and sustained efforts to improve both treatment and prophylaxis. The crystal ball for AMD suggests that the immediate future will be characterized by refinements in today's favored interventions, especially photodynamic therapy, but no one can really hope or believe that the therapeutic status quo will be preserved. Substantial change is a certainty. Physicians and patients appropriately demand more. The intermediate and long-range future will probably include a large number of definitive clinical trials devoted to fascinating new pharmacological agents, many of which are now in the evaluative pipeline, but many of which have not yet even been conceived. Classes of drugs will include antiangiogenic or angiostatic steroids with glucocorticoid and nonglucocorticoid qualities, as well as diverse agents to bind and inactivate cytokines and chemokines at different points in the angiogenic and vasculogenic cascades. Many will involve blockage of the actions of vascular endothelial growth factor (VEGF). Ingenious surgical approaches will also come, and some will then go, as more and more new approaches of this nature undergo clinical evaluation and gain either widespread acceptance or rejection.

Today's requirements for "evidence-based" medical decisions invoke Darwinian selection processes for numerous known, as well as currently unknown, diagnostic and therapeutic approaches to AMD. Outstandingly good techniques, such as fluorescein angiography, will persist—at least for the foreseeable future. Less desirable ones, such as subfoveal thermal photocoagulation, for example, will be supplanted by something better, such as photodynamic therapy—at least for the moment. The accretion of scientific and clinical knowledge is usually an extremely slow process, but that is not necessarily bad because new ideas and techniques are afforded ample opportunity for dispassionate evaluation. Sudden breakthroughs, on the other hand, intellectual or technical epiphanies, are infrequent. When they do occur—such as angiography, photocoagulation, or intravitreal surgery—they abruptly create quantum leaps characterized by dramatic flourishing of new hypotheses, experiments, and clinical procedures. The world of AMD would benefit from such giant steps (such as a new class of drugs or a new physical modality or type of equipment), but, because they are unpredictable in their origin and timing, we are presently faced with the less spectacular, but important, responsibilities of initiating and sustaining more prosaic, but potentially useful research efforts.

Hopefully, more emphasis in the future will be placed on preventive approaches. Modification of relevant risk factors for AMD may prove to be much more effective, from the perspective of the public health, than therapeutic attempts aimed at a disease that has already achieved a threshold for progressive degeneration and visual impairment. Thus far, epidemiological studies have largely been inconclusive and occasionally contradictory, and we now know of only one clear-cut modifiable risk factor, namely, cigarette smoking (and possibly systemic hypertension).

The influences of race and heredity remain tantalizing, and it will be important to understand why some races are protected from severe visual loss in AMD and why others are not. Moreover, the major influence of heredity is inescapable, but we now know only that this influence is complex, and it may be even more complex than anticipated because of a multiplicity of unknown contributory environmental and other genetic factors. We do know the genes responsible for a previously enigmatic group of juvenile forms of inherited macular degeneration, such as the eponymously interesting diseases named for Best, Stargardt, Doyne, and Sorsby, but there appears to be no universally accepted or substantive relationship between any of these single-gene, rare Mendelian traits and the far more common AMD, which has no clear-cut Mendelian transmission pattern, but currently affects millions of aging individuals.

The march of time related to scientific progress is ceaseless, and this is certainly true of research related to AMD. Darwinian selection of the best new ideas will inevitably emerge, allowing an evolutionary approach to enhanced understanding and improved treatment or prophylaxis. Should we be fortunate enough to witness a bona fide revolution or breakthrough in ideas related to AMD, such an advance is likely to emanate from those scientists and clinicians meeting Louis Pasteur's observation that "chance favors the prepared mind." It is toward that goal—the creation of the prepared mind—that Dr. Lim has fashioned this valuable compendium of the way things are—for now!!

Morton F. Goldberg, M.D.
Director and William Holland Wilmer Professor of Ophthalmology
The Wilmer Eye Institute
Baltimore, Maryland

Preface

Age-related macular degeneration (AMD) remains one of the most enigmatic diagnoses for elderly patients. Over the past two decades, there has been significant progress in the pathophysiology and treatment of AMD. These research strides have resulted in novel therapies that offer not only sight-saving, less destructive forms of treatment for exudative AMD but also treatment to prevent progression of nonexudative AMD. The purpose of this book is to summarize and synthesize in a single resource this information for clinicians and scientists involved in AMD patient care and research. I have asked retinal experts first to summarize established information and then to present the recent developments in their specific areas of AMD research.

It is important to understand how the normal eye ages. In Part I, Chapter 1 focuses on aging-related changes of the retina and retinal pigment epithelium and compares them with the retinal findings of AMD. Chapter 2 presents the light and electron microscopic findings of AMD to facilitate understanding of its ultrastructural pathophysiology. Such an understanding is useful in directing future areas of research toward a cure for AMD. Chapter 3 elucidates immunological aspects of AMD. This avenue of research may offer clues to the pathophysiology of AMD and point to potential new treatments.

Part II focuses on clinical features of nonexudative and exudative AMD, which are discussed with respect to the natural history and prognosis for vision. This information is useful for the clinician who frequently must provide information to the patient regarding prognosis.

Evaluation of the patient and planning treatment for AMD is aided by imaging techniques. Part III discusses imaging techniques, such as OCT, which are helpful not only for evaluating the patient but also for making objective assessments of treatment outcome. Application of OCT to animal and clinical research studies helps to determine efficacy outcomes objectively. Continued application of ICG angiography to the evaluation of AMD patients has led to refinements in the diagnosis of AMD and to ICG-based laser treatments for choroidal neovascularization (CNV) lesions. Chapter 7 summarizes the current state of knowledge about the application of ICG angiography to diagnosis and treatment of AMD.

Parts IV to VI of this book present the current and experimental forms of treatment for nonexudative and exudative forms of AMD. Much progress in the area of AMD research has occurred since the MPS study first began over 20 years ago. Thus, the clinical application of the MPS data is updated in light of the availability of newer, less destructive forms of therapy for CNV. Refinements in the application of laser photocoagulation, such as feeder-vessel treatment and subthreshold laser, have contributed to new applications for thermal laser for AMD.

The past decade has witnessed the genesis of novel therapies for CNV, which range from photodynamic therapy, radiation therapy, transpupillary thermotherapy, and anti-angiogenesis drugs to submacular surgery and macular translocation. Discussions of the basic mechanism of action, clinical treatment technique, target patient population, expected outcomes, and both positive and negative aspects of the treatment are included.

When possible, comparisons between the results of the different treatments are drawn. Known risk factors for AMD progression are discussed, as well as the recent Age-Related Eye Disease Study (AREDS) finding of risk reduction through micronutrient supplementation.

Basic science research followed by its application to clinical trials is the mode by which new treatments for AMD are created. Part VII of this book focuses upon active areas of basic science research that may lead to clinical trials in the near future. The future application of genetics research to gene therapy for AMD may be curative and/or preventative for younger patients possessing the gene for AMD. Retinal pigment cell transplantation research may lead to future treatments that reverse damage from AMD. The discussion of these future treatments is intriguing and presents new hope for the future generations afflicted with AMD.

Despite the progress in AMD research and the attendant clinical applications, in reality there still exist patients with visual loss and untreatable disease. For these patients, visual rehabilitation is extremely important. A discussion of the available low-vision devices and the psychosocial aspects of visual loss from AMD is included to help counsel patients with AMD and visual loss. The possibility of using an intraocular retinal prosthesis to restore vision in the future is intriguing and this area of research is presented. The prosthesis may represent the ultimate low-vision device for patients with AMD and vision loss.

Throughout the book, clinical trials data are summarized. Clinical trials remain the gold standard for proving clinical efficacy of a new treatment. Part VIII discusses the design of clinical research trials and quality-of-life assessments. The importance of quality-of-life assessments as part of clinical research outcome measurements is now recognized.

No single volume can present all the existing knowledge about AMD. Thus, only the most clinically useful and exciting research information was included in this book. My goal is for this book to serve as a first-hand resource for researchers and clinicians in the area of AMD. My contributors and I hope we have achieved this and that the information presented herein will inspire inquiry and ignite research that may unearth answers to those enigmatic questions about the etiology of and cure for AMD.

I wish to thank all the outstanding contributors, without whom this book would not be possible. Their eagerness to collaborate and their expertise made my job as editor extremely enjoyable, educational, and satisfying. I am grateful to Onita Morgan-Edwards and Charlotte Kler for their efficient and accurate secretarial assistance, and to the staff at Marcel Dekker, Inc., for their great help in compiling this book.

I dedicate this book to my parents, to my husband, John Miao, and to our daughter, Bernadette, who was with me (in utero) during the preparation and editing of most of this book.

Jennifer I. Lim

Contents

VII. Rehabilitation of the Eye

VIII. Development of Research Protocols in AMD

Contributors

Kah-Guan Au Eong, M.D. Wilmer Eye Institute, Johns Hopkins University School of Medicine, Baltimore, Maryland

Jeffrey W. Berger, M.D. Scheie Eye Institute, University of Pennsylvania Health System, Philadelphia, Pennsylvania

Audina M. Berrocal, M.D. Bascom Palmer Eye Institute, Miami, Florida

Neelakshi Bhagat, M.D. Doheny Eye Institute, University of Southern California Keck School of Medicine, Los Angeles, California

Mark S. Blumenkranz, M.D. Professor and Chairman, Vitreoretinal and Macular Diseases, Department of Ophthalmology, Stanford University School of Medicine, Stanford, California

Peter A. Campochiaro, M.D. George S. and Delores Dore Eccles Professor of Ophthalmology and Neuroscience, Department of Ophthalmology, Wilmer Eye Institute, Johns Hopkins University School of Medicine, Baltimore, Maryland

Thomas S. Chang, M.D., M.H.Sc., F.R.C.S.(C) Associate Professor of Ophthalmology, Doheny Retina Institute of the Doheny Eye Institute, University of Southern California Keck School of Medicine, Los Angeles, California

Lawrence P. Chong, M.D. Associate Professor of Ophthalmology, Doheny Retina Institute of the Doheny Eye Institute, University of Southern California Keck School of Medicine, Los Angeles, California

Antonio P. Ciardella, M.D. Doheny Eye Institute, University of Southern California Keck School of Medicine, Los Angeles, California

Michael J. Cooney, M.D. Assistant Professor, Vitreoretinal Department, Duke University Eye Center, Durham, North Carolina

Scott W. Cousins, M.D. Associate Professor, Department of Ophthalmology, Bascom Palmer Eye Institute, University of Miami, Miami, Florida

Karl G. Csaky, M.D., Ph.D. Investigator, National Eye Institute, National Institutes of Health, Bethesda, Maryland

Eugene de Juan, Jr., M.D. Professor of Ophthalmology, Department of Ophthalmology, Doheny Retina Institute of the Doheny Eye Institute, University of Southern California Keck School of Medicine, Los Angeles, California

Lucian V. Del Priore, M.D., Ph.D. Robert L. Burch III Scholar, Department of Ophthalmology, Columbia University, New York, New York

Joshua L. Dunaief, M.D., Ph.D. Scheie Eye Institute, University of Pennsylvania Health System, Philadelphia, Pennsylvania

Jacque L. Duncan, Ph.D. Scheie Eye Institute, University of Pennsylvania Health System, Philadelphia, Pennsylvania

Stuart L. Fine, M.D. William F. Norris and George E. De Schweinitz Professor and Chairman, Department of Ophthalmology, and Director, Scheie Eye Institute, University of Pennsylvania Health System, Philadelphia, Pennsylvania

Paul Finger, M.D. New York AMDRT Center, New York, New York

Christina J. Flaxel, M.D. Assistant Professor of Ophthalmology, Doheny Retina Institute of the Doheny Eye Institute, University of Southern California Keck School of Medicine, Los Angeles, California

Robert W. Flower, D.Sc. Professor, Department of Ophthalmology, New York University School of Medicine, New York, New York, and Associate Professor, Department of Ophthalmology, University of Maryland School of Medicine, Baltimore, Maryland

K. Bailey Freund, M.D. Manhattan Eye, Ear, and Throat Hospital, New York, New York

Thomas R. Friberg, M.D., F.A.C.S. Professor, Department of Ophthalmology, University of Pittsburgh, Pittsburgh, Pennsylvania

Gildo Y. Fujii, M.D. Doheny Retina Institute of the Doheny Eye Institute, University of Southern California Keck School of Medicine, Los Angeles, California

David R. Guyer, M.D. Manhattan Eye, Ear, and Throat Hospital, New York, New York

Julia A. Haller, M.D. Associate Professor, Department of Ophthalmology, Wilmer Eye Institute, Johns Hopkins University School of Medicine, Baltimore, Maryland

David R. Hinton, M.D., F.R.C.P. (C) Professor, Doheny Eye Institute, University of Southern California Keck School of Medicine, Los Angeles, California

Allen C. Ho, M.D. Associate Professor, Wills Eye Hospital, Thomas Jefferson University School of Medicine, Philadelphia, Pennsylvania

Mark S. Humayun, M.D. Professor, Doheny Retina Institute of the Doheny Eye Institute, University of Southern California Keck School of Medicine, Los Angeles, California

Frances E. Kane, Ph.D. Senior Director, Clinical Sciences, Novartis Ophthalmics, Inc., Duluth, Georgia

Henry J. Kaplan, M.D. Professor and Chairman, Department of Ophthalmology and Visual Sciences, University of Louisville, Louisville, Kentucky

Jennifer I. Lim, M.D. Associate Professor of Ophthalmology, Doheny Retina Institute of the Doheny Eye Institute, University of Southern California Keck School of Medicine, Los Angeles, California

Paul J. Mackenzie, Ph.D. Department of Ophthalmology, University of British Columbia, Vancouver, British Columbia, Canada

Eyal Margalit Wilmer Eye Institute, Johns Hopkins University School of Medicine, Baltimore, Maryland

Adam Martidis, M.D. Assistant Professor of Ophthalmology, Wills Eye Hospital, Thomas Jefferson University School of Medicine, Philadelphia, Pennsylvania

Frank J. McCabe, M.D. Retina Consultants of Worcester, Worcester, Massachusetts

Dennis Orlock, C.R.A. Manhattan Eye, Ear, and Throat Hospital, New York, New York

Dante J. Pieramici, M.D. Co-Director, California Retina Research Foundation, Santa Barbara, California, and Assistant Professor, Wilmer Eye Institute, Johns Hopkins University School of Medicine, Baltimore, Maryland

Susan A. Primo, O.D. Assistant Professor, Department of Ophthalmology, Emory University School of Medicine, Atlanta, Georgia

Narsing A. Rao, M.D. Professor, Doheny Eye Institute, University of Southern California Keck School of Medicine, Los Angeles, California

P. Kumar Rao, M.D. Department of Ophthalmology, Barnes Retina Institute, Washington University, St. Louis, Missouri

Elias Reichel, M.D. Associate Professor of Ophthalmology and Director, Vitreoretinal Diseases and Surgery, New England Eye Center, Tufts University School of Medicine, Boston, Massachusetts

Mark J. Rivellese, M.D. New England Eye Center, Tufts University School of Medicine, Boston, Massachusetts

Adam H. Rogers, M.D. Assistant Professor of Ophthalmology, New England Eye Center, Tufts University School of Medicine, Boston, Massachusetts

Philip J. Rosenfeld, M.D., Ph.D. Assistant Professor, Department of Ophthalmology, Bascom Palmer Eye Institute, University of Miami School of Medicine, Miami, Florida

Brian D. Sippy, M.D., Ph.D.   Associate Professor, Department of Ophthalmology, Emory University, Atlanta, Georgia

Jason S. Slakter, M.D.   Manhattan Eye, Ear, and Throat Hospital, New York, New York

Sharon D. Solomon, M.D.   Retinal Vascular Center, Wilmer Eye Institute, Johns Hopkins University School of Medicine, Baltimore, Maryland

John A. Sorenson, M.D.   Manhattan Eye, Ear, and Throat Hospital, New York, New York

Richard F. Spaide, M.D.   Manhattan Eye, Ear, and Throat Hospital, New York, New York

Janet S. Sunness, M.D.   Associate Professor, Department of Ophthalmology, Wilmer Eye Institute, Johns Hopkins University School of Medicine, Baltimore, Maryland

Tongalp H. Tezel, M.D.   Department of Ophthalmology, Columbia University, New York, New York

Matthew A. Thomas, M.D.   Associate Professor, Department of Ophthalmology, Barnes Retina Institute, Washington University, St. Louis, Missouri

Gretchen B. Van Boemel, Ph.D.   Doheny Retina Institute of the Doheny Eye Institute, Univesity of Southern California Keck School of Medicine, Los Angeles, California

Rohit Varma, M.D., M.P.H.   Associate Professor, Doheny Eye Institute, University of Southern California Keck School of Medicine, Los Angeles, California

A. Frances Walonker, M.P.H.   Clinical Instructor, Department of Ophthalmology, Doheny Eye Institute, University of Southern California Keck School of Medicine, Los Angeles, California

James D. Weiland, Ph.D.   Assistant Professor, Department of Ophthalmology, Doheny Retina Institute of the Doheny Eye Institute, University of Southern California Keck School of Medicine, Los Angeles, California

Kathryn W. Woodburn, M.D.   AP Pharma, Redwood City, California

Lawrence A. Yannuzzi, M.D.   Manhattan Eye, Ear, and Throat Hospital, New York, New York

Jonathan Yoken, M.D.   Scheie Eye Institute, University of Pennsylvania Health System, Philadelphia, Pennsylvania

Ehud Zamir, M.D.   Assistant Professor, Department of Ophthalmology, Hadassah–Hebrew University Medical School, Jerusalem, Israel

1
Aging of Retina and Retinal Pigment Epithelium

Brian D. Sippy
Emory University, Atlanta, Georgia

David R. Hinton
Doheny Eye Institute, University of Southern California Keck School of Medicine, Los Angeles, California

I. INTRODUCTION

It has been said that as soon as we are born, we begin dying. This rather discouraging adage, however, does embody the theory that aging is a chronic process defined by endogenous programming and exogenous factors. It is a challenging task to separate the universal effects of aging on the human condition from those of disease. In extreme age, the boundaries of normal and disease are obscured. This chapter attempts to define the changes that occur with aging in the retina and retinal pigment epithelium (RPE) in the vast majority of humans and that are not specifically found in the diseased eye. Emphasis will be given to the macular region to facilitate the comparison of age-related changes to changes associated with age-related macular degeneration.

To fully understand a disease that seems to be specific to the human macula, it is essential to understand the normal aging processes that affect this tissue. Yet, we are limited by biased population studies representing only certain people and by the ethical restriction associated with the study of human subjects. Animal models have been pursued to elicit the underlying mechanisms of age-related macular degeneration (ARMD), but they are just that, models. Because of the complexities of interspecies differences, data from nonhuman models have been minimized here.

II. EMBRYOLOGY

The primitive eye begins development near the end of the fourth week of embryogenesis. On the rostral end of the neutral tube, two optic pits form and then develop into the optic vesicle and optic stalk. As this outpouching from the neural tube approaches the surface ectoderm, it buckles inward to form the optic cup. The invagination process is quite asymmetrical, allowing for the formation of the choroidal fissure. This choroidal fissure is accompanied by growth of a primitive blood vessel that enters along the underside of the optic stalk and proceeds anteriorly to reach the rim of the cup and primitive lens. This vessel eventually gives rise to the hyaloid artery and later the central retinal artery. The choroidal fissure closes by the end of the fifth or sixth week of gestation, and the basic form of the eye has taken shape. The optic cup and optic stalk represent the beginnings of the future retina and optic nerve, respectively. The inner layer of the optic cup forms the sensory retina, including neurons and glial cells. This inner retinal layer terminates anteriorly at the ora serrata, but it is continuous with the layers of the nonpigmented ciliary body epithelium and the posterior pigmented iris epithelium. The outer layer of the optic cup will form the RPE that extends anteriorly also to the ora serrata, and it is continuous with the pigmented ciliary body epithelium and the anterior pigmented iris epithelium. Posterior to the ora serrata, the sensory retina and the RPE are separated only by a potential space filled with the interphotoreceptor matrix (1).

III. GROWTH AND AGING

A definite challenge exists in separating functional or anatomical changes related to normal aging and those seen in age-associated disease. This is particularly true for the retina and RPE. This highly specialized tissue is exposed to environmental stressors not typically encountered by other neural tissues. By its design to enhance vision, the retina functions to maximize the capture of photon radiation. Lifelong function in this actinic environment may accentuate the normal aging process, a term referred to as photoaging (2, 3). Thus, knowledge we have acquired regarding aging of other neural tissues, such as the central nervous system, may not directly apply to the retina (4).

Many elderly adults experience attenuation in their ability to function effectively and independently. Such a decline is multifactorial and includes impairment of vision. Nearly every assessment of visual function has been shown to diminish later in life. Decreased visual acuity, visual field, contrast sensitivity, motion perception, and dark adaptation are all recognized deficits found in elderly patients (5–7). However, it must be kept in mind that many of the tests commonly employed to assess visual function do not take into account age-related decline. The aging nervous system appears to recover more slowly from the effects of visual stimulation, compatible with an overall slowing in processing time (8).

A. Sensory Retina

The human neural retina is almost fully developed at birth. The fovea contains most of the retinal layers but is incompletely differentiated. The fovea and macula complete their maturation in the first few months of life. The peripheral retina, especially near the ora serrata, is slower to develop and sometimes displays a Lange's fold histologically in premature or newborn infants (9). Macular pigments are essentially absent during the first 2 years of life. As the pigment accrues, the macula takes on a yellow hue, giving this area a distinct clinical appearance. Relative hypofluorescence of the macular region on fluorescein angiography may be partly due to these pigments (10). Macular pigment consists primarily of lipid-soluble carotenoids, including lutein and zeaxanthin. These substances are photically inert and have antioxidant properties (11–14).

The mature sensory retina is a delicate, transparent structure firmly attached at the ora serrata anteriorly and at the optic nerve head posteriorly. The neural retina is composed of nine layers, from the outside inward, of (1) the photoreceptor cell outer and inner segments; (2) the external limiting membrane; (3) the outer nuclear layer containing photoreceptor nuclei; (4) the outer plexiform layer; (5) the inner nuclear layer containing nuclei of horizontal cells, bipolar cells, amacrine cells, and Müller cells; (6) the inner plexiform layer; (7) the ganglion cell layer; (8) the nerve fiber layer; and (9) the internal limiting membrane (ILM) (Fig. 1).

The ILM is the innermost layer of the sensory retina that is in direct contact with the vitreous. The ILM is normally attenuated or absent over the optic nerve head. The vitreous

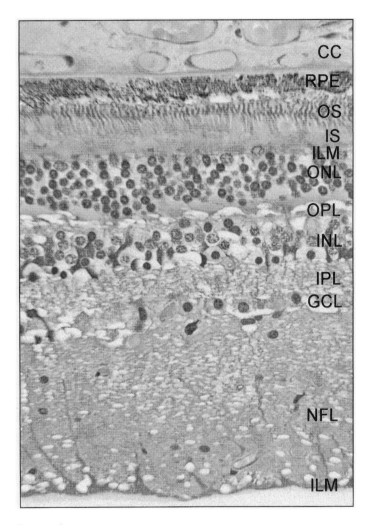

Figure 1 Photomicrograph of normal retina obtained from 59-year-old with no known ocular disease. Tissue embedded in glycol methacrylate and cut at 3 microns. Section stained with 1% toluidine blue. The identified retinal layers are the internal limiting membrane (ILM), nerve fiber layer (NFL), ganglion cell layer (GCL), inner plexiform layer (IPL), inner nuclear layer (INL), outer plexiform layer (OPL), outer nuclear layer (ONL), inner limiting membrane (ILM), inner segments of photoreceptors (IS), and outer segments of photoreceptors (OS). External to the retina is the retinal pigment epithelial cell layer (RPE) and choriocapillaris (CC), separated by Bruch's membrane.

is attached to and blends with the ILM through fine collagenous fibrils. This attachment is firm in young persons, but with increasing age and vitreous liquefaction, the connections become tenuous, leading to posterior vitreous detachment (PVD) in 63% of individuals over 70 years of age (15). The ILM is primarily composed of basement membrane formed by Müller cell footplate processes. Occasionally, this basal lamina is composed of astrocytic processes and broad, flat cells containing rod-shaped nuclei. The latter probably represent vitreous hyalocytes that have migrated into the ILM. Müller cells hypertrophy with age with associated thickening of their basal lamina. Heegaard has reported that fetal ILM is very thin, being thickest in the macular region, and that adult ILM is slightly thicker with regional differences (16). Others have shown that ILM increases in thickness to age 57 years, and then decreases in thickness and increases in density to age 82 years (17).

The nerve fiber layer is primarily composed of axons from the retinal ganglion cells, but it does contain a few neuroglial cells. The axons radiate toward the optic disk, and the nerve fiber layer thickens as axons converge. With increasing age, there is a progressive reduction in nerve fiber layer thickness (18, 19). This thinning is coincident with the loss of ganglion cells with age; thus, it may represent loss of axons (20). In addition, degenerated cellular material accumulates in the nerve fiber layer with increasing age. Corpora amylacea are small, noncalcified, occasionally laminated spheroids that stain poorly with hematoxylin and eosin (H&E) and stain prominently with periodic acid-Schiff (PAS) and Alcian blue. Corpora amylacea have been found in the peripapillary nerve fiber layer. Electron microscopy has shown that these inclusions are intra-axonal organelles consisting of neurotubules, mitochondria, and dense bodies (21, 22).

The retinal ganglion cell layer contains the cell bodies, including nuclei, of the ganglion cells. These third-order afferent neurons extend axons into the nerve fiber layer and extend dendrites into the inner plexiform layer that synapse with neurons of the inner nuclear layer. Between 14 and 24 weeks of gestation the ganglion cell layer and inner nuclear layer undergo precise differentiation to create a topography that maximizes macular function (23). In the fovea, ganglion cell nuclei and inner nuclear layer cells are displaced circumferentially to enhance the transmission of light into the outer retina. In the parafoveal area, the ganglion cells are numerous, forming a layer up to eight cells deep. Elsewhere in the retina, the ganglion cell layer is mostly a single-cell layer. Lipofuscin, the so-called pigment of aging, is a complex matrix of partially degraded cellular elements that accrues within aging cells. Lipofuscin has been shown to accumulate in retinal neurons, including ganglion cells (24). Because lipofuscin is capable of photogenerating a variety of reactive oxygen species, accrual of this substance in cells exposed to light could potentially lead to neuronal demise (25, 26). Indeed, Barreau et al. have demonstrated mitochondrial DNA deletions consistent with oxidative damage within the adult neural retina but not the fetal retina (27). Others have not confirmed an age-related increase in mitochondrial DNA deletions in retina but have noted that the level of these deletions in retina is less than in optic nerve or susceptible regions of brain (28). With increasing age, there is evidence for up to 25% loss in the number of ganglion cells in certain retinal locations (20).

The inner plexiform layer is composed of a fine reticulum of axons and dendrites. The primary synapses found in this layer are those of bipolar cells and amacrine cells with ganglion cells. Age changes found in the ganglion cell layer and the inner nuclear layer would likely impact the delicate inner plexiform layer; however, no human studies have addressed this phenomenon.

The inner nuclear layer is a uniformly dense mass of cells consisting of neuronal and glial cell bodies and nuclei. Three types of neurons have been identified in this layer.

Amacrine cells are pear-shaped cells that lie at the inner aspect of the inner nuclear layer. Their processes extend primarily into the inner plexiform layer where they synapse with bipolar cells and dendrites of ganglion cells. Bipolar cells are found throughout the inner nuclear layer; and, as their name implies, they send processes both to the inner plexiform layer to synapse with ganglion cells and to the outer plexiform layer to synapse with photoreceptor cells. In the fovea, the ratio of photoreceptor cell, bipolar cell and ganglion cell synapses approaches 1:1:1 to enhance resolution of spatial and temporal stimulation. The horizontal cells reside in the outer aspect of the inner nuclear layer and have complex arborizing processes that extend primarily into the outer plexiform layer, where they synapse with bipolar cells and spherules and peduncles of rod and cone axons. Complex signaling and editing converts photic stimulation into reportable imagery (29). Müller cells, which are also found in the inner nuclear layer, send processes to the inner aspect of the retina to form the ILM and to the outer aspect of the retina to form the external limiting membrane. The inner nuclear layer specifically has not been studied with regard to aging. However, neurons in this layer have demonstrated accumulation of lipofuscin and, therefore, may be susceptible to oxidative damage.

The outer plexiform layer consists of fine processes of photoreceptor cells and bipolar and horizontal cell synapses. In the macular region, this layer takes on a specialized architecture to enhance visual resolution. The axons and dendrites are elongated and radiate outward from the fovea to form the fiber layer of Henle. This allows for lateral displacement of nuclei that could scatter light entering the foveal region.

The outer nuclear layer is composed of eight or nine layers of densely packed nuclei and cell bodies of the rod and cone photoreceptor cells. With H&E stain, the two kinds of cells can be differentiated by nuclear morphology. The rods tend to have smaller, more densely stained nuclei, and the cones have larger, weakly staining nuclei that tend to reside just internal to the external limiting membrane. Occasionally, the photoreceptor nuclei are displaced outside of the external limiting membrane. This migration may represent a normal variant associated with age-related change (30), but it has been suggested that this displacement may be associated with cellular demise (31).

Curcio and colleagues have helped define normal human photoreceptor topography and changes in this mosaic that occur with age. They have reported that the number of rods in the human retina ranges from 78 to 107 million and that there is a preferential loss of rods with aging (32, 33). A loss of up to 30% of rods in the central retina was seen in grossly normal eyes (34). Cone numbers in the macula remain relatively stable between the ages of 40 and 65 years (35). With progressing age, cone numbers eventually decline. By the age of 90 years, a 40% reduction in cones has been reported (36). Theoretically, however, this reduction in the number of photoreceptors would not be sufficient to account for age-associated decline in visual acuity. In the foveal region, photoreceptor density approximates 200,000 cells/mm^2. These densely packed cells are primarily cones, but with a specialized architecture that resembles rods. The density of these cones in the fovea causes an inward bowing of the sensory retina, anatomically referred to as the umbo (37).

The external limiting membrane is not a true membrane. It is, instead, formed by adhesions that fuse Müller cells with photoreceptor inner segments. A junctional complex of this nature is referred to as the zonula adherens. Age-related cellular changes may lead to weakening of this pseudomembrane, allowing for subtle architectural and perhaps functional variation.

Photoreceptor inner and outer segments extend beyond the external limiting membrane and represent the outermost aspect of the neural retina. The inner segments of cones are large and contain organelles and numerous mitochondria, whereas rods have long cylindrical inner segments with fewer mitochondria. Scanning electron microscopy clearly demonstrates the morphological differences between cone and rod inner segments, and it has been used to evaluate photoreceptor populations and distribution.

Rod photoreceptors possess long outer segments that reach the apex of the RPE cells. The outer segments consist of stacked disks. These disks are formed near the junction of the inner and outer segments and mature as they approach the distal tip of the outer segment. Disks are shed at the end of the outer segment and are phagocytosed by RPE cells (38). Morphological changes in rod outer segments have been demonstrated in the aging human retina (39). Aged rod outer segments undergo hypertrophy and an increase in length secondary to the buildup of mismanaged disks. At the distal tip of the outer segment, the disks fold back into the outer segment, leading to a disorganization of the internal structure. Rod outer-segment disks contain rhodopsin that is responsible for photon capture. Recent studies have shown that rhodopsin content in the human retina increases from preterm to approximately 6 months of age and then is stable (40). Despite the loss of rod photoreceptors with age, rhodopsin levels remain stable, perhaps as a result of the hypertrophy and convolution of disks in the remaining rods.

The outer segments of cones are typically shorter than rods and do not extend to the apical surface of the RPE. Instead, the RPE cells send long apical processes or microvilli to encompass the cone outer segments. Outer segments of the specialized foveal cones are long and approach the apex of underlying RPE cells. As with rods, cone outer segments are composed of stacked disks. Cone disks taper in diameter as they approach the distal end, where they are shed. Cone outer segments and, to a lesser extent, rod outer segments accumulate lipofuscin material after the age of 30 years (41). In contrast to rods, foveal cone outer segments show no alteration in outer-segment length with age. And unlike rhodopsin in rods, there is a decline in cone visual pigments after the fifth decade of life (42, 43).

B. Retinal Circulation

The retinal circulation is derived from a primitive fibrovascular ingrowth within the choroidal fissure. As the hyaloid artery regresses, the primary vascular arcade of the retina remains. The vascular architecture achieves an adult pattern approximately 5 months after birth. Retinal vessels provide oxygen and nutrients to the inner aspect of the neural retina. Capillary beds have been demonstrated in layers from the nerve fiber layer outward to the inner nuclear layer (44). On the contrary, the outer retina derives its oxygen and nutrients from the choroid and choriocapillaris.

Aging changes in retinal vessels, including arteriosclerosis, are similar to those found elsewhere in the body. But the retinal circulation is analogous to the cerebral circulation in that it maintains a functional barrier, the blood-retinal barrier. Within the retina, at the capillary level, there is a diffuse loss of cellularity with age. Typically, endothelial cells maintain a one-to-one relationship with pericytes; however, in the aged eye, there is a loss of endothelial cells followed by a loss of pericytes, leading in some cases to an acellular vascular channel (45). In a rigid acellular state, there could be perturbation in the autoregulation of retinal circulation, as seen with the cerebral blood flow in elderly patients (46).

Cellular loss combined with hyalinization and thickening of the pericyte basement membrane leads to narrowing of vascular lumens. Narrowing diminishes retinal microcirculatory flow and thus tissue perfusion (47, 48). In the macular region, blood flow may decline as much as 20% in people more than 50 years old (49).

In the center of the macula, there is a capillary-free zone functioning to enhance visual acuity. This area typically measures 300–500 μm and is an important landmark on fluorescein angiography. There is a decrease in total capillary number in the macula with age, and this corresponds with an increase in size of the foveal capillary-free zone (50, 51).

C. Interphotoreceptor Matrix

The interphotoreceptor matrix (IPM) fills the potential space between the photoreceptor cells and the RPE. It is an exceptionally stable and unusual extracellular matrix (ECM) that actively supports retinal function by housing specialized molecules involved in retinoid exchange, disk phagocytosis, and stabilization of the photoreceptor mosaic. The IPM contains no collagen, elastin, laminin, or fibrocytes. It does contain an abundance of interphotoreceptor retinoid binding protein (IRBP), synthesized by RPE cells. Enzymes responsible for turnover of the IPM, such as matrix metalloproteinases (MMP) and tissue inhibitor of metalloproteinases (TIMPs), have been recently described in human IPM. These enzymes may be impacted by aging, resulting in perturbed function of the adjacent neural retina or RPE (52). Hyaluronan has recently been detected in human IPM and displays unique properties of resistance to degradation by hyaluronidase digestion (53). Rod and cone outer segments are encased with cell-specific sheaths of ECM, which implies an active role for the photoreceptors in creating and maintaining the IPM (54, 55). Müller cells extend fine processes external to the external limiting membrane to reside between the inner segments of rods and cones. These glial extensions may also contribute to the formation of the IPM (56).

D. Retinal Pigment Epithelium

In contrast to the structural and cellular complexity of sensory retina, the RPE represents a unicellular tissue that is easily identified grossly and histologically based on its innate pigmentation and sheet-like integrity. The hardy nature of the RPE cell also allows for predictable culturing and in vitro experimentation. Most of this report thus far has minimized discussion of animal or cell culture models. However, in recent years, there has been an explosion of research conducted to improve our understanding of function and dysfunction in the context of macular degeneration pathophysiology. To be more inclusive, although we risk speculation, we have included below references to works that address some of the current interests in RPE culture research.

Polarity provides the RPE cell with a foundation of function (57). The apical surfaces of the RPE cells are tightly bound by junctional complexes, also known as zonulae occludentes (58). This pseudomembrane limits the movement of molecules to and from the sensory retina and the choroidal circulation, making the RPE the most essential effector of controlled exchange between these two compartments. In the inner aspect of the zonulae occludentes, the RPE cell membrane is bathed in IPM. Just to the outer aspect of the zonulae occludentes, there is a narrow space along the lateral aspect of the RPE cells. The basal surface of the RPE cells contains prominent infoldings that increase membrane surface area.

The RPE is a monolayer of regularly arranged hexagonal cells that spans the retina from the margin of the optic disk anteriorly to the ora serrata. Several studies have evaluated the morphology and density of RPE cells within the human retina. Harman et al. have recently reviewed the literature and have suggested various pitfalls in evaluating the human RPE (59). They conclude that there is an increase in retinal area until approximately 30 years of age, no change in RPE cell number between the ages of 12 and 89 years, and an overall decrease in RPE cell density between the ages of 12 and 40 years. These find-ings of a stable cell number and decreased cell density imply that early in life the RPE monolayer uniformly underlies the sensory retina and that as the eye grows and the sensory retina expands to cover the increased surface area, the RPE cells spread out rather than di-vide to cover the increased area. This spreading phenomenon appears to be heterogeneous with preservation of central macular density and dramatic change in the peripheral areas (Fig. 1) (59, p. 2020).

RPE cells establish higher density in the macula early in development and reach adult levels by 6 months of age (60, 61). No mitotic figures have been observed in the macular RPE after birth, so density preservation is likely secondary to differential spreading and not replenishment through replication. Actually, RPE cell density in the human macula may in-crease with extreme age, representing a structural change in the RPE monolayer that allows tissue contraction and a change in cell morphology from regular hexagons to less regular polygons (59, 62). RPE cell culture models from young and old donors have suggested that extracellular matrix enzymes may be influenced by age (52). Recent molecular studies us-ing microarray analysis on senescent human RPE cell culture suggest that these cells may have diminished capacity to form and maintain extracellular matrix and structural proteins with a potential impact on monolayer architecture (63).

The individual RPE cell architecture reflects the complexity of functions that these cells perform. An extensive review of RPE cellular structure and function is presented in *The Retinal Pigment Epithelium: Function and Disease* (64). As mentioned earlier, the api-cal surface of the RPE cell extends microvilli to encompass the rod and cone outer seg-ments. The microvilli function to increase cellular surface area and to maintain biochemi-cal relations with the photoreceptor cells. In particular, the apex of the RPE cells is responsible for the phagocytosis of shed photoreceptor outer-segment disks, forming phagosomes in the apical RPE cell cytoplasm. The eventual fate of the phagosome is to be incorporated into the lysosomal system for degradation and partial recycling. Cathepsin D is an important protease involved in digestion of the rhodopsin-rich disk membranes. Age-associated change in enzymatic activity within the lysosomal system could adversely affect processing of the shed photoreceptor membrane material. Perturbation of cathepsin D, or other catabolic enzyme systems such as ubiquitination, may lead to the buildup of intracel-lular and extracellular debris (65, 66).

The apical cytoplasm also contains numerous pigment granules, primarily consisting of melanin. The RPE appears to be completely melanized at birth with minimal to no melanin granule formation thereafter (67). Melanin density is greatest in the macula and particularly in the fovea, and this concentrated pigment is believed to contribute to the rel-ative hypofluorescence of the macula and fovea in angiography (10, 68). Melanin, inde-pendent of or together with phagosomes, may become incorporated into the lysosomal sys-tem, creating melanolysosomes or melanolipofuscin, respectively (69). With age, there would be an expected decrease in melanin concentration if no new granules were produced while some granules were modified or degraded. Clinically, the RPE of aged eyes appears less pigmented than that of younger eyes. Feeney-Bums et al. reported a progressive de-pletion of RPE melanin in all topographical areas of the human retina, including the mac-ula (70). Two years later, it was reported that melanin concentrations in the human macula were stable from 14 to 97 years of age (71). Controversy still surrounds the topic of RPE pigmentary changes associated with aging.

The outer compartment of the cytoplasm houses the nucleus, abundant mitochondria, extensive endoplasmic reticulum, and lysosomal storage deposits, including lipofuscin or lipofuscin-like material (72). With increasing age, lipofuscin accumulates in the RPE in an apparent biphasic pattern, with one peak occurring between 10 and 20 years of age and the second peak occurring around 50 years of age (70, 73). Lipofuscin buildup is greatest in the posterior pole, especially the macula but sparing the fovea (69). Macular pigments composed of lutein and zeaxanthin may influence the accumulation of lipofuscin in the fovea (74). Also, specialized cones that reside in the fovea may have cellular membrane properties or differing visual pigments that preclude the formation of lipofuscin.

Lipofuscin is contained within granules of relatively uniform size. It is a lipid-protein aggregate that autofluoresces when excited by short-wavelength light. The composition of RPE lipofuscin is controversial, but most believe that partially degraded outer-segment disks and autophagy processes contribute to the bulk of lipofuscin (75–77). A growing body of evidence suggests that lipofuscin may actually induce oxidative damage by acting as a photosensitizing agent generating reactive oxygen species (14, 78, 79). As a design of function, the macula is exposed to a lifetime of light radiation, including blue light wavelengths that have been shown to induce reactive oxygen intermediates (25). In addition, biochemical properties of lipofuscin may actually interfere with the enzymatic pathways of degradation by influencing lysosomal pH (80, 81). Thus, as lipofuscin accumulates with age, the cellular catabolic machinery may be damaged or inhibited, leading to more accumulation. This cycle would theoretically continue thoughout life until the RPE cell is overwhelmed.

Senescence of the RPE may be another factor contributing to compromised function later in life. Senescence differs from quiescence in that senescent cells cannot be provoked to reenter the replicative cell cycle. The telomere hypothesis of senescence proposes that cells become senescent when progressive telomere shortening secondary to cell division reaches a threshold level. In culture, RPE cells have been shown to reach replicative failure with as few as 15 doublings (82). With introduction of a telomerase that rebuilds telomere length, replicative potential of RPE cells has been restored (83). However, it has been stated previously that the human RPE in vivo is nonmitotic. The RPE, therefore, should not be susceptible to senescence by this mechanism. Hjeimeland et al. have proposed that RPE telomeres may suffer from oxidative damage and that this may lead to senescence without true replicative exhaustion (84, 85). Senescent RPE may exhibit altered function leading to diseased states later in life (86).

Underlying the entire RPE is a basal lamina, or basement membrane, generated by the basal surface of the RPE cells. This membrane joins tightly with the inner collagen layers of Bruch's membrane. The convoluted basal surface of the RPE creates pockets where the cells are not in direct contact with the basement membrane. With age, extracellular debris, such as drusen and basal laminar deposits, accumulates in this space and may represent early pathophysiological changes within the RPE machinery. Bruch's membrane is also structurally and functionally impacted with age, including thickening and decreased permeability (87).

IV. SUMMARY

A continuum of structural, phenotypic, and molecular changes, that have only been partially characterized, is involved in retinal development, growth, and aging. Retinal ganglion cells accumulate lipofuscin with aging; there is evidence for up to 25% loss in ganglion cell number in certain retinal locations. There is preferential loss of rods in the retina with aging, but with progressive aging cone numbers eventually decline. RPE cells show numerous aging changes including accumulation of lipofuscin, alterations in cell shape, density, pigmentation, lysosomal activity, and extracellular matrix formation. Bruch's membrane shows thickening and decreased permeability with age. Arteriosclerotic aging changes occur in the retinal vessels while the macular choriocapillaris shows a decrease in total capillary number with age.

Normal aging changes may result in altered retinal function and, in cooperation with environmental and genetic factors, predispose to age-related diseases such as AMD.

ACKNOWLEDGMENTS

The authors thank Susan Clarke for her editorial assistance and Ernesto Barron for preparation of the figure.

REFERENCES

1. Oyster CW. Formation of the human eye. In: Oyster CW, ed. The Human Eye: Structure and Function. Sunderland, MA: Sinauer Associates, 1999:64–73.
2. Weale RA. Retinal senescence. In: Weale RA, ed. The Senescence of Human Vision. Oxford: Oxford University Press, 1992:112–168.
3. Organisciak DT, Darrow RM, Barsalou L, Darrow RA, Kutty RK, Kutty G, Wiggert B. Light history and age-related changes in retinal light damage. Invest Ophthalmol Vis Sci 1998;39:1107–1116.
4. McCann SM, Licinio J, Wong ML, Yu WH, Karanth S, Rettorri V. The nitric oxide hypothesis of aging. Exp Gerontol 1998;33:813–826.
5. Hogan RN. The eye in aging. In: Albert DM, Jacobiec FA, eds. Principles and Practice of Ophthalmology, 2nd ed. Philadelphia: WB Saunders, 2000:4813.
6. Willis A, Anderson SJ. Effects of glaucoma and aging on photopic and scotopic motion perception. Invest Ophthalmol Vis Sci 2000;41:325–335.
7. Schefrin BE, Tregear SJ, Harvey LO Jr, Werner JS. Senescent changes in scotopic contrast sensitivity. Vision Res 1999;39:3728–3736.
8. Rizzo M, Barton JJS. Central disorders of visual function. In: Miller NR, Newman NJ, eds. Walsh and Hoyt's Clinical Neuro-Ophthalmology, 5th ed. Baltimore: Williams & Wilkins, 1998:469.
9. Gartner S, Henkind P. Lange's folds: a meaningful ocular artifact. Ophthalmology 1981;88:1307–1310.
10. Boyer MM, Poulson GL, Nork TM. Relative contributions of the neurosensory retina and retinal pigment epithelium to macular hypofluorescence. Arch Ophthalmol 2000;118:27–31.
11. Kilbride PE, Alexander KR, Fishman M, Fishman GA. Human macular pigment assessed by imaging fundus reflectometry. Vision Res 1989;29:663–674.
12. Bone RA, Landrum JT, Fernandez L, Tarsis SL. Analysis of the macular pigment by HPLC: retinal distribution and age study. Invest Ophthalmol Vis Sci 1988;29:843–849.
13. Werner JS, Donnelly SK, Kliegl R. Aging and human macular pigment density. Appended with translations from the work of Max Schultze and Ewald Hering. Vision Res 1987;27:257–268.
14. Winkler BS, Boulton ME, Gottsch JD, Sternberg P. Oxidative damage and age-related macular degeneration. Mol Vis 1999;5:32.
15. Foos RY. Posterior vitreous detachment. Trans Am Acad Ophthalmol Otolaryngol 1972;76:480–497.

16. Heegaard S. Structure of the human vitreoretinal border region. Ophthalmologica 1994;208:82–91.
17. Balazs EA. Functional anatomy of the vitreous. In: Jakobiec FA, ed. Ocular Anatomy, Embryology, and Teratology. Philadelphia: Harper & Row, 1982:433.
18. Poinoosawmy D, Fontana L, Wu JX, Fitzke RW, Hitchings RA. Variation of nerve fiber layer thickness measurements with age and ethnicity by scanning laser polarimetry. Br J Ophthalmol 1997;81:350–354.
19. Chen HJ, Lee YM, Woung LC, Jou JR, Lin HJ. Scanning laser polarimetry in evaluation of retinal nerve fiber layer thickness for normal Taiwanese. Kaohsiung J Med Sci 2000;16:223–232.
20. Curcio CA, Drucker DN. Retinal ganglion cells in Alzheimer's disease and aging. Ann Neurol 1993;33:248–257.
21. Avendano J, Riodrigues MM, Hackett JJ, Gaskins R. Corpora amylacea of the optic nerve and retina: a form of neuronal degeneration. Invest Ophthalmol Vis Sci 1980;19:550–555.
22. Woodford B, Tso MOM. An ultrastructural study of the corpora amylacea of the optic nerve head and retina. Am J Ophthalmol 1980;90:492–502.
23. Georges P, Madigan MC, Provis JM. Apoptosis during development of the human retina: relationship to foveal development and retinal synaptogenesis. J Comp Neurol 1999;18:198–208
24. Green RW. Retina. In: Spencer WH, ed. Ophthalmic Pathology: An Atlas and Textbook, 4th ed. Philadelphia: WB Saunders, 1996:681.
25. Riozanowska M, Jarvis-Evans J, Korytowski W, Boulton ME, Burke JM, Sarna T. Blue light-induced reactivity of retinal age pigment. In vitro generation of oxygen-reactive species. J Biol Chem 1995;270:18825–18830.
26. Gaillard ER, Atherton SJ, Eldred G, Dillon J. Photophysical studies on human retinal lipofuscin. Photochem Photobiol 1995;61:448–453.
27. Barreau E, Brossas JY, Courtois Y, Treton JA. Accumulation of mitochondrial DNA deletions in human retina during aging. Invest Ophthalmol Vis Sci 1996;37;384–391
28. Soong NW, Dang MT, Hinton DR, Arnheim N. Mitochondrial DNA deletions are rare in the free radical-rich retinal environment. Neurobiol Aging 1996;17:827–831.
29. Oyster CW. Retina II: editing photoreceptor signals. In: Oyster CW, ed. The Human Eye: Structure and Function. Sunderland, MA: Sinauer Associates, 1999:595–647.
30. Gartner S, Henkind P. Aging and degeneration of the human macula. 1. Outer nuclear layer and photoreceptors. Br J Ophthalmol 1981;65:23–28.
31. Lai YL, Masuda K, Mangum MD, Lug R, Macrae DW, Fletcher G, Liu YP. Subretinal displacement of photoreceptor nuclei in human retina. Exp Eye Res 1982;34:219–228.
32. Curcio CA, Sloan KR, Kalina RE, Hendrickson AE. Human photoreceptor topography. J Comp Neurol 1990;292:497–523.
33. Curcio CA, Saunders PL, Younger PW, Malek G. Peripapillary chorioretinal atrophy: Bruch's membrane changes and photoreceptor loss. Ophthalmology 2000;107:334–343.
34. Curcio CA, Millican CL, Allen KA, Kalina RE. Aging of the human photoreceptor mosaic: evidence for selective vulnerability of rods in the central retina. Invest Ophthalmol Vis Sci 1993;34:3278–3296.
35. Gao H, Hollyfield JG. Aging of the human retina. Differential loss of neurons and retinal pigment epithelial cells. Invest Ophthalmol Vis Sci 1992;33:1–17.
36. Feeney-Burns L, Burns RP, Gao CL. Age-related macular changes in human over 90 years old. Am J Ophthalmol 1990;109:265–278.
37. Green RW. Retina. In: Spencer WH, ed. Ophthalmic Pathology: An Atlas and Textbook, 4th ed. Philadelphia: WB Saunders, 1996:674–676.
38. Young RW, Bok D. Participation of the retinal pigment epithelium in the rod outer segment renewal process. J Cell Biol 1969;42:392–403.

39. Marshall J, Grindle J, Ansell PL, Borwein B. Convolution in human rods: an ageing process. Br J Ophthalmol 1979;63:181–187

40. Fulton AB, Dodge J, Hansen RM, Williams TP. The rhodopsin content of human eyes. Invest Ophthalmol Vis Sci 1999;40:1878–1883.

41. Iwasaki M, Inomata H. Lipofuscin granules in human photoreceptor cells. Invest Ophthalmol Vis Sci 1988;29:671–679.

42. Keunen JE, van Nooren D, van Meel GJ. Density of foveal cone pigments at older age. Invest Ophthalmol Vis Sci 1987;28:985–991.

43. Kilbride PE, Hutman LP, Fishman M, Read JS. Foveal cone pigment density difference in the aging human eye. Vision Res 1986;26:321–325.

44. Green RW. Retina. In: Spencer WH, ed. Ophthalmic Pathology: An Atlas and Textbook, 4th ed. Philadelphia: WB Saunders, 1996:679.

45. Kuwabara T, Cogan DG. Retinal vascular patterns. VII. Acellular change. Invest Ophthalmol 1965;4:1049–1064.

46. Miller NR. Anatomy and physiology of the cerebral vascular system. In: Miller NR, Newman NJ, eds. Walsh and Hoyt's Clinical Neuro-Ophthalmology, 5th ed. Baltimore: Williams & Wilkins, 1998:2970.

47. Lee WR, Blass GE, Shaw DC. Age-related retinal vasculopathy. Eye 1987;2:296–303.

48. Groh MJ, Michelson G, Langhans MJ, Harazny J. Influence of age on retinal and optic nerve head blood circulation. Ophthalmology 1996:103:529–534.

49. Grunwald JE, Piltz J, Patel N, Bose S, Riva CE. Effect of aging on retinal macular microcirculation: a blue field simulation study. Invest Ophthalmol Vis Sci 1993;34:3609–3613.

50. Laatikainen L, Larinkari J. Capillary-free area of the fovea with advancing age. Invest Ophthalmol Vis Sci 1997;16:1154–1157.

51. Kornzweig AL, Eliasoph I, Feldstein M. Retinal vasculature in the aged. Bull NY Acad Med 1964;40:116–129.

52. Padgett LC, Lui GM, Werb Z, LaVail MM. Matrix metalloproteinase-2 and tissue inhibitor of metalloproteinases-1 in the retinal pigment epithelium and interphotoreceptor matrix: vectorial secretion and regulation. Exp Eye Res 1997;64:927–938.

53. Hollyfield JG, Rayborn ME, Tammi M, Tammi R. Hyaluronan in the interphotoreceptor matrix of the eye: species differences in content, distribution, ligand-binding and degradation. Exp Eye Res 1998;66:241–248.

54. Tien L, Rayborn ME, Hollyfield JG. Characterization of the interphotoreceptor matrix surrounding rod photoreceptors in the human retina. Exp Eye Res 1992;55:297–306.

55. Hageman GS, Johnson LV. Structure, composition and function of the retinal interphotoreceptor matrix. Prog Retin Res 1991;10:207–249.

56. Green RW. Retina. In: Spencer WH, ed. Ophthalmic Pathology: An Atlas and Textbook, 4th ed. Philadelphia: WB Saunders, 1996:672.

57. Burke JM. Determinants of retinal pigment epithelial cell phenotype and polarity. II. Fundamental properties. In: Marmor MF, Wolfensberger TJ, eds. The Retinal Pigment Epithelium: Function and Disease, 2nd ed. Oxford: Oxford University Press, 1998:86–102.

58. Verhoeff FH. A hitherto undescribed membrane of the eye and its significance. Boston Med Surg J 1903;149:456–458.

59. Harman AM, Fleming PA, Hoskins RV, Moore SR. Development and aging of cell topography in the human retinal pigment epithelium. Invest Ophthalmol Vis Sci 1997;38:2016–2026.

60. Robb RM. Regional changes in retinal pigment epithelial cell density during ocular development. Invest Ophthalmol Vis Sci 1985;26:614–620.

61. Streeten BW. Development of the human retinal pigment epithelium and the posterior segment. Arch Ophthalmol 1969;81:383–384.

62. Watzke RC, Soldevilla JD, Trune DR. Morphometric analysis of human retinal pigment epithelium: correlation with age and location. Curr Eye Res 1993;12:133–142.

63. Shelton DN, Chang E, Whittier PS, Choi D, Funk WD. Microarray analysis of replicative senescence. Curr Biol 1999;9:939–945.

64. Marmor MF. Structure, function, and disease of the retinal pigment epithelium. In: Marmor MF, Wolfensberger TJ, eds. The Retinal Pigment Epithelium: Function and Disease, 2nd ed. Oxford: Oxford University Press, 1998:3–12.

65. Verdugo ME, Ray J. Age-related increase in activity of specific lysosomal enzymes in the human retinal pigment epithelium. Exp Eye Res 1997;65:231–240.

66. Loeffler KU, Mangini NJ. Immunolocalization of ubiquitin and related enzymes in human retina and retinal pigment epithelium. Graefes Arch Clin Exp Ophthalmol 1997;235:248–254.

67. Miyamoto L, Fitzpatrick TB. On the nature of the pigment in retinal pigment epithelium. Science 1957;126:449–450.

68. Ts'o MO and Friedman E. The retinal pigment epithelium. I. Comparative histology. Arch Ophthalmol 1967;78:641–649.

69. Weiter JJ, Delori FC, Wing GL, Fitch KA. Retinal pigment epithelial lipofuscin and melanin and choriodal melanin in human eyes. Invest Ophthalmol Vis Sci 1986;27:145–152.

70. Feeney-Burns L, Hilderbrande ES, Eldridge S. Aging human RPE: morphometric analysis of macular, equatorial and peripheral cells. Invest Ophthalmol Vis Sci 1984;25:195–200.

71. Schmidt SY, Peisch RD. Melanin concentration in normal human retinal pigment epithelium. Regional variation and age-related reduction. Invest Ophthalmol Vis Sci 1986;27:1063–1067.

72. Eldred GE. Lipofuscin and other lysosomal storage deposits in the retinal pigment epithelium. In: Marmor MF, Wolfensberger TJ, eds. The Retinal Pigment Epithelium: Function and Disease, 2nd ed. Oxford: Oxford University Press, 1998:651–668.

73. Wing GL, Blanchard GC, Weiter JJ. The topography and age relationship of lipofuscin concentration in the retinal pigment epithelium. Invest Ophthalmol Vis Sci 1978;17:601–607.

74. Hammond BR JR, Wooten BR, Snodderly DM. Individual variations in the special profile of human macular pigment. J Opt Soc Am A 1997;14:1187–1196.

75. Dorey CK, Wu G, Ebenstein D, Garsd A, Weiter JJ. Cell loss in the aging retina. Relationship to lipofuscin accumulation and macular degeneration. Invest Ophthalmol Vis Sci 1989;30:1691–1699.

76. Burke JM, Skumatz CMB. Autofluorescent inclusions in long-term postconfluent cultures of retinal pigment epithelium. Invest Ophthalmol Vis Sci 1998;39:1478–1486.

77. Wassell J, Ellis S, Burke J, Boulton M. Fluorescence properties of autofluorescent granules generated by cultured human RPE cells. Invest Ophthalmol Vis Sci 1998;39:1487–1492.

78. Beatty S, Koh H, Phil M, Henson D, Boulton M. The role of oxidative stress in the pathogenesis of age-related macular degeneration. Surv Ophthalmol 2000;45:115–134.

79. Frank RN. "Oxidative protector" enzymes in the macular retinal pigment epithelium of aging eyes and eyes with age-related macular degeneration. Trans Am Ophthalmol Soc 1998;96:634–689.

80. Holz FG, Schutt F, Kopitz J, Eldred GE, Kruse FE, Volcker HE, Cantz M. Inhibition of lysosomal degradative functions in RPE cells by a retinoid component of lipofuscin. Invest Ophthalmol Vis Sci 1999;40:737–743.

81. Sparrow JR, Parrish CA, Hashimoto M, Nakanishi K. A2E, a lipofuscin fluorophore, in human retinal pigmented epithelial cells in culture. Invest Ophthalmol Vis Sci 1999;40:2988–2995.

82. Rawes V, Kipling D, Kill IR, Faragher RG. The kinetics of senescence in retinal pigmented epithelial cells: a test for the telomere hypothesis of ageing? Biochemistry (Mosc) 1997;62:1291–1295.

83. Bodnar AG, Ouellette M, Frolkis M, Holt SE, Chiu CP, Morin GB, Hartley CB, Shay JW, Lichtsteiner S, Wright WE. Extension of life-span by introduction of telomerase into normal human cells. Science 1998;279:349–352.

84. Hjelmeland LM, Cristofolo VJ, Funk W, Rakoczy E, Katz ML. Senescence of the retinal pigment epithelium. Mol Vis 1999;5:33–36.

85. Sitte N, Saretzki G, von Zglinicki T. Accelerated telomere shortening in fibroblasts after extended periods of confluency. Free Radic Biol Med 1998;24:885–893.

86. Matsunaga H, Handa JT, Gelfman CM, Hjelmeland LM. The mRNA phenotype of a human RPE cell line at replicative senescence. Mol Vis 1999;5:39–45.
87. Marshall J et al. Aging and Bruch's membrane. In: Marmor MF, Wolfensberger TJ, eds. The Retinal Pigment Epithelium: Function and Disease, 2nd ed. Oxford: Oxford University Press, 1998:669–692.

2

Histopathological Characteristics of Age-Related Macular Degeneration

Ehud Zamir
Hadassah–Hebrew University Medical School, Jerusalem, Israel

Narsing A. Rao
Doheny Eye Institute, University of Southern California Keck School of Medicine, Los Angeles, California

I. INTRODUCTION

Age-related macular degeneration (AMD) is common among the elderly, and its incidence increases progressively with advancing age. According to the Beaver Dam Eye Study, 11% of the population are affected by AMD at age 65–74, and this number increases to 28% after age 74. Therefore, postmortem studies have been a source of extensive histopathological information on this disease. Large series have been presented and analyzed in multiple studies, and the result is a significant body of well-established histopathological data that is available at present. Additional information derives from the availability of subretinal neovascular membranes removed by a variety of increasingly popular subretinal surgery techniques (1). AMD is currently well characterized at both the light microscopic and the electron microscopic level.

The histopathological hallmark of early, nonexudative AMD is the occurrence of drusen, as well as basal deposits along the basement membrane of the retinal pigment epithelium, with degeneration of the overlying retinal pigment epithelium (RPE) and photoreceptor cells. Drusen are classified into three main categories: small, hard drusen (also termed nodular drusen), soft drusen, and large, confluent drusen. Small, hard drusen are the most common type. They are, by definition, smaller than 63 microns, and may be present in the eyes of patients with or without AMD, including young individuals. They are not considered to be a risk factor for AMD (2–5). Hard drusen can be detected clinically when they reach the size of 25–30 microns (2), and they tend to hyperfluoresce on fluorescein angiography. Histologically, they appear as globular, hyaline structures external to the RPE basement membrane. The overlying RPE cells may be atrophic (5) (Fig. 1). Ultrastructurally, hard drusen contain membrane-bound bodies that are found in what Sarks and associates have described as "entrapment sites," in which coated, membrane-bound bodies are "trapped" between the RPE basement membrane and the inner collagenous layer of Bruch's membrane (2). This material is currently presumed to derive from the RPE (5).

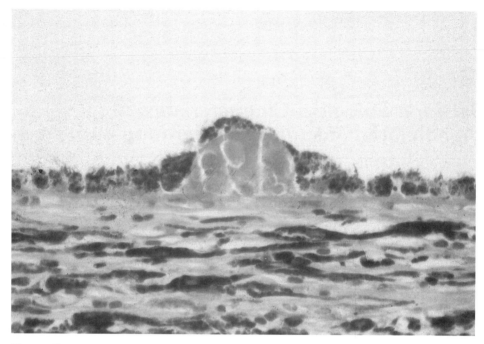

Figure 1 A hard druse. A globular hyaline deposit with overlying RPE atrophy. The retina is artifactually detached, thus not shown in this picture (H&E). See also color insert, Fig. 2.1.

Bruch's membrane normally contains five layers, in the following order: Innermost is the basement membrane of the RPE, followed by the inner collagenous layer of Bruch's membrane, the elastic lamina, the outer collagenous layer, and the basement membrane of the choriocappillaris. Basal deposits (6) are collections of acellular debris in different planes in and along Bruch's membrane (Fig. 2, 3). Most authors define two different types of basal deposits as follows: Amorphous, acellular debris accumulating between the basal plasma membrane of the retinal pigment epithelium and the basement membrane of the RPE is referred to as basal laminar deposits (BLamD) (3). In contrast, deposition of material external to the BM of the RPE, e.g., between the latter and the inner collagenous layer of Bruch's membrane, is termed basal linear deposits (BlinD). The two types differ not only in their anatomical distribution, but also with regard to their chemical characteristics and pathological significance, as will be explained below. Differentiation of these two findings on light microscopic grounds is difficult, and there may be significant morphological overlap (4). Transmission electron microscopy is the main tool in detecting and analyzing those deposits. It demonstrates that BLamD are composed of fibrous long-spacing collagen (possibly type IV collagen); amorphous, basement membrane-like deposits are features of normal aging that appear after age 60 and are not markers of AMD.

BlinD, also termed diffuse or confluent drusen (3,7,8), are composed of membraneous material and this was found to be a sensitive and specific feature of AMD, although the association between the two does not necessarily indicate causality. Rather, both could reflect damage to the RPE (6). While BLamD only appear after age 60, they are not specific to AMD, and are also present in non-AMD, aging eyes. In contrast, the prevalence of BlinD and large, soft drusen is 24 times higher in eyes with AMD compared to age-

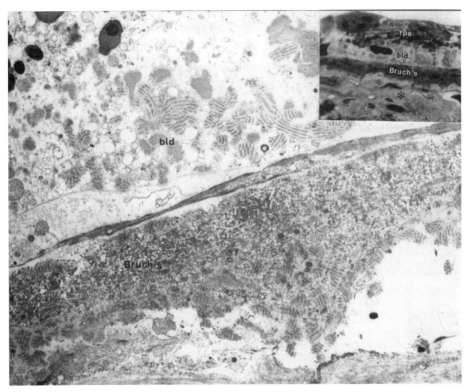

Figure 2 Basal laminar deposit (bld) lies between the retinal pigment epithelium (rpe) and the inner aspect of Bruch's membrane in this choroidal neovascular membrane excised from a patient with age-related macular degeneration. Wide-spaced collagen is in the basal laminar deposit and scarred choroid versus a component of the choroidal neovascular membrane (asterisk) are present within Bruch's membrane (original magnification, × 10,440; inset, original magnificaton, × 400). Reprinted with permission from Ref. 14.)

matched controls (6). BlinD are composed of granular, vesicular, or membranous material, with foci of wide-spaced collagen. The origin of that membranous debris is thought to be membranes of photoreceptor outer segments, delivered by the RPE in the form of vacuoles and vesicles (6,7,9). Soft drusen (large, poorly delineated drusen) may represent focal accentuation of that basal linear material, while its diffuse deposition forms BlinD (3,8). Soft drusen are seen by light microscopy as localized deposition of granular, pale material with sloping edges (4). They can also represent areas of detachment of BlinD or BLamD by proteinatious material. Larger detachments of basal deposits correspond to serous pigment epithelial detachments. Unlike hard drusen, large, soft, and confluent drusen (Fig. 4) are a sign of AMD (4). In Green and Enger's series of 760 globes with AMD, 10.9% showed soft drusen by histopathology, and 27.6% had basal linear deposits (3).

All forms of drusen may show calcification in the process of regression (5). It was shown to be present in nodular (hard) and soft drusen in 0.8% and 7.7% of eyes with AMD, respectively (3).

Calcification and fragmentation of Bruch's membrane were shown to be associated with AMD, and to be more severe in eyes with exudative AMD compared to dry AMD (4). Calcification was mostly found in the elastic layer of Bruch's membrane, and both calcification and fragmentation were more common in the macular, compared to the extramacular,

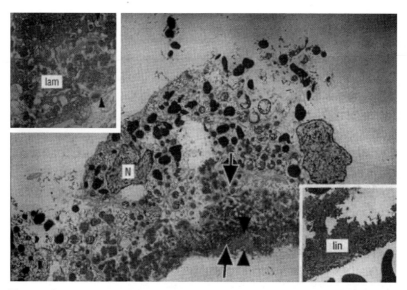

Figure 3 A retinal pigment epithelial cell with a bland nuceus (N) displays basal laminar deposit (between arrows) and basal linear deposit (between arrowheads) (transmission electron microscopy, original magnification × 3610). Close inspection shows that the basal laminar deposit (lam, upper inset, transmission electron microscopy, original mangnification × 5365) is located between the plasma membrane and basement membrane (arrowheads) of the retinal pigment epithelium, and the basal linear deposit (lin, lower inset, transmission electron microscopy, original magnification × 2600) is external to the basement membrane. (Reprinted with permission from Ref. 17).

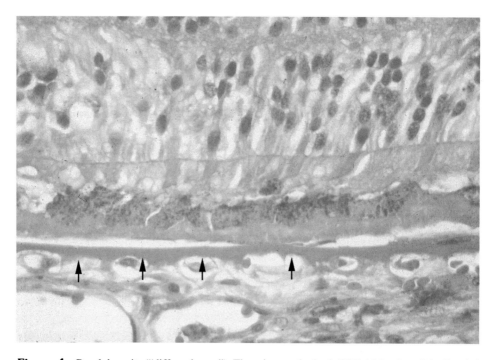

Figure 4 Basal deposits ("diffuse drusen"). There is a marked sub-RPE thickening of the Bruchs' membrane (arrows) (PAS). See also color insert, Fig. 2.4.

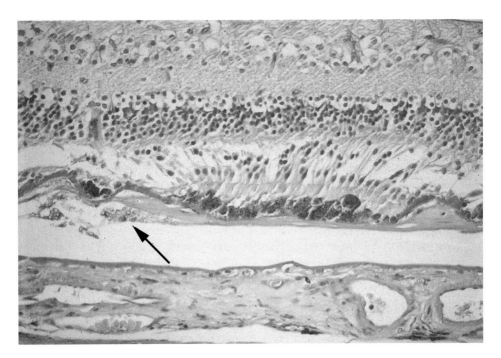

Figure 5 Diskiform scarring, low magnification. Notice dystrophic calcification. Calcium crystals are seen within the substance of the sub-RPE fibrous plaque (arrow). See also color insert, Fig. 2.5.

area (4). The authors suggested that such changes in Bruch's membrane play a role, together with diseased RPE and basal deposits, in facilitating growth of fibrovascular membranes.

II. GEOGRAPHICAL (AREOLAR) AGE-RELATED MACULAR DEGENERATION

This form, also called "dry AMD," is more common than the "wet," neovascular form. Its main features include atrophy, migration, and degeneration of the RPE cells. There is a tendency for sparing of the foveal area early on, with eventual foveal involvement and more severe visual loss. This fact was attributed by Weiter et al. (10) to the higher concentration of xanthophyll pigment. There is secondary degeneration and loss of the photoreceptors that overlie the degenerating RPE cells, including their inner segments in severe cases (Fig. 5). This condition may follow serous RPE detachments or large drusen (11). In Green and Enger's series (3), 37% of the eyes had RPE atrophy.

III. THE "WET" (NEOVASCULAR) FORM OF AMD

This form is characterized by growth of choroidal neovascular membranes into the sub-RPE or subretinal areas. These membranes can distort the macular topography and later produce hemorrhagic or serous RPE and retinal detachments. The latter are the major sources of visual loss in AMD. Later in the process, these lesions may scar to form a fibrovascular, "diskiform" scar (Fig. 5–7). In the early stages, choroidal capillaries are seen growing into the Bruch's membrane. The proliferating choroidal vessels start as capillaries and develop into arteries and veins over time. Exudation of lipid under the RPE or into the subretinal space may be seen. Bleeding into the sub-RPE space is common, and blood may gain access into the subretinal space, and even into the vitreous cavity. At a later stage, this serous or hemorrhagic detachment evolves into a dense fibrous scar, clinically described as a "diskiform" scar. Such lesions were found in 40.6% of 760 globes studied by Green and Enger (3). The scar may contain hyperplastic RPE cells and basement membrane, as well as hemosiderin and calcifications. It may have a single subretinal component, or three components separated by RPE basement membrane and basal deposits. The larger the diskiform scar, the more likely it is to find degenerated photoreceptors in the overlying retina. RPE tears were found in 6.8% of eyes (3). A rare finding in diskiform scars is the occurrence of granulomatous reaction with giant cells (12,13). Dastgheib and Green (12) described a diskiform scar of at least 11 years' duration, which had a prominent foreign-body giant cell response located at the Bruch's membrane, with cytoplasmic extensions from some of the cells in the inner and outer layers of Bruch's membrane. These cells seemed to be actively breaking down Bruch's membrane and engulfing it. The authors hypothesized that inflammatory response may take part in the pathogenesis of breaks in Bruch's membrane and the ensuing choroidal neovascularization. By this theory, the diseased RPE as well as the basal deposits induce a local inflammatory response that includes macrophages, T-cell activation, and formation of multinucleated giant cells. These in turn may cause damage to the Bruch's membrane and secrete angiogenic factors, both contributing to the development of choroidal neovascular membranes (CNVM). Excised neovascular membranes from eyes with AMD, but not from other underlying etiologies, also contained foreign-body giant

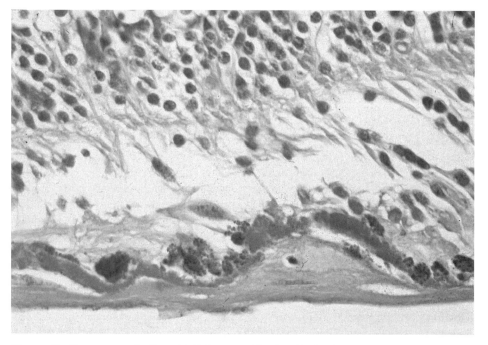

Figure 6   Same case as in Figure 5, higher magnification. Notice degenerated outer segments of photoreceptors and atrophic RPE. There is a sub-RPE fibrous sheet. See also color insert, Fig. 2.6.

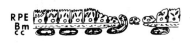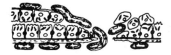

EARLY OCCULT STAGE

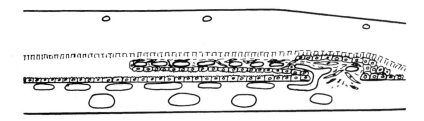

SYMPTOMATIC STAGE

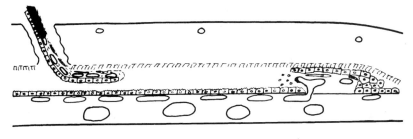

SURGICAL EXCISION

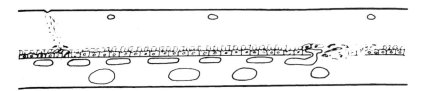

Figure 7 Diagram of the stages of development and surgical excision of type 2 choroidal neovascularization. Closed arrows indicate growth of new capillaries from the choriocapillaris (cc), through a defect in the focally damaged Bruch's membrane (Bm), and into the subsensory retinal space accompanied by proliferating retinal pigment epithelial cells (RPE) at their advancing border and along their posterior surface. Open arrow shows how the neovascular membrane was removed through retinotomy site using forceps. (Reprinted with permission from Ref. 21.)

cells and basal deposits (14). These findings have been suggested as evidence for CNVM representing a stereotypical, nonspecific wound repair-like process that is analogous to granulation tissue (15).

IV. EXCISED SUBRETINAL MEMBRANES AND ANGIOGRAPHIC CORRELATIONS

Studies of excised subretinal membranes reveal that their most common constituents are RPE cells, vascular endothelium, and fibrocytes. Less common are inflammatory cells, macrophages, photoreceptors, myofibroblasts, pericytes, and choroidal tissue (14,16,17). The anatomical level at which CNVM grow has been a subject of interest of a large number of studies. Evidence from different authors has suggested a predominant sub-RPE growth pattern (3,18–20). In Green and Enger's series, 39/44 early (small) membranes grew under the RPE, and only 5/44 were subretinal (3). However, of 310 disciform scars, 80% had subretinal involvement. Gass (21) has suggested two types of CNVM: Type I, common in AMD, grows under the RPE, while type 11, seen in other pathologies such as the presumed ocular histoplasmosis syndrome (POHS), grows under the neurosensory retina (Fig. 8,9). Gass postulated that, since there is a generalized weakening of normal adhesion between the RPE and Bruch's membrane in AMD, the proliferating choroidal vessels are growing unimpeded in the sub-RPE space. In contrast, POHS includes only focal defects in the RPE–Bruch's membrane integrity, and therefore, the vascular proliferation cannot easily grow under the RPE. According to this theory, these anatomical differences would explain the less favorable visual results after excision of membranes in AMD, compared to POHS. In the former, the membrane does not grow in a potential space, but rather within the inner layers of Bruch's membrane. Therefore, its removal would cause more destruction to the overlying RPE, limiting final visual acuity.

Evidence from histopathological studies of excised membranes has been accumulating in recent years. Grossniklaus et al. (14) studied 90 excised membranes from eyes with AMD, and correlated their anatomical localization and other histopathological features with their fluorescein angiographic characteristics (all membranes with interpretable FA were classic, and were subdivided into well-demarcated versus poorly demarcated). Approximately 60% of the membranes were classic, well demarcated, while the other 40% were classic and poorly demarcated. Well-demarcated membranes had a "bull's-eye" appearance on FA, with a hyperfluorescent center that histologically corresponded to the sub-RPE fibrovascular core of the membrane. The rim of blocked fluorescence corresponded to hypertrophied RPE, and the outer rim of faint hyperfluorescence corresponded to subretinal fibrin. Conversely, membranes that histologically seemed to break through the RPE into the subretinal space were mostly poorly demarcated in the preoperative FA, showing a pattern of scalloped net with late obscuration. The authors suggest that well-demarcated, sub-RPE membranes may evolve into "breakthrough," poorly demarcated, subneurosensory retinal membranes. Results from the Submacular Surgery Trial, reported by Grossniklaus and Green (17), showed that of 32 excised AMD membranes that could be anatomically oriented, 16 were subretinal. Sixteen had a sub-RPE component, and all the non-AMD membranes were subretinal. Surprisingly, this study showed that a significant number (50%) of AMD membranes could be localized to the subretinal space and had no sub-RPE component. This is in contrast to earlier reports showing predominantly sub-RPE location of CNVM (3,18–21).

Lafaut et al. (22) described a different correlation between the location of membranes relative to the RPE and their fluorescein angiographic features. The study included 35 AMD membranes that were preoperatively classified as classic or occult, based on the definitions of

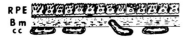 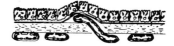

RPE
B m
c c

EARLY OCCULT STAGE

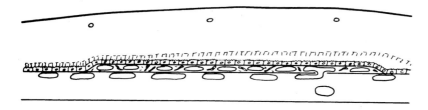

SYMPTOMATIC STAGE

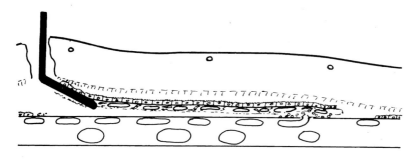

SURGICAL EXCISION

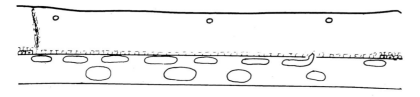

POST-OPERATIVE STAGE

Figure 8 Diagram of stages of development and surgical excision of type 1 choroidal neovascularization. Closed arrows indicate growth of new capillaries from choriocapillaris (cc) through Bruch's membrane (Bm) and between the basement membrane of the retinal pigment epithelium (RPE) and the thickened and degenerated inner collagenous zone of Bruch's membrane. Open arrow shows how the neovascular membrane was removed through a retinotomy by using forceps. (Reprinted from Ref. 21.)

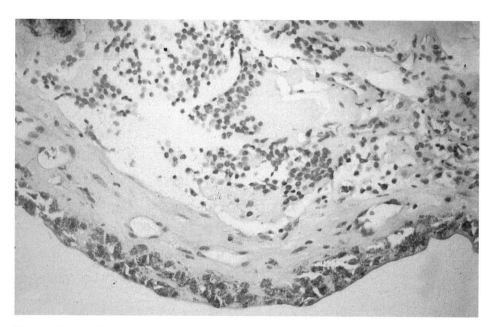

Figure 9 Surgically excised subfoveal choroidal neovascular membrane specimen from an 82-year-old man with AMD. Outer retinal elements were included in the excised specimen. Notice a dense fibrovascular membrane above the RPE and underneath the photoreceptor nuclei. This is a type II, or subretinal, membrane, which, according to Gass' theory, is more typical of non-AMD membranes (21). See also color insert, Fig. 2.9.

the Macular Photocoagulation Study (23). This is in contrast to earlier studies that only included classic membranes, as described above. Histopathological features were studied by light microscopy. Classic membranes had a predominant subretinal fibrovascular component, while occult membranes predominantly involved the sub-RPE space. Mixed (classic and occult) membranes had both subretinal and sub-RPE histopathological components. It was also found that the vascular pattern of classic membrane included presence of both capillaries and large-caliber vessels, whereas occult membranes contained mostly capillaries. The authors therefore suggested that CNVM usually starts at the sub-RPE level, and appears classical on fluorescein angiography (FA) if it breaks through the RPE, into the subretinal space. Otherwise, if it remains sub-RPE, it has FA features of "occult" membranes. Part of this inconsistency of results between different studies stems from the inherent difficulty in properly orienting the excised specimens to determine whether they are from the sub-RPE or the subretinal space. Grossniklaus et al. (14) have noted that the presence of RPE in the membrane, although usually used to indicate a sub-RPE location, may be misleading. Membranes removed from the subretinal space also contain RPE cells, lining their external surface (Fig. 10). This may simulate a sub-RPE membrane and hence prohibit proper orientation. Overall, only about half the specimens studied in another publication from the same group could be oriented, owing to folds or lack of landmarks (17).

Grossniklaus et al. have suggested that the lack of vascular endothelium in excised membranes may represent inadequate surgical removal and may be a predictor of recurrence (14). This was based on the observation that approximately 50% of the membranes that recurred did not show vascular endothelium.

A study by Lee et al. (24) examined the light microscopic features of 14 surgically

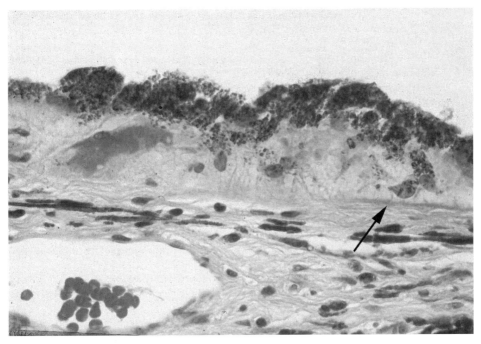

Figure 10   A choroidal neovascular membrane breaking through the Bruch's membrane and into the sub-RPE plane ("type II" membrane). Notice intact Bruch's membrane at the right side of the picture (arrow). Elements seen in the membrane include a capillary, a few mononuclear leukocytes, endothelial cells, RPE cells, and collagen (PAS). See also color insert, Fig. 2.10.

removed subretinal neovascular membranes related to AMD. One membrane was studied by TEM. All were well-defined membranes smaller than 3.5 disk areas as seen by preoperative FA. In addition, ICG angiography was performed in all patients before and after surgery. Cellular elements found in the excised membranes included RPE cells, vascular endothelium, inflammatory cells (including rare foreign-body giant cells), red blood cells, smooth muscle cells, and fibrocytes (spindle-shaped cells). Acellular constituents included basal laminar deposits, Bruch's membrane, collagen, and fibrin. No correlation was found between the anatomical location of the membranes (sub-RPE vs. subretinal) and the ICG angiographic features (well demarcated vs. poorly demarcated). However, this study only included membranes with well-demarcated membranes on FA, while ICG angiography is more useful in cases of occult membranes, which are often poorly demarcated.

REFERENCES

1. de Juan E, Machemer R. Vitreous surgery for hemorrhagic and fibrous complications of age-related macular degeneration. Am J Ophthalmol 1988;105:25–29.
2. Sarks SH, Arnold JJ, Killingsworth MC, Sarks JP. Early drusen formation in the normal and aging eye and their relation to age related maculopathy: a clinicopathological study. Br J Ophthalmol 1999;83:358–368.
3. Green WR, Enger C. Age-related macular degeneration histopathologic studies. The 1992 Lorenz E. Zimmerman Lecture. Ophthalmology 1993;100:1519–1535.
4. Spraul CW, Grossnildaus HE. Characteristics of Drusen and Bruch's membrane in postmortem eyes with age-related macular degeneration. Arch Ophthalmol 1997;115:267–273.

5. Abdelsalam A, Del Priore L, Zarbin MA. Drusen in age-related macular degeneration: pathogenesis, natural course, and laser photocoagulation-induced regression. Surv Ophthalmol 1999;44:1–29.

6. Curcio CA, Millican CL. Basal linear deposit and large drusen are specific for early age-related maculopathy. Arch Ophthalmol 1999;117:329–339.

7. Sarks JP, Sarks SH, Killingsworth MC. Evolution of geographic atrophy of the retinal pigment epithelium. Eye 1988;2:552–577.

8. Bressler NM, Silva JC, Bressler SB, Fine SL, Green WR. Clinicopathologic correlation of drusen and retinal pigment epithelial abnormalities in age-related macular degeneration. Retina 1994;14:130–142.

9. van der Schaft TL, de Bruijn WC, Mooy CM, de Jong PT. Basal laminar deposit in the aging peripheral human retina. Graefes Arch Clin Exp Ophthalmol 1993;231:470–475.

10. Weiter JJ, Delori F, Dorey CK. Central sparing in annular macular degeneration. Am J Ophthalmol 1988;106:286–292.

11. Willerson DJ, Aaberg TM. Senile macular degeneration and geographic atrophy of the retinal pigment epithelium. Br J Ophthalmol 1978;62:551–553.

12. Dastgheib K, Green WR. Granulomatous reaction to Bruch's membrane in age-related macular degeneration. Arch Ophthalmol 1994;112:813–818.

13. Penfold PL, Killingsworth MC, Sarks SH. Senile macular degeneration. The involvement of giant cells in atrophy of the retinal pigment epithelium. Invest Ophthalmol Vis Sci 1986;27:364–371.

14. Grossniklaus HE, Hutchinson AK, Capone A, Jr., Woolfson J, Lambert HM. Clinicopathologic features of surgically excised choroidal neovascular membranes. Ophthalmology 1994;101:1099–1111.

15. Grossniklaus HE, Martinez JA, Brown VB, Lambert HM, Sternberg P, Capone A, Aaberg TM, Lopez PF. Immunohistochemical and histochemical properties of surgically excised subretinal neovascular membranes in age-related macular degeneration. Am J Ophthalmol 1992;114:464–472.

16. Lopez PF, Grossniklaus HE, Lambert HM, Aaberg TM, Capone A, Sternberg P, L'Hernavlt N. Pathologic features of surgically excised subretinal neovascular membranes in age-related macular degeneration. Am J Ophthalmol 1991;112:647–656.

17. Grossniklaus HE, Green WR. Histopathologic and ultrastructural findings of surgically excised choroidal neovascularization. Submacular Surgery Trials Research Group. Arch Ophthalmol 1998;116:745–749.

18. Bressler SB, Silva JC, Bressler NM, Alexander J, Green WR. Clinicopathologic correlation of occult choroidal neovascularization in age-related macular degeneration. Arch Ophthalmol 1992;110:827–832.

19. Small ML, Green WR, Alpar JJ, Drewry RE. Senile mecular degeneration. A clinicopathologic correlation of two cases with neovascularization beneath the retinal pigment epithelium. Arch Ophthalmol 1976;94:601–607.

20. Sarks JP, Sarks SH, Killingsworth MC. Morphology of early choroidal neovascularisation in age-related macular degeneration: correlation with activity. Eye 1997;11:515–522.

21. Gass JD. Biomicroscopic and histopathologic considerations regarding the feasibility of surgical excision of subfoveal neovascular membranes. Am J Ophthalmol 1994;118:285–298.

22. Lafaut BA, Bartz-Schmidt KU, Vanden Broecke C, Aisenbrey S, De Laey JJ, Heimann K. Clinicopathological correlation in exudative age related macular degeneration: histological differentiation between classic and occult choroidal neovascularisation. Br J Ophthalmol 2000;84:239–243.

23. Subfoveal neovascular lesions in age-related macular degeneration. Guidelines for evaluation and treatment in the macular photocoagulation study. Macular Photocoagulation Study Group. Arch Ophthalmol 1991;109:1242–1257.

24. Lee BL, Lim JI, Grossniklaus HE. Clinicopathologic features of indocyanine green angiography-imaged, surgically excised choroidal neovascular membranes. Retina 1996;16:64–69

3
Immunology of Age-Related Macular Degeneration

Scott W. Cousins
Bascom Palmer Eye Institute, University of Miami, Miami, Florida

Karl G. Csaky
National Eye Institute, National Institutes of Health, Bethesda, Maryland

I. INTRODUCTION

Traditionally, immune and inflammatory mechanisms of disease pathogenesis were applied only to disorders characterized by acute onset and progression associated with obvious clinical signs of inflammation. Recently, however, it has become clear that many chronic degenerative diseases associated with aging demonstrate important immune and inflammatory components. Perhaps similar immune mechanisms participate in age-related macular degeneration (AMD). Unfortunately, scant information is available on this topic, and if this chapter were restricted to published findings for AMD, it would be quite brief.

Nevertheless, the potential scientific merit of this topic is important enough to justify "informed speculation." Accordingly, this chapter will attempt to achieve three goals. First, a brief overview will be provided of the biology of the low-grade inflammatory mechanisms relevant to chronic degenerative diseases of aging, excluding the mechanisms associated with acute severe inflammation. Innate immunity, antigen-specific immunity, and amplification systems will be differentiated. Second, the immunology of AMD will be discussed in the context of three age-related degenerative diseases with immunological features, including atherosclerosis, Alzheimer's disease, and glomerular diseases. Since these disorders share epidemiological, genetic, and physiological associations with AMD, the approach will attempt to delineate the scope of the subject based on analysis of other age-related degenerative diseases, and to highlight areas of potential importance to future AMD research. Finally, this chapter will introduce the paradigm of "response to injury" as a model for AMD pathogenesis. This paradigm proposes that immune mechanisms not only participate in the initiation of injury, but also significantly contribute to abnormal reparative responses resulting in disease pathogenesis and complications. The response to injury paradigm, emerging as a central hypothesis in the pathogenesis of atherosclerosis, Alzheimer's disease, glomerular diseases, provides a connection between immunological mechanisms of disease and the biology of tissue injury and repair in chronic degenerative disorders.

II. OVERVIEW OF BIOLOGY OF IMMUNOLOGY RELEVANT TO AMD

A. Innate Versus Antigen-Specific Immunity

In general, an immune response is a sequence of cellular and molecular events designed to rid the host of an offending stimulus, which usually represents a pathogenic organism, toxic substance, cellular debris, neoplastic cell, or other similar signal. Two broad categories of immune responses have been recognized: innate and antigen-specific immunity (1–3).

1. Innate Immunity

Innate immunity (also called "natural" immunity) is a pattern recognition response by certain cells of the immune system, typically macrophages and neutrophils, to identify broad groups of offensive stimuli, especially infectious agents, toxins, or cellular debris from injury (4–6). Additionally, many stimuli of innate immunity can directly interact with parenchymal cells of tissues (i.e., the retinal pigment epithelium) to initiate a response. Innate immunity is triggered by a preprogrammed, antigen-independent cellular response, determined by the preexistence of receptors for a category of stimuli, leading to generation of biochemical mediators that recruit additional inflammatory cells. These cells remove the offending stimulus in a nonspecific manner via phagocytosis or enzymatic degradation. The key concept is that the stimuli of innate immunity interact with receptors on monocytes, neutrophils, or parenchymal cells that have been genetically predetermined by evolution to recognize and respond to conserved molecular patterns or "motifs" on different triggering stimuli. These motifs often include specific amino acid sequences, certain lipoproteins, certain phospholipids or other specific molecular patterns. Different stimuli often trigger the same stereotyped program. Thus, the receptors of innate immunity are identical among all individuals within a species in the same way that receptors for neurotransmitters or hormones are genetically identical within a species.

   The classic example of the innate immune response is the immune response to acute infection (7). For example, in endophthalmitis, bacterial-derived toxins or host cell debris stimulates the recruitment of neutrophils and monocytes, leading to the production of inflammatory mediators and phagocytosis of the bacteria. Bacterial toxins can also directly activate receptors on retinal neurons, leading to injury. The triggering mechanisms and subsequent effector responses to bacteria such as *Staphylococcus* are nearly identical to those of other organisms, determined by nonspecific receptors recognizing families of related toxins or molecules in the environment.

2. Antigen-Specific Immunity

Antigen-specific immunity (also called "adaptive" or "acquired" immunity) is an acquired host response, generated in reaction to exposure to a specific "antigenic" molecule, and is not a genetically predetermined response to a broad category of stimuli (1–3). The response is initially triggered by the "recognition" of a unique foreign "antigenic" substance as distinguished from "self" by cells of the immune system (and not by nonimmune parenchymal cells). Recognition is followed by subsequent "processing" of the unique antigen by specialized cells of the immune system. The response results in unique antigen-specific immunologic effector cells (T and B lymphocytes) and unique antigen-specific soluble effector molecules (antibodies) whose aim it is to remove the specific stimulating antigenic substance from the organism, and to ignore the presence of other irrelevant antigenic stimuli. The key concept is that an antigen (usually) represents an alien, completely foreign substance against which specific cells of the immune system must generate, de novo, a specific receptor, which, in turn, must recognize a unique molecular structure in the antigen for which no preexisting gene was present. Thus, the antigen-specific immune system has evolved a way for an individual's B and T lymphocytes to continually generate new antigen receptor genes through recombination, rearrangement, and mutation of the germline genetic structure to create a "repertoire" of novel antigen receptor molecules that vary tremendously in spectrum of recognition among individuals within a species.

The classic example of acquired immunity is the immune response to a mutated virus. Viruses (such as adenovirus found in epidemic keratoconjunctivitis) are continuously evolving or mutating new "antigenic" structures. The susceptible host could not have possibly evolved receptors for recognition to these new viral mutations. However, these new mutations do serve as "antigens" that stimulate an adaptive antigen-specific immune response by the host to the virus. The antigen-specific response recognizes the virus in question and not other organisms (such as the polio virus).

3. Amplification Mechanisms for Both Forms of Immunity

Although innate or antigen-specific immunity may directly induce injury or inflammation, in most cases, these effectors initiate a process that must be amplified to produce overt clinical manifestations. Molecules generated within tissues that amplify immunity are termed "mediators," and several categories of molecules qualify including: (1) cytokines (growth factors, angiogenic factors, others); (2) oxidants (free radicals, reactive nitrogen); (3) plasma-derived enzyme systems (complement, kinins, and fibrin); (4) vasoactive amines (histamine and serotonin); (5) lipid mediators (prostaglandins, leukotrienes, other eicosanoids, and platelet-activating factors); and (6) neutrophil-derived granule products. A detailed discussion of all of these factors is beyond the scope of this chapter, especially since minimal evidence exits for the participation of many of these amplification systems in the pathogenesis of AMD (1–6). However, since complement, cytokines, and oxidants seem to be relevant to many degenerative diseases of aging and AMD, these will be discussed below.

a. Complement. Components and fragments of the complement cascade, accounting for approximately 5% of plasma protein concentration and over 30 different protein molecules, represent important endogenous amplifiers of innate and antigen-specific immunity as well as mediators of injury responses (8–10). All complement factors are synthesized by the liver and released into blood. However, some specific factors can also be synthesized locally within tissues, including within cornea, sclera, and retina. Upon activation, the various proteins of the complement system interact in a sequential cascade to produce different fragments and products capable of effecting a variety of functions. Three pathways have been identified to activate the complement cascade: classical pathway, alternative pathway, and the lectin pathway (Fig. 1).

Antigen-specific immunity typically activates complement via the classic pathway with antigen/antibody (immune) complexes, especially those formed by IgM, IgG1, and IgG3 (8–10). Innate immunity typically activates complement via the alternative pathway using certain chemical moieties on the cell wall of microorganisms (e.g., LPS) or activated surfaces (e.g., implanted medical devices) (11). However, some innate stimuli, such as DNA, RNA, insoluble deposits of abnormal proteins (e.g., amyloid P), or apoptotic cells, can also trigger the classic pathway (11–14). Recently, a new innate activational pathway, the lectin pathway, has been identified (15). This pathway utilizes mannose-binding lectin (MBL) to recognize sugar moieties, such as mannose and *N*-acetylglucosamine, on

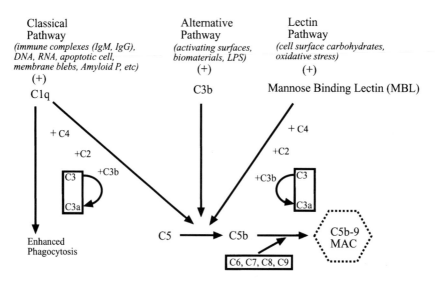

Figure 1 Schematic of the components and fragments of the complement cascade indicating three primary sources of activation via the classic, alternative, or lectin pathway.

cell surfaces. While MBL does not normally recognize the body's own tissue, oxidant injury, as can occur in AMD, may alter surface protein expression and glycosylation causing MBL deposition and complement activation (16–19). The activation of complement is also regulated by inhibitors, such as decay-accelerating factor, factor H, and others that serve to block, resist, or modulate the induction of various activation pathways (8–10).

Each activation pathways results in generation of the same complement by-products that amplify injury or inflammation by at least three mechanisms: (1) a specific fragment of the third component, C3b, can coat antigenic or pathogenic surfaces to enhance phago-cytosis by macrophages or neutrophils; (2) activation of terminal complement components C5–9, called the membrane attack complex (MAC), forms pores or leaky patches in cell membranes leading to activation of the cell, entrance of extracellular chemicals, loss of cy-toplasm, or lysis of the cell; (3) generation of small proinflammatory polypeptides, called anaphylatoxins (C3a, C4a, and C5a), can induce many inflammatory mediators and lead to the recruitment of inflammatory cells.

In addition, individual complement components (especially C3) can be produced locally by cells within tissue sites rather than derived from the blood (9). C3 and other com-plement proteins can be cleaved into biologically activated fragments by various enzyme systems, in the absence of the entire cascade, to activate certain specific cellular functions. Further, complement activation inhibitors can be produced by cells within tissues, including the RPE, serving as a local protective mechanism against complement-mediated injury (20,21). Recently several components of the complement system have been identified within Bruch's membrane and drusen indicating a potential role for complement in AMD (22).

b. Cytokines. "Cytokine" is a generic term for any soluble polypeptide mediator (i.e., protein) synthesized and released by cells for the purposes of intercellular signaling and communication. Cytokines can be released to signal neighboring cells at the site (paracrine action), to stimulate a receptor on its own surface (autocrine action), or in some cases, released into the blood to act upon a distant site (hormonal action). Traditionally, investigators have used terms like "growth factors," "angiogenic factors," "interleukins," "lymphokines," "interferon, "monokines," and "chemokines" to subdivide cytokines into families with related activities, sources, and targets. Nevertheless, research has demonstrated that, although some cytokines are cell-type specific, most cytokines have such multiplicity and redundancy of source, function, and target that excessive focus on specific terminology is not particularly conceptually useful for the clinician. The reader is directed to several recent reviews (23–25). RPE as well as cells of the immune system can produce many different cytokines relevant to AMD such as monocyte chemoattractant protein-1 (MCP-1) and vascular endothelial growth factor (VEGF).

c. Oxidants. Under certain conditions, oxygen-containing molecules can accept an electron from various substrates to become highly reactive products with the potential to damage cellular molecules and inhibit functional properties in pathogens or host cells. Four of the most important oxidants are singlet oxygen, superoxide anion, hydrogen peroxide, and the hydroxyl radical. In addition, various nitrogen oxides, certain metal ions, and other molecules can become reactive oxidants or participate in oxidizing reactions. A detailed description of the chemistry of oxidants is beyond the scope of this chapter, but can be found in several recent reviews (26–28).

Oxidants are continuously generated as a consequence of normal noninflammatory cellular biochemical processes, including electron transport during mitochondrial respiration, autooxidation of catecholamines, cellular interactions with environmental light or radiation, or prostaglandin metabolism within cell membranes. During immune responses, however, oxidants are typically produced by neutrophils and macrophages by various enzyme-dependent oxidase systems (29). Some of these enzymes (e.g., NADPH oxidase) are bound to the inner cell membrane and catalyze the intracellular transfer of electrons from specific substrates (like NADPH) to oxygen or hydrogen peroxide to form highly chemically reactive compounds meant to destroy internalized, phagocytosed pathogens (30). Other oxidases, like myeloperoxidase, can be secreted extracellularly or released into phagocytic vesicles to catalyze oxidant reactions between hydrogen peroxide and chloride to form extremely toxic products that are highly damaging to bacteria, cell surfaces, and extracellular matrix molecules (31). Finally, several important oxidant reactions involve the formation of reactive nitrogen species (32).

Oxidants can interact with several cellular targets to cause injury. Among the most important are damage to proteins (i.e., enzymes, receptors) by crosslinking of sulfhydryl groups or other chemical modifications, damage to the cell membrane by lipid peroxidation of fatty acids in the phospholipid bilayers, depletion of ATP by loss of integrity of the inner membrane of the mitochondria, and breaks or crosslinks in DNA due to chemical alterations of nucleotides (26,27). Not surprising, nature has developed many protective antioxidant systems including soluble intracellular antioxidants (i.e., glutathione or vitamin C), cell membrane-bound lipid-soluble antioxidants (i.e., vitamin E), and extracellular antioxidants (26,27).

In the retina, oxidation-induced lipid peroxidation and protein damage in RPE and photoreceptors have been proposed as major injury stimuli (33–37). Relevant sources of oxidants in AMD might include both noninflammatory biochemical sources (e.g., light interactions between photoreceptors and RPE, lysosomal metabolism in RPE, prostaglandin biosynthesis, oxidants in cigarette smoke) and innate immunity (e.g., macrophage release of myeloperoxidase).

B. Cells of the Immune Response

Both innate and antigen-specific immune system use leukocytes as cellular mediators to effect and amplify the response (i.e., immune effectors). In general, leukocyte subsets include lymphocytes (T cells, B cells), monocytes (macrophages, microglia, dendritic cells), and granulocytes (neutrophils, eosinophils, and basophils). A complete overview is beyond the scope of this chapter, especially since no evidence exists that all of these cellular effectors participate in AMD. Thus, this section will focus only upon leukocyte subsets potentially relevant to AMD, including monocytes, basophils/mast cells, and B lymphocytes/antibodies.

1. Monocytes and Macrophages

The monocyte (the circulating cell) and the macrophage (the tissue-infiltrating equivalent) are important effectors in all forms of immunity and inflammation (38–40). Monocytes are relatively large cells (12–20 μm in suspension, but up to 40 μm in tissues) and traffic through many normal sites. Most normal tissues have at least two identifiable macrophage populations: tissue-resident macrophages and blood-derived macrophages. Although many exceptions exist, in general, tissue-resident macrophages represent monocytes that migrated into a tissue weeks or months previously, or even during embryological development of the tissue, thereby acquiring tissue-specific properties and specific cellular markers. In many tissues, resident macrophages have been given tissue-specific names (e.g., microglia in the brain and retina, Kupffer cells in the liver, alveolar macrophages in the lung) (41–43). In contrast, blood-derived macrophages usually represent monocytes that have recently migrated from the blood into a fully developed tissue site, usually within a few days, still maintaining many generic properties of the circulating cell.

Macrophages serve three primary functions: as scavengers to clear cell debris and pathogens without tissue damage, as antigen-presenting cells for T lymphocytes, and as inflammatory effector cells. Conceptually, macrophages exist in different levels or stages of metabolic and functional activity, each representing different "programs" of gene activation and synthesis of mediators. Three different stages are often described: (1) scavenging or immature macrophages; (2) "primed" macrophages; and (3) "activated" macrophages. Activated macrophages often undergo a morphological change in size and histological features into a cell called an epithelioid cell. Epithelioid cells can fuse into multinucleated giant cells. Only upon full activation are macrophages most efficient at synthesis and release of mediators to amplify inflammation and to kill pathogens. Typical activational stimuli include bacterial toxins (such as lipopolysaccharides), antibody-coated pathogens, complement-coated debris, or certain cytokines (44–46) (Fig. 2).

A fourth category of macrophage, often called "reparative" or "stimulated," is used by some authorities to refer to macrophages with partial or intermediate level of activation (47–50). Reparative macrophages can mediate chronic injury in the absence of inflammatory cell infiltration or widespread tissue destruction. For example, reparative macrophages contribute to physiological processes such as fibrosis, wound repair, extracellular matrix turnover, and angiogenesis (51–59). Reparative macrophages play important roles in the pathogenesis of atherosclerosis, glomerulosclerosis, osteoarthritis, keloid formation, pulmonary fibrosis, and other noninflammatory disorders, indicating that the "repair" process is not always beneficial to delicate tissues with precise structure-function requirements. In eyes with AMD, choroidal macrophages and occasionally choroidal epithelioid cells have been observed underlying areas of drusen, geographic atrophy, and CNV (60–64). Also, cell culture data suggest that blood monocytes from patients with AMD can

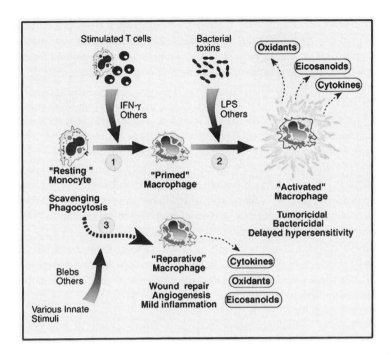

Figure 2 Overview of macrophage biology indicating process to "primed" macrophage (step 1) by IFN and subsequent activation through the exposure to LPS (step 2). Alternatively, via scavenging and phagocytosis (step 3), macrophages can become "reparative" resulting in local tissue rearrangement.

become partially activated into reparative macrophages by growth factors and debris released by oxidant-injured RPE (65).

2. Dendritic Cells (DC)

DC are terminally differentiated, bone-marrow-derived circulating mononuclear cells distinct from the macrophage-monocyte lineage and comprise approximately 0.1–1% of blood mononuclear cells (66). However, in tissue sites, DC become large (15–30 µm) with cytoplasmic veils that form extensions 2–3 times the diameter of the cell, resembling the dendritic structure of neurons. In many nonlymphoid and lymphoid organs, dendritic cells become a system of antigen-presenting cells. These sites recruit DC by defined migration pathways, and in each site, DC share features of structure and function. DC cells function as accessory cells that play an important role in processing and presentation of antigens to T cells, and their distinctive role is to initiate responses in naive lymphocytes. Thus, DC serve as the most potent leukocytes for activating T-cell-dependent immune responses. However, DC do not seem to serve as phagocytic scavengers or effectors of repair or inflammation. Both the retina and the choroid contain a high density of dendritic cells (67,68), and some data suggest that choroidal dendritic cells may insert processes into drusen in early AMD (69).

3. Basophils and Mast Cells

Basophils are the blood-borne equivalent of the tissue-bound mast cell. Mast cells exist in two major subtypes: connective tissue versus mucosal types, both of which can release preformed granules and synthesize certain mediators de novo (70,71). Connective tissue mast cells contain abundant granules with histamine and heparin, and synthesize PGD2 upon stimulation. In contrast, mucosal mast cells require T-cell cytokine help for granule formation, and therefore normally contain low levels of histamine. Also, mucosal mast cells synthesize mostly leukotrienes after stimulation. Importantly, the granule type and functional activity can be altered by the tissue location, but the regulation of these important differences is not well understood. Basophils and mast cells differ from other granulocytes in several important ways. The granule contents are different from those of PMN or eosinophils and mast cells express high-affinity Fc receptors for IgE. They act as the major effector cells in IgE-mediated immune-triggered inflammatory reactions, especially allergy or immediate hypersensitivity. Mast cells also participate in the induction of cell-mediated immunity, wound healing, and other functions not directly related to IgE-mediated degranulation (72,73). Other stimuli, such as complement or certain cytokines, may also trigger degranulation (74). Mast cells are also capable of inducing cell injury or death through their release of TNF-α. For example, mast cells have been associated with neuronal degeneration and death in thiamine deficiency and toxic metabolic diseases. Recent reports have demonstrated the presence of mast cells in atherosclerotic lesions and the colocalization of mast cells with the angiogenic protein, platelet-derived endothelial growth factor (74–80).

Mast cells are widely distributed in the connective tissue, are frequently found in close proximity to blood vessels, and are present in abundance in the choroid (81,82). Mast cells may play important roles in the pathogenesis of AMD since they have an ability to induce angiogenesis and are mediators of cell injury (83). Mast cells have also been shown to accumulate at sites of angiogenesis and have been demonstrated to be present around Bruch's membrane during both the early and late stages of choroidal neovascularization in AMD. Mast cells can interact with endothelial cells and induce their proliferation through the release of heparin, metalloproteinases, and VEGF (84–86). Interestingly, oral tranilast, an antiallergic drug that inhibits the release of chemical mediators from mast cells, has been shown to suppress laser-induced choroidal neovascularization in the rat (87).

4. T Lymphocytes

Lymphocytes are small (10–20 μm) cells with large, dense nuclei also derived from stem cell precursors within the bone marrow (1–3). However, unlike other leukocytes, lymphocytes require subsequent maturation in peripheral lymphoid organs. Originally characterized and differentiated based upon a series of ingenious but esoteric laboratory tests, lymphocytes can now be subdivided based upon detection of specific cell surface proteins (i.e., surface markers). These "markers" are in turn related to functional and molecular activity of individual subsets. Three broad categories of lymphocytes have been determined: B cells, T cells, and non-T, non-B lymphocytes.

Thymus-derived lymphocytes (or T cells) exist in several subsets (88,89). Helper T cells function to assist in antigen processing for antigen-specific immunity within lymph nodes, especially in helping B cells to produce antibody and effector T cells to become sensitized. Effector T-lymphocyte subsets function as effector cells to mediate antigen-specific inflammation and immune responses. Effector T cells can be distinguished into two main types. CD8 T cells (often called cytotoxic T lymphocytes) serve as effector cells for killing tumors or virally infected host cells via release of cytotoxic cytokines or specialized pore-forming molecules. It is possible, but unlikely, that these cells play a major role in AMD.

CD4 T cells (often called delayed-hypersensitivity T cells) effect responses by the release of specific cytokines such as interferon gamma and TNF-beta (90). They function by homing into a tissue, recognizing antigen and APC, becoming fully activated, and releasing cytokines and mediators that then amplify the reaction. Occasionally, CD4 T cells can also become activated in an antigen-independent manner, called bystander activation (91–93), a process that may explain the presence of T lymphocytes identified in CNV specimens surgically excised from AMD eyes.

5. B Lymphocytes and Antibody

B lymphocytes mature in the bone marrow and are responsible for the production of antibodies. Antibodies (or immunoglobulins) are soluble antigen-specific effector molecules of antigen-specific immunity (1–3). After appropriate antigenic stimulation with T-cell help, B cells secrete IgM antibodies, and later other isotypes, into the efferent lymph fluid draining into the venous circulation. Antibodies then mediate a variety of immune effector activities by binding to antigen in the blood or in tissues.

Antibodies serve as effectors of tissue-specific immune responses by four main mechanisms. Intravascular circulating antibodies can bind antigen in the blood, thereby form circulating immune complexes. Then the entire complex of antigen plus antibody can deposit into tissues. Alternatively, circulating B cells can infiltrate into a tissue and secrete antibody locally to form an immune complex. Third, antibody can bind to an effector cell (especially mast cell, macrophage, or neutrophil) by the Fc portion of the molecule to produce a combined antibody and cellular effector mechanism. It is unlikely that any of these mechanisms play a major role in AMD.

However, one possible antibody-dependent mechanism relevant to AMD is the capacity for circulating antibodies, usually of the IgG subclasses previously formed in lymph nodes or in other tissue sites, to passively leak into a tissue with fenestrated capillaries (like the choriocapillaris). Then, these antibodies form an immune complex with antigens trapped in the extracellular matrix, molecules expressed on the surface of cells, or even antigens sequestered inside the cell to initiate one of several types of effector responses described below (1–3, 94–97) (Fig. 3).

a. Immune Complexes with Extracellular-Bound Antigens. When free antibody passively leaks from the serum into a tissue, it can combine with tissue-bound antigens

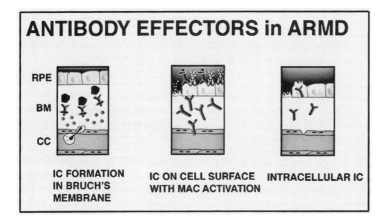

Figure 3 Possible antibody effects in AMD with subsequent immune complex (IC) formation at variation locations in the subretinal space, on or within the retinal pigment epithelium.

(i.e., antigen trapped in the extracellular matrix). These "in situ" or locally formed complexes sometimes activate the complement pathway to produce complement fragments called anaphylatoxins. This mechanism should be differentiated from deposition of circulating immune complexes, which are preformed in the blood. Typically, the histology is dominated by neutrophils and monocytes, but at low level of activation minimal cellular infiltration may be observed. Many types of glomerulonephritis and vasculitis are thought to represent this mechanism.

b. Immune Complexes with Cell-Surface Antigen. If an antigen is associated with the external surface of the plasma membrane, antibody binding might activate the terminal complement cascade to induce cell injury via formation of specialized pore-like structures called the membrane attack complex. Hemolytic anemia of the newborn due to Rh incompatibility is the classic example of this process. Hashimoto's thyroiditis, nephritis of Goodpasture's syndrome, and autoimmune thrombocytopenia are other examples.

c. Immune Complex with Intracellular Antigen. Circulating antibodies can cause tissue injury by mechanisms different from complement activation, using pathogenic mechanisms not yet clearly elucidated (96,97). For example, some autoantibodies in systemic lupus erythematosus appear to be internalized by renal cells independent of antigen binding, but then combine with intracellular nuclear or ribosomal antigens to alter cellular metabolism and signaling pathways. This novel pathway of intracellular antibody/antigen complex formation may cause some cases of nephritis in the absence of complement activation. This pathway has also been implicated in paraneoplastic syndromes, especially cancer-associated retinopathy (CAR), in which autoantibodies to intracellular photoreceptor-associated antigens may mediate rod or cone degeneration (98).

C. Mechanisms for the Activation of the Immune Responses in Degenerative Diseases

1. Activation of Innate Immunity

a. Cellular Injury as a Trigger of Innate Immunity. Not only can immune responses cause cellular injury, but cellular responses to nonimmune injury are also common initiators of innate immunity (1–4,99,100). Injury can be defined as tissue exposure to any physical and/or biochemical stimulus that alters preexisting homeostasis to produce a physiological cellular response. In addition to injury stimuli produced by the immune effector and amplification systems described above, nonimmune injurious stimuli include physical injury (heat, light, mechanical) or biochemical stimulation (hypoxia, pH change, oxidants, chemical mediators, cytokines) (100). Typical cellular reactions to injury include a wide spectrum of responses, including changes in intracellular metabolism, plasma membrane alterations, cytokine production and gene upregulation, morphological changes, cellular migration, proliferation, or even death. Some of these cellular responses, in turn, can result in the recruitment and activation of macrophages or activation of amplification systems, especially if they include upregulation of cell adhesion molecules, production of macrophage chemotactic factors, or release of activational stimuli.

Two important injury responses relevant to AMD that commonly activate innate immunity include vascular injury and extracellular deposit accumulation (100,101). Vascular injury induced by physical stimuli (i.e., mechanical stretch of capillaries or arterioles by hydrostatic expansion induced by hypertension or thermal injury from laser) or biochemical stimuli (i.e., hormones associated with hypertension and aging) can upregulate cell adhesion molecules and chemotactic factors that lead to macrophage recruitment into various vascularized tissues. Extracellular deposit accumulation can also contribute to activation of innate immunity by serving as a substrate for scavenging and phagocytosis, especially if the deposits are chemically modified by oxidation or other processes (see below).

b. Infection as a Trigger of Innate Immunity. Infection can also activate innate immunity, usually by the release of toxic molecules (i.e., endotoxins, exotoxins, cell wall components) that directly interact with receptors on macrophages, on neutrophils, or, in some cases, on parenchymal cells. Active infection is differentiated from harmless colonization by the presence of invasion and replication of the infectious agent (102). However, active infections do not always trigger innate immunity, illustrated by some retinal parasite infections in which inflammation occurs only when the parasite dies.

Recently, the idea has emerged that certain kinds of chronic infections might cause (or at least contribute to) degenerative diseases that are not considered to be truly inflammatory (99–102). One of the most dramatic examples is peptic ulcer disease, recently recognized to be caused by infection of the gastric subepithelial mucosa with a gram-positive bacterium called *Helicobacter pylori* (103). Accordingly, ulcer disease is now treated by antibiotics and not with diet or surgery. Recently, chronic bacterial or viral infection of vascular endothelial cells has been suggested as an etiology for coronary artery atherosclerosis, and infection with an unusual agent called prion has been shown as a cause of certain neurodegenerative diseases. The relevance to AMD is discussed below.

2. Activation of Normal and Aberrant Antigen-Specific Immunity

a. Activation of Antigen-Specfic Immunity. This is often expressed as the concept of the "immune response arc," which proposes that interaction between antigen and the antigen-specific immune system at a peripheral site (such as the skin) can conceptually be subdivided into three phases: afferent (at the site), processing (within the immune system), and effector (at the original site completing the arc) (1–3,7) (Fig. 4.) Antigen within the skin or any other site is recognized by the afferent phase of the immune response, which conveys the antigenic information to the lymph node in one of two forms. Antigen-presenting cells (APC), typically DC, can take up antigen (almost always in the form of a protein) at a site, digest the antigen into fragments, and carry the digested fragments to the lymph node to interact with T cells (88–90). Alternatively, the natural, intact antigen can directly flow into the node via lymphatics where it interacts with B cells (1–3).

In the lymph node, *processing* of the antigenic signal occurs where antigen, APC, T cells, and B cells interact to activate the immune response. For tissues without draining lymph nodes (such as the retina and choroid), the spleen is often a major site of processing. Immunological, processing has been the topic of extensive research and the details are too complex to discuss in this brief review. Processing results in release of immune effectors (antibodies, B cells, and T cells) into efferent lymphatics and venous circulation, which conveys the intent of the immune system back to the original site where an effector re-

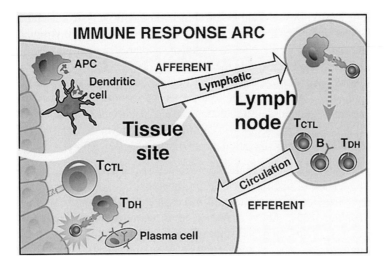

Figure 4 The immune response arc indicating cross-talk between the tissue site, where antigen recognition and effector processes take place, and the lymph node, the site of antigen processing.

sponse occurs (i.e., immune complex formation or delayed hypersensitivity reaction). Compared to that of the skin, the immune response arcs of the retina and choroid express many similarities as well as important differences (i.e., immune privilege, anatomy), which are discussed in recent reviews (104,105).

b. Aberrant Activation of Antigen-Specific Immunity. The inappropriate activation of antigen-specific immunity may play a role in the pathogenesis of chronic degenerative diseases. Autoimmunity is the activation of antigen-specific immunity to normal self-antigens, and two different mechanisms of autoimmunity may be relevant to AMD: molecular mimicry and desequestration. Additionally, immune responses directed at "neo-antigens" or foreign antigens inappropriately trapped within normal tissues may also play a role in AMD.

Molecular mimicry is the immunological cross-reaction between antigenic regions (epitopes) of an unrelated foreign molecule and self-antigens with similar structures (106). For example, immune system exposure to foreign antigens, such as those present within yeast, viruses, or bacteria, can induce an appropriate afferent, processing, and effector immune response to the organism. However, antimicrobial antibodies or effector lymphocytes generated to the organism can inappropriately cross-react with similar antigenic regions of a self-antigen. A dynamic process would then be initiated, causing tissue injury by an autoimmune response that would induce additional lymphocyte responses directed at other self-antigens. Thus, the process would not require the ongoing replication of a pathogen or the continuous presence of the inciting antigen. Molecular mimicry against antigens from a wide range of organisms, including *Streptococcus*, yeast, *Escherichia coli*, and various viruses, has been shown to be a potential mechanism for antiretinal autoimmunity (107).

A second mechanism for aberrant autoimmunity is desequestration (108–110). For most self-antigens, the immune system is actively "tolerized" to the antigen by various mechanisms, preventing the activation of antigen-specific immune effector responses even when the self-antigen is fully exposed to the immune system. For some other antigens, however, the immune system relies on sequestration of the antigen within cellular compartments that are isolated from antigen-presenting cells and effector mechanisms. If the sequestered molecules are allowed to escape their protective isolation, they can become recognized as foreign, thereby initiating an autoimmune reaction. For example, certain nuclear or ribosomal-associated enzymes are apparently sequestered, and if organelles become extruded into a location with exposure to dendritic cells or macrophages, an immune response can be triggered against these antigens (109). Accordingly, some RPE and retina-associated peptides appear to be sequestered from the immune system and could potentially serve as antigens if RPE injury or death leads to their release into the choroid (104,110).

Another mechanism for aberrant activation of antigen-specific immunity is the formation of "neo-antigens" secondary to chemical modification of normal self-proteins trapped or deposited within tissues (111). For example, oxidation or acetylation of peptides in apolipoproteins trapped within atherosclerotic plaques can induce new antigenic properties resulting in specific T cells and antibodies immunized to the modified protein.

A final mechanism for aberrant antigen-specific immunity is antigen trapping (112). Antigen trapping is the immunological reaction to circulating foreign antigens inappropriately trapped within the extracellular matrix of a normal tissue site containing fenestrated capillaries. Typically occurring after invasive infection or iatrogenically administered drugs, this mechanism may be very important in glomerular diseases (112) and has been postulated to induce ocular inflammation (113). Physical size and charge of the antigen are important. For example, antigen trapping within the choriocapillaris may contribute to ocular histoplasmosis syndrome (114).

III. EXAMPLES OF IMMUNE AND INFLAMMATORY MECHANISMS OF NONOCULAR DEGENERATIVE DISEASES

A. Immune Mechanisms in Atherosclerosis

Myocardial infarction due to thrombosis of atherosclerotic coronary arteries is the major cause of death in Western countries, and epidemiological studies suggest a possible association with AMD (115,116). The pathology of atherosclerosis suggests a spectrum of changes whose pathogenesis may be relevant to the understanding of AMD (117,118). The fatty streak, representing the earliest phase of atherosclerosis, is characterized by lipid deposition and macrophage infiltration within the vessel wall (111,118,119). Some investigators have suggested similarities in pathogenesis between fatty streak formation and early AMD (120). The fatty streak can progress into the fibrous plaque, characterized by the proliferation of smooth muscle cells, increasing inflammation, and formation of connective tissue with neovascularization within the vessel wall. The fibrous plaque predisposes to the complications of atherosclerosis such as thrombosis, dissection, or plaque ulceration (111,118,119). The pathogenesis of the fibrous plaque may share similarity with mechanisms for the late complications of AMD, including formation of CNV and disciform scars (Fig. 5).

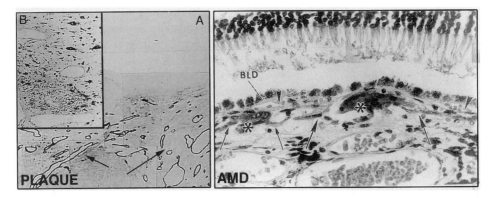

Figure 5 Micrographs of an atheromatous plaque (left) and a choroidal neovascular membrane (right) indicating similar histological components of intrastromal neovascularization (arrows) and macrophages (left, B) and (right, asterisk). (From Jeziorska M, Woolley, DE. Local neovascularization and cellular composition within vulnerable regions of atherosclerotic plaques of human carotid arteries. J Pathol 1999; 188:189–196 [left] and Green WR, Enger C. Age-related macular degeneration histopatholgic studies. The 1992 Lorenz E. Zimmerman Lecture. Ophthalmology 1993; 100:1519–153 [right].)

Many mechanisms contribute to the pathogenesis of atherosclerosis, including genetic predisposition and physiological risk factors such as high blood cholesterol, smoking, diabetes, and hypertension. However, most authorities now believe that chronic low-grade inflammation, induced by a wide variety of injury stimuli, followed by a fibroproliferative (wound healing) response within the vessel wall, is central to the pathogenesis of atherosclerosis. Thus, various immune mechanisms implicated in atherosclerosis might be relevant to AMD.

1. Innate Mechanisms

a. Injury and Atherosclerosis. The "response to injury" hypothesis for the initiation and progression of atherosclerosis has been supported by numerous investigators who cite many different participating injury stimuli (111,118,119). For example, hemodynamic injury by blood flow turbulence can directly injure endothelial cells at bifurcations of major vessels (121). Biochemical injury secondary to exposure to polypetide mediators associated with hypertension (i.e., angiotensin II or endothelin-1) can stimulate the endothelial and smooth muscle responses. Oxidized LDL cholesterol particles in the blood, advanced glycosylation endproducts in diabetes, or toxic chemicals secondary to smoking are other potential sources of injury (122). The interested reader is referred to several recent reviews on these topics.

b. Macrophages in Atherosclerosis. Blood-derived macrophages are major contributors to the pathogenesis of atherosclerosis (111,118,123). In the fatty streak phase of atherosclerosis, lipids accumulate in the subendothelial vascular wall at sites of vascular injury. Injury results in the oxidation of lipids or endothelial production of specific macrophage chemotactic signals, such as macrophage chemotactic protein-1, recruiting circulating monocytes to sites of endothelial injury. There, they migrate into the subendothelial extracellular matrix to scavenge the extracellular lipid-rich deposits (i.e., scavenging macrophages). Macrophages may also contribute to the solubilization of lipid deposits by the release of apolipoprotein B (ApoE), which may facilitate uptake and scavenging of lipids. Genetic polymorphisms of ApoE have been associated with variations in the severity of atherosclerosis and AMD (124).

Foam cells and macrophages are very numerous in fibrous plaques, and probably play a major role in lesion progression. Although overly simplistic, experimental data suggest that scavenging macrophages can become activated into reparative "foam" cells by numerous stimuli, including by phagocytosis of oxidized lipoproteins (123,124). Reparative macrophages secrete amplifying mediators, including platelet-derived growth factor (PDGF), VEGF, matrix metalloproteinases, or others that contribute to fibrosis, smooth muscle proliferation, or vascularization of the plaque (125–128).

c.   Infectious Etiology of Atherosclerosis.   Although numerous risk factors are associated with the initiation and progression of atherosclerosis, an infectious etiology has been suggested by recent data. Many patients with atherosclerosis exhibit signs of mild systemic inflammation, especially elevated serum C-reactive protein and erythrocyte sedimentation rate (129). Statistical evidence has been generated to suggest that infection with various infectious agents, especially *Chlamydia pneumoniae* or cytomegalovirus (CMV), might initiate vascular injury and explain the systemic inflammatory signs (130–133).

Numerous epidemiological studies have revealed a statistical correlation between atherosclerosis and serological evidence of infection with *C. pneumoniae* (130). Follow-up studies have demonstrated the presence of *C. pneumoniae* by histochemical methods within atherosclerotic plaques and organisms have been cultured from the lesions (131). Additionally, pilot studies using appropriate antibiotic therapy have demonstrated a beneficial effect in patients with severe atherosclerosis (132,133). Several proposed mechanisms for the role of *C. pneumoniae* in atherosclerosis may be relevant to AMD. Chronic infection of vascular endothelial cells may upregulate cell surface molecules that recruit macrophages or alter responses to injury. For instance, *C. pneumoniae* endothelial infection can enhance endotoxin binding to LDL particles that might induce various inflammatory cascades at the site of uptake (134). Additionally, chlamydial heat shock proteins (HSPs) can directly stimulate macrophages and other cellular amplification systems (135). Also, antigen-specific immune responses directed against chlamydial HSPs may cross-react with host cellular HSP including those expressed in the retina (136).

Similar but less extensive data have been generated to support a role of CMV infection in atherosclerosis (137–139). Cytomegalovirus infects 60–70% of adults in the United States. Several studies have linked serological evidence of prior CMV infection to atherosclerosis. Although the association is mild, studies have elucidated possible mechanisms for this association such as enhanced scavenging of LDL particles by virally infected endothelial cells.

2.   Antigen-Specific Immunity

The potential importance of antigen-specific immune mechanisms in atherosclerosis is illustrated by the observation of accelerated atherosclerosis in heart transplant patients who experience vascular injury associated with mild, chronic allograft rejection (140). In normal patients with atherosclerosis, T lymphocytes are numerous in fibrous plaques and a role for lymphocyte-mediated antigen-specific immunity has been proposed for progression of atherosclerotic fibrous plaques (111). Experimental data suggest that oxidized lipoproteins can become neo-antigens to activate an immune response arc (141). Scavenging macrophages may become antigen-presenting cells at the site, serving to restimulate recruited T cells, thereby activating the effector phase of the immune response. Immune responses to bacterial or viral antigens, especially chlamydial heat shock proteins, trapped in tissues after occult infection may also stimulate antigen-specific immunity, or autoimmunity by cross-reactive molecular mimicry (142). Alternatively, T cells may be recruited by innate responses and become activated by antigen-independent bystander mechanisms. Interestingly, vaccination against oxidized LDL produces antibodies that seem to prevent or reduce formation of atherosclerotic plaques (143), similar to those observed in AD (see below).

3. Nonspecific Amplification Cascades

a.   Complement Activation in Atherosclerosis.   In atherosclerotic lesions, several complement components and inhibitory proteins have been detected including MAC complexes (144–146). Cholesterol is also a potent activator of the complement system in vitro. Alternatively, MAC complex concentration has been shown to induce macrophage chemotactic factor production in smooth muscle cells, and studies have shown MAC deposition in the arterial wall prior to monocyte infiltration and foam cell formation. Interestingly, in addition to its cytotoxic function, limited complement activation and deposition of the complement precursor protein C1q on apoptotic cells, cell debris, and cell membrane blebs can enhance phagocytosis by C1q-receptor-bearing macrophages and may play a role in tissue repair.

b.   Oxidants and Cytokines in Atherosclerosis.   Oxidation is considered to be a major injury stimulus in the initiation and progression of atherosclerosis. The role of oxidized lipoproteins in circulating LDL cholesterol as an initiating injury stimulus as well as in oxidation of lipid deposits within vessel walls as an amplifier of foam cell activation has been discussed above (122,123,147). Numerous cytokines, especially PDGF and TGF-beta, have also been implicated as major mediators of atherosclerosis progression (125–128).

B. Immune Mechanisms in Alzheimer's Disease

Alzheimer's disease is a progressive neurodegenerative disease affecting up to 25% of Americans older than age 80. The pathology is characterized by the atrophic loss of selective cortical neurons and the presence of neurofibrillary tangles and senile plaques (148). An epidemiological association between AD and AMD has been suggested (149). The pathogenesis of Alzheimer's disease is multifactorial, including both genetic predisposition and physiological factors. Recently, increasing evidence has become available to suggest an important role for a "response to injury" mechanism with major immunological contributions (150–154).

1. Innate Immunity in AD

a.   Injury and Monocyte Function in Alzheimer's Disease.   Accumulation of senile plaques formed from extracellular release and aggregation of abnormally processed amyloid β-protein is an early event associated with neural degeneration in Alzheimer's disease (155,156). Although the abnormal processing of amyloid may be genetically determined in some forms of Alzheimer's disease, the subsequent events leading to neural degeneration probably represent physiological responses to injury involving

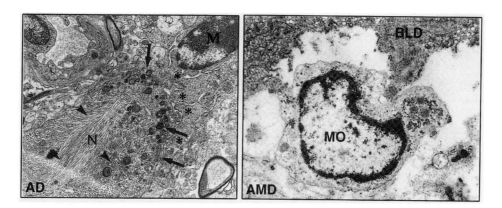

Figure 6 Electron micrographs from a patient with Alzheimer's disease (AD) and age-related macular degeneration (AMD) indicating similar appearance of scavenging of cellular debris by immune cells. Figure AD shows microglia (M) with cellular processes (asterisks) around extracellular debris (arrows) from a dying neuronal cell (N) while figure AMD indicates digestion of basal laminar deposits (BLD) by subretinal macrophage (MO). (From el Hachimi KH, Foncin JF. Do microglial cells phagocyte the beta/A4-amyloid senile plaque core of Alzheimer disease? CR Acad Sci III 1994; 317:445–451 [left] and Sarks JP Sarks SH. Macrophages related to Bruch's membrane in age-related macular degeneration. Eye 1990; 4:613–621 [right].)

innate immunity (150–154). For example, new evidence suggests that accumulation of amyloid plaques can activate microglia, the tissue-resident monocytes of the brain (157). Like blood-derived macrophages, microglia exhibit scavenging of extracellular deposits, and phagocytosis of abnormal amyloid deposits in Alzheimer's disease might lead to inappropriate cellular activation (158,159). Activated microglia can cause neuronal death by the secretion of mediators like interleukin-1, interleukin-6, TNF, and prostaglandin. Nonsteroidal anti-inflammatory agents, which block enzymes responsible for the production of certain prostaglandin derivatives, appear to slow the progression of Alzheimer's disease (160). Microglia are also involved in the regulation of extracellular ApoE. As in atherosclerosis and AMD, increased deposition of ApoE has been demonstrated in specimens from patients with Alzheimer's disease (152,161–163). Since the retina contains abundant microglia with similar properties, some investigators have proposed that microglia might contribute to photoreceptor death in AMD (164). Thus, Alzheimer's disease, like atherosclerosis, illustrates a disease in which monocyte scavenging of abnormal deposits inadvertently induces activation of these cells, a mechanism potentially relevant to drusen scavenging by monocytes in AMD (Fig. 6).

b. Infectious Etiology of Neurodegenerative Diseases.   A link between infectious agents and chronic degenerative diseases of the elderly was established many decades ago with the understanding that *Treponema pallidum* is the causative agent for some cases of dementia, including Alzheimer's disease (165). A new paradigm for infection-induced neurodegeneration has been established based on the identification of brain infection with an unusual agent called a prion (166). Prion infection induces neuronal protein misfolding leading to the accumulation of extracellular protein deposits. Prions have been identified as causative agents in certain neurodegenerative diseases, especially Creutzfeld-Jacob disease and related spongiform encephalopathies in animals (i.e., mad cow disease). Several studies have indicated that prion infection can produce amyloid aggregates similar in appearance to those seen in Alzheimer's disease (167).

2. Antigen-Specific Immunity in Alzheimer's Disease

In general, the brain, like the retina, is considered to be immune privileged in the sense that the blood-brain barrier resists passive deposition of antibodies and reduces the recruitment of antigen-specific lymphocytes (168). Consistent with this observation is the absence of lymphocyte infiltration or widespread antibody deposition in Alzheimer's disease. However, antiphospholipid autoantibodies have been shown to be present in Alzheimer's disease serum and can induce brain pathology (169). Further, antibodies purified from serum from patients with Alzheimer's disease causes Alzheimer's disease–like lesions when injected into the brains of experimental rats (170).

Paradoxically, antigen-specific immunity might actually function to protect against degenerative diseases. As mentioned above, amyloid accumulation in Alzheimer's disease is caused by an abnormally cleaved variant of the amyloid protein that is two amino acids longer than the normal form. Recently, immunization with the abnormal amyloid, or passive administration of antibodies against the abnormal protein, greatly reduced the quantity of deposition in the brain of genetically modified mice with Alzheimer's disease, and improved their performance in laboratory tests of memory and cognitive function (171,172). The mechanisms are unclear, but may be related to enhance phagocytosis, neutralization of toxic moieties on deposits, or interference with amyloid fibril aggregation. In Alzheimer's disease patients, however, individuals may be immunologically tolerant to amyloid preventing protective autoimmunization to the abnormally processed protein (173).

3. Nonspecific Amplification Cascades in AD

Complement activation has been implicated in the pathogenesis of Alzheimer's disease (174–176). Cerebral astrocytes and resident microglia are both capable of secreting all the components of the classical and alternative pathway; thus deposition from the blood is not absolutely necessary. Additionally, amyloid has been shown to activate C3 and lead to the formation of MAC in the brain with subsequent damage to the adjacent neurons (176). Not surprisingly, oxidants have also been implicated as injury stimuli and amplification mechanisms in AD (177,178).

C. Immune Mechanisms in Glomerular Diseases

Glomerular diseases account for 70% of chronic renal failure in the United States. Many glomerular diseases are primarily mediated by inflammatory mechanisms, and are usually classified as glomerulonephritis. Other glomerular diseases are mediated by a mixture of degenerative and inflammatory mechanisms, and these are often classified as glomerulosclerosis (179,180). Genetic and systemic health factors contribute to the pathogenesis of both groups (178–182).

The glomerulus shares some anatomical similarities with the outer retina and inner choroid, so analysis of the mechanism of deposit formation and extracellular matrix changes of glomerular disorders might be informative in terms of AMD (179). For instance, both the glomerulus and inner choroid/outer retina can be described as containing capillary lobules with endothelium on one side of an extracellular matrix and epithelium on the other.

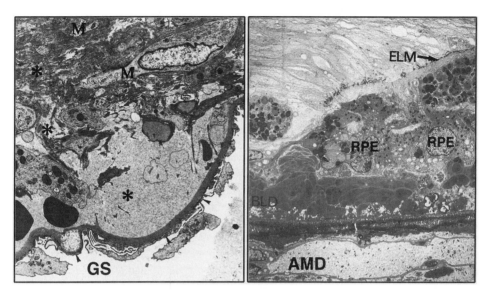

Figure 7 Electron micrographs from glomerulosclerosis and geographic atrophy from age-related macular degeneration showing appearance of excessive extracellular material and cellular loss. In GS there is accumulation of glomerular extracellular material (asterisks) and loss of cellular structure (M), while in AMD there is accumulation of BLD and loss of RPE cells under the external limiting membrane (ELM). (From Tisher CC, Hostetter TH. Diabetic nephropathy. In Tisher CC, Brenner BM. Renal Pathology with Clinical and Functional Correlations. Philadelphia: JB Lippincott, 1994 [left] and Sarks JP, Sarks SH, Killingsworth MC. Evolution of geographic atrophy of the retinal pigment epithelium. Eye 1988;2:552–577 [right].)

In the glomerulus, endothelial cells (conceptually corresponding to the choriocapillaris) cover the internal surface of an extracellular matrix, whose external surface is covered by an epithelial layer (the podocyte). External to the podocyte is Bowman's capsule (conceptually corresponding to the subretinal space). Smooth muscle cells located internally to the endothelium, called mesangial cells, are responsible for regulating contractility and maintaining the glomerular matrix. These cells may share analogies with choroidal pericytes underlying and surrounding the choriocapillaris.

1. Innate Immunity in Glomerular Diseases

a. Chronic Injury. As is the case for atherosclerosis, a "response to injury" hypothesis has been substantiated for glomerulosclerosis due to aging, hypertension, or diabetes (179–186). Glomerulosclerosis is characterized by progressive thickening of the glomerular extracellular matrix ultimately associated with loss of glomerular capillaries and epithelial cells. If enough glomeruli are involved, renal impairment occurs. In some ways, glomerulosclerosis resembles geographic atrophy in AMD (Fig. 7).

The response to injury hypothesis has been thoroughly evaluated for renal hypertension, a major cause of glomerulosclerosis (182–187). The hemodynamic injury hypothesis proposes that glomerular capillary hypertension causes excessive flow through the glomerulus or hydraulic stretching of the capillary wall to activate injury responses in glomerular cells. The humoral hypothesis proposes that hypertension-associated hormones or cytokines associated with low-grade systemic inflammation induced by hypertensive vascular injury activate cellular injury responses. In either case, the injured endothelium, podocytes, and mesangial cells demonstrate abnormal production and turnover of collagen and other matrix molecules, leading to collagenous thickening of the matrix with degeneration of the glomerulus (187–189). Genetic background and gender can influence the rate of progression. Since hypertension is a risk factor associated with AMD and glomerular disease, hypertension-associated inflammation may also injure the choriocapillaris endothelium or RPE in an analogous fashion.

b. Macrophage-Mediated Injury. Macrophages contribute significantly to glomerular damage in renal diseases (190–200). Not surprisingly, infiltration with activated inflammatory macrophages is a significant histological feature in inflammatory glomerulonephritis caused by antigen-specific immune mechanisms (i.e., immune complex disease or allograft rejection) (200), and blockade of macrophage infiltration or function ameliorates glomerular damage (193). Perhaps of more relevance to AMD is the contribution of reparative macrophages to glomerulosclerosis. Recruitment of blood-derived reparative macrophages develops early in the course of glomerulosclerosis in proportion to the severity of the injury (190,191). Various innate injury stimuli, including renal hypertension, hyperlipidemia, and glomerular capillary endothelial injury by oxidized LDL, can upregulate macrophage chemotactic factors and adhesion molecules in the capillaries to induce macrophage recruitment (194–197). Experimental data suggest that reparative macrophages release mediators that induce mesangial cell proliferation, amplify the accumulation of extracellular matrix, and might induce killing of endothelial cells.

2. Antigen-Specific Immunity in Glomerular Diseases

Antigen-specific immunity contributes significantly to inflammatory glomerular disorders. Lymphocyte-mediated immunity clearly contributes to glomerulonephritis, especially in renal allograft rejection (200). However, the relevance of this mechanism to AMD is probably minimal. Many forms of chronic glomerulonephritis are caused by antibody-dependent mechanisms, and some of these disorders are characterized by subendothelial or subepithelial deposit formation (112,178–180). Direct deposition of circulating antibodies targeted at antigens uniformly expressed within the glomerular matrix is a well-defined, but rare, form of glomerulonephritis, especially in Goodpasture's syndrome. Deposition of preformed circulating antigen/antibody complexes in the blood has been proposed as another major mechanism in many types of glomerulonephritis associated with deposit formation. Nevertheless, it is unlikely that deposition of either anti-basement membrane antibodies or circulating immune complexes plays an important role in AMD.

However, another interpretation of the clinical and experimental data is that some forms of glomerulonephritis may actually represent antigen trapped or "planted" within the glomerular matrix, followed by the subsequent formation of in situ immune complexes. This alternative explanation is probably especially relevant to glomerulonephritis associated with subepithelial deposits rather than subendothelial deposits (since it is unlikely that large immune complexes would be able to filter through the matrix). For example, glomerulonephritis that occurs 10–20 days after streptococcal pharyngitis or streptococcal skin infections is characterized by subepithelial deposits (similar to homogeneous basal laminar deposits). These do not stain for immune complexes (201).

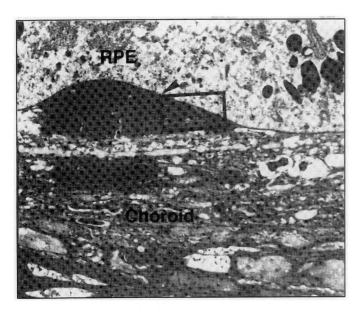

Figure 8 Electron micrograph of dense deposit disease of the retina demonstrating subretinal deposit (box) located between the retinal pigment epithelium and its basement membrane. (From Duvall-Young J, MacDonald MK, McKechnie NM. Fundus changes in [type II] mesangiocapillary glomerulonephritis simulating drusen: a histopathological report, Br J Ophthalmol 1989; 73:297–302.)

3. Nonspecific Amplification Cascades in Glomerular Diseases

Complement deposition plays a major primary role in many glomerular diseases associated with deposits, especially those mediated by antigen-specific immune complexes. In these disorders, various fragment of the complement cascade, including C3, C5, and others, are usually identified within extracellular deposits in association with immunoglobulin and acute cellular inflammation (178–181).

Complement seems to participate as a secondary amplification mechanism in some glomerular diseases. Type II membranoproliferative glomerulonephritis (or dense deposit disease) is especially relevant to AMD since these patients also develop drusen-like changes in the retina (202–207). Clinically, the retina demonstrates whitish drusen-like changes, and some eyes develop choroidal neovascularization.

Histologically, the subretinal deposits appear to be localized between the RPE and its basement membrane (similar to basal laminar deposits) (Fig. 8). The glomerular deposits are characterized as electron-dense linear deposits within the glomerular extracellular matrix, occasionally demonstrating dome-shaped subepithelial "humps" under the podocyte. Complement 3 is present within the deposits, but the presence of other complement proteins, immunoglobulins, and fibronectin is highly variable. Systemic complement is usually normal. The source of complement (i.e., locally synthesis or blood-derived) as well as the mechanisms for activation (typical cascades versus enzymatic cleavage) remain unknown. Finally, oxidants have been implicated as important mediators and amplifiers in progression of renal disease (208).

IV. EVIDENCE FOR IMMUNE AND INFLAMMATORY
MECHANISMS IN AMD

A. Direct Evidence for Innate or Antigen-Specific Immune Effectors

Direct evidence for the role of immune mechanism in AMD is scant. The best data suggest an important role for macrophage-mediated innate immunity (60–69). Investigators have observed that choroidal macrophages appear to be important in the pathogenesis of both early and late AMD. However, macrophage involvement is clearly different than their participation in overt inflammatory disorders characterized by widespread cellular infiltration.

In early AMD, macrophages have been detected along the choriocapillaris side of Bruch's membrane underlying areas of thick deposits. Processes from choroidal monocytes have been noted to insert into Bruch's membrane deposits, presumably for the purpose of scavenging debris. The identity of these cells is uncertain, but they seem to lack typical phagocytic vacuoles and express HLA DR, suggesting that the cells may represent dendritic cells or nonactivated macrophages (69).

In late AMD, macrophages and giant cells have been observed around CNVM and are numerous in excised CNVM, suggesting a role in promoting choroidal angiogenesis (60,63,210). Also, macrophages are present underlying zones of geographic atrophy, suggesting a role in RPE or endothelial death (61). These observations imply a potential pathogenic role for cytokines, chemical mediators, MMPs, mitogens, or angiogenic factors released by macrophages from the choroid. In support of this concept, numerous investigators have demonstrated that macrophage-derived cytokines (especially TNF-α) induce major functional and morphological changes in RPE cells (211–215). Further, macrophage involvement may be underestimated in AMD. Choroidal macrophages are often difficult to detect by routine histopathology in noninflammatory disorders because they typically acquire very flattened profiles. Finally, evidence from several recent clinical trials has shown a benefit from intravitreal corticosteroid therapy in the treatment of choroidal neovascularization in AMD patients (216,217). Corticosteroids are potent modulators of macrophage function (218) and these studies suggest that more research should explore the therapeutic potential of nonspecific anti-inflammatory therapy in AMD.

Evidence for antigen-specific immunity has not been described in AMD. The possible contribution of antibody-dependent mechanisms is suggested by recent understanding of the mechanism for CAR (see Sec. IV.B). In AMD, one group has identified IgG and MAC association with RPE overlying drusen (219). However, another study has identified only antibody light chains within drusen, but not the presence of associated heavy chains to indicate an intact immunoglobulin molecule (22,220). Lymphocytes, especially T cells, have been identified within some CNV (63). It remains unknown whether these cells are recruited as part of bystander activation or are responding to antigen-specific immunity. However, bystander recruitment of T cells occurs in many other forms of pathological neovascularization and wound healing.

Nonspecific amplification mechanisms may also play a role in AMD. Recently, several groups have identified complement components in drusen (22,219,220). Fragments of C5 and MAC were identified in most specimens, and C3 was present in some.

The activation pathway remains unknown. The RPE express specific and nonspecific complement inhibitors such as decay-accelerating factor and vitronectin to suggest intrinsic defense mechanisms to prevent against complement-mediated injury (221,222).

B. Ocular Immune and Inflammatory Disorders Resulting in Atrophic Retinal Degeneration or CNV

1. Presumed Ocular Histoplasmosis Syndrome (POHS)

POHS may represent a condition suggesting a role for infection-triggered immunity as a mechanism for RPE injury and CNV formation. The syndrome is presumed to be induced by the inhalation of live *histoplasma capsulatum*, which infects the lung and hilar lymph nodes (223). In some patients, systemic dissemination of the organism occurs, including into the choroid, but the organism is rapidly recognized and killed by the immune response. According to data from a primate model, the acute phase of immune response can induce clinically detectable, small, multifocal creamy lesions in the deep retina and choroid caused by localized choriocapillaris inflammation mediated by CD4 T cells (presumably delayed hypersensitivity) (224,225). However, many other areas of active choroidal inflammation are clinically inapparent. Ultimately the overlying RPE become atrophic "histo spot." Chronic, persistent low-grade inflammation apparently triggers CNV formation (226,227). Additionally, many other forms of chronic chorioretinitis are also associated with RPE atrophy and CNV formation, and some of these may represent occult infection of the choroid or RPE with virus or other infectious agents (228).

  The role of infection in AMD remains entirely speculative. Although it is unlikely that histoplasmosis contributes to AMD, trapping of antigens related to other common organisms conceivably could occur. Based on analogies to the role of infection in fibrous plaque progression, investigation of possible contributions from choroidal endothelial infection with *Chlamydia* or cytomegalovirus might be informative. Finally, as new unusual infectious agents, such as prions, are being discovered, the potential role of retinal or RPE infection in AMD should at least be considered.

2. Cancer-Associated Retinopathy

CAR may serve as a model disease to suggest how antigen-specific autoimmunity can induce retinal degeneration. CAR is a paraneoplastic syndrome in which some patients with carcinoma, especially small cell carcinoma of the lung or occasionally cutaneous melanoma, develop antibodies against a tumor-associated antigen that happens to cross-react with an ocular autoantigen (229,230). For example, some small cell carcinomas aberrantly synthesize recoverin (a normal protein in photoreceptors) (230). The immune system inappropriately recognizes, processes, and produces an antibody effector response, releasing antirecoverin antibodies into the circulation. These antibodies passively permeate into the retina, are taken up by photoreceptors, and cause slowly progressive photoreceptor degeneration by a novel, poorly understood cytotoxic mechanism. Current research speculation proposes induction of programmed cell death caused by intracellular antibody/antigen complex formation after photoreceptor uptake of antirecoverin antibodies (98). Recently, a subset of CAR patients have been shown to also express antibodies to an RPE-derived protein and demonstrate physiological evidence of RPE dysfunction to suggest anti-RPE autoimmunity (231).

V. IMMUNE MECHANISMS IN AMD: FINAL
QUESTIONS AND FUTURE DIRECTIONS

A. Is the "Response to Injury" Hypothesis Applicable
to AMD?

As discussed above, the response-to-injury hypothesis has become one of the central paradigms for the pathogenesis of atherosclerosis, Alzheimer's disease, and glomerulosclerosis. The response-to-injury paradigm proposes that pathological features of degenerative diseases can be explained by exaggerated or abnormal cellular reparative responses induced by exposure to chronic, recurrent injurious stimuli. Both genetic and physiological factors can contribute to injury or repair. This chapter has focused on the physiological role of innate immunity, antigen-specific immunity, and immune amplification systems as potential triggers of injury and as modulators of abnormal repair.

In terms of AMD, response to injury is implicit in pathogenic models that propose a role for various injurious stimuli, such as oxidants, lipofuscin cytotoxicty, and other factors. Injury stimuli relevant to other systemic diseases associated with AMD have not been carefully evaluated, including hyperlipidemia, oxidized lipoproteins, hormonal changes associated with aging, or hypertension (232). Presumably, photoreceptors, RPE, choricapillaris endothelium, and/or choroidal pericytes may all be relevant targets. However, to exploit the full power of the response to injury paradigm, AMD investigators must more precisely delineate the relevant cellular responses to injury to explain the specific pathological changes in AMD. Cellular repair responses are manifested by a wide spectrum, ranging from transient metabolic changes to cell death (233,234). The appropriate cellular response must be matched to a specific pathological change. For example, analysis of programmed cell death in response to lethal injury is relevant to the understanding of geographic atrophy of the RPE (235). However, it is unlikely that analysis of cell death will explain the formation of sub-RPE deposits, recruitment of macrophages, or CNV formation. RPE can react to nonlethal injury by many responses relevant to deposit formation, including by extruding patches of cell membranes and cytosol (i.e., blebs) (234); by altering the synthesis of collagen, matrix metalloproteinases, and other matrix molecules; by increasing production of chemotactic signals or angiogenic factors; and many other responses (236). These other specific responses need to be correlated with specific injury stimuli.

Recent studies of RPE injury responses may serve as an example of how immunity can induce deposits or promote abnormal repair. RPE can be injured by myeloperoxidase-mediated lipid peroxidation of the cell membrane, which represents a physiologically relevant macrophage-derived oxidative stimulus. Such oxidant-injured RPE undergo significant blebbing of cell membrane (Fig. 9), cytosol, and organelles, but without activation of programmed cell death or nuclear fragmentation. However, oxidant-injured cells downregulate another response, matrix metalloproteinase production (Cousins and Csaky, personal communication).

Regardless of the stimulus, accumulation of blebs can lead to deposit formation, which, in turn, can activate an immune response that interferes with healthy repair. For example, under certain conditions, blebs might serve as an innate stimulus for recruitment and activation of reparative macrophages (see below). In addition to innate immunity, blebbing might cause desequestration of intracellular antigens to provide a target for antigen-specific immunity or blebs might provide a substrate for nonspecific activation of complement or other amplification systems, as described for atherosclerosis, AD, and glomerular diseases.

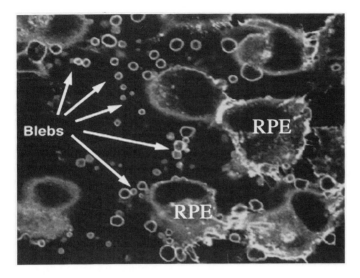

Figure 9   Image of retinal pigment epithelial cells in culture exhibiting extensive cell membrane blebbing following sublethal oxidative injury.

Response to injury may also be relevant to formation of CNV. All blood vessels, including the choriocapillaris, must continuously repair endothelial and vessel wall damage following injury. Increasing evidence suggests that aging is associated with dysregulated vascular repair after injury (237–239). For example, abnormal and exaggerated repair following acute vascular injury is a well-defined mechanism for accelerated restenosis after coronary artery angioplasty in older patients (237). A similar phenomenon may exist in the choroid in terms of CNV. Aging mice exposed to laser injury of the choroid develop much larger CNV than do younger animals. Investigation of differences between younger and aging individuals in terms of activation of immune and reparative responses after vascular injury may be an important topic for research in AMD (Cousins and Csaky, personal communication).

B.   What Is the Role of Choroidal Monocytes?

Although the presence of choroidal monocytes in AMD has been established, their identity and function remain uncertain. If analogies with atherosclerosis are correct, then these cells are probably scavenging macrophages recruited to remove lipids and deposits within Bruch's membrane. As is the case for atherosclerosis or Alzheimer's disease, the function of scavenging monocytes in AMD can be protective or pathogenic depending upon the activation status. Scavenging macrophages probably can remove sub-RPE deposits safely and assist in healthy repair of Bruch's membrane. However, activation into reparative macrophages may result in the production of mediators that can damage Bruch's membrane, injury choriocapillaris, and promote CNV. Recently, it has been shown that blood monocytes from some patients with AMD can become stimulated into reparative macrophages after phagocytosis with RPE-derived cell debris and membrane blebs. Analysis of interaction between sub-RPE deposits and scavenging macrophages may address this topic.

C. Does Antigen-Specific Immunity Participate in the Progression of AMD?

If the identification of dendritic cells in association with drusen is confirmed, this observation implies an entirely different function for choroidal monocytes and suggests a role for T-cell-mediated antigen-specific immunity. DC lack scavenging and inflammatory effector function. However, they might sample antigens within drusen (perhaps inappropriately de-sequestered or chemically modified proteins), and then might initiate the afferent phase of the immune response by presenting these antigens to T lymphocytes within lymphoid tissues.

The participation of antibody-dependent immune responses in AMD is intriguing but remains speculative. Typically, B cells require exposure to the natural, intact antigen within lymph nodes to become activated, not exposure to antigens that were processed and presented by dendritic cells. It is possible, but unlikely, that intact retina-specific antigens in AMD can diffuse into the choroid, gain access to lymphoid compartments, and trigger a "de novo" retina-specific immune antibody response. Nevertheless, as in CAR, circulating antibodies, perhaps produced in response to immunity triggered elsewhere in the body by molecular mimicry, desequestration, or neoantigen formation, might cross-react with similar antigens trapped within subretinal deposits or expressed within ocular cells. A similar mechanism has been described in atherosclerosis. Finally, investigators should explore the idea that protective immunization may improve the clearance of extracellular deposits, as observed in Alzheimer's disease and atherosclerosis.

D. Do Inflammatory Amplification Cascades Contribute to Injury or Progression?

Ongoing research indicates that various cytokines and growth factors are crucial in the development of AMD complications. However, the contribution of macrophages, mast cells, or lymphocytes as potential sources for these factors in AMD remains unexplored. The identification of terminal complement components C5–9 (i.e., MAC) within drusen and near RPE is intriguing and suggests that complement-mediated cell injury may play a role in AMD. However, investigators must demonstrate intact MAC in association with endothelial or RPE cell membranes as well as local activation of these complement fragments. Further, a clear mechanism must be established to link this injury stimulus to relevant cellular responses involved in deposit formation.

The role of immune- and nonimmune-derived oxidants as potential injury stimuli and amplifiers of injury responses was briefly described above and reviewed elsewhere. Evidence to demonstrate an age-related loss of protective antioxidants in AMD patients is controversial, but is currently being evaluated by several groups (240).

E. Can Anti-Inflammatory Therapy Play a Role in the Treatment of AMD?

Recently, intravitreal corticosteroids were found to be partially effective in improving vision and decreasing exudation due to CNV, suggesting the possibility that anti-inflammatory therapy might be effective in AMD treatment. Clinical medicine is on the verge of a revolution in anti-inflammatory therapy based on drugs and other therapeutics developed from knowledge of the molecular basis of effector mechanisms and amplification systems described above. Perhaps some of these new approaches may be relevant to the treatment of AMD.

One anti-inflammatory approach might be to block the upregulation of amplification systems discussed above. For instance, various complement inhibitors are in development, especially inhibitors of C3 activation and the MAC formation (241). The potential role for vitronectin as an inhibitor of MAC was mentioned above (242). The role of specific antioxidant agents, rather than generic antioxidant cocktails, must also be better evaluated. Relatively high doses of the lipophilic antioxidant vitamin E, which inserts into the plasma membrane to quench cell membrane lipid peroxidation, have been shown to diminish complications of myocardial infraction and stroke, in part by diminishing secondary inflammation-mediated oxidant injury (243). However, recent research suggests that dosing and bioavailability will be important issues for the eye. For example, exogenous supplementation with soluble antioxidants, such as glutathione, may be inadequate because the compound is not taken up by RPE (240). Effective treatment may require the use of agents that upregulate intracellular synthesis. Biosynthesis of prostaglandins by immune or parenchymal cells also results in the generation of oxidants. Accordingly, the use of nonsteroidal anti-inflammatory agents slows the progression of AD, although they have not been evaluated in AMD (244).

Another anti-inflammatory approach is to block mast cell or macrophage recruitment to the choroid, or inhibit their local activation. In this regard, blockade of endothelial cell adhesion molecule expression to prevent the recruitment of macrophages or other leukocytes to injured sites is an active area of research (245). Pentoxifylline has been shown to diminish macrophage adhesiveness and cell activation in arthritis, suggesting a rationale for use in AMD (246). The mast cell inhibitor tranilast was observed to be effective in experimental CNV. Other areas of drug development are inhibitors of cytokines, their intracellular signaling cascades, and/or transcription factor expression (247). These approaches might not only target macrophage-derived cytokines, like TNF-alpha, which can injure RPE or endothelium, but also RPE-derived cytokines, like MCP-1, which serve to activate macrophages. Finally, should an infectious etiology be determined, specific anti-infective agents for *Chlamydia* or CMV might be considered.

VI. BIOLOGY OF THE IMMUNE RESPONSE IN AMD

To summarize: Innate immunity involves activation by retinal or choroidal injury or infection. Antigen-specific immunity invovles normal activation by foreign antigens and aberrant activation in AMD by molecular mimicry, antigen desequestration, neo-antigen formation, or antigen trapping.

Amplification mechanisms include complement, cytokines, oxidants, and others. Immune cells include monocytes, macrophages, dendritic cells, mast cells, and lymphocytes.

Innate immunity, antigen-specific immunity, and amplification cascades contribute to the pathogenesis of atherosclerosis, AD, and glomerular diseases. Innate immunity, antigen-specific immunity, and amplification cascades may contribute to AMD.

REFERENCES

1. Janeway CA, Travers P, Walport M. Immunobiology. London: Academic Press, 1999.
2. Roitt IM. Roitt's Essential Immunology. Oxford: Blackwell Science, 1999.

3. Male D, Cooke A, Owen M, Trowsdale J, Champion B. Advanced Immunology, London: Mosby, 1996.
4. Rosenberg HF, Gallin JI. Inflammation. In: WE Paul, ed. Fundamental Immunology, 4th ed. Philadelphia: Lippincott-Raven, P. 1999.
5. Wright SD. Innate recognition of micropbial lipids. In: Gallin JI, Snyderman R, eds. Inflammation: Basic Principles and Clinical Correlates, 3rd ed. Philadelphia: Lippincott Williams & Wilkins, 1999.
6. Hamrick TS, Havell EA, Horton JR, Orndorff PE. Host and bacterial factors involved in the innate ability of mouse macrophages to eliminate internalized unopsonized *Escherichia coli*. Infect Immun 2000 J; 68:125–132.
7. Intraocular Inflammation and Uveitis, section 9. In: Basic and Clinical Science Course, American Academy of Ophthalmology, San Francisco, 1999.
8. Cooper NR Biology of complement. In: Gallin JI, Snyderman R, eds. Inflammation: Basic Principles and Clinical Correlates, 3rd ed. Philadelphia: Lippincott Williams & Wilkins, 1999.
9. Prodinger WM, Wurzner R, Erdei A, Dietrich, MP. Complement. In: Paul WE, ed. Fundamental Immunology, 4th ed. Philadelphia: Lippincott-Raven, 1999.
10. Gasque P, Dean YD, McGreal EP, VanBeek J, Morgan BP. Complement components of the innate immune system in health and disease in the CNS. Immunopharmacology 2000;49:171–186.
11. Gewurz H, Ying SC, Jiang H, Lint TF. Nonimmune activation of the classical complement pathway. Behring Inst Mitt 1993;93:138–147.
12. Preissner KT, Seiffert D. Role of vitronectin and its receptors in haemostasis and vascular remodeling. Thromb Res 1998;89:1–21.
13. Hogasen K, Mollnes TE, Harboe M. Heparin-binding properties of vitronectin are linked to complex formation as illustrated by in vitro polymerization and binding to the terminal complement complex. J Biol Chem 1992;267:23076–23082.
14. Sorensen IJ, Nielsen EH, Andersen O, Danielsen B, Svehag SE. Binding of complement proteins C1q and C4bp to serum amyloid P component (SAP) in solid contra liquid phase. Scand J Immunol 1996;44:401–407.
15. Turner MW. Mannose-binding lectin: the pluripotent molecule of the innate immune system. Immunol Today 1996;17:532–540.
16. Ogawa S, Clauss M, Kuwabara K, Shreeniwas R, Butura C, Koga S, Stern D. Hypoxia induces endothelial cell synthesis of membrane-associated proteins. Proc Natl Acad Sci USA 1991;88:9897–9901.
17. Weinhouse GL, Belloni PN, Farber HW. Effect of hypoxia on endothelial cell surface glycoprotein expression: modulation of glycoprotein IIIa and other specific surface glycoproteins. Exp Cell Res 1993;208:465–478.
18. Collard CD, Lekowski R, Jordan JE, Agah A, Stahl GL. Complement activation following oxidative stress. Mol Immunol 1999;36:941–948.
19. Collard CD, Vakeva A, Morrissey MA, Agah A, Rollins SA, Reenstra WR, Buras JA, Meri S, Stahl GL. Complement activation after oxidative stress: role of the lectin complement pathway. Am J Pathol 2000;156:1549–1556.
20. Bardenstein DS, Cheyer C, Okada N, Morgan BP, Medof ME. Cell surface regulators of complement, 512 antigen, and CD59, in the rat eye and adnexal tissues. Invest Ophthalmol Vis Sci 1999;40:519–524.
21. Lass JH, Walter EI, Burris TE, Grossniklaus HE, Roat MI, Skelnik DL, Needham L, Singer M, Medof ME. Expression of two molecular forms of the complement decay-accelerating factor in the eye and lacrimal gland. Invest Ophthalmol Vis Sci 1990;31:1136–1148.
22. Mullins RE, Russell SR, Anderson DH, Hageman GS. Drusen associated with aging and age-related macular degeneration contain proteins common to extracellular deposits associated with atherosclerosis, elastosis, amyloidosis, and dense deposit disease. FASEB J 2000;14(7):835–846.

23. Thompson A, ed. The Cytokine Handbook. London: Academic Press, 1998.
24. Oppenheim JJ, Feldman, M. Cytokine Reference: A compendium of cytokines and other mediators of host defense. London: Academic Press, 2000.
25. Sundy JS, Patel DD, Haynes BF. Cytokines in normal and pathogenic inflammatory responses. Gallin JI, Snyderman R, eds. Inflammation: Basic Principles and Clinical Correlates, 3rd ed. Philadelphia: Lippincott Williams & Wilkins, 1999.
26. Halliwell B, Gutteridge JMC. Free Radicals in Biology and Medicine. Oxford: Clarendon Press, 1999.
27. Knight JA. Free radicals: their history and current status in aging and disease. Ann Clin Lab Sci 1998;28:331-346.
28. Halliwell B. Free radicals and antioxidants: a personal view. Nutr Rev 1994;52(8 Pt 1):253–265 (review).
29. Khodr B, Khalil Z. Modulation of inflammation by reactive oxygen species: implications for a tissue repair. Free Radic Biol Med 2001;30:1–8.
30. Leto TL. Respiratory burst oxidase. In: Gallin JI, Snyderman R, eds. Inflammation: Basic Principles and Clinical Correlates, 3rd ed. Philadelphia: Lippincott Williams & Wilkins, 1999.
31. Heinecke JW. Mechanisms of oxidative damage by myeloperoxidase in atherosclerosis and other inflammatory disorders. J Lab Clin Med 1999;133:321–325.
32. Moilanen W, Whittle B, Moncada S. Nitric oxide as a factor in inflammation. In: Gallin JI, Snyderman R, eds. Inflammation: Basic Principles and Clinical Correlates, 3rd ed. Philadelphia; Lippincott Williams and Wilkins, 1999.
33. Rao NA, Wu GS. Free radical mediated photoreceptor damage in uveitis. Prog Retin Eye Res 2000 Jan; 19:41–68.
34. Winkler BS, Boulton ME, Gottsch JD, Sternberg P. Oxidative damage and age-related macular degeneration. Mol Vis 1999;5:32.
35. Rozanowska M, Jarvis-Evans J, Korytowski W, Boulton ME, Burke JM, Sarna T. Blue light-induced reactivity of retinal age pigment. In vitro generation of oxygen-reactive species. J Biol Chem 1995;270:18825–18830.
36. Gottsch JD, Bynoe LA, Harlan JB, Rencs EV, Green WR. Light-induced deposits in Bruch's membrane of protoporphyric mice. Arch Ophthalmol 1993;111:126–129.
37. Boulton M, Dontsov A, Jarvis-Evans J, Ostrovsky M, Svistunenko D. Lipofuscin is a photo-inducible free radical generator. J Photochem Photobiol B 1993;19:201–204.
38. Gordon S. Macrophages and the Immune Response. In: Paul WE, ed. Fundamental Immunology, 4th ed. Philadelphia: Lippincott-Raven, 1999.
39. Gordon, S. Development and distribution of mononuclear phagocytes. In: Gallin JI, Snyderman R, eds. Inflammation: Basic Principles and Clinical Correlates, 3rd ed. Philadelphia: Lippincott Williams & Wilkins, 1999.
40. Ali H, Haribabu B, Richardson RM, Snyderman R. Mechanisms of inflammation and leukocyte activation. Med Clin North Am 1997;81:1–28.
41. Wozniak W. Origin and the functional role of microglia. Folia Morphol 1998; 57:277–285.
42. Naito M, Umeda S, Yamamoto T, Moriyama H, Umezu H, Hasegawa G, Usuda H, Shultz LD, Takahashi K Development, differentiation, and phenotypic heterogeneity of murine tissue macrophages. J Leukoc Biol 1996;59:133–138.
43. Faust N, Huber MC, Sippel AE, Bonifer C. Different macrophage populations develop fromembryonic/fetal and adult hematopoietic tissues. Exp Hematol 1997; 25:432–444.
44. Jiang Y, Beller DI, Frendl G, Graves DT. Monocyte chemoattractant protein-1 regulates adhesion molecule expression and cytokine production in human monocytes. 1998;767–793.
45. Schumann RR, Latz E. Lipopolysaccharide-binding protein. Chem Immunol 2000;74:42–60.
46. Schlegel RA, Krahling S, Callahan MK, Williamson P. CD14 is a component of multiple recognition systems used by macrophages to phagocytose apoptotic lymphocytes. Cell Death Differ 1999;6:583–592.

47. Hammerstrom J. Human macrophage differentiation in vivo and in vitro. A comparison of human peritoneal macrophages and monocytes. Acta Pathol Microbiol Scand 1979;87:113–120.
48. Takahashi K, Naito M, Takeya M. Development and heterogeneity of macrophages and their related cells through their differentiation pathways. Pathol Int 1996;46:473–485.
49. Blackwell JM, Searle S. Genetic regulation of macrophage activation: understanding the function of Nramp1 (=Ity/Lsh/Bcg). Immunol Lett 1999; 65:73–80.
50. Rutherford MS, Witsell A, Schook LB. Mechanisms generating functionally heterogeneous macrophages: chaos revisited. J Leukoc Biol 1993;53:602–618.
51. Everson MP, Chandler DB. Changes in distribution, morphology, and tumor necrosis factor-a secretion of alveolar macrophage subpopulations during the development of bleomycin-induced pulmonary fibrosis. Am J Pathol 1992;140.
52. Chettibi S, Ferguson MJ. Wound repair: an overview. In: Gallin JI, Snyderman R, eds. Inflammation: Basic Principles and Clinical Correlates, 3rd ed. Philadelphia: Lippincott Williams & Wilkins, 1999.
53. Arenberg DA, Strieter RM. Angiogenesis. In: Gallin JI, Snyderman R, eds. Inflammation: Basic Principles and Clinical Correlates; 3rd ed. Philadelphia: Lippincott Williams & Wilkins, 1999.
54. Postlewaite AE, Kang AH. Fibroblasts and matrix proteins. In: Gallin JI, Snyderman R, eds. Inflammation: Basic Principles and Clinical Correlates, 3rd ed. Philadelphia: Lippincott Williams & Wilkins, 1999.
55. Jackson JR, Seed MP, Kircher CH, Willoughby DA, Winkler JD. The codependence of angiogenesis and chronic inflammation. FASEB J 1997; 11:457–465.
56. Polverini PJ. How the extracellular matrix and macrophages contribute to angiogenesis-dependent diseases. Eur J Cancer 1996;32A(14):2430–2437.
57. Laking DL, Laskin JD. Macrophages, inflammatory mediators, and lung injury. Methods 1996;10:61–70.
58. Hauser CJ. Regional macrophage activation after injury and the compartmentalization of inflammation in trauma. New Horiz 1996;4:235–251.
59. Raines EW, Russell R. Is overamplification of the normal macrophage defensive role critical to lesion development? Ann NY Acad Sci 1997; 811:76–85.
60. Penfold PL, Killingsworth MC, Sarks SH. Senile macular degeneration: the involvement of immunocompetent cells. Graefe's Arch Clin Exp Ophthalmol 1985;223:69–76.
61. Killingsworth MC, Sarks JP, Sarks SH. Macrophages related to Bruch's membrane in age-related macular degeneration. Eye 1990;4:613-621.
62. Penfold P, Killingsworth M, Sarks S. An ultrastructural study of the role of leucocytes and fibroblasts in the breakdown of Bruch's membrane. Aust Ophthalmol 1984;12:23–31.
63. Lopez PF, Grossniklaus HE, Lambert MH, Aaberg TM, Capone A, Steinberg D, L'Hernault N. Pathologic features of surgically excised subretinal neovascular membranes in age-related macular degeneration. Am J Ophthalmol 1991;112:647–656.
64. Oh H, Takagi H, Takagi C, Suzuma K, Otani A, Ishida K, Matsumura M, Ogura Y, Honda Y. The potential angiogenic role of macrophages in the formation of choroidal neovascular membranes. Invest Ophthalmol Vis Sci 1999;40(9):1891–1898.
65. Cousins SW, Sall J, Dix R, Csaky KG. High responsive macrophages in patients with age-related macular degeneration. IOVS 1999;40:S922 (abs).
66. Steinman RM. Dendritic cells. In: Paul WE, ed. Fundamental Immunology, 4th ed. Philadelphia: Lippincott-Raven, 1999.
67. McMenamin PG. The distribution of immune cells in the uveal tract of the normal eye. 1997;11:183–193.
68. Forrester JV, Liversidge J, Andrew D, McMenamin P, Kuppner M, Crane I, Hossain P. What determines the site of inflammation in uveitis and chorioretinitis? Eye 1997;11: 162–166.

69. Mullins RE, Aptsiauri N, Hageman GS. Dendritic cells and proteins involved in immune-mediated processes are associated with drusen and may play a central role in drusen biogenesis. IOVS 2000;41:S (abstract).

70. Nilsson G, Costa JJ, Metcalfe DD. Mast cells and basophils. In: Gallin JI, Snyderman R, eds. Inflammation: Basic Principles and Clinical Correlates, 3rd ed. Philadelphia: Lippincott Williams & Wilkins, 1999.

71. Dines KC, Powell HC. Mast cell interactions with the nervous system: relationship to mechanisms of disease. J Neuropathol Exp Neurol 1997;56:627–640.

72. Meininger CJ. Mast cells and tumor-associated angiogenesis. Chem Immunol 1995;62:239–257.

73. Hagiwara K, Khaskhely NM, Uezato H, Nonaka S. Mast cell "densities" in vascular proliferations: a preliminary study of pyogenic granuloma, portwine stain, cavernous hemangioma, cherry angioma, Kaposi's sarcoma, and malignant hemangioendothelioma. J Dermatol 1999;26:577–586.

74. Costa, JJ, Galli SJ. Mast cells and basophils. In: Rich R, Flesher TA, Schwartz BD, Shearere WT, Strober W, eds. Clinical Immunology: Principles: and Practice, vol. 1. St Louis: Mosby, 1996.

75. Kovanen PT. Role of mast cells in atherosclerosis. Chem Immunol 1995;62:132–170.

76. Ignatescu MC, Gharehbaghi-Schnell E, Hassan A, Rezaie-Majd S, Korschineck I, Schleef RR, Glogar HD, Lang IM. Expression of the angiogenic protein, platelet-derived endothelial cell growth factor, in coronary atherosclerotic plaques: in vivo correlation of lesional microvessel density and constrictive vascular remodeling. Arterioscler Thromb Vasc Biol 1999;19:2340–2347.

77. Kaartinen M, van der Wal AC, van der Loos CM, Piek JJ, Koch KT, Becker AE, Kovanen PT. Mast cell infiltration in acute coronary syndromes: implications for plaque rupture. J Am Coll Cardiol 1998;32:606–612.

78. Boesiger J, Tsai M, Maurer M, Yamaguchi M, Brown LF, Claffey KP, Dvorak HF, Galli SJ. Mast cells can secrete vascular permeability factor/ vascular endothelial cell growth factor and exhibit enhanced release after immunoglobulin E-dependent upregulation of fc epsilon receptor I expression. J Exp Med 1998; 188:1135–1145.

79. Kanbe N, Tanaka A, Kanbe M, Itakura A, Kurosawa M, Matsuda H. Human mast cells produce matrix metalloproteinase 9. Eur J Immunol 1999;29:2645–2649.

80. Johnson JL, Jackson CL, Angelini GD, George SJ. Activation of matrix-degrading metalloproteinases by mast cell proteases in atherosclerotic plaques. Arterioscler Thromb Vasc Biol 1998;18:1707–1715.

81. May CA. Mast cell heterogeneity in the human uvea. Histochem Cell Biol 1999; 112:381–386.

82. McMenamin PG. The distribution of immune cells in the uveal tract of the normal eye. Eye 1997;1 1(Pt 2):183–193.

83. Penfold P, Killingsworth M, Sarks S. An ultrastructural study of the role of leucocytes and fibroblasts in the breakdown of Bruch's membrane. Aust J Ophthalmol 1984;12:23–31.

84. Tonnesen MG, Feng X, Clark RA. Angogenesis and wound healing. J Invest Dermatol Symp Proc 2000;5:40–46.

85. Azizkhan RG, Azizkhan JC, Zetter BR, Folkman J. Mast cell heparin stimulates migration of capillary endothelial cells in vitro. J Exp Med 1980;152:931–944.

86. Tharp MD. The interaction between mast cells and endothelial cells. J Invest Dermatol 1989;93(Suppl 2):107S–112S.

87. Takehana Y, Kurokawa T, Kitamura T, Tsukahara Y, Akahane S, Kitazawa M, Yoshimura N. Suppression of laser-induced choroidal neovascularization by oral tranilast in the rat. Invest Ophthalmol Vis Sci 1999;40:459–466.

88. Benoist C, Mathis, D. T-lymphocyte differentiation and biology. In: Paul WE, ed. Fundamental Immunology, 4th ed. Philadelphia: Lippincott-Raven, 1999.

89. Seder RA, Mosmann TM. Differentiation of effector phenotypes of CD4+ and CD8+ T cells. In Paul WE, ed. Fundamental Immunology, 4th ed. Philadelphia: Lippincott–Raven, 1999.

90. Weiss, A. T-lymphocyte activation. In: Paul WE, ed. Fundamental Immunology, 4th ed. Philadelphia: Lippincott-Raven, 1999.

91. Lee KP, Harlan DM, June CH. Role of costimulation in the host response to infection. In: Gallin JI, Snyderman R, eds. Inflammation: Basic Principles and Clinical Correlates, 3rd ed. Philadelphia: Lippincott Williams & Wilkins, 1999.

92. Augustin AA, Julius MH, Losenza, H. Antigen-specific and trans-stimulation of T cells in long term culture. Eur J Immunol 1979;9:665.

93. Dunn, DE, Jin J, Lancki DW, Fitch FW. An alternative pathway of induction of lymphokine production by T lymphocyte clones. J Immunol 1989;142:3847.

94. Clark MR. IgG effector mechanisms. Chem Immunol 1997;65:88–110.

95. Dwyer JM. Immunoglobulins in autoimmunity: history and mechanisms of action. Clin Exp Rheumatol 1996;14 (Suppl 15):S3–7.

96. Shoenfeld Y, Alarcon-Segovia D, Buskila D, Abu-Shakra M, Lorber M, Sherer Y, Berden J, Meroni PL, Valesini G, Koike T, Alarcon-Riquelm. Frontiers of SLE: review of the 5th International Congress of Systemic Lupus Erythematosus, Cancun, Mexico, April 20–25. Semin Arthritis Rheum 1999;29:112–130.

97. Reichlin M. Cellular dysfunction induced by penetration of autoantibodies into living cells; cellular damage and dysfunction mediated by antibodies to dsDNA and ribosomal P proteins. J Autoimmun 1998;11:557–561.

98. Adamus G, Machnicki M, Elerding H, Sugden B, Blocker YS, Fox DA. Antibodies to recoverin induce apoptosis of photoreceptor and bipolar cells. J Autoimmun 1998;11:523–533.

99. Descotes J, Choquet-Kastylevsky G, Van Ganse E, Vial T. Responses of the immune system to injury. Toxicol Pathol 2000;28:479–481 (review).

100. Cotran RS, Kumar V, Collins T, Robbins SL. Robbins Pathologic Basis of Disease. Philadelphia: WB Saunders, 1999.

101. Silverstein RL. The vascular endothelium. In: JI Gallin, R Snyderman, eds. Inflammation: Basic Principles and Clinical Correlates, 3rd ed. Philadelphia: Lippincott Williams & Wilkins, 1999.

102. Mims CA, Nash A, Stephen J. Mims Pathogenesis of Infectious Diseases. London: Academic Press, 2001.

103. Blaser MJ, Smith, PD. Persisten mucosal colonization by Helicobacter pylori and the induction of inflammation. In: Gallin JI, Snyderman R, eds. Inflammation: Basic Principles and Clinical Correlates, 3rd ed. Philadelphia: Lippincott Williams & Wilkins, 1999.

104. Gregerson DS. Immune privilege in the retina. Ocular Immunol Inflamm 1998;6:257–267.

105. Cousins SW, Dix RD. Immunology of the eye. In: Keane RW, Hickey WF, eds. Immunology of the Nervous System. New York: Oxford University Press, 1997.

106. Shevach EM. Organ-specific autoimmunity. In: Paul WE, ed. Fundamental Immunology, 4th ed. Philadelphia: Lippincott–Raven, 1999.

107. Singh VK, Kalra HK, Yamaki K, Abe T, Dopnosos LA, Shinohara T. Molecular mimicry between a uveitopathogenic site of S-antigen and viral peptides. J Immunol 1990;144:1282–1287.

108. Levine JS, Koh JS. The role of apoptosis in autoimmunity: immunogen, antigen, and accelerant. Semin Nephrol 1999;19:34–47 (review).

109. Berden JH, Van Bruggen MC. Nucleosomes and the pathogenesis of lupus nephritis. Kidney Blood Press Res 1997;20:198–200. Review.

110. Gregerson DS, Torseth JW, McPherson SW, Roberts JP, Shinohara T, Zack DJ. Retinal expression of a neo-self antigen, beta-galactosidase, is not tolerogenic and creates a target for autoimmune uveoretinitis. J Immunol 1999;163:1073–1080.

111. Ross R. Atherogenesis. In: Gallin JI, Snyderman R, eds. Inflammation: Basic Principles and Clinical Correlates, 3rd ed. Philadelphia: Lippincott Williams & Wilkins, 1999.

112. Adler S, Couser W. Immunologic mechanisms of renal disease. Am J Med Sci 1985;289:55–60.
113. Dick AD. Immune mechanisms of uveitis: insights into disease pathogenesis and treatment. Int Ophthalmol Clin 2000;40:1–18.
114. Smith RE. Commentary on histoplasmosis. Ocul Immunol Inflamm 1997;5:69–70.
115. Klein R, Klein BE, Jensen SC. The relation of cardiovascular disease and its risk factors to the 5-year incidence of age-related maculopathy: the Beaver Dam Eye Study. Ophthalmology 1997;104:1804–1812.
116. Hyman L, Schachat AP, He Q, Leske MC. Hypertension, cardiovascular disease, and age-related macular degeneration. Age-Related Macular Degeneration Risk Factors Study Group. Arch Ophthalmol 2000;118:351–358.
117. Vingerling JR, Dielemans I, Bots ML, Hofman A, Grobbee DE, de Jong PT. Age-related macular degeneration is associated with atherosclerosis. The Rotterdam Study. Am J Epidemiol 1995;142:404–409.
118. Ross R. Atherosclerosis–an inflammatory disease. N Engl J Med 1999;340:115–126.
119. Masuda J, Ross R. Atherogenesis during low level hypercholesterolemia in the nonhuman primate. I. Fatty streak formation. Arteriosclerosis 1990;10:164–177.
120. Curcio CA, Millican CL, Bailey T, Kruth HS. Accumulation of cholesterol with age in human Bruch's membrane. Invest Ophthalmol Vis Sci 2001 Jan; 42:265–274.
121. Hariri RJ, Alonso DR, Hajjar DP, Coletti D, Weksler ME. Aging and arteriosclerosis. I. Development of myointimal hyperplasia after endothelial injury. J Exp Med 1986;164:1171–1178.
122. Napoli C. Low density lipoprotein oxidation and atherogenesis: from experimental models to clinical studies. G Ital Cardiol 1997 Dec; 27:1302–1314.
123. Nagornev VA, Maltseva SV. The phenotype of macrophages which are not transformed into foam cells in atherogenesis. Atherosclerosis 1996;121:245–251.
124. Klaver CC, Kliffen M, van Duijn CM, Hofman A, Cruts M, Grobbee DE, van Broeckhoven C, de Jong PT. Genetic association of apolipoprotein E with age-related macular degeneration. Am J Hum Genet 1998 Jul; 63:200–206.
125. George SJ. Tissue inhibitors of metalloproteinases and metalloproteinases in atherosclerosis. Curr Opin Lipidol 1998;9:413–423.
126. Ross R, Masuda J, Raines EW, Gown AM, Katsuda S, Sasahara M, Malden LT, Masuko H, Sato H. Localization of PDGF-B protein in macrophages in all phases of atherogenesis. Science 1990;248(4958):1009–1012.
127. Rajavashisth TB, Xu XP, Jovinge S, Meisel S, Xu XO, Chai NN, Fishbein MC, Kaul S, Cercek B, Sharifi B and others. Membrane type 1 matrix metalloproteinase expression in human atherosclerotic plaques: evidence for activation by proinflammatory mediators. Circulation 1999;99:3103–3109.
128. Clinton SK, Underwood R, Hayes L, Sherman ML, Kufe DW, Libby P. Macrophage colony-stimulating factor gene expression in vascular cells and in experimental and human atherosclerosis. Am J Pathol 1992;1 40:301–316.
129. de Boer OJ, van der Wal AC, Becker AE. Atherosclerosis, inflammation, and infection. J Pathol 2000;190:237–243.
130. Saikku P. Epidemiologic association of Chlamydia pneumoniae and atherosclerosis: the initial serologic observation and more. J Infect Dis 2000;81(Suppl 3):S411–413.
131. Leinonen M. Chlamydia pneumoniae and other risk factors for atherosclerosis. J Infect Dis 2000 181 (Suppl 3):S414–416.
132. Taylor-Robinson D, Thomas BJ. Chlamydia pneumoniae in atherosclerotic tissue. J Infect Dis 2000;181(Suppl 3):S437–440.
133. Meier CR. Antibiotics in the prevention and treatment of coronary heart disease. J Infect Dis 2000;181(Suppl 3):S558–562.
134. Kol A, Lichtman AH, Finberg RW, Libby P, Kurt-Jones EA. Cutting edge: heat shock protein (HSP) 60 activates the innate immune response: CD14 is an essential receptor for HSP60 activation of mononuclear cells. J Immunol 2000; 164:13–17.

135. Kol A, Bourcier T, Lichtman AH, Libby P. Chlamydial and human heat shock protein 60s activate human vascular endothelium, smooth muscle cells, and macrophages. J Clin Invest 1999;103:571–577.

136. Tezel G, Wax MB. Mechanism of hsp27 antibody mediated apoptosis in retinal cells. J Neurosci 2000;20:3552–3562.

137. Leinonen M, Saikku P. Infections and atherosclerosis. Scand Cardiovasc J 2000;34:12–20.

138. High KP. Atherosclerosis and infection due to Chlamydia pneumoniae or cytomegalovirus: weighing the evidence. Clin Infect Dis 1999; 28:746–749.

139. Epstein SE, Zhou YF, Zhu J. Potential role of cytomegalovirus in the pathogenesis of restenosis and atherosclerosis. Am Heart J 1999; 138(5 Pt 2):5476–478.

140. Weis M, Pehlivanli S, Von Scheidt W. Heart allograft endothelial cell dysfunction. Cause, course, and consequence. Z Kardiol 2000;89(Suppl 9):58–62.

141. Silverman GJ, Shaw PX, Luo L, Dwyer D, Chang M, Horkos S, Witztam JL. Neo-self antigens and the expansion of B-1 cells: lessons from atherosclerosis prone mice. Curr Top Microbiol Immunol 2000;252:189–200.

142. Wick G, Perschinka H, Xu Q. Autoimmunity and atherosclerosis. Am Heart J 1999;138(5 Pt 2):S444–449.

143. Zhoux X, Caligiuri G, Hamsten A, Hanson GR. LDL Immunization induces Tcell-dependent antibody formation and protection against atherosclerosis. Atheroscler Thromb Vasc Biol 2001;21:108–114.

144. Seifert PS, Hugo F, Hansson GK, Bhakdi S. Prelesional complement activation in experimental atherosclerosis. Terminal C5b-9 complement deposition coincides with cholesterol accumulation in the aortic intima of hypercholesterolemic rabbits. Lab Invest 1989;60:747–754.

145. Benzaquen LR, Nicholson-Weller A, Halperin JA. Terminal complement proteins C5b-9 release basic fibroblast growth factor and platelet-derived growth factor from endothelial cells. J Exp Med 1994;179:985–992.

146. Torzewski M, Torzewski J, Bowyer DE, Waltenberger J, Fitzsimmons C, Hombach V, Gabbert HE. Immunohistochemical colocalization of the terminal complex of human complement and smooth muscle cell alpha-actin in early atherosclerotic lesions. Arterioscler Thromb Vasc Biol 1997;17:2448–2452.

147. Hazen SL. Oxidation and atherosclerosis. Free Radic Biol Med 2000;28:1683–1684.

148. Vickers JC, Dickson TC, Adlard PA, Saunders HL, King CE, McCormack G. The cause of neuronal degeneration in Alzheimer's disease. Prog Neurobiol 2000; 60:139–165 (review).

149. Klaver CC, Ott A, Hofman A, Assink JJ, Breteler MM, de Jong PT. Is age-related maculopathy associated with Alzheimer's Disease? The Rotterdam Study. Am J Epidemiol 1999;150:963–968.

150. Eikelenboom P, Roxemuller JM, Van Muiswinkel FL. Inflammation and Alzheimer's disease: relationships between pathogenic mechanisms and clinical expression. Exp Neurol 1998;154:89–98 (review).

151. King CE, Adlard PA, Dickson TC, Vickers JC. Neuronal response to physical injury and its relationship to the pathology of Alzheimer's disease. Clin Exp Pharmacol Physiol 2000;27:548–552.

152. Graham DI, Horsburgh K, Nicoll JA, Teasdale, GM. Apolipoprotein E and the response of the brain to injury. Acta Neurochir Suppl (Wein) 1999;73:89–92 (review).

153. Akiyama H, Barger S, Barnum S, Bradt B, Bauer J, Cole GM, Cooper NR, Eikelenboom P, Emmerling M, Fiebich BL, et al. Inflammation and Alzheimer's disease. Neurobiol Aging 2000;21:383–421.

154. Lukiw WJ, Bazan NG. Neuroiniflammatory signaling upregulation in Alzheimer's disease. Neurochem Res 2000;25:1173–1184.

155. Games D. Alzheimer-type neuropathology in transgenic mice overexpressing V717F-amyloid protien. Nature 1995;373:523–527.

156. Duff K. Increased amyloid-42(43) in brains of mice expressing mutant presenilin 1. Nature 1996;383:710–713.

157. Giulian D. Microglia and the immune pathology of Alzheimer disease. Am J Hum Genet 1999;65:13–18.

158. McGeer EG, McGeer PL. Brain inflammation in Alzheimer disease and the therapeutic implications. Current Pharm Des 1999;5:821–836.

159. Tan J, Town T, Paris D, Mori T, Suo Z, Crawford F, Mattson MP, Flavell RA, Mullan M. Microglial activation resulting from CD40-CD40L interaction after beta-amyloid stimulation. Science 1999;286(5448):2352–2355.

160. Cole GM, Beech W, Frautschy SA, Sigel J, Glasgow C, Ard MD. Lipoprotein effects on Abeta accumulation and degradation by microglia in vitro. J Neurosci Res 1999;57:504–520.

161. Samatovicz RA. Genetics and brain injury: apolipoprotein E. J Head Trauma Rehabil 2000;15:869–874 (review).

162. Laskowitz DT, Horsburgh K, Roses AD. Apolipoprotein E and the CNS response to injury. J Cereb Blood Flow Metab 1998;18:465–471 (review).

163. Sanders AM. Apolipoprotein E and Alzheimer disease: an update on genetic and functional analyses. J Neuropathol Exp Neurol 2000;59:751–758.

164. Adler R, Curcio C, Hicks D, Price D, Wong F. Cell death in age-related macular degeneration. Mol Vis 1999;5:31.

165. Miklossy J. Alzheimer's disease-a spirochetosis? Neuroreport 1993;4:841–848.

166. Hope J. Prions and neurodegenerative diseases. Curr Opin Gent Dev 2000;10:568–574.

167. Thompson A, White AR, McLean C, Masters CL, Cappai R, Barrow CJ. Amyloidogenicity and neurotoxicity of peptides corresponding to the helical regions of PrP(C). J Neurosci Res 2000;62:293–301.

168. Cserr HF, Knopf PM. Cervical lymphatics, the blood brain barrier and immunoreactivity of the brain. In: Keane RW, Hickey WF, eds. Immunology of the Nervous System. New York; Oxford University Press, 1997.

169. Mosek A, Yust I, Treves TA, Vardinon N, Korczyn AD, Chapman J. Dementia and antiphospholipid antibodies. Dementia Geriat Cogn Dis 2000; 11:36–38.

170. Engelhardt JI, WD L, Siklos L, Obal I, Boda K, Appel SH. Steriotaxic injection of IgG from patients with Alzheimer disease initiates injury of cholinergic neurons of the basal forebrain. Arch Neurol 2000;57:681–686.

171. Schenk. Immunization with amyloid-beta attenuates Alzheimer disease-like pathology in the PDAPP mouse. Nature 1999;40: 173–177.

172. Younkin S. Amyloid- vaccination: reduced plaques and improved cognition. Nature Med 2001;7:18–19.

173. Schmitt TL, Steger MM, Pavelka M, Grubeck-Loebenstein B. Interactions of the alzheimer beta amyloid fagment (25–35) with peripheral blood dendritic cells. Mech Ageing Dev 1997;94:223–232.

174. Morgan BP, Gasque P. Expression of complement in the brain: role in health and disease. Immunol Today 1996;17:461–466.

175. Bradt BM, Kolb WP, Cooper NR. Complement-dependent proinflammatory properties of the Alzheimer's disease beta-peptide. J Exp Med 1998;188:431–438.

176. Pasinetti GM, Johnson SA, Rozovsky I, Lampert-Etchells M, Morgan DG, Gordon MN, Morgan TE, Willoughby D, Finch CE. Complement C1qB and C4 mRNAs responses to lesioning in rat brain. Exp Neurol 1992;118:117–125.

177. Owen AD, Schapira AH, Jenner P, Marsden CD. Indices of oxidative stress in Parkinson's disease, Alzheimer's disease and dementia with Lewy bodies. J Neural Transm 1997;51 (Suppl): 167–173.

178. Frolich L, Riederer P. Free radical mechanisms in dementia of Alzheimer type and the potential for antioxidative treatment. Arzneimittel-Forschung 1995; 45(3A):443–446.

179. Brenner BM, Rector FC. Brenner and Rector's the Kidney, 6th ed. Philadelphia: WB Saunders, 2000.
180. Makker SP. Mediators of immune glomerular injury. Am J Nephrol 1993; 13:324–336.
181. Olson JL, Heptinstall RH. Nonimmunologic mechanisms of glomerular injury. Lab Invest 1988;59:564–578.
182. Johnson RJ. The glomerular response to injury: progression or resolution? Kidney Int 1994 45:1769–1782.
183. Neuringer JR, Brenner BM. Glomerular hypertension: cause and consequence of renal injury. J Hypertens 1992;10 (Suppl): S91-97 (review).
184. Suzuki D. Metalloproteinases in the pathogenesis of diabetic nephropathy Nephron 1998;80:125–133.
185. Anderson S, Vora JP. Current concepts of renal hemodynamics in diabetes. J Diab Complic 1995;9:304–307.
186. O'Bryan GT, Hostetter TH. The renal hemodynamic basis of diabetic nephropathy. Semin Nephrol 1997;17:93–100.
187. Luft FC, Mervaala E, Muller DN, Gross V, Schmidt F, Park JK, Schmitz C, Lippoldt A, Breu V, Dechend R, Dragun D, Schneider, W. Hypertension-induced end-organ damage: A new transgenic approach to an old problem. Hypertension 1999;33 (Pt): 212–218.
188. Peten EP, Garcia-Perez A, Terada Y, Woodrow D, Martin BM, Striker GE, Striker LJ. Age-related changes in alpha 1- and alpha 2-chain type IV collagen mRNAs in adult mouse glomeruli: competitive PCR. Am J Physiol 1992;263:F951–957.
189. Ungar A, Castellani S, Di Serio C, Cantini C, Cristofari C, Vallotti B, La Cava G, Masotti, G. Changes in renal autacoids and hemodynamics associated with aging and isolated systolic hypertension. Prostaglandins Other Lipid Mediat 2000; 62:117–133.
190. Yang N, Wu LL, Nikolic-Patterson DJ, Ng YY, Yang WC, Mu W, Gilbert RE, Cooper ME, Atkins RC, Lan HY. Local macrophage and myofibroblast proliferation in progressive renal injury in the rat remnant kidney. Nephrol Dial Transplant 1998;13:1967–1974.
191. Suto TS, Fine LG, Shimizu F, Kitamura M. In vivo transfer of engineered macrophages into the glomerulus: endogenous TGF-beta-mediated defense against macrophage-induced glomerular cell activation. J Immunol 1997; 159:2476–2483.
192. Pawluckzyk IZ, Harris KP. Macrophages promote prosclerotic responses in cultured rat mesangial cells: a mechanism for the initiation of glumerolusoclerosis. J Am Soc Nephrol 1997 8:1525–1536.
193. Dsouza MJ, Oettinger CW, Shah A, Tipping PG, Huang XR, Milton GV. Macrophage depletion by albumin microencasulated clodronate: attenuation of cytokine release in macrophage-dependent glomerulonephritis. Drug Dev Ind Pharm 1999;25:591–596.
194. Kamanna VS, Pai R, Kirshenbauum MA, Roh DD. Oxidized low-density lipoprotein stimulates monocyte adhesion to glomerular endothelial cells. Kidney Int 1999;55:2192–2202.
195. Hattori M, Nikolic-Paterson DJ, Miyazaki K, Isbel NM, Lan HY, Atkins RC, Kawaguchi H, Ito K. Mechanisms of glomerular macrophage infiltration in lipid-induced renal injury. Kid Int 1999 71 (Suppl): S47–50.
196. Pauluczyk IZ, Harris KP. Cholesterol feeding activates macrophages to upregulate rat mesangial cell fibronectin production. Nephrol Dial Trans 2000; 15:161–166.
197. Duffield JS, Erwig LP, Wei X, Liew Fy, Rees AJ, Savill JS. Activated macrophages direct apoptosis and suppress mitosis of mesangial cells. J Immunol 164:2110–2119.
198. Kitamura M. Adoptive transfer of nuclear factor-kappaB-inactive macrophages to the glomerulus. Kidney Int 2000;57:709–716.
199. Lan HY, Yang N, Brown FG, Isbel NM, Nikolic-Paterson DJ, Mu W, Metz CN, Bacher M, Atkins RC, Bucala R. Macrophage migration inhibitory factor expression in human renal allograft rejection. Transplantation 1998; 66:1465–1471.
200. Ponticelli C. Progression of renal damage in chronic rejection. Kidney Int 2000; S75:62–70.

201. Nordstrand A, Norgren M, Holm SE. Pathogenic mechanism of acute post-streptococcal glomerulonephritis. Scand J Infect Dis 1999;31:523–527.
202. Bennett WM, Fassett RG, Walker RG, Fairley KF, D'ApiceAJF, Kincaid-Smith P. Mesangio-capillary glomerulonephritis type II (dense-deposit disease): clinical features of progressive disease. Am J Kidney Dis 1989;8(6):469–476.
203. Joh K, Aizawa S, Matsuyama N, Yamaguchi Y, Kitajima T, Sakai O, Mochizuki H, Usui N, Hamaguchi K-I, Mitarai T. Morphologic variations of dense deposit disease: Light and electron microscopic, immunohistochemical and clinical finding in 10 patients. Acta Pathol Jpn 1993;43:552–565.
204. Leys A, Vanrenterghem Y, Van Damme B, Snyers B, Pirson Y, Leys M. Fundus changes in membranoproliferative glomerulonephritis type II: A fluorescein angiographic study of 23 patients. Graefe's Arch Clin Exp Ophthalmol 1991; 229:406–410.
205. Michielsen B, Leys A, Van Damme B, Missotten L. Fundus changes in chronic membranopro-liferative glomerulonephritis type II. Doc Ophthalmol 1991;76:219–229.
206. Jansen JH, Hogasen K, Mollness T. Extensive complement activation in hereditary porcine membranoproliferative glomerulonephritis type II (porcine dense deposit disease). Am J Pathol 1993;143:1356–1365.
207. Leys A, Michielsen B, Leys M, Vanrenterghem Y, Missotten L, Van Damme B. Subretinal neo-vascular membranes associated with chronic membranoproliferative glomerulonephritis type II. Graefe's Arch Clin Exp Ophthalmol 1990;228:499–504.
208. Baud L, Fouqueray B, Philippe C, Ardaillou R. Reactive oxygen species as glomerular auto-coids. J Am Soc Nephrol 1992;10 (Suppl): S132–138.
209. Jaffe GJ, Roberts WL, Wong HL, Yurochko AD, Cianciolo GJ. Monocyte-induced cytokine expression in cultured human retinal pigment epithelial cells.
210. Gross N, Klaus HE, Cingle KA, Voon YD, Ket Kar N, L'Hernault N, Brown S. Correlation of histologic 2-D reconstruction and confocal scanning laser microscopic imaging of CNV in ARMD. Arch Ophthalmol 2000;118:625–629.
211. Osusky R, Soriano D, Ye J, Ryan SJ. Cytokine effect on fibronectin release by retinal pigment epithelial cells. Curr Eye Res 1994;13:569–764.
212. Nagineni CN, Kutty RK, Detrick B, Hooks JJ. Inflammatory cytokines induce intercellular ad-hesion molecule-1 (ICAM-1) mRNA synthesis and protein secretion by human retinal pigment epithelial cell cultures. Cytokine 1996; 8:622–630.
213. Platts KE, Benson MT, Rennie IG, Sharrard RM, Rees RC. Cytokine modulation of adhesion molecule expression on human retinal pigment epithelial cells. Invest Ophthalmol Vis Sci 1995;36:2262–2269.
214. Kurtz RM, Elner VM, .Bian ZM, Strieter RM, Kunkel SL, Elner SG. Dexamethasone and Cyclosporin A Modulation of Human Retinal Pigment Epithelial Cell Monocyte Chemotactic Protein-1 and Interleukin-8. Invest Ophthalmol Vis Sci 1997;38:436–445.
215. Osusky R, Malik P, Yoush A, Stephen JR. Monocyte-macrophage differentiation induced by co-culture of retinal pigment epithelium cells with monocytes. Ophthal Res 1997;29:124–129.
216. Danis RP, Ciulla TA, Pratt LM, Anliker W. Intravitreal triamcinolone acetonide in exudative age-related macular degeneration. Retina 2000;20:244–250.
217. Challa JK, Gillies MC, Penfold PL, Gyory JF, Hunyor AB, Billson FA. Exudative macular de-generation and intravitreal triamcinolone: 18 months. Aust NZ J Ophthalmol 1998 Nov; 26:277–281.
218. Adcock IM. Molecular mechanisms of glucocorticosteroid actions. Pulm Pharmacol Ther 2000;13:115–126.
219. Johnson LV, Ozaki S, Staples MK, Erickson PA, Anderson DH. A potential role for immune complex pathogenesis in drusen formation. Exp Eye Res 2000; 70:441–449.
220. Van Der Schaft TL, Mooy CM, de Bruijn WC, de Jong PT. Early stages of age-related macular degeneration: an immunofluorescence and electron microscopy study. Br J Ophthalmol 1993;77(10):657–661.

221. Delcourt C, Cristol JF, Tessier F, Leger CL, Descomps B, Papoz L. Age-related macular degeneration and antioxidant status in the POLA study. POLA Study Group. Pathologies Oculaires Liees a l'Age. Arch Ophthalmol 1999; 117(10):1384–1390.

222. Bora NS, Gobleman CL, Atkinson JP, Pepose JS, Kaplan HJ. Differential expression of the complement regulatory proteins in the human eye. Invest Ophthalmol Vis Sci 1993;34(13):3579–3584.

223. Anderson A, Taylor C, Azen S, Jester JV, Hagerty C, Ormerod LD, Smith RE. Immunopathology of acute experimental histoplasmic choroiditis in the primate. Invest Ophthalmol Vis Sci 1987;28:1195–1199.

224. Anderson A, Clifford W, Palvolgi I, Rife L, Taylor C, Smith RE. Immunopathology of chronic experimental histoplasmic choroiditis in the primate. Invest Ophthalmol Vis Sci 1992, 33:1637–1641.

225. Palvolgi I, Anderson A, Rife L, Taylor C, Smith RE. Immunopathology of reactivation of experimental ocular histoplasmosis. Exp Eye Res 1993; 57:169–175.

226. Smith RE, Dunn S, Jester JY. Natural history of experimental histoplasmic choroiditis in the primate. Invest Ophthalmol 1984;25:810–819.

227. Jester JV, Smith RE. Subretinal neovascularization after experimental ocular histoplasmosis in a primate. Am J Ophthalmol 1985;100:252–258.

228. Smith RE. The uvea: questions of pathogenesis and treatment. Eye 1997;11(Pt 2): 145–147.

229. Goldstein SM, Syed NA, Milam AH, Maguire AM, Lawton TJ, Nichols CW. Cancer-associated retinopathy. Arch Ophthalmol 1999;117(12):1641–1645.

230. Ohguro H, Ogawa K, Maeda T, Maeda A, Maruyama I. Cancer-associated retinopathy induced by both anti-recoverin and anti-hsc7 antibodies in vivo. Invest Ophthalmol Vis Sci 1999;40(13):3160–3167.

231. Thirkill CE. Retinal pigment epithelial hypersensitivity, an association with vision loss: RPE hypersensitivity complicating paraneoplastic retinopathies. Ocular Immunol Inflamm 2000;8(1):25–37.

232. Kain HL, Reuter U. Release of lysosomal protease from retinal pigment epithelium and fibroblasts during mechanical stresses. Graefe's Arch Clin Exp Ophthalmol 1995;233:236–243.

233. Malorni WD. Cell death: general features and morphological aspects. Ann NY Acad Sci 1992;663:218.

234. Malorni W. Cytoskeleton as a target in menadione-induced oxidative stress in cultured mamalian cells: alterations in underlying surface bleb formation. Chemico-biol Invest 1991;80:217.

235. Ruben A, Curcio C, Hicks D, Price D, Fulton W. Cell death in age-related macular degeneration. Mol Vis 1999;5:31.

236. Campochiaro PA, Soloway P, Ryan SJ, Miller JW. The pathogenesis of choroidal neovascularization in patients with age-related macular degeneration. Mol Vis 1999;5:34.

237. Bilato C, Crow MT. Atherosclerosis and the vascular biology of aging. Aging (Milano) 1996;8:221–234.

238. Hariri RJ, Alonso DR. Hajjar DP, Coletti D, Weksler ME. Aging and arteriosclerosis. I. Development of myointimal hyperplasia after endothial injury. J Exp Med 1986;164:1171–1178.

239. Spagnoli LG, Sambuy Y, Palmieri G, Mauriello A. Age-related modulation of vascular smooth muscle cells proliferation following arterial wall damage. Artery 1985;13:187–198.

240. Cai J, Nelson KC, Wu M, Sternberg P Jr, Jones DP. Oxidative damage and protection of the RPE. Prog Retinal Eye Res 2000;19(2):205–221.

241. Makrides SC. Therapeutic inhibition of the complement system. Pharmacol Rev 1998;50:59–87.

242. Hageman GS, Mullins RE, Russell SR, Johnson LV, Anderson DH. Vitronectin is a constituent of ocular drusen and the vitronectin gene is expressed in human retinal pigmented epithelial cells. FASEB J 1999;13:477–484.

243. Rimm EB, Stampfer MJ. Antioxidants for vascular disease. Med Clin North Am 2000; 84:239–249.

244. Hull M, Lieb K, Fiebich BL. Anti-inflammatory drugs: a hope for Alzheimer's disease? Expert Opin Invest Drugs 2000;9:671–683.
245. Penfold PL, Wen L, Madigan MC, Gillies MC, King NJ, Provis JM. Triamcinolone acetonide modulates permeability and intercellular adhesion molecule-1 (ICAM-1) expression of the ECV304 cell line: implications for macular degeneration. Clin Exp Immunol 2000;121:458–465.
246. Graninger W, Wenisch C. Pentoxifylline in severe inflammatory response syndrome. J Cardiovasc Pharmacol 1995;25(Suppl 2): S134–138.
247. Simon LS, Yocum D. New and future drug therapies for rheumatoid arthritis. Rheumatology (Oxford) 2000;39(Suppl 1): 36–42.

4

Nonexudative Macular Degeneration

Neelakshi Bhagat and Christina J. Flaxel

Doheny Eye Institute, University of Southern California Keck School of Medicine, Los Angeles, California

I. INTRODUCTION

Age-related macular degeneration (AMD) is the leading cause of blindness in the Western world (1). The severity of AMD increases with age. The highest prevalence of AMD is found in individuals over 75 years of age; 7.1% in this age group have late AMD (2–4). The Beaver Dam Eye Study, a population-based report, evaluated the incidence and progression of AMD and found the 5-year incidence of late AMD was 0.9%, with exudative AMD in at least one eye in 0.6% and pure geographic atrophy in 0.3% (4). The Chesapeake-Waterman study had previously reported a lower incidence of 0.2% (5). A total of 11.7% of patients with early AMD will develop late AMD over 5 years, with 7.1% developing an exudative component (4).

The prevalence of early and late age-related maculopathy increases with age as shown in population-based studies all over the world (Table 1). Soft indistinct reticular drusen or soft distinct drusen with retinal pigment epithelial (RPE) abnormalities form early age-related maculopathy (6,7).

II. NONEXUDATIVE VERSUS EXUDATIVE AMD

Age-related macular degeneration is either nonexudative or exudative. Nonexudative or dry maculopathy is the most common form of AMD, accounting for 80–90% of cases overall (10). Drusen with associated visual acuity loss due to overlying RPE atrophy constitutes nonexudative AMD. There is absence of subretinal hemorrhage, subretinal fluid, and hard exudates (2). Choroidal neovascularization heralds the onset of exudative macular degeneration. Clinically this is associated with subretinal fluid, subretinal hemorrhage, hard exudates, pigment epithelium irregularity, pigment epithelium detachment, or subretinal greenish-gray lesion. Fluorescein angiography will delineate the exact location (subfoveal, juxtafoveal, or extrafoveal), the size, and the pattern of leakage (classic versus occult).

67

Table 1 Prevalence of Age-Related Macular Degeneration (AMD)

		Age (years)	AMD prevalence (%)		
			Early	Late	Early or late
1	Chesapeake Bay	<50	4.0		
	(2)	50–59	6.0		
		60–69	13.0		
		70–79	26.0	4.3	
		80+		13.6	
2	Beaver Dam Study	43–54	8.4	0.1	
	(2)	55–64	13.8	0.6	
		65–74	18.0	1.4	
		65–74	18.0	1.4	
		75+	29.7	7.1	
		75+	29.7	7.1	
3	Klein and Klein	45–64			2.3
	(3)	65–74			9.0
4	Blue Mountains Eye Study (6)	49–54	1.3	0.0	
		55–64	2.6	0.2	
		65–74	8.5	0.7	
		75–84	15.5	5.4	
		85+	28.0	18.5	
5	Copenhagen	60–69			4.1
	(9)	70–80			20.0
6	Framingham	52–64			1.6
	(10)	65–74			11.0
		75–85			27.9

The patients who develop exudative AMD are older, with an average age of 70.5 years, than the patients with nonexudative AMD, with an average age of 56.8 years as noted in the study by Smiddy and Fine in 1984 (12).

III. ASSOCIATED FACTORS

Epidemiological, clinical, and histological studies suggest different factors are associated with macular degeneration (5,7,13–18). Hereditary influence, photic injury, nutritional deficiency, toxic insult, and systemic cardiovascular factors have been implicated in epidemiological studies (10,19,20). We can group these risk factors into the following categories: (1) personal characteristics, which include age, sex, race, eye color, smoking, and genetic predisposition.(21–23); (2) systemic disease, especially hypertension, cardiovascular disease, and blood lipid levels (1,10,15,24–26); and (3) environmental influences such as sunlight and nutrition (15,24,27–29).

A. Personal Characteristics

1. Age

The prevalence of AMD increases after 65 years of age; 27.9% of individuals between the age of 75 and 85 have macular degeneration (1,7,22). The number of drusen and the presence of confluent drusen correlates with increasing age (12,13).

2. Sex

AMD has been reported to be more prevalent in females (25,30). The Beaver Dam Study, after adjusting for age, revealed that the incidence of early AMD was 2.2% higher in women 75 years of age and older than in men in this age group (25). The prevalence of early age-related maculopathy was higher in men than women in each age category in the Blue Mountains Eye Study (6). Others have not noted such a difference between males and female (3).

3. Race

Drusen and pigmentary changes have been reported to be twice more common in whites than blacks (31).

4. Family History

AMD is known to run in families (1). Stone and co-workers have reported a genetic mutation that predisposes to drusen formation in malatia Leventinese and certain patients with macular degeneration (21,22,32). Further studies are needed.

5. Hyperopia

Hyperopia has been associated with AMD (23,33). Persons with brown iris color were shown to have a lower risk of developing AMD (33).

B. Systemic Diseases

1. Hypertension and Cardiovascular Disease

The Framingham Eye Study (1) and other studies (34) including the Macular Photocoagulation Study (MPS) (26) found a positive correlation between AMD and hypertension. This was, however, not seen in the studies by Hyman et al. (24), the Beaver Dam Study (3), and the Eye Disease Case-Control Study (35). Hyman et al. (33), on the other hand, found positive association of AMD with stroke, arteriosclerosis, and ischemic attacks. In their most recent case-control series, a strong association was found between neovascular AMD and moderate to severe hypertension, particularly in patients on antihypertensive therapy (24,26,30).

2. Hypercholesterolemia

The association between lipid profile and AMD has been inconsistent in various studies. The Beaver Dam Eye Study (28) noted a positive correlation between high intake of saturated fat and cholesterol and early AMD. A positive relationship was found with high-density lipoprotein (HDL) levels in men, and total serum cholesterol was inversely related to early AMD in women (25). Hyman and colleagues recently reported a positive association between dietary cholesterol and high levels of HDL with neovascular AMD (24).

C. Environmental Influences

1. Photic Injury

Although not scientifically proven, it has been suggested that accumulative exposure to light may cause gradual loss of photoreceptor cells in the macula (36).

2. Nutrition

It has been suggested that oxidative stress may play an important role in the etiology of AMD. Light induces the superoxide radicals to form that can damage the outer segments of photoreceptors (27,29). Antioxidants may prevent this damage (27). Antioxidants like ascorbate and vitamin E (alpha-tocopherol) may be deficient in elderly individuals, which may increase their susceptibility to light damage. It is also known that the retina and particularly the macula is highly susceptible to oxidative stress due to a high polyunsaturated fatty acid content that is prone to lipid peroxidation (27). One study tested the hypothesis that ascorbate could protect the retina from oxidative damage in rats: rats fed supplementary vitamin C were noted to have much milder damage to the retina than the rats that were exposed to the same amount of light but no supplementary ascorbate (37). In the POLA Study (27), an inverse association was found between AMD and levels of plasma alpha-tocopherol. This study and the Eye Disease Case-Control Study found no association between AMD and plasma ascorbate levels (27,38). Obviously, further randomized studies are needed to evaluate completely the role of antioxidants in the prevention of neovascular AMD. The Age-Related Eye Diseases Study (AREDS) (39) is an ongoing study looking at the effects of antioxidant and zinc supplementation. No results are available.

The Carotene and Retinol Efficacy Trial (CARET) Study (40) found that individuals who smoked and were assigned to beta-carotene and retinol were developing lung cancer at a rate of about 28% more than those assigned to placebo. This study was stopped after 4 years. A trial study in Finland (41) also suggested an increase in mortality from cancer and cardiovascular disease in patients on beta-carotene supplements. These studies did not take into account AMD but they do implicate possible adverse effects of high-dose vitamin intake in AMD patients who smoke (40,41).

Recently, much attention has been given to the dietary importance of carotenoids specially lutein and zeaxanthine (38). Seddon et al. reported the results of further investigations from the Eye Disease Case-Control Study (EDCCS), which showed that a high dietary intake of carotenoids, in particularly dark-green leafy vegetables, was associated with a 43% lower risk of AMD (38). A recent report in the *British Journal of Ophthalmology* analyzed various fruits and vegetables to establish which ones contain lutein and/or zeaxanthine and can serve as possible dietary supplements for these two carotenoids (15).

IV. DRUSEN

Drusen were first described in 1854 by Donders (42). These are deposits of membranous debris, extracellular material between the RPE and its basement membrane (basilar laminar drusen) or between the RPE basement layer and the inner collagenous layer of Bruch's membrane (basilar linear drusen) (17), (43–46). Drusen lead to secondary Bruch's membrane thickening and RPE degeneration. Visual loss due to macular degeneration is the result of degeneration of photoreceptor cells and the choriocapillaris, which ensues soon after RPE atrophy (47).

A. Etiology

Drusen form as a deposition of membranous material between the plasma membrane and the basement membrane of the RPE and are found as early as the second decade of life. They thus may represent a normal aging change (48). Stone and colleagues have identified a genetic mutation in patients with Malattia Leventinese, which also has been attributed to drusen formation in Best's disease and macular degeneration (32). Experimental and postmortem human studies show that the drusen are RPE-derive (49–51). Different theories have been entertained regarding the pathogenesis of the drusen.

Ishibashi et al. described the formation of drusen using electron microscopy as follows: (1) evagination or budding of the RPE cell in the subepithelial space; (2) separation of the evaginated portion from the parent RPE cell; (3) degeneration and disintegration of this evaginated cell components devoid of a nucleus; (4) accumulation of granular, vesicular, tubular, and linear material in the sub-RPE space (16). The etiology of the evagination is unknown.

The pathology of the aging changes in the retina is discussed in other chapters.

B. Types

Different types of drusen are noted in the retina: (1) hard, nodular drusen, (2) soft drusen, (3) crystalline drusen, and (4) cuticular or basal laminar drusen (14).

1. Hard Drusen

Hard drusen are discrete, small, round, yellow, nodular hyaline deposits found in the sub-RPE space, between the basement membrane of RPE and the inner collagenous layer of the Bruch membrane (52). These drusen are smaller than 50 microns in diameter (Fig. 1).

Focal densifications of Bruch's membrane, termed microdrusen, may precede the formation of hard drusen (53). Preclinical drusen appear ultrastructurally as "entrapment sites" with coated membrane-bound bodies that form adjacent to the inner collagenous layer of Bruch's membrane (53). These are structurally different from basal linear deposit.

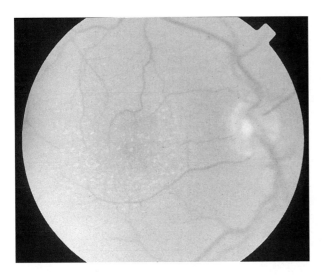

Figure 1 Color photograph of hard drusen in a 65-year-old asymptomatic man. See also color insert, Fig. 4.1.

Hard drusen are common in young people and do not lead to macular degeneration (43). Small, hard, indistinct drusen were found in the macula of 94% of the Beaver Dam population (2). These were not noted to increase in number with age. However, if present in excessive number, they may predispose to RPE atrophy (11).

Hard drusen act as window defects on fluorescein angiograms with early hyperfluorescence and fading on late frames (Fig. 2).

2. Basal Laminar Drusen

Basal laminar drusen are tiny, white multiple deposits found between the plasma membrane of retinal pigment epithelium and its basement membrane (43) (Fig. 3). These are found in normal aging eyes and do not predispose to macular degeneration.

(A)   **(B)**

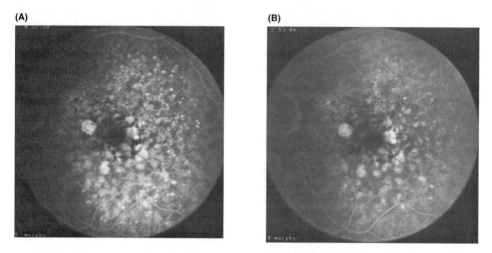

Figure 2   Fluorescein angiogram: early (A) and late (B) frames of hard drusen demonstrating window defects (early hyperfluorescence and fading late) and areas of geographic atrophy.

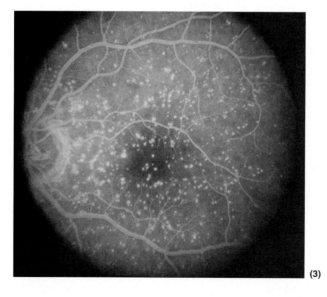

(3)

(4)

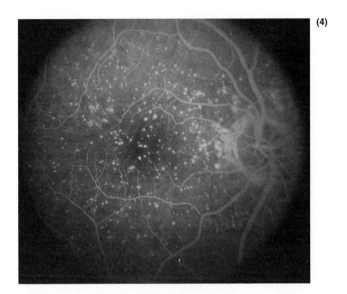

(5)

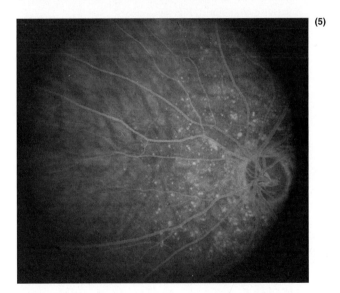

Figures 3, 4, and 5 Fluorescein angiogram: early form of basal laminar drusen from a 35-year-old asymptomatic patient. Fluorescein angiogram: mid and late frames demonstrating "starry night" appearance.

Basal laminar deposit is composed mainly of collagen, laminin, membrane-bound vesicles and fibronectin. It tends to accumulate over thickened Bruch's membrane suggesting that the accumulation of the debris may be a local response to altered filtration at these sites (52). These hyperfluoresce early on fluorescein angiography and give an appearance of "starry night" as discussed by Gass (54). They have been reported to be anatomically and histologically similar to soft drusen (Figs 4 and 5).

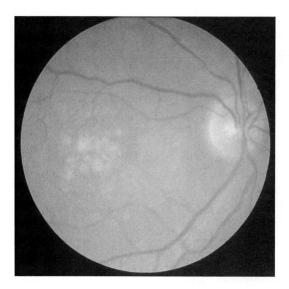

Figure 6   Color photograph showing soft drusen in a mildly symptomatic 70-year-old patient (mild distortion on Amsler grid testing). See also color insert, Fig. 4.6.

3. Soft Drusen

Soft drusen appear clinically as yellowish lesions with poorly defined edges. Histologically, they represent small, shallow RPE detachments. They are usually greater than 50 microns and are found after age 55 (Fig. 6). On fluorescein angiography, soft drusen show early hypofluorescence or hyperfluorescence with no late leakage.

Clinical and histological studies show that soft drusen precede macular degeneration (55,56). Drusen lead to secondary Bruch's membrane thickening and RPE degeneration and subsequent overlying retinal photoreceptor loss and predispose to the ingrowth of choroidal neovascularization (CNV) (14,46,57).

4. Crystalline Drusen

Crystalline drusen are discrete calcific refractile drusen (Fig. 7). These are dehydrated soft drusen that predispose to geographical atrophy (11,54).

C. High-Risk Drusen Characteristics

Drusen characteristics associated with a high risk of progression to exudative age-related maculopathy include drusen type (soft), drusen number (greater than five), large size ($>$ 63 microns), confluence, and associated findings such as hyperpigmentation (8,17,30,55–57). The risk of developing exudative maculopathy increases if there is a history of CNV in the fellow eye and with a positive family history (4,21,30,58).

The 5-year risk of eyes with bilateral drusen and good visual acuity to develop CNV is 0.2–18% (5,12,47,57). This risk increases to 7%–87% if the fellow eye has CNV (30,46,55,58). Bressler et al., in their age-adjusted analysis, showed that greater than 20 drusen, the presence of soft drusen, confluent drusen, and focal RPE hyperpigmentation were more often noted in the fellow eyes with unilateral exudative maculopathy than in eyes with bilateral drusen (56). Focal hyperpigmentation and confluence of drusen are

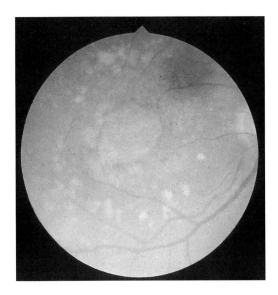

Figure 7 Color photograph of geographic atrophy and drusen. See also color insert, Fig. 4.7.

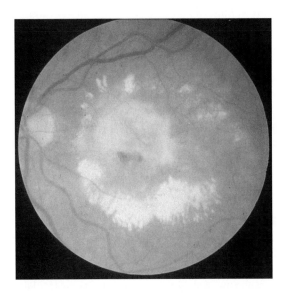

Figure 8 Color photograph showing the end-stage appearance of the fellow eye of the patient in Figure 6 with high-risk drusen. See also color insert, Fig. 4.8.

associated with an increased risk of progression to exudative AMD (7). In his discussion of Smiddy and Fine, Jampol explains that focal hyperpigmentation may be associated with subclinical subretinal neovascularization that cannot be detected by fluorescein angiography (59). It may also reflect that changes have occurred already in the RPE, Bruch's membrane, and choriocapillaris, which facilitate future development of CNV and may simply suggest the chronicity of the disease process (59) (Fig. 8).

V. DISAPPEARANCE OF DRUSEN

A. Natural History

Various reports have described the spontaneous disappearance of drusen (5,60). Bressler et al. noted in their Waterman study that large drusen disappeared in 16 (34%) of 47 individuals in 5 years of follow-up (55).

Areolar atrophy may ensue as drusen disappear (12). With loss of the RPE, photoreceptor and choriocapillaris loss follows quickly. Atrophy of overlying RPE is noted as drusen disappear.

B. Laser to Drusen Studies

Various pilot studies have shown mixed results in an attempt to answer the question regarding the risk of exudative AMD and the disappearance of drusen (61,62). Two multicenter trials of laser to drusen have been undertaken, the Choroidal Neovascularization Prevention Trial (CNVPT) and the Prophylactic Treatment of AMD Study (PTAMD). The two subsets of AMD patients are: (1) patients with bilateral soft large drusen and good visual acuity and (2) patients with soft large drusen and good visual acuity in the fellow eye of those with exudative AMD in one eye. Results from the CNVPT study demonstrated an increased risk of exudative AMD in the fellow eye randomized to light argon laser treatment (61,63). The PTAMD trial, using subthreshold diode laser, has shown similar findings of increased risk of exudative maculopathy in fellow eyes of patients treated with laser. A recent paper in the *British Journal of Ophthalmology* by Guymer et al. (64) looked at the effect of laser photocoagulation on choroidal capillary cytoarchitecture and found that qualitative differences were seen following laser. They postulate that these changes brought on by laser at just suprathreshold levels may carry a risk of inducing choroidal neovascularization as these processes may play a part in the clearance of debris from Bruch's membrane, and represent an early stage of angiogenesis (64). This side effect is discussed in another chapter. The bilateral drusen arms of both trials are still in progress though the pilot subthreshold paper by Olk et al. does show efficacy of diode laser for drusen (62) (Fig. 9).

VI. NONEXUDATIVE MACULAR DEGENERATION

Clinical and histological studies show that soft drusen precede macular degeneration (47,55).

The mere presence of drusen does not account for significant loss of vision (45). Soft drusen lead to RPE atrophy with resultant overlying photoreceptor atrophy and vision loss. When the vision falls below or equal to 20/30, the disease process is termed nonexudative or dry macular degeneration.

Subretinal fluid, subretinal hemorrhage, retinal pigment epithelium detachment, hard exudates, subretinal fibrosis, all signs of exudative maculopathy, are absent in dry macular degeneration.

Focal hyperpigmentation along with the increased number (> 5) and confluence of soft, large (> 63 microns) drusen is associated with increased risk of progression of RPE atrophy and choroidal atrophy. These eyes have a higher incidence of developing CNV (45,46).

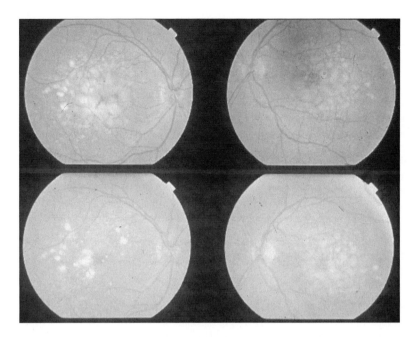

Figure 9 Example of pre (upper left and upper right) and post (lower left and lower right) subthreshold diode laser showing drusen disappearance in a 45-year-old man with a hereditary form of AMD. See also color insert, Fig. 4.9.

Geographic atrophy (GA) is a form of advanced dry macular degeneration. This involves marked choriocapillaris and small choroidal vessel atrophy along with the RPE atrophy. This progresses slowly over years and often spares the center of the foveal avascular zone until late in the course of the disease (65). Almost 3.5% of individuals older than 75 years of age suffer from GA, which causes visual loss of 20/200 or worse. This severe form of GA accounts for at least 20% of all patients with 20/200 or worse vision from advanced macular degeneration (66).

Although nonexudative AMD is more prevalent, it accounts for only 10% of the severe vision loss due to AMD (25,66). Bressler et al. reported a prevalence of 1.8% of AMD in men 50 years of age or older in the Chesapeake Bay study. Of these, almost 75% had the nonexudative maculopathy (8).

The Beaver Dam Eye Study (4) and Chesapeake Bay Waterman Study (5) were population-based eye studies that provided data on 5-year incidence and progression of AMD. Soft drusen and retinal pigmentary changes were found to increase with age. In the 5-year period of the Beaver Dam Eye Study, people 75 years or older were 3.3–8.4 times as likely to develop large drusen between 63 microns and 250 microns in diameter and 40.7 times more likely to develop drusen greater than or equal to 250 microns in diameter as compared to persons 43–54 years of age. Also, persons 75 years of age or over were 16 times more likely to develop confluent drusen when compared to people 43–54 years of age (4). There was a much higher incidence of dry macular degeneration clinical findings in people over 75 years of age (Table 2). This was consistent with the results of the Blue Mountains Australian (6), Rotterdam (67), and Colorado-Wisconsin (68) studies of AMD.

Table 2 The Beaver Dam Eye Study, 5-Year Incidence of Nonexudative AMD Findings

		p-value	>75 years of age	43–54 years of age
1	Large drusen (125–249 microns)	<0.05	17.6%	2.1%
2	Large drusen (>250 microns)	<0.05	6.5%	0.2%
3	Soft indistinct (drusen)	<0.05	16.3%	1.8%
4	Retinal pigment (abnormalities)	<0.05	12.9%	0.9%
5	Pure geographic atrophy	<0.05	1.7%	0%

Source: Ref. 4.

VII. MONITORING NONEXUDATIVE AMD

Amsler-grid testing is a sensitive indicator of progression of the disease process. Straight door and window frames may be crude ways to check for any metamorphopsia.

Patients are encouraged to seek medical help if visual distortion, metamorphopsia, loss of central vision, or any new symptoms occur. These herald the growth of choroidal neovascular membranes. The early detection of the choroidal neovascular membranes may facilitate treatment with either laser photocoagulation, photodynamic therapy, transpupillary thermotherapy, or macular translocation, as described in other chapters.

VIII. SUMMARY

Prevalence of AMD increases with age. Nonexudative AMD is the most common form of AMD. Factors associated with AMD include increased age, heredity, photic injury, nutrition, toxic insults, and cardiovascular risk factors. High-risk characteristics of drusen for development of CNV include: soft drusen, large drusen, greater than five drusen, confluence, and focal hyperpigmentation. Disappearance of drusen can occur sponta- neously or may follow laser to drusen (CNVPT and PTAMD). Disappearance of drusen may result in geographic atrophy. Monitoring visual acuity and visual symptoms for the progression of AMD is of utmost importance in applying timely treatment.

REFERENCES

1. Leibowitz HM, Krueger DE, Maunder LR, Milton RC, Kini MM, Kahn HA, Nickerson RJ, Pool J, Colton TL, Ganley JP, Loewenstein JI, Dawber TR. The Framingham Eye Study monograph: an ophthalmological and epidemiological study of cataract, glaucoma, diabetic retinopathy, macular degeneration, and visual acuity in a general population of 2631 adults, 1973–1975. Surv Ophthalmol 1980;24(suppl):335–610.
2. Klein R, Klein BE, Linton KL. Prevalence of age-related maculopathy. The Beaver Dam Eye Study. Ophthalmology 1992;99:933–943.
3. Klein BE, Klein R. Cataracts and macular degeneration in older Americans. Arch Ophthalmol 1982;100:571–573.

4. Klein R, Klein BEK, Jensen SC, Meuer SM. The five-year incidence and progression of age-related maculopathy: the Beaver Dam Eye Study. Ophthalmology 1997;104:7–21.

5. Bressler NM, Munoz B, Maguire MG, Vitale SE, Schein OD, Taylor HR, West SK. Five-year incidence and disappearance of drusen and retinal pigment abnormalities. Waterman study. Arch Ophthalmol 1995;113:301–308.

6. Mitchell P, Smith W, Attebo K, Wang JJ. Prevalence of age-related maculopathy in Australia. The Blue Mountains Eye Study. Ophthalmology 1995;102:1450–1460.

7. Sarraf D, Gin T, Yu F, Brannon A, Owens SL, Bird AC. Long-term drusen study. Retina 1999;19:513–519.

8. Bressler NM, Bressler SB, West SK, Fine SL, Taylor HR. The grading and prevalence of macular degeneration in Chesapeake Bay watermen. Arch Ophthalmol 1989;107:847–852.

9. Vinding T. Age related macular degeneration. Macular changes, prevalence and sex ratio. An epidemiological study of 1000 aged individuals. Acta Ophthalmol (Copenh) 1989;67:609–616.

10. Kahn HA, Leibowitz HM, Ganley JP, Kini MM, Colton T, Nickerson RS, Dawber TR. The Framingham Eye Study. II. Association of ophthalmic pathology with single variables previously measured in the Framingham Heart Study. Am J Epidemiol 1977;106:33–41.

11. Sarks SH. Drusen patterns predisposing to geographic atrophy of the retinal pigment epithelium. Aust J Ophthalmol 1982;l0:91–97.

12. Smiddy WE, Fine SL: Prognosis of patients with bilateral macular drusen. Ophthalmology 1984;91:271–277.

13. Gragoudas ES, Chandra SR, Friedman E, Klein ML, Van Buskirk M. Disciform degeneration of the macula. II. Pathogenesis. Arch Ophthalmol 1976;94:755–757.

14. Green WR, McDonnell PJ, Yeo JH. Pathologic features of senile macular degeneration. Ophthalmology 1985;92:615–627.

15. Sommerburg O, Keunen JE, Bird AC, van Kuijk FJ. Fruits and vegetables that are sources for lutein and zeaxanthin: the macular pigment in human eyes. Br J Ophthalmol 1998;82:907–910.

16. Ishibashi T, Patterson R, Ohnishi Y, Inomata H, Ryan SJ. Formation of drusen in the human eye. Am J Ophthalmol 1986;101:342–353.

17. Abdelsalam A, Del Priore L, Zarbin MA. Drusen in age-related macular degeneration: pathogenesis, natural course, and laser photocoagulation-induced regression. Surv Ophthalmol 1999;44:1–29.

18. Gregor Z, Bird AC, Chisholm IH. Senile disciform macular degeneration in the second eye. Br J Ophthalmol 1977;61:141–147.

19. Goldberg J, Flowerdew G, Smith E, Brody JA, Tso MO. Factors associated with age related macular degeneration. An analysis of data from the first National Health and Nutrition Examination Survey. Am J Epidemiol 1988;128:700–710.

20. Vinding T, Appleyard M, Nyboe J, Jensen G. Risk factor analysis for atrophic and exudative age related macular degeneration. An epidemiological study of 1000 aged individuals. Acta Ophthalmol (Copenh) 1992;70:66–72.

21. Klein ML, Mauldin WM, Stoumbos VD. Hereditary and age related macular degeneration. Observations in monozygotic twins. Arch Ophthalmol 1994;112:932–937.

22. Klein ML, Schultz DW, Edwards A, Matise TC, Rust K, Berselli CB, Trzupek K, Weleber RG, Ott J, Wirtz MK, Acott TS. Age-related macular degeneration: clinical features in a large family and linkage to chromosome 1q. Arch Ophthalmol 1998;116:1082–1088.

23. Maltzman BA, Mulvihill MN, Greenbaum A. Senile macular degeneration and risk factors: a case-control study. Ann Ophthalmol 1979;11:1197–1201.

24. Hyman L, Schachat AP, He Q, Leske MC. Hypertension, cardiovascular disease, and age-related macular degeneration. Age-Related Macular Degeneration Risk Factors Study Group. Arch Ophthalmol 2000;118:351–358.

25. Klein R, Klein BE, Jensen SC. The relation of cardiovascular disease and its risk factors to the 5-year incidence of age-related maculopathy: the Beaver Dam Eye Study. Ophthalmology 1997;104:1804–1812.

26. Laser photocoagulation for juxtafoveal choroidal neovascularization. Five-year results from randomized clinical trials. Macular Photocoagulation Study group. Arch Ophthalmol 1994;112:500–509.

27. Delcourt C, Cristol JP, Tessier F, Leger CL, Descomps B, Papoz L. Age-related macular degeneration and antioxidant status in the POLA Study. POLA Study Group. Pathologies Oculaires Liees a l'Age. Arch Ophthalmol 1999;117:1384–1390.

28. Mares-Perlman JA, Brady WE, Klein R, VandenLagenberg GM, Klein BE, Palta M. Dietary fat and age-related maculopathy. Arch Ophthalmol 1995;113:743–748.

29. Tso MO. Pathogenetic factors of aging macular degeneration. Ophthalmology 1985;92:628–635.

30. Risk factors for choroidal neovascularization in the second eye of patients with juxtafoveal or subfoveal choroidal neovascularization secondary to age-related macular degeneration. Macular Photocoagulation Study Group. Arch Ophthalmol 1997;115:741–747.

31. Gregor Z, Joffe L. Senile macular changes in black African. Br J Ophthalmol 1978;62:547–550.

32. Stone EM, Lotery AJ, Munier FL, Heon E, Piguet B, Guymer RH, Vandenburgh K, Cousin P, Nishimura D, Swiderski RE, Silvestri G, Mackey DA, Hageman GS, Bird AC, Sheffield VC, Schorderet DF. A single EFEMP1 mutation associated with both Malattia Leventinese and Doyne honeycomb retinal dystrophy. Nat Genet 1999;22:199–202.

33. Hyman LG, Lilienfeld AM, Ferris FL, Fine SL. Senile macular degeneration: a case-control study. Am J Epidemiol 1983;118:213–227.

34. Delaney WV, Oates RP. Senile macular degeneration: a preliminary study. Ann Ophthalmol 1982;14:21–24.

35. The Eye Disease Case-Control Study Group. Risk factors for neovascular age related macular degeneration. Arch Ophthalmol 1992;110:1701–1708.

36. Gartner S, Henkind P. Aging and degeneration of the human macula. 1. Outer nuclear layer and photoreceptors. Br J Ophthalmol 1981;65:23–28.

37. Li ZY, Tso MOM, Woodford BJ, Wang HM, Organisciak DT. Amelioration of photic injury in rat retina by abscorbic acid. ARVO abstract. Invest Ophthalmol Vis Sci 1984;25(suppl):90.

38. Seddon JM, Ajani UA, Sperduto RD, Hiller R, Blair N, Burton TC, Farber MD, Gragoudas ES, Haller J, Miller DT, et al. Dietary carotenoids, vitamins A, C, and E and advanced age-related macular degeneration. Eye Disease Case-Control Study Group. JAMA 1994;272:1413–1420.

39. The Age-Related Eye Disease Study (AREDS): design implications AREDS report no. 1. The Age-Related Eye Diseases Study Research Group. Control Clin Trials 1999;20:573–600.

40. Omenn GS, Goodman GE, Thornquist MD, Balmes J, Cullen MR, Glass A, Keogh JP, Meyskens FL, Valanis B, Williams JH, Barnhart S, and Hammar S. Effects of a combination of beta carotene and vitamin A on lung cancer and cardiovascular disease. N Engl J Med 1996;334:1150–5.

41. The Alpha-Tocopherol, Beta Carotene Cancer Prevention Study Group. The effect of vitamin E and beta carotene on the incidence of lung cancer and other cancers in male smokers. N Engl J Med 1994;330:1029–1035.

42. Donders FC. Beitrage zur pathologischen Anatomie des Auges. Arch Ophthalmol 1854;1(II):106–118.

43. Spraul CW, Grossniklaus HE. Characteristics of Drusen and Bruch's membrane in postmortem eyes with age-related macular degeneration. Arch Ophthalmol 1997;115:267–273.

44. Green WR, Enger C. Age-related macular degeneration histopathologic studies. The 1992 Lorenz E. Zimmerman Lecture. Ophthalmology 1993;100:1519–1535.

45. Gass JD. Drusen and disciform macular detachment and degeneration. Trans Am Ophthalmol Soc 1972;70:409–36.

46. Sarks SH. Council Lecture. Drusen and their relationship to senile macular degeneration. Aust J Ophthalmol 1980;8:117–130.

47. Gass JD. Drusen and disciform macular detachment and degeneration. Arch Ophthalmol 1973;90:206–17.

48. Sarks JP, Sarks SH, Killingsworth MC. Evolution of geographic atrophy of the retinal pigment epithelium. Eye 1988;2:552–77.

49. Sarks JP, Sarks SH, Killingsworth MC. Evolution of soft drusen in age-related maular degeneration. Eye 1994;8:269–83.

50. Green WR, Key SN. Senile macular degeneration: a histopathologic study. Trans Am Ophthalmol Soc 1977;75:180–254.

51. Coffey AJ, Brownstein S. The prevalence of macular drusen in postmortem eyes. Am J Ophthalmol 1986;102:164–171.

52. Sarks SH. Ageing and degeneration in the macular region: a clinicopathologic study. Br J Ophthalmol 1976;60:324–41.

53. Sarks SH, Arnold JJ, Killingsworth MC, Sarks JP. Early drusen formation in the normal and aging eye and their relation to age-related maculopathy: a clinicopathological study. Br J Ophthalmol 1999;83:358–68.

54. Gass JD. Stereoscopic atlas of macular diseases: Diagnosis and treatment. Vol. 1. St. Louis: CV Mosby, 1987.

55. Bressler SB, Maguire MG, Bressler NM, Fine SL. Relationship of drusen and abnormalities of the retinal pigment epithelium to the prognosis of neovascular macular degeneration. The Macular Photocoagulation Study Group. Arch Ophthalmol 1990;108:1442–1447.

56. Bressler NM, Bressler SB, Seddon JM, Gragoudas ES, Jacobson LP. Drusen characteristics in patients with exudative versus non-exudative age-related macular degeneration. Retina 1988;8:109–114.

57. Holz FG, Wolfensberger TJ, Piguet B, Gross-Jendroska M, Wells JA, Minassian DC, Chisholm IH, Bird AC. Bilateral macular drusen in age-related macular degeneration. Prognosis and risk factors. Ophthalmology 1994;101:1522–1528.

58. Strahlman ER, Fine SL, Hillis A. The second eye of patients with senile macular degeneration. Arch Ophthalmol 1983;101:1191–1193.

59. Smiddy WE, Fine SL. Prognosis of patients with bilateral macular drusen. Ophthalmology 1984;91:271–277.

60. Javornik NB, Hiner CJ, Marsh MJ, Maguire MG, Bressler NM for the MPS Group. Changes in drusen and RPE abnormalities in age-related macular degeneration. Invest Ophthalmol Vis Sci 1992;33:1230.

61. Laser treatment in eyes with large drusen. Short-term effects seen in a pilot randomized clinical trial. Choroidal Neovascularization Trial Research Group. Ophthalmology 1998;105:11–23.

62. Olk RJ, Friberg TR, Stickney KL, Akduman L, Wong KL, Chen MC, Levy MH, Garcia CA, Morse LS. Therapeutic benefits of infrared (810-nm) diode laser macular grid photocoagulation in prophylactic treatment of non-exudative age-related macular degeneration: two-year results of a randomized pilot study. Ophthalmology 1999;106:2882–2090.

63. Kaiser RS, Berger JW, Shin DS, Maguire MG. CNVPT Study Group. Laser burn intensity and the risk for choroidal neovascularization in the CNVPT Fellow Eye Study (abstr). Invest Ophthalmol Vis Sci 1999;40(suppl):S377.

64. Guymer RH, Hageman GS, Bird AC. Influence of laser photocoagulation on choroidal capillary cytoarchitecture. Br J Ophthalmol 2001;85:40–46.

65. Sunness JS, Rubin GS, Applegate CA, Bressler NM, Marsh MJ, Hawkins BS, Haselwood D. Visual function abnormalities and prognosis in eyes with age-related geographic atrophy of the macula and good visual acuity. Ophthalmology 1997;104:1677–1691.

66. Ferris FL, Fine SL, Hyman LG. Age-related macular degeneration and blindness due to neovascular maculopathy. Arch Ophthalmol 1984;102:1640–1642.

67. Vingerling JR. Dielemans I, Hofman A, Grobbee DE, Hijmering M, Kramer CF, de Jong PT. The prevalence of age-related maculopathy in the Rotterdam study. Ophthalmology 1995;102:205–210.

68. Cruickshanks KJ, Hamman RE, Klein R, Nondahl DM, Shetterly SM. The prevalence of age-related maculopathy by geographic region and ethnicity. The Colorado-Wisconsin Study of Age-Related Maculopathy. Arch Ophthalmol 1997;115:242–250.

5
Geographic Atrophy

Sharon D. Solomon and Janet S. Sunness
Wilmer Eye Institute, Johns Hopkins University School of Medicine, Baltimore, Maryland

Michael J. Cooney
Duke University Eye Center, Durham, North Carolina

I. INTRODUCTION

Geographic atrophy (GA) of the retinal pigment epithelium (RPE) is the advanced form of nonneovascular age-related macular degeneration (AMD) and is associated with the gradual, progressive loss of central vision. Dense scotomas have been shown to correspond to the retinal areas affected by GA (1). These scotomas involve the parafoveal and perifoveal retina early in the course of the disease, sparing the foveal center until late in the course of the disease (2–5). Consequently, GA is only responsible for approximately 20% of the legal blindness secondary to AMD, compared to choroidal neovascularization (CNV), which tends to involve the foveal center much earlier in the course of the disease and accounts for nearly 80% of the legal blindness secondary to AMD (6). However, the parafoveal and perifoveal scotomas, in the early stages of GA, compromise the ability to read and to recognize faces, often despite the retention of good visual acuity, and account for a much larger percentage of moderate visual loss in those affected (7). The prevalence of GA in the population 75 years of age or older is approximately 3.5%, half that of neovascular AMD (8,9), and increases to 22% in those 90 years of age or older (22). While there are treatments for some forms of choroidal neovascularization, at present no treatment is available for GA. As our understanding of GA grows, it is hoped that medical and surgical interventions will be developed to slow or completely halt its progression rate and prevent subsequent moderate and severe visual loss.

II. CLINICAL FEATURES OF GEOGRAPHIC ATROPHY

GA is easily recognized clinically, as it appears as a well-demarcated area of decreased retinal thickness, compared to the surrounding retina, with a relative change in color that allows for increased visualization of the underlying choroidal vessels. Both the location and pattern of the atrophy may vary in appearance. Forty percent of eyes with macular GA also have peripapillary GA, which may become confluent with the macular atrophy (7). There may be pigmentary alteration, either hypopigmentation or hyperpigmentation, surrounding the macular atrophy. Peripheral reticular degeneration of the pigment epithelium is present in about 41% of eyes (7). Drusen, usually a mixture of the soft and calcific types, are present in most eyes until the GA becomes so extensive as to resorb the macular drusen (2). The increased choroidal vessel detail in the area of GA is usually the most easily identified fundus change and further reflects the extent of RPE attenuation. On fluorescein angiography, this translates into an area of hyperfluorescence that corresponds to the ophthalmoscopic borders of the GA, secondary to transmission defect and staining. The intensity of hyperfluorescence from choroidal flush may vary depending on the presence or absence of the underlying choriocapillaris (4). Fluorescein angiography may also aid in distinguishing GA from occult choroidal neovascularization, which may otherwise appear clinically indistinguishable.

Hemorrhage may occur in eyes with GA. Though this may be a reflection of the development of CNV and the likelihood of a more precipitous decline in visual function secondary to neovascular maculopathy, often the small areas of CNV that develop are transient and may become clinically inapparent a few months later (11). Hemorrhages have also been described in GA in the complete absence of any CNV (11,12). In general, however, the presence of hemorrhage, especially when associated with a sudden change in vision, warrants an angiographic evaluation for the presence of CNV (13).

Though there are frequently small areas of retinal sparing within the GA, especially at the center of the macula, foveal localization may still prove challenging on clinical examination, on the color fundus photograph, and on the angiogram. Clinically, the location of xanthophyll, if visible, is helpful in determining the location of the foveal center. On fluorescein angiography, the intense hyperfluorescence associated with the GA may obscure the view of the entire foveal avascular zone, making foveal localization a less certain task. Under such circumstances, the red-free photographs can often be of significant help. The presence of xanthophyll may suggest that the fovea has visual function, even if the retina appears atrophic and nonfunctional (14). Testing with devices such as the scanning laser ophthahnoscope (SLO) may help to ascertain the central visual potential that remains (1,5).

III. HISTOPATHOLOGY AND PATHOGENESIS

Histopathological examination of eyes with GA demonstrates a loss of RPE cells in the area of atrophy with a secondary loss of overlying photoreceptor cells (15). The choriocapillaris may also be absent, and there is indeed some experimental evidence to suggest that when the RPE is removed or has atrophied, the choriocapillaris involutes secondarily (16,17). GA is associated with thickening of Bruch's membrane secondary to the deposition of basal laminar and basal linear deposits in the surrounding retina (18). Therefore, histologically, GA has been thought of as the end-stage of the AMD process if CNV does not develop (19). GA may also occur following the flattening of a RPE detachment (20).

There is controversy as to whether the loss of RPE cells, perhaps related to the deposits in and near Bruch's membrane, is the primary event in the evolution of GA, or whether this RPE atrophy develops secondary to choroidal vascular insufficiency. Green and Key have argued that the presence of choroidal vascular insufficiency should result in the subsequent degeneration of all the outer retinal layers (15). This is not seen in eyes with GA. Friedman et al. suggest that choroidal vascular resistance may predispose to the development of AMD, specifically high-risk drusen and CNV (21). However, a causal association between choroidal vascular resistance and GA has not been established to date.

IV. PREVALENCE AND EPIDEMIOLOGY OF GEOGRAPHIC ATROPHY

Population-based studies, such as the Beaver Dam Eye Study and the Rotterdam Study, have examined the prevalence of GA in the elderly and compared it to the prevalence of CNV in the same groups. The prevalence of GA is approximately 3.5% for people age 75 and above in the United States and other developed nations, half that of CNV (8,9). The prevalence of GA increases with age and is actually more common than CNV in older age groups. In the population over age 90, the prevalence of GA can reach levels of 20–35% (10,22). The studies indicate that there is a lower prevalence of GA in African-Americans (23). There does not appear to be a gender difference in prevalence across the populations studied.

In the Beaver Dam Eye Study, 8% of eyes with drusen larger than 250 microns went on to develop GA over a 5-year period. Eyes that developed GA all had pigmentary abnormalities and at least 0.2 Macular Photocoagulation Study (MPS) disk areas of drusen at baseline (24). Of the eyes with GA, 42% had a visual acuity of 20/200 or worse. This was similar to the 48% of eyes with neovascular AMD that had a comparable level of severe visual loss (24).

GA is bilateral in 48–65% of cases (39). While the rate of bilateral severe vision loss is lower from GA than from CNV, GA is still responsible for a full 20% of the binocular legal blindness secondary to AMD (6). These statistics for severe visual loss measure only the incidence of legal blindness and significantly underestimate the disability associated with GA. A patient with GA may not be able to read or to recognize faces because the object being visualized does not "fit" into the spared central island of vision (5).

A. Systemic Risk Factors

A number of population-based studies have attempted to identify possible risk factors for the development of GA and neovascular AMD. The Beaver Dam Eye Study did not demonstrate a relationship between GA and cholesterol level or alcohol intake (8,25). While current or past smoking was a significant risk factor for the presence of GA for women in the Blue Mountains Eye Study, the same association did not reach statistical significance for men (26). In Sunness' study, there was a trend for current smokers to have a more rapid progression of GA than nonsmokers (7). The same study suggested that patients who are pseudophakic or aphakic do not have more rapid progression of GA than their phakic counterparts (7).

More recently, the Age-Related Eye Disease Study (AREDS), an ongoing multicenter study of the natural history of AMD and cataract, has reported its findings on possible risk factors for the development of GA and neovascular AMD. The presence of GA was found to be associated with increasing age and smoking, confirming the findings of previous population-based studies (27). In addition, there appeared to be a positive association between the use of antacids and the use of thyroid hormones and the presence of GA (27). These two associations have not been previously reported and will certainly prompt further investigation. Level of education was found to be inversely proportional to the presence of GA in that persons with more years of formal schooling seemed to be at lower risk for GA (27).

B. Heredity

Several studies have suggested that genetic factors may also be important in the pathogenesis of AMD. Hereditary retinal dystrophies, with clinical manifestations similar to AMD, may share potential candidate susceptibility genes. For example, a mutation of the RDS/peripherin gene has been shown to be associated with Zermatt macular dystrophy, which is a dominant, age-related, progressive macular dystrophy that resembles GA in its later stages (28). Particular interest has focused on the ABCR gene, which is responsible for autosomal recessive Stargardt macular dystrophy. One study reported that 16% of patients with AMD had a mutation in this gene, compared with 13% of Stargardt's patients and 0.5% of the general population (29). The mutation was identified primarily in eyes affected by atrophic AMD, on the continuum between early and advanced disease (30,31). There is some disagreement with these findings, however.

Pedigree studies have included families in which GA and CNV occur in different members as well as twin studies, where both twins are affected by GA or where one twin has GA and the other has an earlier atrophic form of AMD. In one large AMD family, linkage has been reported to markers in 1q25–q31 (32). Recent data also suggest that the ApoE epsilon 4 allele may be associated with a reduced risk for the development of AMD (32). Identification of those genetic factors that play a role in the pathogenesis of AMD may aid with the recognition of those at risk and permit possible lifestyle modifications to prevent or decrease the severity of disease.

V. NATURAL HISTORY OF GEOGRAPHIC ATROPHY

Over the last three decades, several studies have described the progression of GA with respect to visual acuity loss and actual enlargement of the atrophy in populations of patients. Their observations form the foundation of our knowledge of the natural history of GA.

GA typically develops in eyes that, at baseline, have drusen or pigmentary alteration. As drusen fade, focal areas of atrophy may develop in their place, enlarge, and evolve into GA (2,33,34). Alternatively, areas of mottled hypopigmentation may also predispose to the development of GA (2). The progression goes through a number of stages. Initially, single or multifocal areas of GA may be found in the region around the fovea. As these areas enlarge and coalesce over time, they can form a horseshoe of atrophy that spares the foveal center (Fig. 1). This horseshoe of atrophy may close off into a ring of atrophy that still permits foveal preservation. In the late stages of GA, the fovea itself becomes atrophic and nonseeing, from further coalescence of the GA, requiring the patient to use eccentric retinal loci for fixation and seeing (2). GA may also occur secondary to an RPE detachment. Elman and others have reported RPE detachments flattening and evolving into GA in about 20% of cases (20,35–37). Whether the GA was extrafoveal or foveal depended on the preceding location of the RPE detachment. Because visual loss tends to be gradual and subtle, and takes place over a period of years, patients may not seek medical attention until the solid central GA is present.

GA continues to enlarge over time with a median rate of enlargement over a 2-year period of 1.8 MPS disk areas (7). The amount of enlargement of total atrophic area has been

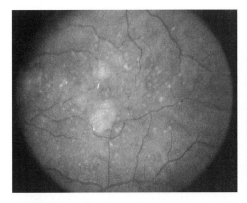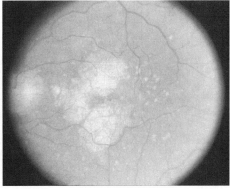

Figure 1 Four-year progression in geographic atrophy. (Left) There are multifocal areas of geographic atrophy, along with drusen and pigmentary alteration. (Right) Four years later, the areas of geographic atrophy have enlarged and coalesced, forming a horseshoe of atrophy surrounding the fovea. See also color insert, Fig. 5.1.

shown to increase with increasing baseline size of atrophy up to approximately 5 MPS disk areas of baseline, after which there appears to be a plateau at a high rate of increase. For eyes with more than 10 MPS disk areas, it is difficult to measure enlargement because the borders of the GA often extend past the photographic field. Baseline level of visual acuity did not appear to significantly affect the degree of enlargement of total atrophy (7). The only risk factor that has been linked to more rapid enlargement of the total atrophic area was a baseline total atrophy area greater than 3 MPS disc areas (7). Neither the phakic status of the study eye nor a history of hypertension in the patient was shown to be a risk factor for the enlargement of total atrophy (7). Though the number of smokers in the study was small, there was an apparent trend for smokers to have a more rapid enlargement of atrophy (7).

GA is associated with a significant decline in visual acuity over time in many eyes. Sunness et al. demonstrated that the median visual acuity tended to be worse in eyes with larger total atrophic areas, with the most dramatic difference in median acuity occurring between eyes with less than 3 MPS disk areas of central atrophy (i.e., within 4 MPS disk areas of the foveal center) and those with greater than three MPS disk areas of central atrophy (7). Overall, 31% of all study eyes lost three or more lines of visual acuity, doubling the visual angle, by 2 years of follow-up, and 53% lost 3 or more lines of visual acuity by 4 years of follow-up (7). Rates of severe vision loss, i.e., a quadrupling of the visual angle or at least six lines of visual acuity loss, were 13% for all study eyes by 2 years and 29% by 4 years (7). There was a significantly larger rate of moderate and severe vision loss for eyes with a baseline visual acuity of better than 20/50. At 2 years of follow-up, 41% of these eyes with good acuity at baseline lost three or more lines of visual acuity and 21% lost six or more lines of visual acuity (7). Those numbers grew to 70% at 4 years of follow-up for moderate vision loss and 45% at 4 years for severe vision loss (7). Twenty-seven percent of the eyes with visual acuity of 20/50 or better at baseline had visual acuity of 20/200 or worse at 4 years of follow-up (7). The presence of CNV in the fellow eye did not appear to affect the rate of visual acuity loss in the GA study eye (7). Risk factors that have thus far been identified for moderate vision loss include baseline visual acuity of better than 20/50 and lightest iris color (7). Among eyes with visual acuity better than 20/50, the

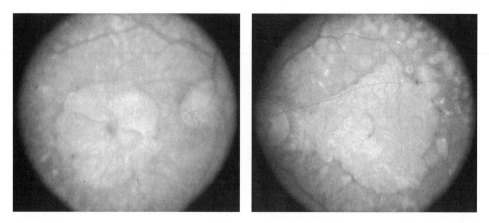

Figure 2 Bilateral geographic atrophy. (Left) This eye had 20/30 visual acuity, and the patient was able to read 80 words per minute, using the spared central area. (Right) The fellow eye did not have a usable spared region and had 20/400 visual acuity. See also color insert, Fig. 5.2.

presence of GA within 250 microns of the foveal center was a strong risk factor for a three-line visual acuity loss (7). No apparent association between phakic status of the study eye, hypertension, or smoking, and moderate vision loss, was demonstrated in the study by Sunness et al. (7).

During the 4-year follow-up period, GA appeared to progress through various stages, including the small, multifocal, horseshoe, ring, and solid stages described in previous studies (2,3,7). For eyes that did not have the solid pattern of atrophy at baseline and that did not develop CNV during the course of the study, 61% advanced to a different configuration over the 2-year follow-up period (7). However, those eyes that had the same configuration at the 2-year follow-up as at baseline still had visual acuity loss, most notably in the ring group where 50% of eyes lost three or more lines of visual acuity (7).

The size and rate of progression of atrophy are highly correlated between the two eyes of patients with bilateral GA. This includes the baseline area of total atrophy, the baseline area of central atrophy, the presence of peripapillary atrophy, and the progression of total atrophy. However, the correlation between eyes for baseline acuity, for acuity at 2 years, and for 2-year change in acuity is significantly smaller, reflecting the importance of the difference in foveal sparing between eyes. (Fig. 2) (7).

The two parameters used to describe the progression of GA in the Sunness study, namely the enlargement of the atrophic area and visual acuity loss, do not completely gauge the actual impact of GA on visual function and performance. Maximum reading rate can be significantly affected by encroachment of GA on the fovea, even while there may still be little change in visual acuity (5). Some patients may be able to read single letters on acuity charts but are unable to read words because of the size of the preserved foveal island (5). The median maximum reading rate decreased from 110 words per minute (wpm) to 51 wpm over a 2-year period in patients with visual acuity better than 20/50, where the normal median rate for the reading test used in elderly people without advanced AMD is 130 wpm. Eighty-three percent of eyes that lost three or more lines of visual acuity had maximum reading rates less than 50 wpm at 2-year follow-up. However, even in the group that maintained good acuity at 2 years, one-third had maximum reading rates below 50 wpm (5). For eyes with visual acuity between 20/80 and 20/200, when the fovea is already involved at baseline, there is evidence to suggest that the maximum reading rate is inversely related to the size of the total atrophic area (38). This may mean that an intervention that could slow the rate of enlargement of atrophy could have a significant impact on preserving visual function, even in the presence of a central scotoma.

VI. DEVELOPMENT OF NEW GEOGRAPHIC ATROPHY

The relatively high prevalence of bilaterality of GA, reported to be anywhere from 48% to 65% (39) in the literature, would suggest that patients with GA in one eye and only drusen or pigmentary change in the fellow eye are at significant risk for developing GA in the fellow eye. In the Beaver Dam Eye Study, 12 patients had GA in one eye at baseline. After 5 years of follow-up, 3 of these patients (25%) had developed GA in the fellow eye (24). Patients with GA in only 1 eye were found to be 2.8 times more likely to develop advanced AMD in the fellow eye than were patients with only early changes from age-related maculopathy in either eye at baseline. This is in contrast to patients with neovascular AMD in only 1 eye where the relative risk of developing advanced AMD in the fellow eye, 1.1, was not significantly different from the rate at which advanced AMD developed in the fellow eye of those patients with only early changes from age-related maculopathy at baseline (24). In Sunness' progression study of GA, 2 of 9 patients (22%) with GA in one eye and only drusen or pigmentary changes in the fellow eye developed new GA in the fellow eye during the 2-year follow-up period (7).

There is limited information available on the rate of development of GA in the eyes of patients who have only drusen and pigmentary alteration bilaterally at baseline. In the Beaver Dam Study population, there was a 5-year incidence of new GA of 0.3%. (24) Eyes with only drusen less than 125 microns in linear dimension at baseline were not observed to go on to develop GA. Of the eyes with drusen between 125 and 250 microns at baseline, 1% were described as developing GA. In comparison, 8% of eyes with drusen 250 microns or larger in linear dimension developed GA over a 5-year period. Similarly, only those eyes with greater than 0.2 MPS disk areas of drusen had a tendency toward developing GA. All eyes that developed GA had pigmentary abnormalities at baseline as well (24). In addition to drusen size, there may be some correlation between the type of drusen present in eyes with early age-related maculopathy and the eventual development of GA. Both calcific drusen (40) and clusters of small, hard drusen have often been observed to be present in eyes with GA. Finally, other potential risk factors that have been identified in the development of GA include delayed choroidal filling on fluorescein angiography (41,42) and diminished foveal dark-adapted sensitivity (43).

VII. DEVELOPMENT OF CHOROIDAL NEOVASCULARIZATION IN EYES WITH GEOGRAPHIC ATROPHY

Population-based studies have confirmed that the incidence of CNV in an eye with GA depends, in part, upon the status of the fellow eye. In patients with GA and no CNV in one eye, and CNV in the fellow eye, the eye affected with only GA follows a course that is essentially identical to that of patients with bilateral GA with respect to foveal preservation, rate of acuity loss, and rate of enlargement of atrophy, so long as it does not develop CNV

(7). However, when the incidence of developing CNV in these eyes with baseline GA is assessed, it is found to be significantly higher if the fellow eye has CNV at baseline as opposed to GA. Of the patients enrolled in the extrafoveal Macular Photocoagulation Study with CNV in the study eye, 11 were found to have only GA in the nonstudy eye at baseline. During the next 5 years of follow-up, 45% of these eyes went on to develop CNV (44). More recent findings from the Macular Photocoagulation Study Group's juxtafoveal and subfoveal CNV trials support this incidence. Forty-nine percent of patients with CNV in the study eye and only GA in the fellow eye at baseline went on to develop CNV over the 5-year follow-up period (45). A prospective study by Sunness et al. in which 31 patients had GA and no CNV in the study eye and CNV in the fellow eye reported a 2-year rate of 18% and a 4-year rate of 34% for developing CNV in the GA study eye (11). This is in contrast to the results reported by Sunness et al. for patients with bilateral GA at baseline, who had a 2-year rate of developing CNV in one eye of 2% and a 4-year rate of 11%. Also, none of the patients with GA in one eye and drusen in the fellow eye developed CNV over the 2-year period (11). These data all demonstrate that there is a higher incidence of CNV in eyes with GA at baseline that have fellow eyes with CNV.

When CNV does develop in an eye with GA, it seems to have a propensity for areas of preserved retina surrounding the GA or in spared foveal regions. In a study by Schatz and McDonald, 8 of 10 patients who developed CNV in eyes that had only GA previously at baseline developed the CNV at the edge of the atrophy. In the two cases where the CNV developed over the atrophy, fluorescein angiography was able to demonstrate evidence of intact choriocapillaris in those areas (4). Sunness et al. observed the development of CNV over areas of GA only when there were areas of sparing within the atrophy. Otherwise, patients developed CNV in areas that were adjacent to atrophy (11). Some histological work likewise suggests that CNV does not develop where the choriocapillaris is absent (15).

CNV that is newly developing in eyes with baseline GA may be difficult to detect by both clinical examination and fluorescein angiography. In the absence of subretinal hemorrhage, it may be difficult to detect subretinal fluid that is shallow and overlying an area of atrophy. On fluorescein angiography, the hyperfluorescence already present from transmission defects and staining due to the GA may obscure any new hyperfluorescence that is secondary to CNV. Because GA does not generally cause an abrupt loss in vision, a patient who presents with subjective and objective evidence of significant changes in baseline visual function should undergo evaluation for the presence of CNV (13). Although GA itself has been associated with subretinal hemorrhages without evidence of CNY (11,12), the presence of hemorrhage should certainly prompt further evaluation to detect newly developing CNV. In some patients, the CNV may spontaneously involute and have an appearance identical to that of GA or may leave small areas of fibrosis as remnants of earlier CNV (11).

VIII. IMPAIRMENT OF VISUAL FUNCTION IN EYES WITH GEOGRAPHIC ATROPHY

Visual acuity alone is an inadequate marker of visual function in patients with GA. In addition to central and paracentral scotoma, eyes with GA have other visual function abnormalities that may be secondary to changes in the function of retina that is not yet atrophic (5). Eyes with GA have marked loss of function in dim environments and benefit greatly from increased lighting (5). Aside from delayed and decreased dark adaptation for both rods and cones (5,46–48), eyes with atrophic AMD may also be compromised by reduced contrast sensitivity (5,49,50). Therefore, despite good visual acuity, the patient's ability to read may be significantly impaired by a combination of factors.

A. Central and Paracentral Scotomas

Many patients with GA have difficulty reading because of an inability to see a full enough central field. Even in the presence of good visual acuity, scotomas near the fovea and involving the foveal center compromise visual performance. Patients may complain that they can read small newsprint but not larger news headlines. On clinical examination, it may be apparent that the foveal center remains intact but with only a tiny preserved foveal island, which cannot accommodate the larger headline letters. For this reason, it is important to take into account that such patients may be able to read smaller letters on an eye chart even if they are unable to read the 20/400 letter (5).

The impact that GA has on a patient's lifestyle is not limited solely to the ability to read. Patients with GA may also describe having great difficulty recognizing faces stemming from their inability to assimilate all the features simultaneously (51). Some find themselves assuming a more reclusive lifestyle after having repeatedly encountered friends and family that they fail to recognize and to greet. Moreover, the same small central islands of preserved retina that impair visual function in the first place also complicate low-vision treatment in these patients. By magnifying the object of interest, these low-vision devices can result in even fewer characters or features being seen by the patient within the spared area.

Conventional visual field measurement is unreliable when an eye lacks steady, central fixation, and can result in plotting scotomas in the wrong location and of the wrong size (1). The scanning laser ophthalmoscope (SLO) provides direct and real-time viewing of stimuli on the retina and permits the precise correlation of visual function with retinal location. SLO macular perimetry has demonstrated that areas of GA are indeed associated with dense scotomas with surrounding retinal sensitivity that may be near normal (1). The fixation behaviors adopted by patients and observed during SLO evaluation may explain the inherent variation in visual acuity in eyes with central scotomas from GA.

In order for a patient with scotomas that involve the foveal center to realize his visual potential, he has to place the object of regard on functioning retina by adopting an extrafoveal location for fixation, referred to as a preferred retinal locus (PRL). Sunness et al. found that in a study of eyes with central GA and visual acuities ranging from 20/80 to 20/200, all patients who were able to adopt an extrafoveal location for fixation placed their PRL immediately adjacent to the area of atrophy. Most patients fixated with the scotomas to their right or above fixation invisual field space (38). In another study of GA patients by Sunness et al., patients reported improvement in the acuity of their worse-seeing eye when their better-seeing eye worsened somewhat. At baseline, it was noted that these patients had not developed eccentric PRLs in the worse-seeing eye so that they placed the object of regard into their scotoma where it could not be seen. Over 3 years of follow-up, these patients, with visual acuities ranging from 20/80 to 20/500, did demonstrate a spontaneous mean improvement of 3.2 lines in visual acuity in the worse-seeing eye. This improvement in the worse-seeing eye was concomitant with the deterioration of vision in the previously better-seeing eye. At follow-up with SLO macular perimetry, the patients were observed to have adopted eccentric PRLs, which appeared to account for the improvement in the vision of the previously worse-seeing eye (52).

Awareness of the presence and location of scotomas can aid in the effective utilization of the remaining functional retina, lessening the searching eye movements some patients make when they have no strategy for moving the object of regard away from the scotomas. For example, having the patient fixate superior to the area of atrophy on the retina, that is, placing the scotoma above fixation, is a good strategy because it moves the blind spot out of the most important part of the visual field. Similarly, fixating with the scotoma to the right, that is to the left of the atrophy in a fundus photograph, allows the patient to anchor himself at the beginning of a line while reading (38,53).

With the aid of a fundus photograph, a physician can help facilitate the patient's development of a PRL. A fundus photograph has the same left-to-right orientation as visual field space since it was already reversed by being viewed from the photographer's perspective. Therefore, an area of atrophy to the left of the fovea, or of fixation, corresponds with a scotoma to the left of fixation. The fundus photograph is inverted in superior-inferior orientation relative to visual field space, such that a patient fixating above an area of atrophy in a fundus photograph has the scotoma above fixation in visual field space. If the fundus photograph indicates the likely location of fixation relative to the scotoma, the physician can then instruct the patient to look toward the scotoma in visual field space. This will have the effect of moving the scotoma farther out of the way. For example, if there is a scotoma to the right of fixation, as when a patient neglects the last letters on each line of an eye chart, having the patient look farther to the right should allow the object of regard to come into view.

B. Difficulties in Dimly Lit Environments

Regardless of their level of visual acuity, most patients with GA have difficulties with reading and with performing other visually related tasks in dimly lit environments. A review of Sunness' questionnaire response found that at least two-thirds of their patients with GA and good enough visual acuity to drive during the day had stopped driving at night (51).

Visual function testing objectively confirms the presence of reduced function in dim illumination in eyes with GA, as demonstrated by Sunness et al. in a study of eyes with GA and visual acuity better than 20/50. When a control group of elderly patients with ocular findings limited to only drusen or pigmentary alteration, without advanced AMD, had a 1.5-log unit neutral density filter placed over the study eye, the median worsening in acuity was 2.2 lines on the ETDRS acuity chart. No eye worsened more than 5 lines (5). For the study group, there was a median worsening in acuity of 4.6 lines on the ETDRS acuity chart when a 1.5-log unit neutral density filter was placed over the study eye (5). When foveal dark-adapted sensitivity was measured by gauging the patient's ability to see a small red target light in the dark after dark adaptation, eyes with GA and good visual acuity had a median sensitivity that was 1.2 log units lower than the sensitivity of the control group of elderly eyes with only early changes from AMD (5).

There is less worsening of visual acuity in dim illumination for eyes that have lost foveal fixation, suggesting that dark-adapted changes may be a sensitive marker for foveal changes even before clinically apparent atrophy of the fovea develops from encroachment of surrounding GA (5). These changes in dark-adapted function may also help to predict which patients with high-risk drusen and pigmentary alteration are more likely to eventually develop GA. In a small prospective study of eyes with drusen, Sunness et al. found that the eyes with the most reduced foveal dark-adapted sensitivity were those most likely to develop advanced AMD, including GA (43). Steinmetz et al. observed similar outcomes.

Eyes with drusen that had associated delayed choroidal filling and dark-adaptation abnormalities were more likely to develop GA with time (41,42).

To maximize the remaining retinal function in these patients, low-vision management of these patients should include an evaluation of lighting needs and appropriate recommendation for the necessary degree of lighting for reading and other tasks. For example, a GA patient may gain an increased sense of independence with the use of a small, handheld penlight to use in a dimly lit restaurant to read a menu. Sloan demonstrated, in a study of visual acuity as a function of chart luminance, that normal eyes reach a plateau and then do not improve further in visual acuity beyond a certain threshold luminance. Though GA was not specifically assessed, she found that eyes with AMD in general continued to improve in acuity with increased luminance for the values tested (54). Eyes with GA and some preservation of central vision likely follow a similar pattern.

C. Other Visual Function Abnormalities

Several other abnormalities in visual function may occur in eyes affected with GA. Contrast sensitivity has been found to be reduced in eyes with GA and visual acuity better than 20/50 compared to eyes of elderly patients with only drusen and pigmentary alteration. Specifically, contrast sensitivity is reduced at low spatial frequencies, and is even more markedly reduced at higher spatial frequencies (5) Despite the presence of good acuity from preserved foveal islands in eyes affected with GA, the reading rate may be dramatically decreased secondary to paracentral scotomas. In Sunness et al.'s study of visual function in eyes with GA and visual acuity better than 20/50, 50% of eyes had maximum reading rates less than 100 words per minute (wpm) while 17% had maximum reading rates less than 50 wpm. In a comparison group of eyes with only the earliest manifestations of AMD, the median maximum reading rate was found to be 130 wpm, no eye having a maximum reading rate less than 100 wpm (5). For this reason, visual acuity alone is an inadequate measure of a patient's ability to read.

Patients with small, functional foveal islands may have to find an acceptable compromise between using their central fixation and their eccentric PRL to optimize their visual capacity. While the small foveal region has good acuity, it by definition has a limited visual field extent. Moreover, before the foveal center is frankly atrophic, it may still be affected by reduced retinal sensitivity, reduced contrast sensitivity, and a substantial worsening of function in dim illumination. An eccentric, preferred, retinal locus for fixation positioned outside the area of GA will inherently have a lower visual acuity but may be able to offer a larger area of functional retina less affected by dim illumination and reduced contrast sensitivity. Patients may therefore find themselves switching back and forth from foveal to eccentric fixation depending upon the visual tasks at hand, illumination conditions, and other factors (5,13,55,56).

The combination of variables that can ultimately affect a GA patient's ability to perform visually related tasks can make it difficult to prescribe low-vision magnification devices that can make the object of regard too large to be accommodated by the intact central region. Evaluation of low-vision requirements should always keep these variables in mind. Good illumination is essential in almost all visually related tasks.

The Motor Vehicle Administration, along with a number of researchers, is currently attempting to develop better ways to evaluate the driving ability of patients with GA and compromised visual function. Patients with GA and good acuity are often able to pass the visual acuity test required for their driver's license renewal and continue to drive. Those with more reduced acuity may still be able to secure restricted licenses. Most patients with GA tend to limit their driving only to areas that they are intimately familiar with and during daylight hours. One study of AMD patients that assessed their driving ability with a simulated video-type driving test found that performance was poor compared to age-matched controls without evidence of macular degeneration. However, it was observed that these patients had very few accidents as they tended to limit their driving (57). Specialized driver-training programs for low-vision patients are becoming increasingly available in an attempt to assess the ability of patients with GA to drive and to aid them in improving their driving ability.

IX. CONDITIONS RESEMBLING GEOGRAPHIC ATROPHY

There are other conditions of the eye that in one stage or other of their progression can resemble GA. Some of these are other manifestations of AMD and simply exist on a different part of the continuum from GA. Other conditions would be classified as retinal or macular degenerations that are not age-related.

CNV that has spontaneously involuted can leave an atrophic scar that resembles GA (58,59). Some scars may have small fibrotic areas that are remnants of previous CNV. Other scars appear identical to GA. In such cases, fluorescein angiography may aid in distinguishing CNV from GA.

Old laser photocoagulation scars may also resemble GA. The history, however, should distinguish the two. Again, fluorescein angiography should demonstrate areas of hypofluorescence that correspond to the laser scars. Areas of GA generally show hyperfluorescence on angiography.

An RPE tear may clinically resemble GA. On fluorescein angiography, however, the straight-line border of hyperfluorescence should be characteristic of a rip. It is unclear whether RPE tears develop atrophy in adjacent areas with time (60).

Eyes with pattern dystrophy and vitelliform changes may develop atrophic changes that progress in a fashion similar to AMD-related GA. These patients may have areas of macular GA, and some may be accompanied by pigmentary alterations characteristic of these conditions, and occasionally by reduced electrooculograms. However, other cases may be difficult to distinguish from age-related GA. The atrophy spreads in a parafoveal pattern with early foveal sparing, often resulting in a similar degree of visual compromise (61).

Central areolar choroidal dystrophy is another degenerative, retinal condition that spares the fovea early in the course of disease. This hereditary condition is generally autosomal dominant and causes areas of atrophy in the macular region to develop since early adulthood. Unlike age-related GA, these lesions tend to have early atrophy of the choroidal circulation and choriocapillaris so that involved areas on fluorescein angiography appear hypofluorescent (62).

Disorders that cause central, atrophic lesions and bull's-eye maculopathies may also mimic age-related GA. Stargardt's disease, cone dystrophy, North Carolina macular dystrophy, benign concentric annular macular dystrophy, and chloroquine and other toxic maculopathies may all have manifestations similar to GA from AMD. The history, including age of onset of symptoms and prior medication use, may be helpful in differentiating some of these disorders from GA. Associated clinical findings, such as sensitivity to light and significant electroretinographic or color vision abnormalities in cone dystrophy, or diskiform flecks and an angiographically dark choroid in Stargardt's disease, may also facilitate differentiating the GA that results from these other entities from age-related GA.

X. POTENTIAL TREATMENT FOR GEOGRAPHIC ATROPHY

Because GA can be clinically visualized in many patients before the development of moderate or severe vision loss, unlike CNV, there is greater potential for medical intervention to preserve visual function. However, there is currently no definitive treatment to prevent GA or even to slow its progression once clinically detected.

The notion of treating AMD with nutritional supplements, including vitamins and minerals, has been entertained for some time, despite any definite evidence that such treatment would be beneficial. The National Institutes of Health are currently funding the Age-Related Eye Disease Study to investigate whether vitamins or minerals have the potential to retard the development of AMD. Two treatment trials specifically geared toward GA began in early 2001. The Glutathione Augmentation in Age-Related Macular Degeneration (GAARD) study, a multicenter, double-blind, clinical study sponsored by ThyoGen Pharmaceutical Corporation, is investigating the efficacy of glutathione in slowing the rate of acuity loss and GA enlargement. A second pilot study at Wilmer is looking at whether a Chinese berry, which is a good source of zeaxanthin, can slow the progression of GA.

Pilot studies are currently being conducted to test the hypothesis that healthy fetal retinal pigment epithelium can directly rescue remaining, viable RPE and choriocapillaris, and therefore indirectly salvage the photoreceptors, in patients with GA. The transplanted RPE is thought to produce a humorally related trophic factor that is necessary for RPE survival and to inhibit or slow the progression of GA. However, attempts at transplantation, as reported for example in one case by Weisz et al., have been complicated by rejection of the transplanted cells (63).

Currently, patients with GA and visual compromise can be offered rehabilitation in terms of low-vision intervention and new strategies for maximizing their utilization of remaining, healthy retina through the development of preferred retinal loci (PRLs). More cases of GA will continue to be seen in ensuing years as its prevalence grows in an aging population. It is hoped that as more is learned about GA in the future, we can offer more to the patient with respect to the management and eventually prevention of this form of AMD.

XI. SUMMARY

The prevalence of GA increases with age, being half as common as CNV at age 75, and more common than CNV in older age groups. GA continues to enlarge over time with a median rate of enlargement over a 2-year period of 1.8 MPS disk areas. Scotomas from GA, the advanced form of nonneovascular AMD, involve the parafoveal and perifoveal retina early in the course of the disease, sparing the foveal center until late in the course of the disease. These parafoveal and perifoveal scotomas compromise the ability to read and to recognize faces, often despite the retention of good visual acuity, accounting for a large percentage of moderate visual loss in those affected. Hemorrhage may occur in eyes with GA in the absence of CNV. Small areas of CNV that can be associated with hemorrhage may be transient, becoming clinically inapparent, or appearing as increased atrophy, a few months later. There is a higher incidence of CNV in eyes with GA at baseline that have fellow eyes with CNV. GA is bilateral in more than half of the people with this condition. The size and rate of progression of atrophy are highly correlated between the two eyes of patients with bilateral GA, but the acuities may differ due to central sparing.

Among eyes with GA with visual acuity better than 20/50, there is a 40% rate of three-line visual loss at 2 years. Maximum reading rate can be significantly affected by encroachment of GA on the fovea, even while there may still be little change in visual acuity. Eyes with GA have marked loss of vision in dim environments and benefit greatly from increased lighting. The development of a preferred retinal locus (PRL) can aid in the effective utilization of the remaining functional retina.

ACKNOWLEDGMENTS

This work was supported in part by a fellowship from the Heed Foundation (SDS), by NEI R01 EY 08552 (JSS), the James S. Adams RPB Special Scholar Award (JSS), the Panitch Fund to Stop AMD (JSS, MJC), and the ThyoGen Pharmaceutical Corporation (JSS).

REFERENCES

1. Sunness JS, Schuchard R, Shen N, Rubin GS, Dagnelie G, Haselwood DM. Landmark-driven fundus perimetry using the scanning laser ophthalmoscope (SLO). Invest Ophthalmol Vis Sci 1995;36:1863–1874.
2. Sarks JP, Sarks SH, Killingsworth MC. Evolution of geographic atrophy of the retinal pigment epithelium. Eye 1988;2:552–577.
3. Maguire P, Vine AP. Geographic atrophy of the retinal pigment epithelium. Am J Ophthalmol 1986;102:621–625.
4. Schatz H, McDonald HR. Atrophic macular degeneration: rate of spread of geographic atrophy and visual loss. Ophthalmology 1989;96:1541–1551.
5. Sunness JS, Rubin GS, Applegate CA, Bressler NM, Marsh MJ, Hawkins BS, Haselwood D. Visual function abnormalities and prognosis in eyes with age-related geographic atrophy of the macula and good acuity. Ophthalmology 1997;104:1677–1691.
6. Ferris FL III, Fine SL, Hyman L. Age-related macular degeneration and blindness due to neovascular maculopathy. Arch Ophthalmol 1984;102:1640–1642.
7. Sunness JS, Gonzalez-Baron J, Applegate CA, Bressler NM, Tian Y, Hawkins B, Barron Y, Bergman A. Enlargement of atrophy and visual acuity loss in the geographic atrophy form of age-related macular degeneration. Ophthalmology 1999;106:1768–1779.
8. Klein R, Klein BEK, Franke T. The relationship of cardiovascular disease and its risk factors to age-related maculopathy: the Beaver Dam Eye Study. Ophthalmology 1993;100:406–414.
9. Vingerling JR, Dielemans I, Hofman A, Grobbee DE, Hijmering M, Kramer CF, deJong PT. The prevalence of age-related maculopathy in the Rotterdam Study. Ophthalmology 1995;102:205–210.
10. Hirvela H, Luukinen H, Laara E, Sc L, Laatikainen L. Risk factors of age-related maculopathy in a population 70 years of age or older. Ophthalmology 1996;103:871–877.
11. Sunness JS, Gonzalez-Baron J, Bressler NM, Hawkins B, Applegate CA. The development of choroidal neovascularization in eyes with the geographic atrophy form of age-related macular degeneration. Ophthalmology 1999;106:910–919.
12. Nasrallah F, Jalkh AE, Trempe CL, McMeel JW, Schepens CL. Subretinal hemorrhage in atrophic age-related macular degeneration. Am J Ophthalmol 1988;107:38–41.

13. Sunness JS, Bressler NM, Maguire MG. Scanning laser ophthalmoscopic analysis of the pattern of visual loss in age-related geographic atrophy of the macula. Am J Ophthalmol 1995;119:143–151.

14. Sunness JS, Bressler NM, Tian Y, Alexander J, Applegate CA. Measuring geographic atrophy in advanced age-related macular degeneration. Invest Ophthalmol Vis Sci. 1999;40:1761–1769.

15. Green WR, Key SN III. Senile macular degeneration: a histopathologic study. Trans Am Ophthalrnol Soc 1977;75:180–254.

16. Korte GE, Reppucci V, Henkind P. Retinal pigment epithelium destruction causes choriocapillary atrophy. Invest Ophthalmol Vis Sci 1984;25:1135–1145.

17. Leonard DS, Zhang XG, Panozzo G, Sugino IK, Zarbin MA. Clinicopathologic correlation of localized retinal pigment epithelial debridement. Invest Ophthalmol Vis Sci 1997;38:1094–1109

18. Green WR, Enger C. Age-related macular degeneration histopathologic studies: the 1992 Lorenz E. Zimmerman Lecture. Ophthalmology 1993;100:1519–1535.

19. Sarks SH. Changes in the region of the choriocapillaris in ageing and degeneration. In: XXIII Concilium Ophthalmologicum. Kyoto. Amsterdam-Oxford: Excerpta Medica, 1979.

20. Elman MJ, Fine SL, Murphy RP, Patz A, Auer C. The natural history of serous retinal pigment epithelium detachment in patients with age-related macular degeneration. Ophthalmology 1986;93:224–230.

21. Friedman E, Krupsky S, Lane AM, Oak SS, Friedman ES, Egan K, Gragoudas ES. Ocular blood flow velocity in age-related macular degeneration. Ophthalmology 1995;102:640–646.

22. Quillen D, Blankenship G, Gardner T. Aged eyes: ocular findings in individuals 90 years of age and older. Invest Ophthalmol Vis Sci 1996;47:S111.

23. Friedman DS, Katz J, Bressler NM, Rahmani B, Tielsch JM. Racial differences in the prevalence of age-related macular degeneration: the Baltimore Eye Survey. Ophthalmology 1999;106:1049-1055.

24. Klein R, Klein BE, Jensen SC, Meuer SM. The five-year incidence and progression of age-related maculopathy: the Beaver Dam Eye Study. Ophthalmology 1997;104:7–21.

25. Ritter LL, Klein R, Klein BE, Mares-Perlman JA, Jensen SC. Alcohol use and age-related maculopathy in the Beaver Dam Eye Study. Am J Ophthalmol 1995;120:190–196.

26. Smith W, Mitchell P, and Leeder SR. Smoking and age-related maculopathy: the Blue Mountain Eye Study. Arch Ophthalmol 1996;114:1518–1523.

27. Age-Related Eye Disease Study Research Group. Risk factors associated with age-related macular degeneration: a case-control study in the Age-Related Eye Disease Study: Age-Related Eye Disease Study Report Number 3. Ophthalmology 2000;107:2224–2232.

28. Piguet B, Heon E, Munier FL, Grounauer PA, Niemeyer G, Butler N, Schorderet DF, Sheffield VC, Stone EM. Full characterization of the maculopathy associated with an Arg-12-Trp mutation in the RDS/peripherin gene. Ophthal Genet 1996;17:175–186.

29. Allikmets R, Shroyer NF, Singh N, Seddon JM, Lewis RA, Bernstein PS, Peiffer A, Zabriskie NA, Li Y, Hutchinson A, Dean M, Lupski JR. Leppert M. Mutation of the Stargardt disease gene (ABCR) in age-related macular degeneration. Science 1997;277:1805–1807.

30. Pennisi E. Human genetics: gene found for the fading eyesight of old age. Science 1997;277:1765–1766.

31. Allikmets and International ABCR screening Consortium. Further evidence for an association of the ABCR alleles with age-related macular degeneration. Am J Hum Genet 2000;67:487–491.

32. Yates JR, Moore AT. Genetic susceptibility to age-related macular degeneration. J Med Genet Feb 2000;37(2):83–87.

33. Gass JDM. Drusen and disciform macular detachment and degeneration. Arch Ophthalmol 1973;90:206–217.

34. Peli E, Lahav M. Drusen measurements from fundus photographs using computer image analysis. Ophthalmology 1986;93:1575–1580.

35. Braunstein RA, Gass JDM. Serous detachments of the retinal pigment epithelium in patients with senile macular disease. Am J Ophthalmol 1979;88:652–660.

36. Casswell AG, Kohen D, Bird AC. Retinal pigment epithlial detachments in the elderly: classification and outcome. Br J Ophthalmol 1985;69:397–403.

37. Meredith TA, Braley RE, Aaberg TM. Natural history of serous detachments of the retinal pigment epithelium. Am J Ophthalmol 1979;88:643–651.

38. Sunness JS, Applegate CA, Haselwood D, Rubin GS. Fixation patterns and reading rates in eyes with central scotomas from advanced atrophic age-related macular degeneration and Stargardt disease. Ophthalmology 1996;103:1458–1466.

39. Porter JW, Thallemer JM. Geographic atrophy of the retinal pigment epithelium: diagnosis and vision rehabilitation. J Am Opt Assoc 1981;52:503–508.

40. Sunness JS, Bressler NM, Applegate CA. Ophthalmoscopic features associated with geographic atrophy from age-related macular degeneration. Invest Ophthalmol Vis Sci 1999;40:S314 (abstract).

41. Steinmetz RL, Walter D, Fitzke FW, Bird AC. Prolonged dark adaptation in patients with age-related macular degeneration. Invest Ophthalmol Vis Sci 1991;32:S711.

42. Steinmetz RL, Haimovici R, Jubb C, Fitzke FW, Bird AC. Symptomatic abnormalities of dark adaptation in patients with age-related Bruch's membrane change. Br J Ophthalmol 1993;77:549-554.

43. Sunness JS, Massof RW, Johnson MA, Bressler NM, Bressler SB, Fine SL. Diminished foveal sensitivity may predict the development of advanced age-related macular degeneration. Ophthalmology 1989;96:375–381.

44. Macular Photocoagulation Study Group. Five-year follow-up of fellow eyes of patients with age-related macular degeneration and unilateral extrafoveal choroidal neovascularization. Arch Ophthalmol 1993;111:1189–1199.

45. Macular Photocoagulation Study Group. Risk factors for choroidal neovascularization in the second eye of patients with juxtafoveal or subfoveal choroidal neovascularization secondary to age-related macular degeneration. Arch Ophthalmol 1997;115:741–747.

46. Brown B, Kitchin JL. Dark adaptation and the acuity/luminance response in senile macular degeneration (SMD). Am J Optom Physi Opt 1983;60:645–650.

47. Brown B, Tobin C, Roche N, Wolanowski A. Cone adaptation in age-related maculopathy. Am J Optom Phys Opt 1986;63:450–454.

48. Sunness JS, Massof RW, Johnson MA, Finkelstein D, Fine SL. Peripheral retinal function in age-related macular degeneration. Arch Ophthalmol 1985;103:811–816.

49. Brown B, Lovie-Kitchin J. Contrast sensitivity in central and paracentral retina in age-related maculopathy. Clin Exp Optom 1987;70:145–148.

50. Midena E, Degli Angeli C, Blarzino MC, Valenti M, Segato T. Macular function impairment in eyes with early age-related macular degeneration. Invest Ophthalmol Vis Sci 1997;38:469–477.

51. Applegate CA, Sunness JS, Haselwood DM. Visual symptoms associated with geographic atrophy from age-related macular degeneration. Invest Ophthalmol Vis Sci 1996;37:S112.

52. Sunness JS, Applegate CA, Gonzalez-Baron J. Improvement of visual acuity over time in patients with bilateral geographic atrophy from age-related macular degeneration. Retina 2000;20:162–169.

53. Guez JE, Le Gargasson JF, Rigaudiere F, O'Regan JK. Is there a systematic location for the pseudo-fovea in patients with central scotoma? Vis Res 1993;9:1271–1279.

54. Sloan L. Variation of acuity with luminance in ocular diseases and anomalies. Doc Ophthalmol 1969;26:384–393.

55. Schuchard RA, Raasch TW. Retinal locus for fixation: pericentral fixation targets. Clin Vis Sci 1992:7:511–520.

56. Lei H, Schuchard RA. Using two preferred retinal loci for different lighting conditions in patients with central scotomas. Invest Ophthalmol Vis Sci 1997;38:1812–1818.

57. Szlyk JP, Pizzimenti CE, Fishman GA, Kelsch R, Wetzel LC, Kagan S, Ho K. A comparison of driving in older subjects with and without age-related macular degeneration. Arch Ophthalmol 1995;113:1033–1040.

58. Bressler NM, Frost LA, Bressler SB, Murphy RP, Fine SL. Natural course of poorly defined choroidal neovascularization in macular degeneration. Arch Ophthalmol 1988;106:1537–1542.

59. Jalkh AE, Nasrallah FP, Marinelli I, Van de Velde F. Inactive subretinal neovascularization in age-related macular degeneration. Ophthalmology 1990;97:1614–1619.

60. Yeo JH, Marcus S, Murphy RP. Retinal pigment epithelial tears: patterns and progression. Ophthalmology 1988;95:8–13.

61. Marmor MF, McNamara JA. Pattern dystrophy of the retinal pigment epithelium and geographic atrophy. Am J Ophthalmol 1996;122:382–39.

62. Krill AE, Archer D. Classification of the choroidal atrophies. Am J Ophthalmol 1917;72:562.

63. Weisz JM, deJuan E, Humayun MS. Sunness JS, Dagnelie G, Soylu M, Rizzo L, Nussenblatt RB. Allogenic fetal retinal pigment epithelial cell transplant in a patient with geographic atrophy. Retina 1999;19:540–545.

6

Exudative Age-Related Macular Degeneration

Jennifer I. Lim

Doheny Eye Institute, University of Southern California Keck School of Medicine, Los Angeles, California

I. INTRODUCTION

Exudative age-related macular degeneration was first described and illustrated in the literature in 1875 by Pagenstecher and Genth (1). They termed the condition chorioidioretinitis in regione maculae luteae. Oeller in 1905 first used the name "diskiform" degeneration (degeneratio maculae luteae disciformis) (2). Later, Junius and Kuhnt in 1926 further elaborated on this condition and established it as a disease (3). Holloway and Verhoeff in 1928 described eight eyes with disk-like degeneration of the retina (4), histopathology in some of these eyes was performed and showed choroidal neovascularization (CNV). In 1937, Verhoeff and Grossman also demonstrated and emphasized that blood vessels had erupted through Bruch's membrane in their cases of macular degeneration (5). In 1951 Ashton and Sorsby demonstrated in clinicopathological correlations that CNV with breaks in Bruch's membrane resulted in subretinal fluid (6). It was not until 1967 that Gass implicated CNV as having a primary role in senile diskiform macular degeneration (7,8). In 1971, Blair and Aaberg showed the clinical and fluorescein angiographic characteristics of CNV in senile macular degeneration (9). In 1976, Small et al. published a clinicopathological correlation of the evolution of CNV with a serous pigment epithelial detachment (PED) to a diskiform scar (10). In 1977, Green and Key (11) studied the histopathological features of 176 eyes from 115 patients with age-related macular degeneration (AMD). They correlated the presence of drusen with CNV. Their results supported the view that drusen predispose to development of exudative AMD.

Since the earliest description of AMD, numerous refinements in the categorization of the types of AMD have developed. In fact, even the name AMD is relatively recent in history. Prior to 1990, the term "senile macular degeneration" had been in common usage. The two main types of AMD are nonexudative AMD and exudative AMD, referred to colloquially as dry AMD and wet AMD, respectively. Nonexudative AMD is typically associated with less severe visual disturbances than exudative AMD. Nonexudative AMD includes the broad spectrum of drusen with no visual disturbance to geographic atrophy, with severe visual loss. In contrast, eyes with exudative AMD typically have some visual disturbance.

The nomenclature of exudative AMD was developed through the concerted efforts of the Macular Photocoagulation Group members and other investigators. The exudative or neovascular form of AMD has the most serious prognosis in terms of visual acuity outcomes. Exudative AMD includes eyes with pigment epithelial detachment (serous and hemorrhagic) and those with the presence of abnormal vessels in the subretinal or subretinal pigment epithelial space (sub- RPE). These abnormal vessels are known as CNV. This chapter will focus upon exudative AMD. An overview of the risk factors associated with development of exudative AMD, fundus characteristics in exudative AMD, fluorescein and indocyanine green (ICG) findings, and treatment options for the various types of exudative AMD will be presented.

Exudative AMD, although the less common form of AMD, is the leading cause of new blindness in the older-age population in the United States, accounting for 16% of all new cases of blindness over the age of 65 years. Indeed, the majority of patients with severe visual loss have CNV (12). In fact, 79% of eyes legally blind in the Framingham Study and 90% of legally blind eyes in a large case-control study had neovascular AMD (13,14). With the aging of the U.S. population, AMD is reaching epidemic proportions. In the United States alone, there are 50,000 new cases of CNV due to AMD each year.

II. RISK FACTORS

Numerous candidate risk factors are associated with the development of CNV in AMD. These risk factors are discussed in great depth within this book in another chapter. Of the nonocular risk factors, it appears that the strongest epidemiological associations are age, race, and smoking. There are also ocular risk factors with strong associations for development of CNV as discussed below.

Increased age is associated with increasing risk of neovascular AMD. Patients with exudative AMD have a mean age of 70.5 years versus 56.8 years for non-exudative AMD (15). Gender is not consistently associated with neovascular AMD.

Racial differences in the prevalence of exudative AMD (and also early AMD) exist. Gregor and Joffe (16) reported that diskiform AMD was found in 3.5% of the white patients compared to 0.1% of the black South African patients ($p < 0.001$). The Baltimore Eye Survey found a prevalence ratio of white:black of 8.8 for neovascular AMD (17). The Barbados Eye Study found neovascular AMD in 0.6%, which is comparable to that found in the Maryland Waterman Study but lower than the 1.2% in the Beaver Dam Eye Study (18). In NHANES-III, the odds ratio for late AMD was 0.34 for non-Hispanic blacks compared to non-Hispanic whites and 0.25 for Mexican-Americans compared to non-Hispanic whites (19). Thus, the prevalence is higher in Caucasians.

Family history is a risk factor for the development of AMD, including the exudative form. The Blue Mountain Eye Study showed an odds ratio of 4.30 for neovascular AMD in patients with a family history (20). Klaver and colleagues noted a lifetime risk estimate of late AMD to be 50% for relatives of patients versus 12% for relatives of controls (21).

Smoking is correlated with exudative AMD in most studies, although it was not linked to AMD in the Framingham Study (13) and the NHANES-III Study (22). The Beaver Dam Eye Study (23) linked smoking to exudative AMD with a relative risk of 3.29 for current smokers and a relative risk of 2.50 for former smokers compared to those who had never smoked. In the Blue Mountain Eye Study (24), the odds ratio for exudative AMD was 4.46 when comparing current smokers to those who never smoked and 1.83 when comparing former smokers to those who never smoked. The POLA study showed an increasing odds ratio for exudative AMD when examining the number of pack-years smoked. This higher risk of exudative AMD remained even until 20 years after cessation of smoking.

The association between sunlight exposure and late AMD is not clear at this time. The Chesapeake Bay Waterman Study found an association between late AMD and sunlight (25) as did the Beaver Dam Eye Study (26). Yet, the EDCCS (27) and the Australian case-control study on sun exposure and AMD (28) did not show this same association. Since the use of sunglasses (ultraviolet blocking) is relatively inexpensive and also protective against cataract formation, it is reasonable to recommend sunglass protection for older patients.

There have been reports of progression of early to late AMD following cataract surgery. The Beaver Dam Eye Study showed an odds ratio of 2.80 for progression of AMD to late AMD after cataract surgery (and after controlling for age) (29). Pollack and colleagues also noted that progression to exudative AMD occurred in 19.1% of eyes operated on for cataracts versus 4.3% of the fellow eye (30, 31).

The risk of CNV developing in patients has been linked to the presence of several fundus characteristics, among which are the presence of soft drusen. Lanchoney and associates calculated the risk of CNV developing in patients with bilateral soft drusen to range from 8.6% to 15.9% within 10 years, depending upon the age and sex of the patient (32). These projections were based upon natural history studies of Smiddy and Fine (15) and Holz et al. (33).

The MPS group has determined the ocular risk factors for development of CNV in the fellow eye (when the opposite eye already has CNV) to include the presence of (5) or more drusen, focal hyperpigmentation, one or more large drusen (>63 microns), and systemic hypertension (34). The 5-year incidence rate for development of CNV ranged from 7% if none of these risk factors was present to 87% if all four risk factors were present. This was based upon follow-up of patients with juxtafoveal CNV.

The role of antioxidants and vitamins in the prevention of AMD is being actively researched in multicenter clinical trials. The role of nutritional supplementation with zinc, beta-carotene, and vitamin E and vitamin C was studied in the AREDS study. The Physicians' Health Study II is also evaluating the role of vitamin E, vitamin C, beta-carotene, and a daily multivitamin. The Vitamin E, Cataract and Age-Related Macular Degeneration Trial (VECAT) and the Women's Health Study (WHS) are two other randomized trials assessing the risk and benefits of antioxidant vitamins for AMD. The role of zinc and vitamins A, C, E supplementation for prevention of exudative AMD has been shown to be beneficial in the AREDS study.

Until the risk factors and genetics are determined, prevention of exudative AMD remains an enigma. It is a difficult area for counseling patients. At this time; modifiable risk factors (such as smoking, hypertension) should be addressed. Whether prophylactic therapy such as laser to drusen is determined to be of benefit for prevention of CNV remains to be determined. Future application of genetic therapy and targeted antiangiogenesis treatments will most likely play a role in the prevention of exudative AMD and attendant visual acuity loss.

III. CLINICAL FEATURES OF EXUDATIVE AMD

Patients with exudative AMD may present with complaints of sudden onset of diminished vision, metamorphopsia, central scotoma, or paracentral sootoma (35). Others may present with loss of vision in their previously "good eye" and may not have even recognized any visual symptoms in the fellow eye with a scar (36). Yet others may present with no ocular symptoms and be noted to have ophthalmoscopic evidence of CNV in the second eye despite a prior CNV in the fellow eye (37). Thus, patients who have risk factors for CNV should be periodically examined for development of CNV and should be encouraged to monitor their vision daily, such as by the use of an Amsler grid.

Other patients with cataracts may attribute their visual blurring to the cataract and the treating ophthalmologist may not detect the underlying PED or CNV. These patients may undergo cataract extraction and complain of persistent poor vision postoperatively. Postoperatively, the macular lesion can now be detected. A careful preoperative examination for exudative AMD or advanced nonexudative AMD is therefore of utmost importance in patients with known AMD. Fluorescein angiography preoperatively may help detect CNV. Alternatively, if the cataract totally obscures the view of the fundus, an ultrasound may be useful in detecting macular fluid or subretinal scar formation (38).

A useful test for detecting the early visual symptoms in patients with AMD is the Amsler grid (39). Each box on the grid represents one degree of visual field. Thus, it tests the central 10 degrees straddling fixation. The patient should look at the Amsler grid daily. The patient may note that the Amsler grid is distorted, missing areas, or has black spots. If these findings are present, the patient should be instructed to see an ophthalmologist immediately for an examination for exudative AMD. A newly developed, computer-automated, three-dimensional threshold Amsler grid visual field test is currently being tested and may also show promise in the earlier detection of exudative AMD (personal communication, Alfredo A. Sadun, M.D., Ph.D., and Wolfgang Fink, Ph.D., Los Angeles).

Another useful test is to have the patient look at the thin slit lamp beam during biomicroscopy. The patient is asked if the beam is distorted. Frequently elevation of the RPE or retina (due to underlying CNV) causes distortion of the beam.

The major clinical features of active exudative AMD include subretinal fluid, subretinal hemorrhage, sub-RPE fluid, sub-RPE hemorrhage, RPE pigment alterations, and hard exudates. These features may appear clinically as any one or any combination of the following: a serous or a hemorrhagic PED, grayish subretinal membrane (Fig. 1, Fig. 2) area of RPE alteration (Fig. 3), subretinal hemorrhage (Fig. 4), or hard exudates (Fig. 3). The late manifestation of exudative AMD is a diskiform scar (Fig. 5) or geographic atrophy (Fig. 6), with or without subretinal fluid or subretinal blood.

It is best to examine a patient with suspected CNV and AMD using the best stereo- imaging possible. A fundus contact or non-contact lens in conjunction with slit lamp biomicroscopy should be utilized for the examination. For those less comfortable with the noncontact fundus macular lenses, a fundus contact lens is easiest to use. The fundus contact lens or the 78-diopter lens offers more magnification than the 90-diopter lens.

Using biomicroscopy with a macular lens, the separation of the retina from the underlying RPE, due to underlying subretinal fluid, can be seen. The overlying retina may have cystic changes and may show cystoid macular edema. Sub-RPE fluid appears as a PED and typically has more sharply demarcated borders in comparison to subretinal fluid (Fig. 7). Often, a combination of sub-RPE and subretinal fluid is associated with the CNV (Fig. 8). The CNV itself may be visible as an area of discoloration (Fig. 9). Other times, overlying subretinal blood or lipid may be the only clinical clue to the presence of an acute CNV. The definitive test for the presence of CNV has been fluorescein angiography. This is further discussed below.

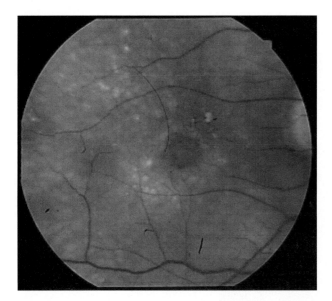

Figure 1 Subfoveal gray pigmented CNV. Soft large drusen surround CNV. See also color insert, Fig. 6.1.

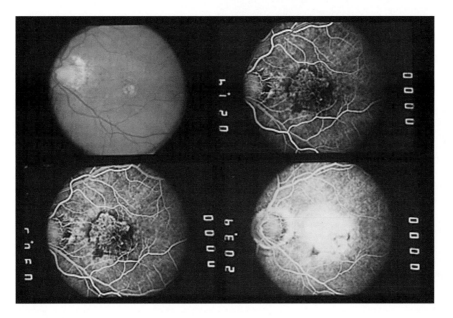

Figure 2 (A) Upper left: Color photo of the left eye shows an atrophic extrafoveal laser scar surrounded by a grayish subretinal lesion. There is overlying subretinal fluid. (B) Upper right: Fluorescein angiogram shows early lacy hyperfluorescence in the subfoveal area surrounding the laser scar. Note the ring of blocked fluorescence around the lacy CNV. There is some extrafoveal occult CNV beyond the blocked fluorescence. (C) Lower left: Occult CNV is present and surrounds the blocked fluorescence around the classic CNV. (D) Lower right: The occult and the classic components show late leakage. See also color insert, Fig. 6.2.

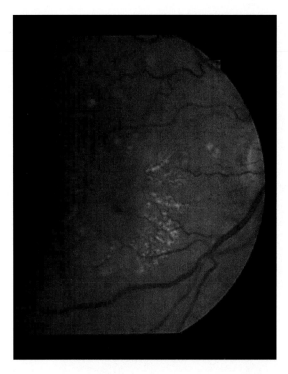

Figure 3 Ring of hard exudates surround an area of turbid fluid with a few spots of intraretinal hemorrhage overlying the central lesion. See also color insert, Fig. 6.3.

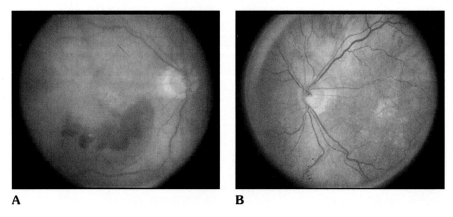

A   B

Figure 4 (A) Right eye shows subretinal blood (red) and sub-RPE blood (gray-green) is seen adjacent to an area of geographic atrophy. There is another area of subretinal blood temporal to the macula. There is overlying subretinal fluid. Visual acuity is 6/200. (B) Left eye showing more advanced geographic atrophy is found in the subfoveal area; visual acuity is 20/200. See also color insert, Fig. 6.4.

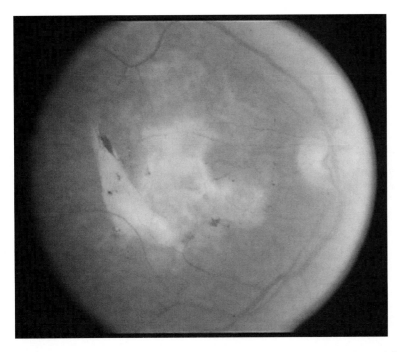

Figure 5 Color photo shows subretinal fibrosis. Note the sharp margins and the whitish color of the scar. See also color insert, Fig. 6.5.

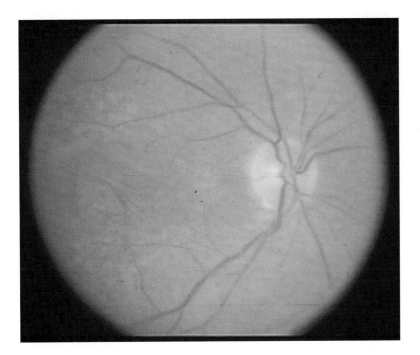

Figure 6 Early geographic atrophy. Note the orange color of the atrophic lesion and the visibility of the deep choroidal blood vessels within the area. There are no drusen in the atrophic area but soft drusen in the area adjacent to the lesion. See also color insert, Fig. 6.6.

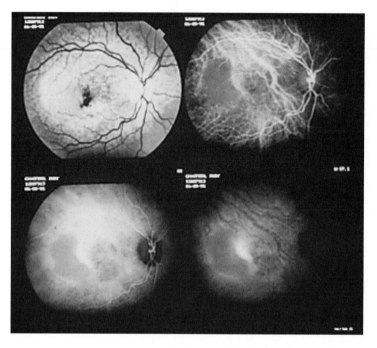

Figure 7 Upper left: Red-free photograph shows the PED as a well-demarcated area adjacent to subretinal blood. Upper right: The PED is hypofluorescent. Lower left and right: There is a hyperfluorescent area adjacent to the blood's location which shows late leakage.

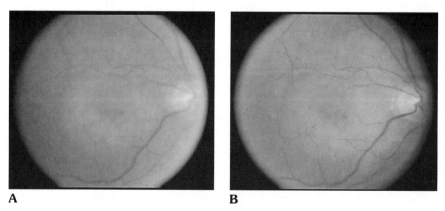

A   B

Figure 8 (A) Left stereo pair. (B) Right stereo pair. Stereoscopic photographs show a pigment epithelial detachment with overlying subretinal fluid and spots of subretinal blood. Visual acuity was 20/300. Three weeks later, the amount of subretinal blood increased and the CNV was more clearly seen as a greenish lesion in the subfoveal area. See also color insert, Fig. 6.8.

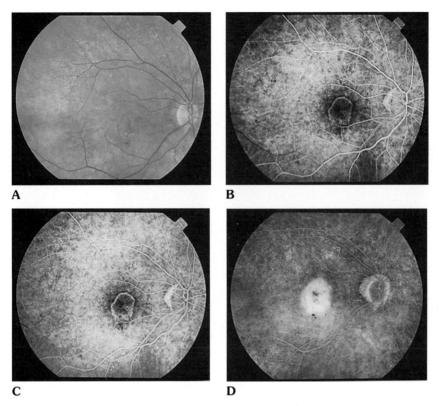

Figure 9 (A) Color fundus photo shows subretinal blood and a subretinal pigmented lesion. (B) Fluorescein angiogram reveals the subfoveal classic CNV. Note the hyperfluorescent border and the central vessels within the membrane. (C) Increasing hyperfluorescence of the CNV. (D) Late leakage of the CNV. See also color insert, Fig. 6.9A.

Spontaneous involution of the CNV may be manifest as any of the above findings with RPE alterations and/or scar formation.

A. Pigment Epithelial Detachment

The borders of a PED are sharply demarcated. Clinically, hemorrhage or hard exudate may or may not be present depending upon the presence or absence of CNV. A fluorescein angiogram (FA) or ICG angiogram is clinically useful to detect the presence of associated CNV. A serous PED shows early hyperfluorescence. The dye pools in the PED on the late phase. The borders remain sharp and the area does not increase in size. On ICG angiography, the PED is hypofluorescent (Fig. 7). Whereas a serous PED will show uniform filling of the PED, a vascularized PED shows irregular filling, notching of the PED, or irregular margins on the FA.

A PED with occult CNV will frequently show associated subretinal fluid, hard exudate, or subretinal blood (Fig. 10). The fluorescein angiogram will demonstrate irregular filling of the PED. The borders may be blurred in the area of the CNV. Leakage on the late frames of the FA is noted. ICG angiography has been shown to be helpful in this regard. ICG can identify areas of CNV associated with the PED. Laser treatment to the hot spots can sometimes cause resolution of the PED and associated subretinal fluid, blood, and lipid (Figs. 10,11) (40–42).

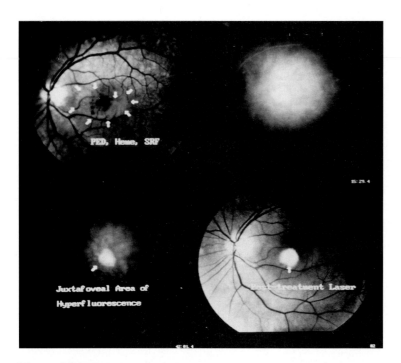

Figure 10 The indocyanine green angiogram was used in treating the presumed area of choroidal neovascularization associated with the pigment epithelial detachment (PED). (Top left) A red-free photograph shows the PED (white arrows) and associated areas of hemorrhage (Heme) and subretinal fluid (SRF). (Top right) A frame from the indocyanine green angiogram shows a well-demarcated area of hyperfluorescence (black arrow) within the PED. (Bottom left) A late-frame indocyanine green photograph shows a juxtafoveal area of leakage (hyperfluorescence; white arrow). (Bottom right) Post-treatment red-free photograph shows the immediate postlaser appearance (white arrow) of the area of leakage. Reprinted by permission from Lim JI, Aaberg TM Sr, Capone A, Jr, Sternberg P Jr. Indocyanine green angiography-guided photocoagulation of choroidal neovascularization associated with retinal pigment epithelial detachment. Am J Ophthalmol 1997;123:524–32 (Fig. 4).

CNV has been associated with 28–58% of PEDs (43). A study by Elman and colleagues showed that 32% of serous PEDs develop CNV at a mean of 19.6 months (44). Risk factors associated with CNV in these eyes included patient age greater than 65 years, associated sensory retinal detachments, and fluorescein findings of hot spots, notches, and late or irregular filling of the PED. The association of CNV with PED increases the chance for visual acuity loss (43,44). In fact, 76% of eyes with macular PEDs and 20/200 or worse visual acuity harbored CNV (44).

In a natural history study by Poliner and associates, the risk of developing CNV was 26% at 1 year, 42% at 2 year, and 49% at 3 years in eyes with PEDs followed up for 12 or more months (45). The risk of 20/200 or worse visual acuity increased from 17% at 1 year to 33% at 2 years and 39% at 3 years; 78% of eyes that developed CNV were 20/200 or worse versus only one of 28 eyes (3%) that did not have CNV.

Even with spontaneous flattening of PEDs, the visual acuity outcome is poor (46,47).

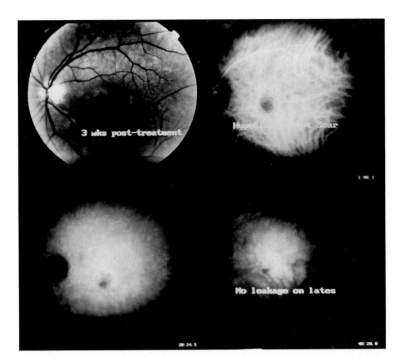

Figure 11 The indocyanine green angiogram was repeated on follow-up visits to search for hyperfluorescent leakage or areas of resolved hyperfluorescence after laser photocoagulation. (Top left) A red-free photograph taken 3 weeks after laser photocoagulation. The hemorrhage is less compared with the previous photograph (Fig. 10). (Top right) An indocyanine green image showing the hypofluorescence (black arrow) of the laser scar. (Bottom left) Absence of leakage (hypofluorescence identified by the black arrow). (Bottom right) Hypofluorescence (black arrow) on a late angiographic frame. Reprinted by permission from Lim JI, Aaberg Tm Sr, Capone A, Jr, Sternberg P Jr. Indocyanine green angiography-guided photocoagulation of choroidal neovascularization associated with retinal pigment epithelial detachment. Am J Ophthalmol 1997;123:524–32 (Fig. 5).

B. Choroidal Neovascularization

The most severe form of exudative AMD remains CNV. The MPS group has defined the various forms and components of CNV (48). The entire complex of components termed a CNV lesion includes the CNV itself, blood, elevated blocked fluorescence due to pigment or scar that obscures the neovascular borders, and any serous detachment of the RPE.

The classic clinical description of a choroidal neovascular membrane is that of a dirty gray, colored membrane (Fig. 12). There is associated subretinal fluid and there may or may not be subretinal blood and lipid. Sometimes the outlines of the CNV are clearly visible with the subretinal vessels readily seen (Fig. 9). Other times, the CNV is manifest only by a neurosensory detachment or even subretinal blood. The fluorescein angiogram is a key test in the evaluation of patients with CNV.

On fluorescein angiography, a well-demarcated area of choroidal hyperfluorescence is seen early (Fig. 9, Fig. 2). The MPS group characterized classic CNV as only occasionally showing a lacy pattern of hyperfluorescence in the early fluorescein phases. In the later

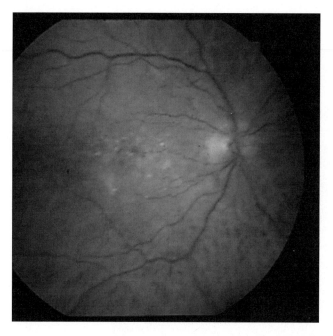

Figure 12 Pigmented CNV with some subretinal blood and surrounding large, soft, confluent drusen. See also color insert, Fig. 6.12.

frames of the angiogram, the boundaries of the CNV are obscured by progressive pooling of dye in the subneurosensory space (Fig. 9).

Occult CNV is classified as either a fibrovascular PED (FVPED) (Fig. 13) or late leakage of undetermined source (LLUS) (Fig. 14). These types of occult CNVs are differentiated on the basis of the fluorescein angiogram. A stereoscopic FA is very helpful in recognizing occult CNV. FVPEDs show early hyperfluorescence with irregular elevation of the RPE. These areas are not as bright or discrete as the classic CNV seen on the transit phases. Within 1–2 min, an area of stippled hyperfluorescence is present. By 10 min there is persistent fluorescein staining or leakage within the subneurosensory detachment. The borders of the occult CNV may be either well demarcated or poorly demarcated (48). Late leakage is present, although it is not as intense as that seen in classic CNV (48).

LLUS in contrast does not show early hyperfluorescence. LLUS appears as speckled hyperfluorescence with pooling of dye in the overlying neurosensory space; choroidal leakage is apparent between 2 and 5 min after fluorescein injection. The boundaries of this type of occult CNV are never well demarcated. In fact, the later frames show hyperfluorescent leakage in an area that showed no hyperfluorescence on the early frames (48).

Finally, there is a slow-filling form of classic CNV in which hyperfluorescence is not seen until 2 min. However, in this form of CNV, the late frames of leakage and pooling of the dye in the subneurosensory space correspond with the area seen at 2 min.

Using ICG angiography, occult CNVs can be further classified into those with hot spots, plaques, combination of these two types, retinal-choroidal anastomosis, and polypoidal-type CNV. Using ICG angiography, about one-third of eyes with occult CNV become eligible for treatment (39). ICG angiography is also useful for evaluating eyes with subretinal hemorrhage for the presence of CNV. Further details of the usefulness of ICG

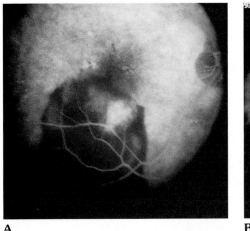

A

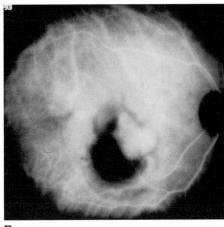

B

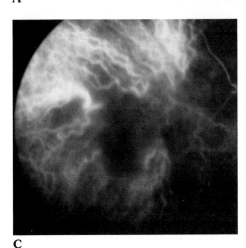

C

Figure 13 Fluorescein angiogram shows a poorly defined area of choroidal neovascularization that was a fibrovascular pigment epithelial detachment (top left). The corresponding indocyanine green angiogram shows a well-demarcated subfoveal area of hyperfluorescence (top right). The indocyanine green angiogram after laser treatment shows resolution of the area of leakage (bottom left). Reprinted by permission from Lim JI, Sternberg P, Capone A Jr, Aaberg TM Sr, Gilman JP. Selective use of indocyanine green angiography for occult choroidal neovascularization. Am J Ophthalmol 1995;120:75–82 (Fig. 1).

angiography and ICG-guided laser photocoagulation of CNV in AMD can be found in another chapter.

CNV lesions are further characterized by their location in relation to the foveal center. The location of the CNV is divided into extrafoveal, juxtafoveal, and subfoveal. These definitions were created by the Macular Photocoagulation Group and are as follows:

Location of CNV	Distance from foveal avascular zone center
Extrafoveal	200–2500 microns
Juxtafoveal	1–199 microns
Subfoveal	0 microns

C. Diskiform Scar

A diskiform scar shows an area of subretinal fibrosis or sub-RPE fibrosis. Dull, white fibrous tissue is seen and may accompany the CNV lesion or replace it over time (Fig. 5). Areas of RPE atrophy may or may not be present. Fluorescein angiography may show

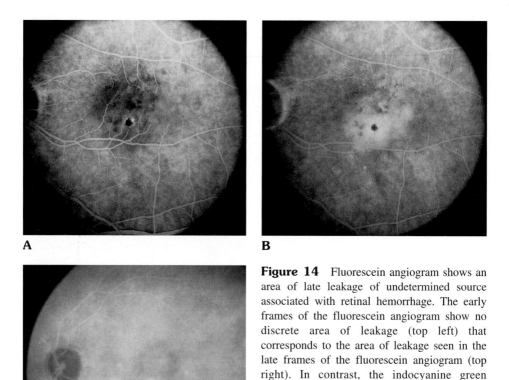

A

B

C

Figure 14 Fluorescein angiogram shows an area of late leakage of undetermined source associated with retinal hemorrhage. The early frames of the fluorescein angiogram show no discrete area of leakage (top left) that corresponds to the area of leakage seen in the late frames of the fluorescein angiogram (top right). In contrast, the indocyanine green angiogram shows a single hyperfluorescent spot of leakage (bottom left). Reprinted by permission from Lim JI, Sternberg P, Capone A Jr, Aaberg TM Sr, Gilman JP. Selective use of indocyanine green angiography for occult choroidal neovascularization. Am J Ophthalmol 1995;120:75–82 (Fig. 2).

leakage associated with the scar if CNV is present. The fibrotic scar may otherwise show only staining of the fibrotic tissue.

Patients with CNV typically present with symptoms of metamorphopsia, decreased vision, uniocular diplopia, Amsler grid distortion, scotoma, or macropsia. The severity of the symptoms varies depending upon the location of the CNV. Obviously lesions closer to fixation will cause more noticeable symptoms in the patient's visual field. Patients complaining of such symptoms require prompt clinical evaluation and fluorescein angiography to detect any CNV or PED and to characterize the CNV by type, location, and size. Treatable lesions should undergo laser photocoagulation within 72 h of the fluorescein angiogram for extrafoveal and juxtafoveal CNV and 96 h of the fluorescein angiogram for subfoveal CNV, or undergo photodynamic therapy (PDT) within 1 week if the lesion is eligible for PDT.

D. Feeder Vessels

A feeder vessel is a choroidal vessel that connects the CNV to the underlying choroidal vasculature thus supplying blood to the CNV membrane. Green and Enger have suggested that there are 2.3 feeder vessels crossing Bruch's membrane per CNV membrane (49). Feeder vessels are sometimes ophthalmoscopically visible within the CNV lesion. Recent work has focused on applying laser photocoagulation to feeder vessels in an attempt to close the CNV. Feeder vessels have been reported to be present in 15% of cases of CNV. Shiraga and co-workers first reported identification and photocoagulation of feeder vessels using ICG videoangiography via a scanning laser ophthalmoscope (50). In 70% of the patients, resolution of the exudative findings was seen and visual acuity improved or stabilized in 68% of patients. Later, Staurenghi and co-workers verified the superiority of dynamic ICG angiography with an SLO system for identifying feeder vessels in subfoveal CNV (51). Dynamic ICG can detect smaller feeder vessels and enables more targeted treatment of these vessels with a 75% success rate.

Most recently, using high-speeed, high-resolution digital angiography, it is possible to detect more feeder vessels in eyes with CNV. Details of this technique are found in another chapter, which describes the combined ICG angiography/dye-enhanced photoco-agulation system. Using this setup, it is possible to synchronize photocoagulation with the arrival of the dye bolus at a targeted vessel site.

E. Pathogenesis of CNV

The pathogenesis of CNV is not fully understood at this time. The primary stimulus for CNV remains unknown. The angiogenesis factors involved in the neovascular response are pre-sented in another chapter. Clues to the pathogenesis of CNV are available from surgically excised membranes. The most consistent pathological finding is accumulation of abnormal extracellular matrix (ECM) resulting in diffuse thickening of Bruch's membrane (49). Fo-cal areas of thickening from drusen and this diffuse thickening suggest altered metabolism of the ECM. There is data to suggest that altered ECM of RPE cells causes increased secretion of angiogenic growth factors that could contribute to the growth of CNV (52).

Iatrogenic breaks of Bruch's membrane in animals have led to animal models of CNV (53). Laser-induced CNV in primates has been used to investigate the mechanisms of CNV production and the role of the RPE (54).

It is known that RPE cells produce vascular endothelial growth factor (VEGF) and fibroblast growth factor 2 (FGF 2). Both are present in fibroblastic cells and in transdiffer-entiated RPE cells of surgically excised CNV (55–57). Healthy photoreceptors are needed to prevent the choriocapillaris from responding to excess VEGF (58).

Blockage of VEGF signaling has been shown to inhibit the development of CNV in mice with laser-induced rupture of Bruch's membrane (59,60). This information and further research will aid in the development of antiangiogenesis drug treatment of CNV in patients with AMD.

F. Idiopathic Polypoidal Choroidal Vasculopathy or Polypoidal Choroidal Vasculopathy

Idiopathic polypoidal choroidal vasculopathy (PCV) has recently been classified as a form of CNV that may occur in elderly patients. A recent study by Yannuzzi and colleagues determined the frequency and nature of PCV in patients suspected of harboring exudative AMD (61). In their prospective study of 167 newly diagnosed patients with exudative AMD, CNV due to AMD was diagnosed in 154 (92.2%) and PCV in 13 (7.8%). Nonwhite race (23.1%), absence of drusen (16.7% had drusen), and peripapillary location were felt to distinguish between PCV and AMD.

IV. PROGNOSTIC IMPLICATIONS OF EXUDATIVE AMD

A. Natural History of Untreated CNV

The natural history of untreated CNV in the setting of AMD is well established in both retrospective reviews and prospective randomized, controlled clinical trials. Untreated, eyes with CNV will often lose visual acuity. The location (extrafoveal, juxtafoveal, subfoveal) of the CNV is linked with the visual acuity prognosis.

B. Natural History of Extrafoveal CNV

The Macular Photocoagulation Study (MPS) gives us important natural history outcome information for eyes with similar (MPS) baseline characteristics and types of CNV. In the MPS untreated group, initial visual acuity was 20/100 or better and patients were symptomatic from the CNV.

When untreated, 50% patients with extrafoveal CNV lesions had, by the time of the first follow-up visit (3 months after enrollment for 98 eyes), already lost two or more lines of visual acuity; 10% had suffered a loss of six or more lines of visual acuity (62). Thus, eyes with classic extrafoveal CNV are at high risk for visual acuity loss without prompt treatment. Patients remain in the treatable phase for only a short time after the onset of symptoms (63).

At the conclusion (18 months after enrollment) of the extrafoveal study, in the untreated (natural history) group, 80% of women and 67% of men lost two or more lines of visual acuity from baseline, 43% of women and 47% of men lost 6 or more lines of visual acuity from baseline (62). Thus, the natural course of extrafoveal CNV may be visually devastating. Although photocoagulation is not a cure for the majority of eyes, the MPS results as summarized below show that there is a statistically significant benefit to photocoagulation versus observation.

C. Natural History of Juxtafoveal CNV

Thirteen percent of patents with juxtafoveal CNV in the natural history arm (249 eyes) of the MPS lost six or more lines of visual acuity by 3 months after enrollment and 58% lost six or more lines by 36 months. The juxtafoveal study included eyes with visual acuity 20/400 or better at entry (64). By 5 years 61% will suffer six or more lines of visual acuity loss. Only 9.6% of eyes remained unchanged and 5.9% of eyes gained ≥2 lines of visual acuity by 5 years (65).

D. Natural History of Subfoveal CNV

The MPS Subfoveal Study is the largest study of the natural history of eyes with subfoveal CNV and initial visual acuity of 20/100 or better. This study found that a majority of eyes will lose significant amounts of visual acuity over time if untreated. In fact, 77% of patients lost four or more lines of visual acuity at 24 months and 64% lost six or more lines. The smaller the lesion at baseline, the better the initial visual acuity (66).

In the MPS subfoveal trials, eyes with subfoveal CNV were enrolled if initial visual acuity was between 20/40 and 20/320. The visual acuity outcomes were dependent upon the baseline visual acuity and the lesion size. For all of the groups (A–D), visual acuity in the natural history group continued to drop during follow-up.

For lesions ≤ 1 disk area with visual acuity 20/125 or worse, lesion >1 or ≤2 disk areas with visual acuity 20/200 or worse (Group A), 14% of untreated eyes lost six or more lines of visual acuity at 3 months after enrollment. By 1 year 25% lost six or more lines of visual acuity. By 4 years, 35% lost six or more lines of visual acuity. These were eyes with small lesions and poor visual acuities.

For lesions ≤1 disk area with visual acuity 20/100 or better and for lesions >1 or ≤ 2 disk areas with visual acuity 20/160 or better (Group B), 11% of the natural history group lost six or more lines of visual acuity at 3 months, 38%, at 6 months, 38% at 1 year, 52% at 2 years and 3 years, and 55% at 4 years after enrollment. Thus these eyes with better initial acuity and smaller lesion size had more to lose over time.

For lesions >2 disk areas and initial visual acuity 20/200 or worse (Group C), 8% lost six or more lines of visual acuity at 6 months, 15% at 1 year, 13% at 2 years, 16% at 3 years and 25% at 4 years. Thus eyes with larger lesions and poorer initial acuity had less visual acuity to lose over time.

For lesions >2 disk areas and initial visual acuity 20/160 or better (Group D), 13% lost six or more lines of visual acuity by 3 months, 26% at 6 months, 31% at 1 year, 54% at 2 years, 45% at 3 years, and 55% at 4 years. Eyes with larger lesions and better visual acuity had more visual acuity to lose over time.

E. Macular Photocoagulation Study

The details of the MPS and the actual treatment techniques are discussed in another chapter. The following is a brief summary of the MPS findings. Treatment recommendations are summarized in Table 1. The MPS inclusion criteria were to enroll patients with classic CNV. However, analysis of the data revealed that there were eyes that had classic CNV associated with occult CNV that had been enrolled. The MPS treatment recommendations, however, should apply only to eyes with classic CNV. Freund et al. have shown that only about 13% of patients with CNV from AMD are eligible for treatment by the MPS criteria(67). Patients treated with laser need to be told about the permanent scotoma (location, size, effect on central vision function such as reading) that results from laser treatment. Patients should also be informed of the high risk of persistent CNV (CNV within 6 weeks of treatment) or recurrent CNV (CNV present after 6 weeks of treatment and initial closure).

1. Extrafoveal CNV

The original MPS report on the efficacy of laser photocoagulation for extrafoveal CNV in the setting of AMD was published in 1982 (62). That study showed an overwhelmingly positive effect of laser treatment for extrafoveal CNV (200–2500 microns from the foveal

Table 1 Table of CNV and Proven Treatments

Type of CNV	Location	Proven treatments
Classic	Extrafoveal	Thermal laser
Classic	Juxtafoveal	Thermal laser
Classic	Subfoveal	PDT
		Thermal laser
Classic and occult	Subfoveal	PDT if CNV is ≥ 50% classic
Occult	Subfoveal	PDT

center). Eligibility criteria included patient age of 50 years or more, best corrected visual acuity at least 20/100, symptoms due to the CNV, no prior laser treatment, drusen, and no other eye diseases that could affect visual acuity. Treatment was required to be given to the entire CNV and all surrounding blocked fluorescence or blood. The treatment, performed with 200-micron spots of 0.5-s duration argon blue-green laser, extended 100–125 microns on all sides of the CNV beyond blood, pigment, or blocked fluorescence. The intention was to treat any occult CNV in those regions.

After 18 months of follow-up, 60% of untreated eyes versus 25% of treated eyes suffered severe visual loss ($p < 0.001$). Severe visual loss was defined as six or more lines of visual acuity loss. The recruitment was halted at 18 months because of the overwhelming treatment benefit of laser treatment. This report, which was the first randomized, controlled multicenter clinical trial for treatment of AMD, led to a firm treatment recommendation of laser photocoagulation for extrafoveal CNV due to AMD (62).

Three-year and 5-year data later confirmed the long-term efficacy of laser photocoagulation. Although the treatment effect was less at subsequent follow-up years owing to the presence of recurrent CNV in the treated eyes, 5-year data showed that treated eyes continued to have better visual acuity outcomes than the control eyes (68). Even though 19% of the original treatment group were actually treated after the early beneficial effects were determined, there was still a difference between the treatment and placebo groups. Recurrent CNV occurred in 54% of the eyes; these eyes had poorer visual acuity outcomes than eyes without recurrences. A follow-up study on recurrent CNV in the argon-treated, extrafoveal, CNV eyes found the recurrence rate to be 59% with the majority of recurrences occurring in the first year (69). Eyes with recurrences had poorer visual acuity outcomes. Cigarette smoking appeared to be related to the rate of recurrence in AMD. At the time of the extrafoveal arm of the MPS, no treatment for the subfoveal recurrences was given. Perhaps, with our current armamentarium of treatment, better visual results would have been seen even in the eyes with the subfoveal recurrences.

2. Juxtafoveal CNV

The MPS AMD juxtafoveal studies showed that krypton laser photocoagulation for juxtafoveal CNV was effective. In this study, krypton red laser was used since it was felt that the red wavelength was not absorbed by the xanthophyll. Eyes were eligible for this study if they had CNV located between 1 and 199 microns of the foveal center or between 200 and 2500 microns of the foveal center if there was associated blood or blocked fluorescence within 200 microns of the foveal avascular zone (FAZ) center. Peripapillary CNV was eligible if the required laser photocoagulation would spare at least 1.5 clock hours along the temporal half of the disk. Patients were required to be 50 years of age or more and to have drusen in the macula with visual acuity no worse than 20/400. Treatment of the entire CNV with a 100-micron border was required on the nonfoveal border and in areas of blood or blocked fluorescence.

Eighty-six of 174 (49%) treated eyes versus 98 of 169 (58%) observed eyes suffered six or more lines of visual acuity loss at 3 years (64). At the 36-month visit, 62% of untreated and 49% of treated eyes had visual acuity worse than 20/200 ($p = 0.02$). The treatment effect depended strongly on the presence or absence of hypertension. Untreated eyes without hypertension were twice as likely to lose six or more lines of visual acuity compared to treated eyes (64% vs. 31%). This treatment effect was only 1.5 times for the eyes with hypertension (70% versus 46%). At 5 years, 71 (52%) of treated eyes versus 83 (61%) of untreated eyes lost six or more lines of visual acuity (65). The effect was greater for normotensive (RR = 1.82) than hypertensive (RR = 0.93) patients.

The MPS found 32% of treated eyes showed persistence and an additional 47% of treated eyes developed recurrent CNV within 5 years after krypton laser to juxtafoveal CNV (70). Eyes without persistent or recurrent CNV maintained 20/80–20/100 visual acuity.

Persistent CNV was twice as high when 10% or more of the foveal side of the CNV was left untreated. Central leakage in the MPS studies was not linked to a worse outcome. Forty-one percent of the eyes in the juxtafoveal group did not have adequate coverage of the CNV on the foveal side. This contrasts with the extrafoveal group, in which the lack of coverage on the foveat side was only 14%. The MPS recommended that the visual loss may be reduced by covering the entire CNV lesion with laser treatment. More than 90% of recurrences are located on the foveal side following laser treatment of extrafoveal and juxtafoveal CNV. Thus, patients should be forewarned of the high risk of persistent/recurrent CNV and the need for more laser therapy or alternative treatment (if subfoveal CNV develops).

Patients with a scar in the fellow eye, 20 or more drusen in the fellow macula, or a fellow eye with non-geographic atrophy at the initial visit had more recurrences than patients without these findings.

3. Subfoveal CNV

Subfoveal CNV was investigated by the MPS group beginning in 1986. Investigators felt that the poor natural history of eyes with subfoveal CNV (71,72) and scattered reports of outcomes of subfoveal laser not resulting in uniformly poor visual acuity warranted trial of photocoagulation of subfoveal CNV lesions (73). In Jalkh et al.'s study of 94 eyes followed up for an average of 15 months, CNV was closed in 88 eyes and visual acuity was stabilized or improved in those eyes (73).

Patients were eligible for inclusion into the MPS subfoveal study if there was some classic CNV, the lesion borders were well defined, the lesion was 3.5 disk areas or less in size, or there were less than six disk areas (new area of treatment plus old scar) if recurrent CNV was present. Visual acuity was required to be at least 20/320 but no better than 20/40. Patients were required to be at least 50 years of age and to be able to return for follow-up for 5 years. Patients were ineligible if they had prior eye disease or laser treatment in the study eye. Treatment was performed to all areas of classic and occult CNV within the lesion. The treatment border was 100 microns beyond the margins or 300 microns into the old treatment scar for recurrent CNV treatment. The treating fluorescein angiogram could be no more than 96 h old.

A total of 373 eyes of 371 patients from 13 clinical centers were randomized to laser treatment (argon green or krypton red as assigned during randomization) versus observation. Visual acuity, contrast sensitivity, and reading speed were measured. Post-treatment photographs were taken to check adherence to the MPS treatment standards (74).

A total of 189 eyes underwent laser treatment (97 argon green laser, 92 krypton laser); 101 (27%) of these eyes were later judged not to meet eligibility criteria primarily owing to poorly demarcated boundaries (36 eyes), CNV comprising less than half of the lesion (35 eyes), lesion component other than CNV (21 eyes), and lesions greater than 3.5 disk areas (14 eyes). For treated eyes, visual acuity usually decreased three lines from baseline within 3 months after treatment and then was stable for 42 months after treatment. In contrast, untreated eyes had less decreased visual acuity initially but continued to have decreases throughout the follow-up period. Treated eyes lost 3.3 lines at 12 months versus 3.7 lines for untreated eyes. At 24 months, treated eyes lost 3.0 lines versus 4.4 lines for untreated eyes. At 3 months, 20% of treated eyes lost six or more lines of visual acuity;

this remained stable at 42 months. For untreated eyes, 11% at 3 months had lost six or more lines of visual acuity; 48% at 42-month follow-up had lost six or more lines of visual acuity ($p = 0.006$). At the 42-month follow-up, reading speed and contrast sensitivity were better for treated than untreated eyes (74).

The persistence rate was 24%; recurrence rate was 32% at 3 years. There was no difference between the argon and the krypton groups. However, persistence and recurrence did not affect visual acuity outcomes, unlike in the extrafoveal and juxtafoveal groups. The 3-year rate for subfoveal persistent/recurrent CNV was 56%.

Subgroup analysis showed that treated eyes with smaller CNV lesions (1 disk diameter or less) experienced an earlier treatment benefit. Eyes with 20/40 to 20/100 visual acuity lost more than four lines on average after treatment and did not experience any treatment benefit until 18 months later. For eyes with 20/200 or worse visual acuity, treatment resulted in less than two lines of vision decrease and the mean decrease was less than for the untreated eyes by 6 months after treatment.

There was no effect of hypertension on the treatment benefit for the subfoveal group. There was no difference in outcome between argon green laser-treated eyes and krypton laser-treated eyes with respect to treatment benefit (visual acuity, contrast sensitivity, reading speed) or any subgroup. (The power of the study could state that the study would have detected a difference greater than 0.7 line.) Thus, investigators feel that either laser wavelength is fine for treatment.

For the recurrent CNV subfoveal group, the MPS found a similar treatment benefit. A total of 206 eyes of 206 patients from 13 clinical centers were enrolled into the study. The lesion had to be well demarcated but could include classic and occult CNV. The CNV had to extend under the foveal center, or if the prior laser scar had extended through the foveal center, the CNV had to be within 150 microns of the foveal center. The randomization was the same as that used for the new subfoveal CNV study.

The treatment extended 100 microns beyond the edge of the lesion and 300 microns into the old scar adjacent to the recurrence. Whenever a feeder vessel was visible, the treatment was to extend 100 microns beyond it on both sides and 300 microns around its base. Retreatment was performed at follow-up as long as some portion of the retina within 1 disk diameter of the foveal center was left untreated and the total scar would not exceed six disc areas.

A total of 97 eyes were treated (49 argon, 48 krypton) and 109 were observed. Seventeen (8%) eyes were later judged to be ineligible (poorly demarcated borders or lesion less than half CNV). Treated eyes had approximately 2.5 lines of visual acuity decrease 3 months after treatment followed by stable vision for 30 months. Untreated eyes continued to lose visual acuity throughout follow-up such that the average loss was 1.1 lines more than the treated eyes at 24 months. Six or more lines of visual acuity were lost in 14% of treated versus 9% of untreated eyes at 3 months. This remained about 10% for the treated group but increased to 32% for the untreated group at 18 months of follow-up. Treated eyes retained contrast sensitivity whereas untreated eyes lost contrast sensitivity.

F. Patient Care After Laser Treatments

After thermal laser photocoagulation, patients require close monitoring consisting of visual acuity, Amsler grid, biomicroscopy, and fluorescein angiography to help detect persistent or recurrent CNV. Usually patients are checked 3 weeks after laser photocoagulation for extrafoveal or subfoveal CNV and 2–3 weeks after laser photocoagulation for juxtafoveal CNV. The 2nd post-treatment visit is typically 4–6 weeks after laser, the third visit is 6–12 weeks after laser, and the fourth visit 3–6 months after laser. Of course, any patient with symptoms should be examined immediately and not wait for the next scheduled visit.

G. Occult Choroidal Neovascularization

1. Natural History

The MPS group reviewed the results of the juxtafoveal study with respect to the presence or absence of occult CNV (75). In this subgroup, they noted that there were eyes with only occult CNV, occult and classic CNV, and only classic CNV. For eyes with occult CNV that were untreated, 41% lost significant visual acuity within 12 months. Of the 26 symptomatic eyes with occult only lesions, classic CNV developed in 23% within 3 months and an additional 23% developed classic CNV by 12 months. For the eyes that developed classic CNV, 58% developed severe visual loss versus 18% in the group that did not develop classic CNV. Overall, 23% of eyes with initially occult CNV-only lesions remained stable or improved at the 36-month follow-up. Of these, 5% of the occult-only group had a two-line or more increase in visual acuity at 36-month follow-up (75).

Bressler et al. performed a natural history study of 84 eyes in 74 patients with poorly defined fluorescein angiographic CNV (76). The lesions were subfoveal in 89% of the eyes. Initial visual acuity averaged 20/80 and 93% had no classic CNV component. Over a follow-up ranging from 6 months to 53 months (mean 28 months), 14% remained stable or improved, 21% lost three to six lines of visual acuity, and 42% lost more than six lines of visual acuity. Including only those 46 eyes with 2 or more years of follow-up yielded similar results: 17% remained stable or improved, 22% lost three to six lines of visual acuity, and 48% lost more than six lines of visual acuity. Eyes that developed diskiform scars had worse visual acuities compared with eyes that had poorly defined CNV and leakage.

Soubrane et al. analyzed visual and angiographic outcomes of 156 patients (82 untreated) with symptomatic occult CNV and initial visual acuity of 20/100 or better. This series excluded eyes with turbid fluid, subretinal blood, PED, or visible CNV. Follow-up ranged from 1 to 8 years. There was no difference between treated and untreated eyes with CNV. Sixty-five percent of eyes with presenting subfoveal CNV had initial visual acuity of 20/50 or better. In this natural history group, visual acuity fell from 20/40 to 20/70. Similar to the results of Bressler et al. (76), when visible new vessels developed, the visual acuity decreased. Treatment did not result in better visual acuity outcomes over time when compared to the natural history group (77).

Bressler et al. investigated the use of macular scatter (grid) laser treatment of symptomatic eyes with poorly demarcated subfoveal CNV and visual acuities of 20/25 to 20/320 (51 treated eyes compared with 52 observation eyes) (78). Observed eyes had a median initial visual acuity of 20/80 and a median visual acuity of 20/320 at 24 months. The difference in visual acuity loss was significant between the treated and observed groups only at 6 months (1.8 lines lost in the observed vs. 3.8 lines lost in the treated group). Treated eyes at 6 months had lost two more lines of visual acuity compared with observed eyes. However, by 24 months approximately 40% of both groups had a mean change of 4.3 lines lost for observed eyes and 4.6 lines lost for treated eyes. At 12 months, 35% observed and 29% treated eyes had improved or remained stable, 37% observed and 30% treated eyes had lost two to five lines, 28% observed and 41% treated eyes had lost six or more lines of visual acuity. At 24 months, 31% observed and 31% treated eyes had improved or remained stable, 31% observed and 28% treated eyes had lost two to five lines, and 38% observed and 42% treated eyes had lost six or more lines of visual acuity.

Thus, conventional laser photocoagulation (either confluent or scatter) is not of benefit for eyes with subfoveal occult CNV and AMD. Recently, photodynamic therapy (PDT) was investigated in the Verteporfin in Photodynamic Therapy (VIP) Study for treatment of subfoveal occult CNV due to AMD. There was a benefit to use of Visudyne in the occult CNV eyes at 2 years as discussed below. Thermotherapy and radiation treatment are also being evaluated for treatment of occult CNV.

V. ALTERNATIVE TREATMENTS TO PHOTOCOAGULATION

Alternatives to laser photocoagulation are mainly for subfoveal CNV. Some physicians feel that PDT may be useful for juxtafoveal CNV in situations in which conventional laser (79) would lead to visual loss in the treating ophthalmologist's opinion.

A. Photodynamic Therapy

PDT initially has been demonstrated to be effective for treatment of subfoveal predominantly classic (greater than 50% classic) choroidal neovascularization. PDT treatment of subfoveal CNV offers an advantage over laser photocoagulation, which causes scotoma formation and hence visual acuity loss. The TAP study demonstrated that PDT using Visudyne for subfoveal CNV due to AMD with visual acuity between 20/40 and 20/200 (ETDRS chart) resulted in a less than 15-letter (approximately three lines of visual acuity) loss in 61% of treated eyes versus 46% of placebo eyes at 1 year. Subgroup analysis showed that eyes with predominantly classic choroidal neovascularization (50% or more classic in composition) had the best treatment benefit (67% treated vs. 39% placebo lost less than three lines of visual acuity). Only a small percentage of patients (16% vs. 7%) gained ≥ 1 line of visual acuity (80). Two-year results continued to show efficacy of PDT (81). For eyes with $\geq 50\%$ classic CNV, 66% of treated versus 32.5% placebo lost <3 lines of visual acuity at 24 months. Thus patients should be told that, although PDT can help prevent severe visual loss, improvement of visual acuity is indeed rare. Despite treatment a significant proportion of patients will still lose visual acuity.

More recently, the VIP study has shown that PDT for occult lesions may be beneficial. The 1-year data showed no statistically significant difference between Visudyne and placebo, but did show a trend in favor of Visudyne therapy (82). The VIP 2-year data, on the other hand, did show a statistically significant dfference between Visudyne and placebo in favor of Visudyne (82). For the occult CNV eyes: avoidance of moderate vision loss was 45% for Visudyne eyes versus 31% for placebo eyes ($p = 0.03$); avoidance of severe vision loss was 71% for Visudyne versus 53% for placebo eyes ($p = 0.004$). The treatment effect was best for eyes with 20/50 or less visual acuity and lesion size smaller than four MPS disk areas. The details of the TAP and VIP studies are given in another chapter.

B. Other Alternative Treatments

Other alternatives to photocoagulation treatment of subfoveal exudative AMD include thermotherapy, radiation therapy, pharmacological (antiangiogenesis) therapy, submacular surgery, submacular surgery with RPE transplantation surgery, and translocation surgery. There are currently ongoing clinical trials evaluating thermotherapy, radiation therapy, antiangiogenesis treatment, submacular surgery and translocation surgery for treatment of CNV secondary to AMD.

Thermotherapy (TTT) is the treatment by which a modified diode laser is used to deliver heat to the choroid and RPE through the pupil. Prior success has been demonstrated for treatment of small choroidal melanoma and retinoblastoma with this method (83–85). Reichel and colleagues (86) performed a pilot study in which 16 eyes of 15 patients with occult CNV were treated with TTT. Over a mean follow-up time of 12 months, 19% improved by two or more lines of visual acuity, 56% remained the same, and 25% lost two or more lines of visual acuity; 94% showed decreased exudation despite the visual acuity results. Reichel and co-workers have since performed a multicenter trial. The results and further findings are elaborated in another chapter in this book. Thermotherapy appears to hold promise in the treatment of AMD eyes with occult CNV.

Radiation therapy has been advocated as a therapy for exudative AMD. Low-dose radiation inhibits neovascularization (87–89). The key factor in the use of radiation therapy is achieving a balance between destruction of abnormal CNV tissue and preservation of normal retinal and choroidal blood vessels (90). Since proliferating tissues are more radiosensitive, this balance is theoretically achievable. The results of radiation therapy for treatment of CNV due to AMD are discussed and reviewed in another chapter. Conflicting data about the efficacy and morbidity of radiation therapy have led to the Age-related Macular Degeneration Radiation Trial (AMDRT), an NEI-sponsored pilot study comparing observation to radiation. The AMDRT is enrolling patients with lesions not amenable to laser treatment (classic, occult, or mixed).

Pilot studies evaluating submacular surgery for CNV due to AMD have shown some promise for use of this technique. The Submacular Surgery Trials (SST) initially were four pilot studies. The recurrent CNV arm showed no difference between surgery or laser treatment and no further study was recommended (91). The other three arms: new subfoveal CNV associated with AMD (Group N), large subfoveal hemorrhage associated with AMD (Group B), and subfoveal histoplasmic and idiopathic CNV (Group H) continue to enroll patients (92). The SST Trials will elucidate long-term visual outcomes and recurrence rates after submacular surgery compared with the natural history of untreated CNV. The techniques of submacular surgery and the results of clinical series are presented in another chapter.

Still others are combining submacular surgery with RPE transplantation. Since the RPE is often removed during submacular surgery and since RPE atrophy often follows submacular surgical procedures, researchers are evaluating the efficacy of transplanting RPE cells to repopulate the RPE layer. Loss of the RPE leads to choriocapillaris loss. The details of this technique and the rationale for RPE transplantation are given in detail in another chapter.

Retinal translocation and limited macular translocation surgery (93–96) have been described for treatment of subfoveal CNV. The rationale behind these surgical techniques is to move the macular area from the underlying CNV to a healthier RPE environment. The underlying CNV is thus moved relative to the foveal center and can be treated with conventional laser. The techniques are described in another chapter.

For patients in whom visual acuity is impaired and no treatment is possible or for whom no treatment possibilities remain, visual rehabilitation is of utmost importance. Low-vision rehabilitation may help these patients best utilize their remaining visual acuity and teach them to utilize ancillary tools such as closed-circuit television (CCTV) and magnifiers. These patients should also be reminded that AMD affects central and not peripheral vision. Expectations of the magnitude benefit of low-vision rehabilitation should be realistically explained to the patient. Further details of the devices and the services available for the low-vision patient are given in other chapters.

Ultimately, prevention of CNV must be our goal to prevent visual loss in patients with AMD. Some experimental approaches include laser to drusen and gene therapy. The next decade will undoubtedly bring more exciting developments in our battle against exudative AMD. Basic science research into the pathophysiology of AMD will, it is hoped, lead to preventive and more innovative treatments such as antiangiogenesis agents targeted against CNV in patients with AMD. Clinical trials into the efficacy of these new treatments are underway and will help us distinguish useful from nonuseful therapy. (The role of clinical studies is further elaborated in another chapter). Pharmacological therapy involving antiangiogenesis agents, gene therapy, and basement membrane stabilizers may one day be the preferred treatment of CNV. It is even possible that such agents may some day be used prophylactically in high-risk eyes.

VI. SUMMARY

The exudative form of AMD is the major cause of visual blindness in patients with AMD. Increased age, Caucasian race, and smoking are closely linked to development of CNV. Large drusen (>5), confluent drusen, hyperpigmentation, and hypertension are associated with an increased risk of CNV in fellow eyes of patients with CNV. Symptoms may be absent in the presence of CNV. Amsler grid testing of patients at risk of CNV may help to detect problems earlier. Prompt evaluation of symptomatic patients is essential for preventing visual loss. Fluorescein angiography is required to characterize the location (extrafoveal, juxtafoveal, subfoveal), type of CNV (classic, occult—FVPED, LLUS), and extent of CNV. Extrafoveal CNV (classic or well-demarcated forms) should be treated with laser photocoagulation as per the MPS guidelines. Conventional laser photocoagulation (either confluent or scatter) is not of benefit for eyes with occult CNV and AMD. ICG is useful for evaluating eyes with occult CNV or PEDs, or subretinal hemorrhage. Occult CNV has a better natural history than that of classic CNV. When classic CNV develops in occult CNV, the visual prognosis is worse than for occult only eyes. Photodynamic therapy is useful: (1) for eyes with subfoveal CNV that are at least 50% or more classic in composition and (2) for eyes with occult CNV with visual acuity less than 20/50 and lesion size less than four MPS disk areas. Persistent and recurrent CNV risk is high for extrafoveal and juxtafoveal CNV treated with thermal laser. Most of these are on the foveal side of the laser treatment. Alternative treatments under investigation include thermotherapy, radiation therapy, antiangiogenesis inhibitors, submacular surgery, RPE transplantation surgery, and translocation surgery.

REFERENCES

1. Pagenstecher H, Genth CP. Atlas der pathofischen Antomie des Augapfels. Wiesbaden: CW Kreiden, 1875.
2. Oeller J. Atlas seltener ophthalmoscopischer Bufunde. Wiesbaden: Bergmann JF, 1905.

3. Junius P, Kuhnt H. Die scheibenfonnige Entartung der Netzhautnfitte (Degeneratio maculae luteae disciformis). Berlin: Karger 1926.
4. Holloway TB, Verhoeff FH. Disk-like degeneration of the macula. Trans Am. Ophth Soc 1928;26:206.
5. Verhoeff FH Grossman HP. Pathogenesis of disciform degeneration of the Macula Arch Ophthalmol1937;18:561–585.
6. Ashton N, Sorsby A. Fundus dystrophy with unusual features: a histological study. Br. J Ophthal 1951;35:751.
7. Gass JDM. Pathogenesis of disciform detachment of the neuroepithelium. III. Senile disciform macular degeneration. Am J Ophthalmol 1967;63:617.
8. Gass JDM. Pathogenesis of disciform detachment of the neuroepithelium. IV. Fluorescein angiographic study of senile disciform macular degeneration. Am J Ophthalmol 1967;63: 645.
9. Blair CJ, Aaberg TM. Massive subretinal exudation associated with senile macular degeneration. Am J Ophthalmol 1971;71:639.
10. Small ML, Green WR, Alpar JJ, Drewry RE. Senile macular degeneration: clinicopathologic correlation of two cases with neovascularization beneath the retinal pigment epithelium. Arch Ophthalmol 1976;94:601–607.
11. Green WR, Key SN. III. Senile macular degeneration: a histopathologic study. Trans Am Ophthalmol Soc 1977;75:180.
12. Ferris FL, Fine SL, Hyman L. Age-related macular degeneration and blindness due to neovascular maculopathy. Arch Ophthalmol 1984;102:1640–1642.
13. Leibowitz HM, Krueger DE, Maunder LR, Milton RC, Kini MM, Kahn HA, et al. The Framingham Eye Study Monography: an ophthalmological and epidemiological study of cataract, glaucoma, diabetic retinopathy, macular degeneration, and visual acuity in a general population of 2631 adults. 1973–1975. Surv Ophthalmol 1980;24(Suppl):335–610.
14. Hyman LG, Lilienfeld AM, Ferris FL, Fine SL. Senile macular degeneration: a case-control study. 1983;2(213):227.
15. Smiddy WE, Fine SL. Prognosis of patients with bilateral macular drusen. Ophthalmology 1984;91:271–277.
16. Gregor Z, Joffe L. Senile macular changes in the black African. Br J Ophthalmol 1978;62(8):547–550.
17. Friedman DS, Katz J, Bressler NM, Rahmani B, Tielsch JM. Racial differences in the prevalence of age-related macular degeneration. Ophthalmology 1999;106(6):1049–1055.
18. Schachat AP, Hyman L, Leske McConnell AMS, Wi SY, and the Barbados Eye Study Group. Features of age-related macular degeneration in a black population. Arch Ophthalmol 1995; 113:728–735.
19. Klein R, Rowland ML, Harris MI. Racial/ethnic differences in age-related maculopathy: Third National Health and Nutrition Examination Survey. Ophthalmology 1995;102(3):371–381.
20. Smith W, Mitchell P. Family history and age-related maculopathy: the Blue Mountain Eye Study. Aust NZ J Ophthalmol 1998;26(3):203–206.
21. Klaver CCW, Wolfs RCW, Assink JM, Duijn CM, Hofman A, deJong PT. Genetic risk of age-related maculopathy: population-based familial aggregation study. Arch Ophthalmol 1998;116(12):1646–1651.
22. Klein R, Klein BEK, Jensen SC, Mares-Perlman JA, Cruickshanks KJ, Palta M. Age-related maculopathy in a multiracial United States population: the National Health and Nutrition Examination Survey III. Ophthalmology 1999;106(6):1056–1065.
23. Klein R, Klein BEK, Linton KLP, Demets DL. The Beaver Dam Eye Study: the relation of age-related maculopathy to smoking. Am J Epidemiol 1993;137(2):190–200.
24. Smith W, Mitchell P, Leeder SR. Smoking and age-related maculopathy: the Blue Mountain Eye Study. Arch Ophthalmol 1996;114(12):1518–1523.

25. Taylor HR, West SK, Munoz B, Rosenthal FS, Bressler SB, Bressler NM. The long-term effects of visible light on the eye. Arch Ophthalmol 1992;110(1):99–104.
26. Cruickshanks KJ, Klein R, Klein BEK. Sunlight and age-related macular degeneration: the Beaver Dam Eye Study. Arch Ophthalmol 1993;111(4):514–518.
27. The Eye Disease Case-Control Study Group (EDCCS). Risk factors for neovascular age-related macular degeneration. Arch Ophthalmol 1992;110(12):1701–1708.
28. Darzins P, Mitchell P, Heller RF. Sun exposure and age-related macular degeneration: an Australian case-control study. Ophthalmology 1997;104(5):770–776.
29. Klein R, Klein BEK, Jensen SC, Cruickshanks KJ. The relationship of ocular factors to the incidence and progression of age-related maculopathy. Arch Ophthalmol 1998; 116(4): 506–513.
30. Pollack A, Marcovich A, Bukelman A, Oliver M. Age-related macular degeneration after extracapsular cataract extraction with intraocular lens implantation. Ophthalmology 1996;103(10):1546–1554.
31. Pollack A, Marcovich A, Bukelman A, Zalish M, Oliver M. Development of exudative age-related macular degeneration after cataract surgery. Eye 1997;11:523–530.
32. Lanchoney DM, Maguire MG, Fine SL. A model of the incidence and consequences of choroidal neovascularization secondary to age-related macular degeneration: comparative effects of current treatment and potential prophylaxis on visual outcomes in high-risk patients. Arch Ophthalmol 1998;116(8):1045–1052.
33. Holz FG, Wolfensberger TJ, Piguet B, Gross-Jendroska M, Wells JA, Minassian DC, Chisholm IH, Bird AC. Bilateral macular drusen in age-related macular degeneration: prognosis and risk factors. Ophthalmology 1994;101(9):1522–1528.
34. Macular Photocoagulation Study Group. Risk factors for choroidal neovascularization in the second eye of patients with juxtafoveal or subfoveal choroidal neovascularization secondary to age-related macular degeneration. Arch Ophthalmol 1997;115:741–747.
35. Bressler NK Bressler SB, Gragoudas ES. Clinical characteristics of choroidal neovascular membranes. Arch Ophthalmol 1987;105:209–213.
36. Bressler NM, Bressler SB, Fine SL. Age-related macular degeneration. Surv Ophthalmol 1988;32:375–413.
37. Moisseiev J, Bressler NM. Asymptomatic neovascular membranes in the second eye of patients with visual loss from age-related macular degeneration. Invest Ophthalmol Vis sci 1990;31(suppl):462.
38. Valencia M, Green RL, Lopez PF. Echographic findings in hemorrhagic disciform lesions. Ophthalmology 1994;101:1379–1383.
39. Fine AM, Elman MJ, Ebert JE, Prestia PA, Starr JS, Fine SL. Earliest symptoms caused by neovascular membranes in the macula. Arch Ophthalmol 1986;104:513–514.
40. Guyer DR, Yannuzzi LA, Slakter JS, Sorenson JA, Hope-Ross M, Orlock DR. Digital indocyanine green videoangiography of occult choroidal neovascularization. Ophthalmology 1994;101:1727–1737.
41. Lim JI, Stemberg P Jr, Capone A Jr, Aaberg TM Sr, Gilman JP. Selective use of indocyanine green angiography for occult choroidal neovascularization. Am J Ophthalmol 1995;120:75–82.
42. Slakter JS, Yannuzzi LA, Sorenson JA, Guyer DR, Ho AC, Orlock D. A pilot study of indocyanine green videoangiography-guided laser photocoagulation of occult choroidal neovascularization in age-related macular degeneration. Arch Ophthalmol 1994;112:465–472.
43. Lim JI Aaberg TM Sr, Capone A Jr, Sternberg P Jr. Indocyanine green angiography-guided photocoagulation of choroidal neovascularization associated with retinal pigment epithelial detachment. Am J Ophthalmol 1997;123:524–532.
44. Elman MJ, Fine SL, Murphy RP, Patz A, Auer C. The natural history of serous retinal pigment epithelium detachment in patients with age-related macular degeneration. Ophthalmology 1986;93:224–230.

45. Poliner LA, Olk RJ, Burgess D, Gordon ME. Natural history of retinal pigment epithelial detachments in age-related macular degeneration. Ophthalmology 1986;93:543–551.
46. Bird AC, Marshall J. Retinal pigment epithelial detachments in the elderly. Trans Ophthalmol Soc UK 1986;105:674–682.
47. Casswell AG, Cohen D, Bird AC. Retinal pigment epithelial detachments in the elderly: classification and outcome. Br J Ophthalmol 1985;69:397–403.
48. Macular Photocoagulation Study Group. Subfoveal neovascular lesions in age-related macular degeneration: guidelines for evaluation and treatment in the macular photocoagulation study. Arch Ophthalmol 1991;109:1242–1257.
49. Green WR, Enger C. Age-related macular degeneration: histopathologic studies. The 1992 Lorenz E Zimmerman lecture. Ophthalmology 1993;100:1519–1535.
50. Shiraga F, Ojima Y, Matsuo T, Takasu I, Matsui N. Feeder vessel photocoagulation of subfoveal choroidal neovascularization secondary to age-related macular degeneration. Ophthalmology 1998;105:662–669.
51. Staurenghi G, Orzalesi N, La Capria A, Aschero M. Laser treatment of feeder vessels in subfoveal choroidal neovascular membranes. A revisitation using dynamic indocyanine green angiography. Ophthalmology 1998;2297–2305.
52. Mousa SA, Lorelli W, Campochiaro PA. 1999. Extracellular matrix-integrin binding modulates secretion of angiogenic growth factors by retinal pigmented epithelial cells. J Cell Biochem 74:135–143.
53. Ryan SJ. 1982. Subretinal neovascularization: natural history of an experimental model. Arch Ophthalmol 100:1804–1809.
54. Miller H, Miller B, Ryan SJ. The role of the retinal pigmented epithelium in the involution of subretinal neovascularization. Invest Ophthalmol Vis Sci 1986;27:1644–1652.
55. Amin R, Puklin JE, Frank RN. Growth factor localization in choroidal neovascular membranes of age-related macular degeneration. Invest Ophthalmol Vis Sci 1994;35:3178–3188.
56. Frank RN, Amin RH, Eliott D, Puklin JE, Abrams GW. Basic fibroblast growth factor and vascular endothelial growth factor are present in epiretinal and choroidal neovascularization membranes. Am J Ophthalmol 1996;122:393–403.
57. Lopez PF, Sippy BD, Lambert HM, Thach AB, Hinton DR. Transdifferentiated retinal pigment epithelial cells are immnunoreactive for vascular endothelial growth factor in surgically excised age-related macular degeneration choroidal neovascular membranes. Invest Ophthalmol Vis Sci 1996;37:855–868.
58. Yamada H, Yamada E, Kwak N, Ando A, Suzuki A, Ensumi N, Zack DJ, Campochiaro PA. Cell injury unmasks a latent proangiogenic phenotype in mice with increased expression of FGF2 in the retina. J Cell Physiol 2000;185:135–142.
59. Seo M-S, Kwak N, Ozaki H, Yamada H, Okamoto N, Fabbro D, Hofmann F, Wood JM, Campochiaro PA. Dramatic inhibition of retinal and choroidal neovascularization by oral administration of a kinase inhibitor. Am J Pathol 1999;54:1743–1753.
60. Kwak N, Okamoto N, Wood JM, Campochiaro PA. VEGF is an important stimulator in a model of choroidal neovascularization. Invest Ophthalmol Vis Sci 2000;41:3158–3164.
61. Yannuzzi LA, Wong DWK, Sforzolini BS, Goldbaum M, Tang KC, Spaide RF, Freund KB, Slakter JS, Guyer DR, Sorenson JA, Fisher Y, Maberley D, Orlock DA. Polypoidal choroidal vasculopathy and neovascularized age-related, macular degeneration. Arch Ophthalmol 1999;117:1503–1510.
62. Macular Photocoagulation Study Group. Argon laser photocoagulation for senile macular degeneration. Results of a randomized clinical trial. Arch Ophthalmol 1982; 100:912–918.
63. Grey RHB, Bird AC, Chisholm IH. Senile disciform macular degeneration: features indicating suitability for photocoagulation. Br J Ophthalmol 1979;63:85–89.
64. Macular Photocoagulation Study Group. Krypton laser photocoagulation for neovascular lesions of age-related macular degeneration. Results of a randomized clinical trial. Arch Ophthalmol 1990;108:816–824.

65. Macular Photocoagulation Study Group. Laser photocoagulation for juxtafoveal choroidal neovascularization. Five year results from randomized clinical trials. Arch Ophthalmol 1994;112:500–509.

66. Guyer DR, Fine SL, Maguire MG, Hawkins BS, Owens SL, Murphy RP. Subfoveal choroidal neovascular membranes in age-related macular degeneration. Visual prognosis in eyes with relatively good initial visual acuity. Arch Ophthalmol 1986;104:702–705.

67. Freund KB, Yannuzzi LA, Sorenson JA. Age-related macular degeneration and choroidal neovascularization. Am J Ophthalmol 1993;115:786–791.

68. Macular Photocoagulation Study Group. Argon laser photocoagulation for neovascular maculopathy: five-year results from randomized clinical trials. Arch Ophthalmol 1991; 109:1109–1114.

69. Macular Photocoagulation Study Group. Recurrent choroidal neovascularization after argon laser photocoagulation for neovascular maculopathy. Arch Ophthalmol 1986;104:503–512.

70. Macular Photocoagulation Study Group. Persistent and recurrent neovascularization after krypton laser photocoagulation for neovascular lesions of age-related macular degeneration. Arch Ophthalmol 1990;108:825–831.

71. Bressler SB, Bressler NM Fine SL, Hillis A, Murphy RP, Olk RJ, Patz A. Natural course of choroidal neovascular membranes within the foveal avascular zone in senile macular degeneration. Am J Ophthalmol 1982;93:157–163.

72. Guyer DR, Fine SL, Maguire MG, Hawkins BS, Owens SL, Murphy RP. Subfoveal choroidal neovascular membranes in age-related macular degeneration: visual prognosis in eyes with relatively good visual acuity. Arch Ophthalmol 1986;104:702–705.

73. Jalkh AE, Avila MP, Trempe CL, Schepens CL. Management of choroidal neovascularization within the foveal avascular zone in senile macular degeneration. Am J Ophthalmol 1993;95:818–825.

74. Macular Photocoagulation Study Group. Laser photocoagulation of subfoveal neovascular lesions in age-related macular degeneration. Results of a randomized clinical trial. Arch Ophthalmol 1991;109:1220–1231.

75. Macular Photocoagulation Study Group. Occult choroidal neovascularization: influence on visual outcome in patients with age-related macular degeneration. Arch Ophthalmol 1996;114:400–412.

76. Bressler NM, Frost LA, Bressler SB, Murphy RP, Fine SL. Natural course of poorly defined choroidal neovascularization associated with macular degeneration. Arch Ophthalmol 1988;106:1537–1542.

77. Soubrane G, Coscas G, Francais C, Koenig F. Occult subretinal new vessels in age-related macular degeneration: natural history and early laser treatment. Ophthalmology 1990;97:649–657.

78. Bressler NM, Maguire MG, Murphy PL, Alexander J, Margherio R, Schachat AP, Fine SL, Stevens TS, Bressler SB. Macular scatter ("grid") laser treatment of poorly demarcated subfoveal choroidal neovascularization in age-related macular degeneration. Arch Ophthalmol 1996;114:1456–1464.

79. Verteporfin Roundtable 2000 Participants, Treatment of Age-related Macular Degeneration with Photodynamic Therapy (TAP) Study Group Principal Investigators, and Verteporfin in Photodynamic therapy (VIP) Study Group Principal Investigators. Guidelines for using Verteporfin (Visudyne™) in photodynamic therapy to treat choroidal neovascularization due to age-related macular degeneration and other causes.

80. Treatment of Age-related Macular Degeneration with Photodynamic Therapy (TAP) Study Group Principal Investigators. Photodynamic therapy of subfoveal choroidal neovascularization in age-related macular degeneration with verteporfin: one-year results of two randomized clinical trials—TAP report 1. Arch Ophthalmol 1999;117:1329–1345.

81. Treatment of age-related macular degeneration with photodynamic therapy (TAP) study group. Photodynamic therapy of subfoveal choroidal neovascularization in age-related macular

degeneration with verteporfin: two-year results of 2 randomized clinical trials— TAP report 2. Arch Ophthalmol 2001;119:198–207.

82. Verteporfin in Photodynamic Therapy (VIP) Study Group. Photodynamic therapy of subfoveal choroidal neovascularization in age-related macular degeneration with Verteporfin: two year results of a randomized clinical trial including lesions with occult but no classic neovascularization—VIP Report #2. Am J Ophthalmol 2001, In press.

83. Godfrey DG, Waldron RG, Capone A Jr. Transpupillary thermotherapy for small choroidal melanoma. Am J Ophthalmol 1999;128(1):88–93.

84. Shields CL, Shields JA, DePotter P, Kheterpal S. Transpupillary thermotherapy in the management of choroidal melanoma. Ophthalmology 1996;103:1542–1650.

85. Shields CL, Santos MC, Diniz W, Gunduz K, Mercado G, Cater JR, Shields JA. Thermotherapy for retinoblastoma. Arch Ophthalmol 1999;117:885–893.

86. Reichel E, Berrocal AM, IP M, Kroll AJ, Desai V, Duker JS, Pulfiafito CA. Transpupillary thermotherapy of occult subfoveal choroidal neovascularization in patients with age-related macular degeneration. Ophthalmology 1999;106:1908–1914.

87. Archambeau JO, Mao XW, Yonemoto LT, Slater JD, Friedrichsen E, Teichman S, Preston W, Slater JM. What is the role of radiation in the treatment of subfoveal membranes?. Review of radiobiologic, pathologic, and other considerations to initiate a multimodality discussion. Int J Radiat Oncol Biol Phys 1998;40:1125–1136.

88. Del Gowin RL, Lewis JW, Hoak JC, Mueller AL, Gibson DP. Radiosensitivity of human endothelial cells in culture. J Lab Clin Med 1974;84:42–48.

89. Hosoi Y, Yamamoto M, Ono T, Sakamoto K. Prostacyclin production in cultured endothelial cells is highly sensitive to low doses of ionizing radiation. Int J Radiat Biol 1993;63:631–638.

90. Sagerman RH, Chung CT, Alterti WE. Radiosensitivity of ocular and orbital structures. In: Alberti WE, Sagerman RH, eds. Radiotherapy of Intraocular and Orbital Tumors. Berlin: Springer-Verlag, 1993.

91. Submacular Surgery Trials Pilot Study Investigators. Submacular Surgery Trials randomized pilot trial of laser photocoagulation versus surgery for recurrent choroidal neovascularization secondary to age-related macular degeneration. I. Ophthalmic outcomes. Am J Ophthalmol 2000;130:387–407.

92. Sternberg P, Capone A. Submacular surgery: a millennium update. Arch Ophthalmol 2000;118:1428–1430.

93. Imai K, Loewenstein A, de Juan E Jr. Translocation of the retina for management of subfoveal choroidal neovascularization I: experimental studies in the rabbit eye. Am J Ophthalmol 1998;125:627–634.

94. De Juan E Jr, Loewenstein A, Bressler NM, Alexander J. Translocation of the retina for management of subfoveal choroidal neovascularization. II. A preliminary report in humans. Am J Ophthalmol 1998;125:635–646.

95. Fujii GY, Pieramici D, Humayun MS, Schachat AP, Reynolds SM, Melia M, de Juan E Jr. Complications associated with limited macular translocation. Am J Ophthalmol 2000;130: 751–762.

96. Lewis H, Kaiser PK, Lewis S, Estafanous M. Macular translocation for subfoveal choroidal neovascularization in age-related macular degeneration: a prospective study. Am J Ophthalmol 1999;128:135–146.

7
Indocyanine Green Angiography

Antonio P. Ciardella
Doheny Eye Institute, University of Southern California Keck School of Medicine, Los Angeles, California

Lawrence A. Yannuzzi, Jason S. Slakter, David R. Guyer, John A. Sorenson, Richard F. Spaide, K. Bailey Freund, and Dennis Orlock
Manhattan Eye, Ear, and Throat Hospital, New York, New York

I. INTRODUCTION

Fluorescein angiography (FA) revolutionized the diagnosis of retinal disorders (1,2). However, there are certain limitations to this technique. Overlying hemorrhage, pigment, or serosanguineous fluid can block underlying pathological changes and prevent adequate visualization by FA. Indocyanine green (ICG) is a tricarbocyanine dye that has several advantageous properties over sodium fluorescein as a dye for ophthalmic angiography. The clinical usefulness of ICG angiography in the past has been limited by our inability to produce high-resolution images. However, enhanced high-resolution ICG angiography can now be obtained owing to the recent technological advance of coupling digital imaging systems to ICG cameras (3,4). Thus, digital ICG videoangiography finally allows the theoretical advantages of ICG as an ophthalmic dye to be realized.

II. SPECIAL PROPERTIES OF INDOCYANINE GREEN DYE

ICG absorbs and fluoresces in the near-infrared range. Owing to the special characteristics of the dye, there is less blockage by the normal eye pigments, which allows enhanced imaging of the choroid and its associated abnormality. For example, Geeraets and Berry (5) have reported that the retinal pigment epithelium (RPE) and choroid absorbs 59–75% of blue-green (500 nm) light, but only 21–38% of near- infrared (800 nm) light. The activity of ICG in the near-infrared range also allows visualization of pathological conditions through overlying hemorrhage, serous fluid, lipid, and pigment that may block the blue-light-exciting fluorescein dye. This property allows enhanced imaging of occult choroidal neovascularization (CNV) and pigment epithelial detachment (PED) (4,6).

A second special property of ICG is that it is highly protein-bound (98%). Therefore, less dye escapes from the choroidal vasculature, which allows enhanced imaging of choroidal abnormalities.

III. HISTORICAL PERSPECTIVES

ICG dye was first used in medicine in the mid-1950s at the Mayo Clinic to obtain blood flow measurements (7). In 1956, ICG was used for determining cardiac output and characterizing cardiac valvular and septal defects. In 1964, studies of systemic arteri-ovenous fistulas and renal blood flow were reported. The finding that exclusively the liver excreted the dye soon led to development of its application for measuring hepatic function.

ICG first became attractive to ophthalmologists interested in better ways to image the choroidal circulation because of its safety and its particular optical and biophysical proper-ties. Kogure and co-workers (8) in 1970 first performed choroidal absorption angiography in monkeys, using intra-arterial ICG injection. The first ICG angiogram in a human patient was performed by David (9) during carotid angiography. In 1971, Hochheimer (10) de-scribed choroidal absorption angiography in cats using intravenous ICG injections and black-and-white infrared film instead of color film. One year later, Flower and Hochheimer performed intravenous absorption ICG angiography for the first time in a human (11,12). These same investigators then described the superior technique of ICG fluorescence an-giography (13,14). Further technological improvements followed (15), and in 1985 Bischoff and Flower (16) reported on their 10-year experience with ICG angiography, which included 500 angiograms of various disorders.

However, the sensitivity of infrared film was too low to adequately capture the low-intensity ICG fluorescence, as the fluorescence efficacy of ICG is only 4% of that of sodium fluorescein. The resolution of ICG angiography was improved in the mid-1980s by Hayashi and co-workers, who developed improved filter combinations and described ICG videoangiography (17–20). However, their video system lacked freeze-frame image recording and possessed cumulative light toxicity potentials owing to its 300-W continu-ous halogen lamp illumination. In 1988, Destro and Puliafito (21) described a similar video system, and in 1989, Scheider and Schroedel (22) reported on the use of the scanning laser ophthalmoscope for ICG videoangiography.

In 1992, Guyer and co-workers (3) and Yannuzzi and associates (4) introduced the use of a 1024-line digital imaging system to produce high-resolution enhanced ICG images. These systems have improved the resolution of ICG videoangiography such that this technique is now of practical clinical value.

IV. PHARMACOLOGY

ICG dye is a water-soluble tricarbocyanine dye, which is an anhdryo-3,3, 3,3-tetramethyl-1,1-di (4-sulfobutyl)-4,5,4,5-dibenzoindotricarbocyanine hydroxide sodium salt. Its empirical formula is $C_{43}H_{47}N_2NaO_6S_2$ and its molecular weight is 775 daltons (23). It is highly protein-bound. Although it has been thought that ICG is primarily bound to albumin in the serum (24), 80% of ICG in the blood is actually bound to globulins, such as al-lipoproteins (25).

ICG special absorption is between 790 and 805 nm (25–27). The dye is excreted by the liver via bile. ICG is not reabsorbed from the liver, is not detected in cerebrospinal fluid (28,29), and does not cross the placenta (30).

V. TOXICITY

ICG is a relatively safe dye. Only a few side effects have been reported with its clinical use (7,24,31–33). In our experience, it is safer than sodium fluorescein. Unlike during FA, nausea and vomiting are extremely uncommon during ICG angiography. However, we have observed two serious vasovagal-type reactions during ICG angiography. Olsen et al. reported a case of anaphylaxis after ICG dye injection (34).

No complications were reported in one study using intravenous ICG doses of 150–200 mg. No side effects were noted in another series of 700 procedures (16). In a study that reported on ICG angiograpby performed on 1226 consecutive patients there were three (0.15%) mild adverse reactions, four (0.2%) moderate reactions, and one (0.05%) severe adverse reaction. There were no deaths (33).

ICG angiography should not be performed on patients allergic to iodide, as it contains approximately 5% iodide by weight. In addition, it should not be performed on patients who are uremic (16) or who have liver disease. Appropriate emergency equipment should be readily available, as with FA.

VI. TECHNIQUE OF INJECTION

ICG videoangiography can be performed immediately before or after FA. We inject intravenously 25 mg of ICG (Cardio-Green: Hynson, Westcott & Dunning Products, Cockeysville, MD) that has been diluted in the aqueous solvent supplied by the manufacturer. Rapid injection is essential. The injection may be immediately followed by a 5-mL normal saline flush.

VII. DIGITAL IMAGING SYSTEMS

The coupling of a digital imaging system with an ICG camera allows production of enhanced high-resolution (1024-line) images, which are necessary for ICG angiography. These systems produce instantaneous images, which decreases patient waiting time and expedites possible laser photocoagulation treatment. Digital imaging systems allow image archiving, hard-copy generation, and direct qualitative comparison between fluorescein and ICG angiography findings. In addition, these systems are useful for planning preoperative laser treatment strategies and for monitoring the adequacy of treatment postoperatively.

Digital imaging systems contain film and video cameras with special antireflective coatings and appropriate excitatory and barrier filters. A video camera is mounted in the camera viewfinder and is connected to a video monitor. The photographer selects the image and activates a trigger, which sends the image to the video adapter. The digitally charged coupling device camera (mega-plus camera) then captures the images and transmits these digitized (1024 × 1024 line resolution) images to a video board within a computer processing unit. Flash synchronization allows high-resolution image capture. These images are captured at one frame per second, stored in buffer memory, and displayed on a high-contrast, high-resolution video monitor. Optical disks are used to store images after editing. Hard-copy photographs can be obtained through a printer, or slides can be produced directly from a slide-making device. Finally, via telecommunications, satellite stations can be placed in laser treatment areas and in other offices.

VIII. INTERPRETATION OF ICG ANGIOGRAPHY FINDINGS IN AMD

A. Definitions

The terminology used to describe the angiographic manifestations of AMD corresponds with certain exceptions described below, to definitions previously reported by the MPS protocols and by our group. Most relevant to the interpretation of ICG angiography in AMD are the definitions of serous retinal pigment epithelium detachment (PED), vascularized PED, classic choroidal neovascularization (CNV), and occult CNV.

1. Serous PED

Serous PED is an ovoid or circular detachment of the RPE. On FA study there is rapid filling with dye of the fluid in the sub-RPE space. This corresponds to early hyperfluorescence beneath the PED, which increases in intensity in the late phase of the study resulting in a bright and homogeneous, well-demarcated pattern. ICG angiography reveals a variable, minimal blockage of normal choroidal vessels, more evident in the midphase of the angiogram (Fig. 1). In simple terms, a serous PED is bright (hyperfluorescent) on FA study and dark (hypofluorescent) on ICG study. This difference is caused by the fact that ICG molecules are larger and almost completely bound to plasma proteins, which prevents free passage of ICG dye throughout the fenestrated choriocapillaris in the sub-RPE space. Also it is important to remember the difference of appearance on ICG angiography between a serous PED in AMD and a serous PED in central serous chorioretinopathy (CSC). In fact, in CSC there is increased permeability of the choriocapillaris that causes leakage of ICG molecules under the PED. As a result a serous PED in CSC appears bright (hyperfluorescent) with ICG angiography. Approximately 1.5% of newly diagnosed patients with exudative AMD present with a pure serous PED.

2. CNV

CNV is defined as a choroidal capillary proliferation through a break in the outer aspect of Bruch's membrane under the RPE and the neurosensory retina. CNV is divided into classic and occult based on the FA angiography appearance.

a. Classic CNV. Classic CNV is an area of bright, fairly uniform hyperfluorescence identified in the early phase of the FA study, fluorescing throughout the transit phase with leakage of dye obscuring the boundaries of this area by the late phase of the angiogram. With ICG angiography, a classic CNV has an appearance similar to that seen with FA angiography, but is usually less well delineated (Fig. 2). Only 12% of newly diagnosed patients with exudative AMD present with classic CNV.

b. Occult CNV. Occult CNV is characterized as either fibrovascular PED (FVPED) or late leakage of undetermined source (LLUS). FVPED consists of irregular elevation of the RPE consisting of stippled hyperfluorescence not as bright or discrete as classic CNV within 1–2 min after fluorescein injection, with persistence of staining of fluorescein dye within 10 min after injection. LLUS consists of areas of leakage at the level of the RPE in the late phase of the angiogram not corresponding to an area of classic CNV

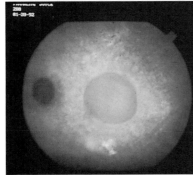

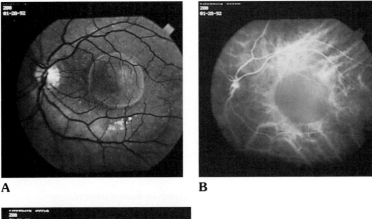

A

B

Figure 1 Serous PED. (A) Red-free clinical photograph of a serous PED in a patient with AMD. (B) Early-phase ICG study demonstrating a hypofluorescent serous PED. The fluid in the sub-RPE space blocks the underlying fluorescence of the choroid. (C) Late-phase ICG study showing the presence of a well-delimited, hypofluorescent serous PED. Note the late staining with ICG dye of confluent drusen inferiorly.

C

or FVPED discernible in the early or middle phase of the angiogram to account for the leakage (35). Also, any area of blocked fluorescence (blood, pigment) contiguous to the CNV is considered occult CNV. More than 85% of newly diagnosed patients with exudative AMD present with occult CNV. Two main types of occult CNV are recognized on ICG angiography.

Without Serous PED. The first type of occult CNV is caused by sub-RPE CNV that is not associated with a PED. The early stages of FA study reveal minimal subretinal hyperfluorescence of undetermined source that slowly increases over a period of several minutes to produce an irregular staining of the sub-RPE tissue. The ICG angiogram reveals early vascular hyperfluorescence and late staining of the abnormal vessels. If the ICG angiographic image has distinct margins, it is considered to be a well-defined CNV on ICG angiography. Two-thirds of newly diagnosed patients with an occult CNV present without an associated serous PED.

With Serous PED. The second type of occult CNV is associated with a serous PED of at least 1 disk diameter in size. Combined CNV and serous PED is called a vascularized PED (V-PED). This lesion is the result of sub-RPE neovascularization associated with a serous detachment of the RPE. One-third of newly diagnosed patients with AMD have an associated serous PED. The determination of whether a serous PED is present is best made on the basis of the FA study. FA may also demonstrate occult vessels as late, indistinct, subretinal staining beneath or at the margin of the serous PED. ICG angiography reveals early vascular hyperfluorescence and late staining of the CNV. The serous PED, as noted previ-

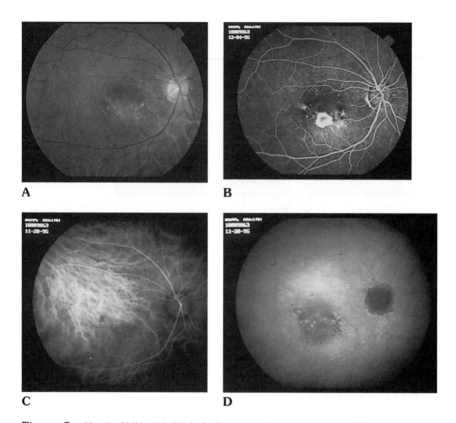

Figure 2 Classic CNV. (A) Clinical photograph demonstrating radial basal laminar drusen and RPE disturbances. There is an overlying neurosensory macular detachment. (B) Midphase FA reveals a well-defined area of classic CNV in the central macula with surrounding occult CNV. (C) Early-phase ICG study demonstrating ill-defined hyperfluorescence corresponding to the neovascular membrane better shown by FA. (D) Late-phase ICG study demonstrating ill-defined staining corresponding to drusen and neovascular vessels. Note the better resolution of the classic CNV by the FA study. See also color insert, Fig. 7.2A.

ously, is comparatively hypofluorescent, because only minimal ICG leakage occurs beneath the serous detachment. ICG is more helpful than FA in differentiating between a serous PED and a V-PED. It also permits better identification of the vascularized and serous component of V-PEDs (Figs. 3,4). These differentiations are not possible with FA alone because both the serous and vascularized portions of a PED demonstrate late hyperfluorescence or leakage. Although fluorescein staining is more intense in the serous portion of the detachment than in the vascularized component, differences in intensity are often too minimal for accurate interpretation. However, the ICG angiographic findings are infinitely more reliable for this differentiation; the serous component of a PED is hypofluorescent and the vascularized component is hyperfluorescent.

Occult CNV is also subgrouped in two types, one with a solitary area of well-defined focal neovascularization (hot spot) and the other with a larger and delineated area of neovascularization (plaque).

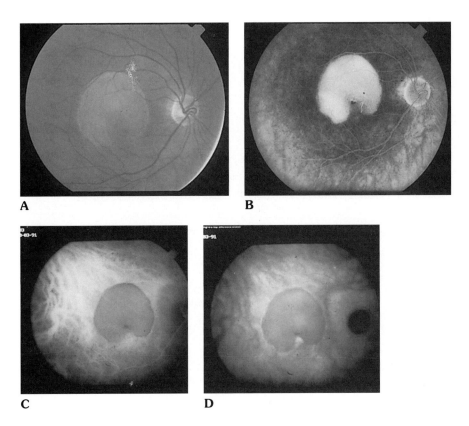

A   B

C   D

Figure 3 Occult CNV with PED (V-PED). (A) Clinical photograph demonstrating an irregularly shaped PED with turbid yellowish sub-RPE fluid. (B) Late-phase FA study demonstrating hyperfluorescence of the serous PED. Note the inferior notch. (C) Early-phase ICG study demonstrating a well-defined hypofluorescent serous PED. Because of the turbidity of the fluid, the underlying choroidal vessel cannot be visualized. (D) Late-phase ICG study demonstrating a persistent hypofluorescent serous PED. A focal area of hyperfluorescence (hot spot) within the notch of the PED is seen, consistent with active CNV. See also color insert, Fig. 7.3A.

Hot Spot (Focal CNV).   Focal CNV or a "hot spot" is an area of occult CNV that is both welldelineated and no more than 1 disc diameter in size on ICG angiography (Figs. 3–5). Also, a hot spot represents an area of actively proliferating and more highly permeable areas of neovascularization (active occult CNV) (Fig. 6). Chorioretnal anastomosis (CRA) and polypoidal-type CNV may represent two subgroups of hot spots (see below).

Plaque.   A plaque is an area of occult CNV larger than 1 disk diameter in size. A plaque often is formed by late-staining vessels, which are more likely to be quiescent areas of neovascularization that are not associated with appreciable leakage (inactive occult CNV) (Fig. 7). Plaques of occult CNV seems to slowly grow in dimension with time (Fig. 8). Well-defined and ill-defined plaques are recognized on ICG study. A well-defined plaque

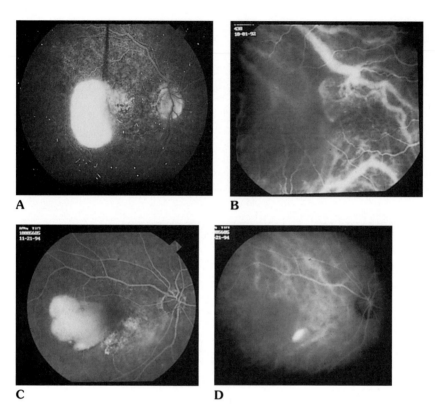

Figure 4 Occult CNV with PED. (A) Late-phase fluorescein study in a patient with AMD demonstrating hyperfluorescence of a serous PED. No classic CNV was identified. (B) High-magnification, early ICG study demonstrating a well-defined area of CNV along the nasal margin of the serous PED. (C) Late-phase fluorescein study demonstrating hyperfluorescence of a serous PED, with irregular mottled hyperfluorescence along its nasal margin. No classic CNV is seen. (D) Early ICG study demonstrating a hot spot of active CNV at the inferior margin of the PED. The PED itself appears hypofluorescent.

has distinct borders throughout the study and the full extent of the lesion can be assessed. An ill-defined plaque has indistinct margins or may be one in which any part of the neo-vascularization is blocked by blood.

In a review of our first 1000 patients with occult CNV by FA that were imaged by ICG angiography, three morphological types of occult CNV were noted: focal CNV or hot spots, plaques (well defined and ill defined), and combination lesions in which both hot spots and plaques were noted. The relative frequency of these lesions was: hot spots 29%, plaques 61%, combined lesions 8%. Combination lesions were further subdivided into *marginal spots* (hot spots at the edge of plaques of neovascularization); *overlying spots* (hot spots on top of plaques of neovascularization); and *remote spots* (hot spots not in contiguity with plaques of neovascularization) (36).

Two other forms of occult CNV are identified by ICG angiography: retinal-choroidal anastomosis (RCA) and polypoidal-type CNV.

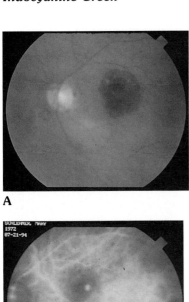

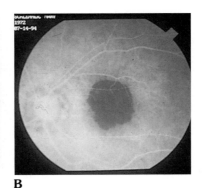

A

B

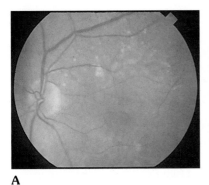

C

Figure 5 Occult CNV with sub-RPE hemorrhage and focal spot. (A) Clinical photograph demonstrating a subretinal hemorrhage in the central macula in a patient with AMD. (B) Late-phase fluorescein study demonstrating blocked fluorescence from the hemorrhage. No CNV could be identified. (C) Early-phase ICG study demonstrating good visualization of choroidal circulation beneath the thin layer of hemorrhage. A focal spot of CNV is seen. See also color insert, Fig. 7.5A.

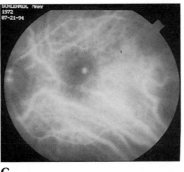

A

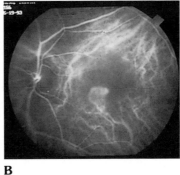

B

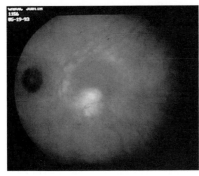

C

Figure 6 Active occult CNV. (A) Clinical photograph demonstrating a serous PED in the central macula. (B) Early-phase ICG study demonstrating intense hyperfluorescence of the CNV along the inferonasal margin of the PED. (C) Late-phase ICG study revealing increased hyperfluorescence and leakage of ICG dye along the active CNV. See also color insert, Fig. 7.6A.

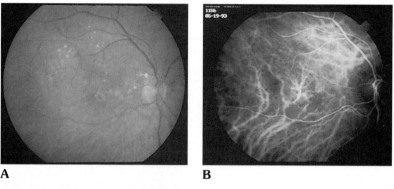

A   **B**

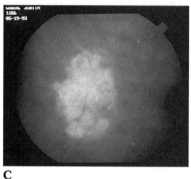

Figure 7 Inactive occult CNV. (A) Clinical photograph demonstrating thickening of the RPE and chronic exudative changes in the central macula. (B) Early-phase ICG study demonstrating hyperfluorescence of a large, well-defined neovascular vessel located in the central macula. (C) Late-phase ICG study demonstrating the full extent of the CNV. The larger vessels of the plaque, which filled early in the study, are now hypofluorescent, appearing in relief against the background of the neovascular lesion. See also color insert, Fig. 7.7A.

C

Retinal-Choroidal Anastomosis.   RCA are present in 20–93% of cases of focal hot spots of CNV noted on ICG study (37,38) (Figs. 9–12). Clinical characteristics helpful in the identification of RCAs are:

1. Presence of intraretinal hemorrhages at the site of the hot spot identified on ICG study.
2. Intraretinal leakage of ICG dye in a cystoid macular edema pattern overlying the area of neovascularization.
3. Presence of a V-PED on ICG study.
4. Highlighting of the RCA with laser treatment (the RCA remains reddish in color and is surrounded by the whitening of the retina after laser treatment).

Stereoscopic view of the ICG study allows direct recognition of the network of vessels that form the RCA. The identification of any of these clinical findings associated with focal hyperfluorescence on the ICG study in association with a PED bodes poorly for successful laser treatment and control of the exudative process (37).

Lafaut et al. recently reported on the clinicopathological correlation of RCA in AMD. They found that RCA represents histologically neovascularization growing out of the neuroretina, into the subretinal space, which mimics choroidal neovascularization (39).

Polypoidal-Type Occult CNV.   A recent observation is the recognition of hot spots of focal CNV with a polypoidal-like appearance on ICG angiography. These areas of focal CNV are more often found near the optic disk, may be associated with a serosanguineous PED, and seem to better respond to direct laser photocoagulation (Figs. 13, 14).

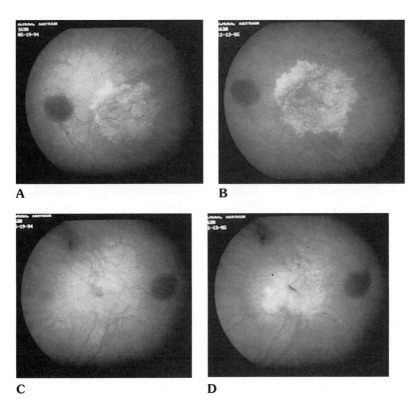

Figure 8 Natural history of occult CNV with plaques. (A) Late-phase ICG study demonstrating a plaque of CNV in the central macula. No laser treatment was performed. (B) Late-phase ICG study obtained 18 months later demonstrates enlargement of the plaque of CNV. (C) Late-phase ICG study of the fellow eye of the same patient on initial presentation demonstrating only minimal irregular hyperfluorescence in the macula. (D) Late-phase ICG study 18 months later demonstrating a larger, well-defined area of plaque of CNV.

IX. CLINICAL APPLICATION OF ICG ANGIOGRAPHY TO THE STUDY OF AMD

Patz and associates (23) were the first to study CNV by ICG videoangiography. They could resolve only two of 25 CNVs with their early model. Bischoff and Flower (16) studied 100 ICG angiograms of patients with age-related macular degeneration. They found "delayed and/or irregular choroidal filling" in some patients. The significance of this finding is unclear, however, because these authors did not include an age-matched control group. Tortuous choroidal vessels and marked dilation of macular choroidal arteries, often with loop formation, were also observed.

Hayashi and associates (17,18,20) found that ICG videoangiography was useful in the detection of CNV. ICG videoangiography was able to confirm the fluorescein angiographic appearance of CNV in patients with well-defined.CNV. It revealed a more well-defined neovascularization in 27 eyes with occult CNV by FA. In a subgroup of patients with poorly defined occult CNV, the ICG angiogram, but not the FA, imaged a well-defined

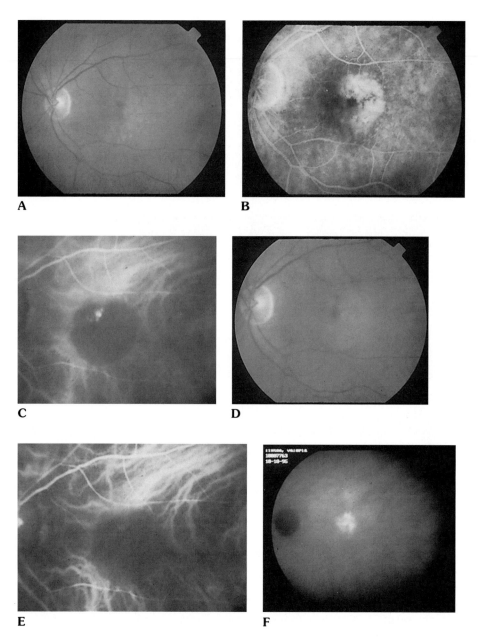

Figure 9 Occult CNV with serous PED and RCA. (A) Clinical photograph demonstrating exudation in the central macula with subretinal hemorrhage, lipid, and a serous PED. (B) Late-phase FA demonstrating occult CNV. There is hyperfluorescence of the PED and blockage by the hemorrhage. No well-defined CNV is seen. (C) Midphase ICG study demonstrating a hot spot in the superonasal portion of the PED. On stereoscopic examination, a RCA was identified in this region. Focal laser treatment of the hot spot was performed. (D) Clinical photograph 3 months following treatment demonstrating persistent turbid detachment of the PED and subretinal hemorrhage. (E) Early-phase ICG study demonstrating multifocal hyperfluorescence at the site of prior laser treatment, indicative of recurrent CNV. (F) Late-phase ICG demonstrating persistent hyper-fluorescence and leakage at the site of the RCA. See also color insert, Fig. 7.9A, D.

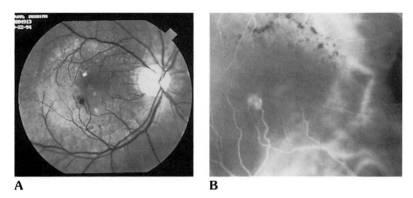

A   B

Figure 10 Occult CNV with serous PED and RCA. (A) Red-free clinical photograph demonstrating a serous PED, submacular exudation, lipid deposition, and intraretinal hemorrhage. (B) Mid-phase ICG study reveals the presence of an anastomosis between two retinal vessels and the underlying neovascular complex.

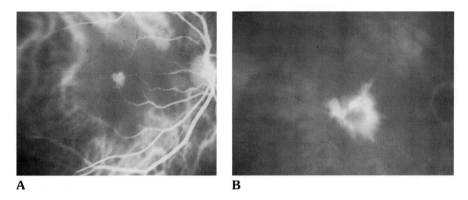

A   B

Figure 11 Occult CNV with serous PED and RCA. (A) Midphase ICG study demonstrating a RCA and an associated serous PED. (B) Late-phase ICG study reveals the presence of intraretinal leakage of ICG dye in a "cystoid macular edema" configuration.

CNV in nine of 12(75%) cases. ICG videoangiography of the other three eyes revealed suspicious areas of neovascularization. Hayashi and co-workers (17, 18, 20) were also the first to show that leakage from CNV with ICG was slow compared to the rapid leakage of sodium fluorescein. While the results of these investigators concerning ICG videoangiographic imaging of occult CNV were promising, the spatial resolution that they could obtain was limited by the 512-line video monitor and analog tape of their ICG system.

Destro and Puliafito (21) reported that ICG videoangiography was particularly useful in studying occult CNV with overlying hemorrhage and recurrent CNV. Guyer and co-workers (3) used a 1024-line digital imaging system to study patients with occult CNV. These authors reported that ICG videoangiography was useful in imaging occult CNV and that this technique could allow photocoagulation of otherwise untreatable lesions. Scheider and co-investigators (40) have reported enhanced imaging of CNV in a study of 80 patients using the scanning laser ophthalmoscope with ICG videoangiography.

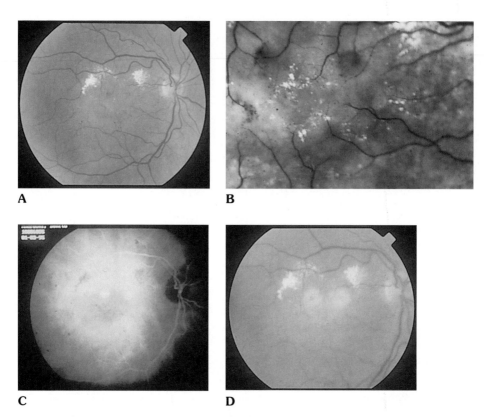

Figure 12 Occult CNV with serous PED and RCA. (A) Clinical photograph demonstrating hemorrhage, subretinal lipid exudates, and a PED in the macula. (B) Red-free photograph reveals the presence of two RCAs in the superior macula. (C) Midphase ICG study shows the presence of a serous PED and two hot spots corresponding to the RCAs. (D) Clinical photograph obtained immediately following laser treatment of the two sites of CNV. The reddish lesion now highlighted within the treatment site represents a network of vessels rather than hemorrhage. See also color insert, Fig. 7.12A.

Yannuzzi and associates (4) have shown that ICG videoangiography is extremely useful in converting occult CNV into classic well-defined CNV. In their study, 39% of 129 patients with occult CNV were converted to well-defined CNV based on information added by ICG videoangiography. These authors reported that ICG videoangiography was especially useful in identifying occult CNV in patients with serous pigment epithelial detachment (SPED) or with recurrent CNV.

Lim et al. found that ICG angiography added useful clinical information to FA by demonstrating well-demarcated areas of hyperfluorescence in 50% of eyes selected because of diagnosis of occult CNV and in 82% of eyes selected because of PED (41).

Yannuzzi et al. studied the ICG atigiograms of 235 consecutive AMD patients with occult CNV and associated vascularized PED. These eyes were divided into two groups, depending on the size and delineation of the CNV. Of the 235 eyes, 89 (38%) had a solitary area of neovascularization that was well delineated, no more than 1 disk diameter in size, and defined as "hot spots" of focal CNV. The other 146 eyes (62%) had a larger area of neovascularization, with variable delineation defined as a plaque CNV (42).

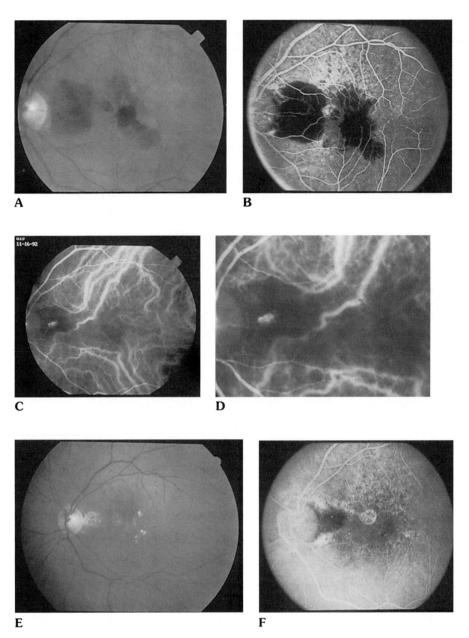

Figure 13 Polypoidal-type occult CNV with subretinal hemorrhage. (A) Clinical photograph demonstrating subretinal hemorrhage secondary to CNV. (B) Late-phase FA study demonstrating blocked fluorescence by the hemorrhage and an area of hyperfluorescence in the nasal juxtafoveal area. (C) Early-phase ICG study demonstrating localized hyperfluorescence in the peripapillary region. This area does not correspond to the hyperfluorescence seen on FA study. (D) High-magnification image of the localized CNV. Note the polypoidal-like appearance of the neovascular complex. This lesion was photocoagulated. (E) Clinical photograph 3 months after laser treatment demonstrating resolution of the subretinal hemorrhage. (F) FA study demonstrating hypo-fluorescence at the site of treatment. The hyperfluorescence noted on the original fluorescein corresponds to an area of RPE atrophy. See also color insert, Fig. 7.13A, E.

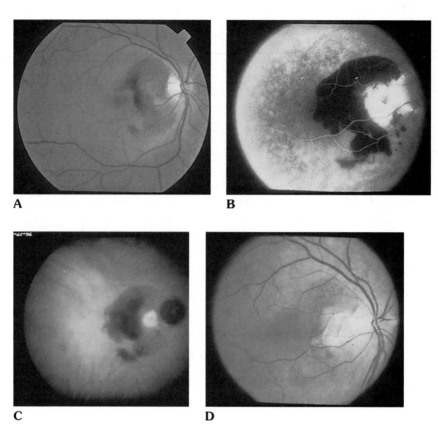

Figure 14 Polypoidal-type occult CNV with subretinal hemorrhage. (A) Color photograph demonstrating hemorrhagic detachment of the macula. Note the absence of drusen at the posterior pole. (B) Late-phase FA study demonstrating blocked fluorescence by the subretinal hemorrhage and intense hyperfluorescence in the papillomacular bundle. (C) Late-phase ICG study demonstrating a hot spot in the papillomacular bundle. On higher magnification the hot spot presented a polypoidal-like appearance. (D) Clinical photograph 1 year after ICG-guide laser treatment demonstrating resolution of the subretinal hemorrhage. Visual acuity improved from 20/200 to 20/25. See also color insert, Fig. 7.14A, D.

In a further report, 657 consecutive eyes with occult CNV by fluorescein angiography were studied with ICG angiography. Of 413 eyes with occult CNV without pigment epithelium detachments, focal areas of neovascularization were noted in 89(22%) Overall, 142 eyes (34.3%) had lesions that were potentially treatable by laser photocoagulation based on additional information provided by ICG angiography. Of the 235 eyes with occult CNV and vascularized PEDs, 98 (42%) were eligible for laser therapy based on ICG angiography findings. The authors calculated that ICG angiography enhances the treatment eligibility by approximately one-third (43).

In an expanded series the same authors reported their results on ICG angiography study of 1000 consecutive eyes with occult CNV by fluorescein angiography (44). They recognized three morphological types of CNV, which included focal spots, plaques (well defined and poorly defined), and combination lesions (in which both focal spots and plaques are noted). Combination lesions were further subdivided into marginal spots (focal spots at the edge of plaque of neovascularization), overlying spots (hot spots overlying plaques of neovascularization), or remote spots (a focal spot remote from a plaque of neo-vascularization).

The relative frequency of these lesions was as follows: focal spots 29%; plaques 61%, consisting 27% of well-defined plaques and 34% of poorly defined plaques; and combination lesions 8%, consisting of 3% of marginal spots, 4% of overlying spots, and 1% of remote spots (44). A follow-up study from the same authors of patients with newly diagnosed unilateral occult CNV secondary to AMD showed that the patients tended to develop the same morphological type of CNV in the fellow eye (45).

Finally, Lee et al. reported on 15 eyes with surgically excised subfoveal CNV that underwent preoperative and postoperative ICG angiography. All excised membranes were examined by light microscopy, and all surgically excised ICG-imaged membranes corresponded to sub-RPE and subneurosensory retinal CNV (46).

Chang et al. (47) reported on the clinicopathological correlation of AMD with CNV detected by ICG angiography. Histopathological examination of the lesion revealed a thick subretinal pigment epithelium CNV corresponding to the plaque-like lesion seen with ICG angiography.

The above studies demonstrate that ICG videoangiography is an important adjunctive study to FA in the detection of CNV. FA appears to be more sensitive than ICG videoangiography in imaging fine capillaries that connect larger vessels and capillaries at the proliferating edge of well-defined CNV. While FA may image well-defined CNV better than ICG videoangiography in some cases, ICG videoangiography can enable treatment of about 30% of occult CNV by the detection of well-defined CNV eligible for ICG-guided laser treatment in about 30% of cases (36,48). Thus, the best imaging strategy to detect CNV is to perform FA and ICG videoangiography.

X. ICG-GUIDED LASER TREATMENT OF CNV IN AMD

Patients potentially eligible for laser photocoagulafion therapy by ICG guidance are the ones with clinical and FA evidence of occult CNV. The technique for ICG-guided laser photocoagulation has been previously described and is illustrated in Figure 15. Of the two types of occult CNV that can be identified by ICG study, hot spots and plaques, we recommend direct laser photocoagulation only of hot spots. In fact, as mentioned above, hot spots represent areas of actively leaking neovascularization that can be obliterated by laser photocoagulation in an attempt to eliminate the associated serosanguineous complications, and stabilize or improve the vision. On the contrary, plaques seem to represent a thin layer of neovascularization that is not actively leaking and may not require laser photocoagulation (Figs. 16–19).

This approach has practical considerations. In the case of a lesion with both a hot spot and a plaque, and in which the hot spot is at the margin of the plaque (which may extend under the fovea), one applies laser photocoagulation to the extrafoveal hot spot and spares the foveal area. This treatment approach was successful in obliterating the CNV and stabilizing the vision in 56% of a consecutive series of AMD patients (48). On the contrary, we have had poor success with direct laser treatment of hot spots overlying plaques, and confluent treatment of the entire plaque.

Two subtypes of hot spots are RCA and polypoidal-type CNV. When a RCA is present, the success of laser photocoagulation is negatively influenced by the presence of an

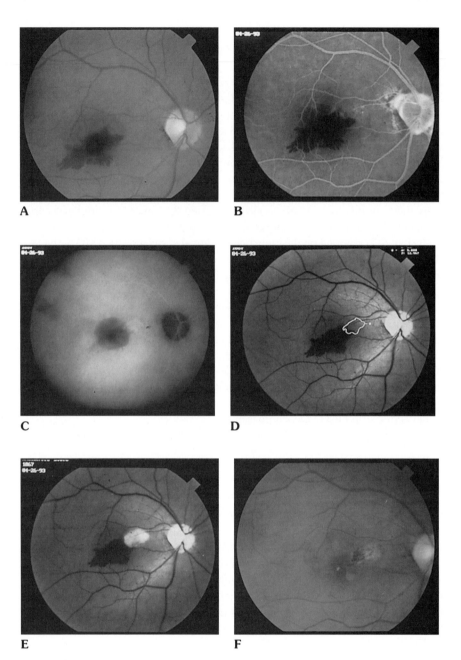

Figure 15 Occult CNV treatment technique. (A) Clinical photograph demonstrating a subretinal hemorrhage in the macular area. (B) Midphase fluorescein study demonstrating blocked fluorescence by the hemorrhage. There is mild staining in the papillomacular bundle and peripapillary region. (C) Late-phase ICG study demonstrating less blocked fluorescence centrally, with a triangular area of faint hyperfluorescence nasal to fixation. (D) Red-free photograph with overlying tracing of the lesion noted on ICG study, used as guide for laser treatment. (E) Red-free photograph immediately after laser treatment demonstrating the extent of the photocoagulation application. (F) Clinical photograph obtained 6 months after treatment demonstrating mottling of the RPE at the site of laser treatment and complete resolution of the subretinal hemorrhage. See also color insert, Fig. 7.15A, D.

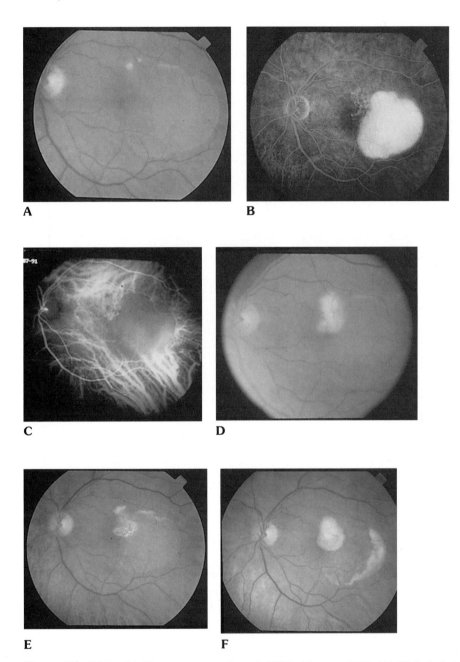

Figure 16 ICG-guided laser treatment of occult CNV with serous PED. (A) Clinical photograph demonstrating a large, lobular serous PED in the temporal macula. (B) Late-phase FA study revealing hyperfluorescence of the serous component of the PED. Nasally there is an area of irregular hyperfluorescence suggesting occult CNV. (C) Early-phase ICG study demonstrating hyperfluorescence of the serous PED, with focal hyperfluorescence corresponding to CNV along the nasal margin of the PED. (D) Clinical photograph immediately after ICG-guided laser treatment of the CNV. (E) Clinical photograph 1 month later demonstrating partial resolution of the PED and a chorioretinal scar at the site of the treatment. (F) Four years later there is flattening of the PED. Fibrous metaplasia is seen temporally at the site of prior exudation. See also color insert, Fig. 7.16A, D, E, F.

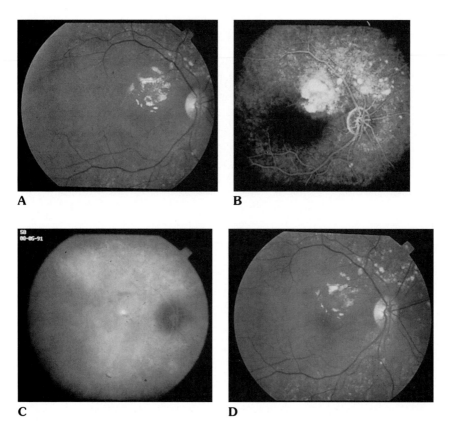

Figure 17 ICG-guided laser treatment of occult CNV. (A) Clinical photograph revealing an exudative macula detachment, with multiple confluent drusen beneath the neurosensory elevation. (B) Late-phase FA study revealing diffuse leakage under the neurosensory retina. Hyperfluorescent drusen are seen nasally. (C) Late-phase ICG study demonstrating a hot spot of focal, active CNV in the juxtafoveal region. (D) Clinical photograph 1 month after ICG-guided laser photocoagulation of the hot spot of focal CNV. There is complete resolution of the neurosensory detachment of the macula. See also color insert, Fig. 7.17A, D.

associated serous PED. In a small series of patients with RCA and associated PED, laser photocoagulation was successful in closing the CNV in only 14% of cases (37). Slakter and associates (49) performed ICG-guided laser photocoagulation in 79 eyes with occult CNV. The occult CNV was successfully eliminated. Visual acuity was stabilized or improved in 29 (66%) of 44 eyes with occult CNV associated with neurosensory retinal elevations, and in 15 (43%) of 35 eyes with occult CNV associated with PED. This study demonstrated that in some cases ICG videoangiography imaging can successfully guide laser photocoagulation of occult CNV.

In another pilot study of ICG-guided laser treatment of occult CNV, Regillo et al. had similar results (50).

Guyer and co-workers reported on a pilot study of ICG-guided laser photocoagulation of 23 eyes that had untreatable occult CNV secondary to AMD with focal spots at the edge of a plaque of neovascularization on the ICG study. ICG-guided laser photocoagulation was applied solely to the focal spot at the edge of the plaque. At 24 months of follow-

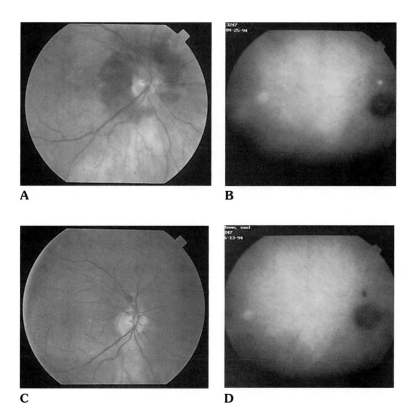

Figure 18 Peripapillary occult CNV with subretinal hemorrhage. (A) Clinical photograph demonstrating subretinal hemorrhage surrounding the optic nerve. (B) Midphase ICG study demonstrating a small hot spot of CNV in the peripapillary area. A large, irregular area of faint hyperfluorescence is seen in the central macula, suggestive of a quiescent plaque of CNV. (C) Posttreatment clinical photograph demonstrating resolution of the subretinal hemorrhage. (D) Posttreatment late-phase ICG study demonstrating an hypofluorescent scar at the site of laser treatment. (Case courtesy of Dr. Kurt Gitter.)

up anatomical success with resolution of the exudative findings was obtained in 6 (37.5%) of 16 eyes (48). Importantly, these studies set the foundation for future prospective studies of ICG-guided laser treatment. In addition, they proved that the presence of a PED is a poor prognostic factor in the treatment of exudative AMD. A recent study prospectively evaluated 185 consecutive eyes with exudative AMD and a well-delineated area (hot spot or focal area) of hyperfluorescence by ICG angiography.

All the patients were divided into two groups (with PED and without PED). Of the 185 eyes, 99 eyes without PED achieved a 71% rate of obliteration at 6 months and 48% rate of obliteration at 12 months. Eyes with PED did significantly worse with an obliteration rate of the CNV of 23% at 12 months. The overall success rate was 36% at 12 months (36). A possible explanation for the high recurrence rate after laser photocoagulation of occult CNV, particularly when a vascularized PED is present, may be found in the peculiar anatomy of the CNV in such cases. It has recently been observed that there is a variant of CNV where the neovascularization is fed both by a choroidal and by a retinal component to create a retinochoroidal anastomosis.

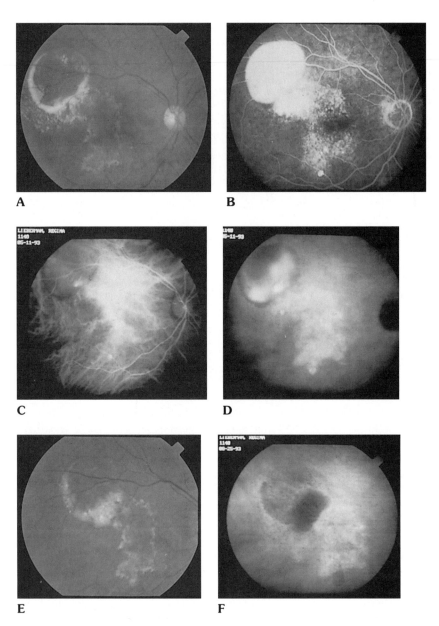

Figure 19   Hot spot at the margin of a plaque. (A) Clinical photograph demonstrating a turbid PED with lipid exudates in the temporal macula. Central RPE mottling and thickening is noted. (B) Late-phase FA study demonstrating the presence of a serous PED and a central are a of diffuse ooze suggestive of occult CNV. No classic CNV is evident. (C) Early-phase ICG study demonstrating two hot spots of CNV in the inferior macula and at the inferonasal edge of the PED. (D) Late-phase ICG study demonstrating leakage of the ICG dye into the PED. A large plaque of "dormant" CNV is now evident in the central macula. Laser treatment was applied only to the two hot spots of active CNV. The large plaque of subfoveal CNV was left untreated. (E) Three months following treatment there is complete flattening of the PED and resolution of the lipids. No change is noted in the central lesion. (F) Late-phase ICG study 3 months after treatment demonstrating hypofluorescence at the site of the active CNV and of the previous PED. The large plaque of CNV is unchanged. See also color insert, Fig. 7.19A, E.

In a recent report by Kuhn et al., RCAs were identified as occurring in 93% of patients with CNV associated with a serous PED. These authors reported a poor success rate from laser treatment as well (38).

Slakter and co-workers followed prospectively 150 patients with newly diagnosed exudative AMD(37). All had clinical and fluorescein angiographic evidence of occult CNV, and each demonstrated focal areas of hyperfluorescence on ICG angiography, felt to be representative of CNV. Thirty-one (21%) of the 150 eyes were found to have a RCA. In 82 eyes the occult CNV was associated with a serous PED. Twenty-two (27%) of these patients were noted to have RCA. In the remaining 68 cases (occult CNV without serous PED), nine eyes (13%) were found to have a RCA. Associated clinical features of RCAs were identified in preretinal or intraretinal hemorrhages at the site of the lesion, dilated tortuous retinal vessels, sudden termination of a retinal vessel, and cystoid macular edema.

The same authors found that the success rate of laser photocoagulation of RCAs without serous PED was 66%, while with serous PED it dropped to 14%. Thus the presence of a RCA may well provide a key to understanding the poor outcome for laser treatment in this subgroup of patients.

In conclusion, from the work of Freund et al. (51), it is known that approximately only 13% of patients with CNV secondary to AMD have a classic or well-defined extrafoveal choroidal neovascularization by fluorescein angiography that is eligible for laser treatment. With a recurrence rate of approximately 50% following laser photocoagulation under fluorescein guidance for classic CNV, only approximately 6.5% of patients will benefit from treatment.

The remaining 87% of patients have occult CNV by fluorescein imaging. About 30% of these eyes have a potentially treatable focal spot by ICG angiography. Therefore, 87% × 29% or 25% of all eyes with exudative maculopathy may be treated by ICG-guided laser photocoagulation. With a success rate of 35%, this means that an additional 9% of patients can be successfully treated using ICG-guided laser photocoagulation. Although this figure significantly increases the 6.5% of patients successfully treated by fluorescein-guided laser photocoagulation, there are still 84.5% of patients who continue to be untreatable or are unsuccessfully treated by thermal laser photocoagulation of the CNV (52).

Lim et al. reported on the visual acuity outcome after ICG angiography-guided laser photocoagulation of choroidal neovascularization associated with pigment epithelial detachment in 20 eyes with age-related macular degeneration. At 3 months after laser photocoagulation, visual acuity had improved two or more Snellen lines in two eyes (10%), worsened by two or more lines in 10 (50%), and remained unchanged in eight of 20 (40%). At 9 months after laser photocoagulation, visual acuity had improved by two or more lines in one eye (9%), worsened by two or more lines in nine (82%), and remained unchanged in one of 11 (9%). Lim et al. concluded that ICG-guided laser photocoagulation may temporarily stabilize visual acuity in some eyes with choroidal neovascularization associated with pigment epithelial detachments, but final visual acuity decreases with time (53).

XI. RECURRENT OCCULT CHOROIDAL NEOVASCULARIZATION

Recurrent CNV following photocoagulation treatment is a major cause of failure of laser therapy. Although most recurrences can be detected and imaged with clinical biomicroscopic examination and FA, a significant number of patients demonstrate new ex-

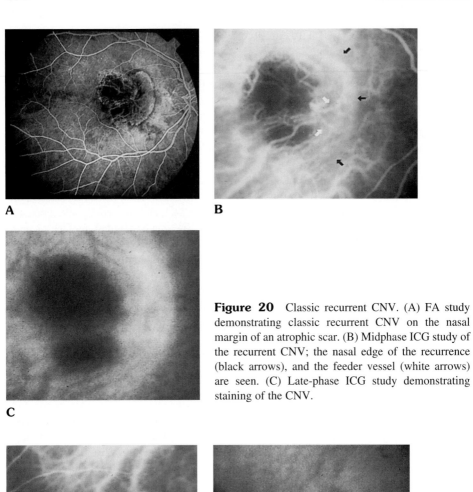

Figure 20 Classic recurrent CNV. (A) FA study demonstrating classic recurrent CNV on the nasal margin of an atrophic scar. (B) Midphase ICG study of the recurrent CNV; the nasal edge of the recurrence (black arrows), and the feeder vessel (white arrows) are seen. (C) Late-phase ICG study demonstrating staining of the CNV.

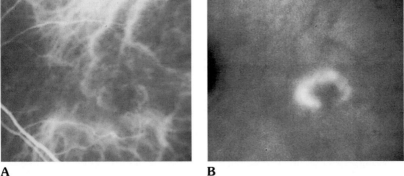

Figure 21 Occult recurrent CNV. (A) Early ICG study demonstrating well-defined hyperfluorescence from recurrent CNV surrounding the photocoagulation site. (B) Late-phase ICG study demonstrating staining and leakage from the area of recurrent CNV.

udative manifestation and visual symptoms without a clearly defined area of recurrent neovascularization identified by FA. These patients may exhibit diffuse staining and leakage at the site of previous treatment or may demonstrate no FA evidence of recurrence despite the new exudative manifestations identified clinically. ICG angiography has often proven to be useful in detecting the recurrent CNV (Figs. 20–30).

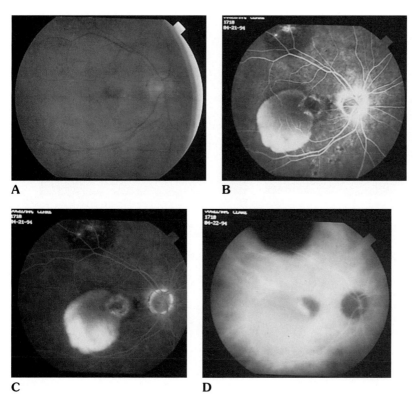

Figure 22 Occult recurrent CNV. (A) Clinical photograph demonstrating a serosanguinous PED at the temporal margin of a laser photocoagulation scar. A choroidal nevus is partially visible superotemporally. (B) Midphase FA study demonstrating hyperfluorescence of the PED and a halo of hyperfluorescence surrounding the photocoagulation scar. (C) Late-phase FA demonstrating further pooling of dye in the sub-RPE space and increased hyperfluorescent halo around the laser photocoagulation scar. (D) Late-phase ICG study revealing the presence of a hot spot of recurrent CNV at the temporal margin of the laser scar. The PED is hypofluorescent. See also color insert, Fig. 7.22A.

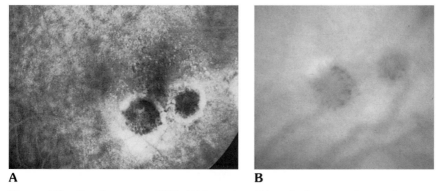

Figure 23 Occult recurrent CNV. (A) Late-phase FA study demonstrating occult recurrent CNV. There is diffuse staining surrounding two previous photocoagulation scars in a patient with recurrence 6 weeks after laser treatment. (B) Late-phase ICG study demonstrating localized hyperfluorescence along the superotemporal margin of one of the previous treatment sites consistent with a localized, well-defined, area of recurrent CNV.

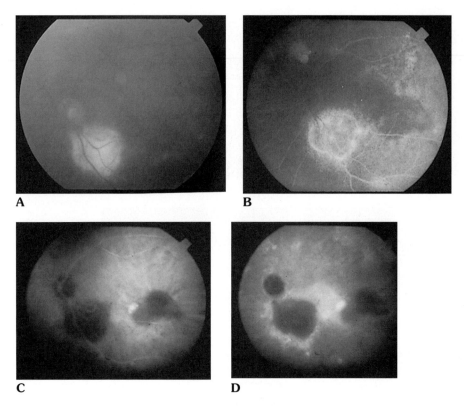

A   B   C   D

Figure 24 Occult recurrent CNV. (A) Clinical photograph demonstrating an exudative macular detachment following two previous laser treatments for CNV—one inferonasally and one inferotemporally to the fovea. (B) FA study revealing staining of the atrophic photocoagulation scar in the inferonasal macula. (C) Midphase ICG study demonstrating a hot spot of recurrent active CNV adjacent to the temporal photocoagulation scar. (D) Late-phase ICG study demonstrating widespread hyperfluorescence bridging and surrounding the previous photocoagulation sites, representing a large plaque of occult CNV. This plaque serves to explain the multiple recurrences. See also color insert, Fig. 7.24A.

Sorenson et al. reported on ICG-guided laser treatment of recurrent occult CNV secondary to AMD. Of 66 eyes that entered in the study, only 29 (44%) were eligible for laser treatment, and of these 29 eyes 18 (62%) had anatomical success with an average follow-up of 6 months (54). Interestingly, 56% of the patients remained untreatable by ICG angiography guidance, and even with treatment, 11 of 29 patients had incomplete resolution or worsening of the exudative manifestations.

XII. IDIOPATHIC POLYPOIDAL CHOROIDAL VASCULOPATHY

Idiopathic polypoidal choroidal vasculopatby (IPCV) is a primary abnormality of the choroidal circulation characterized by an inner choroidal vascular network of vessels end-

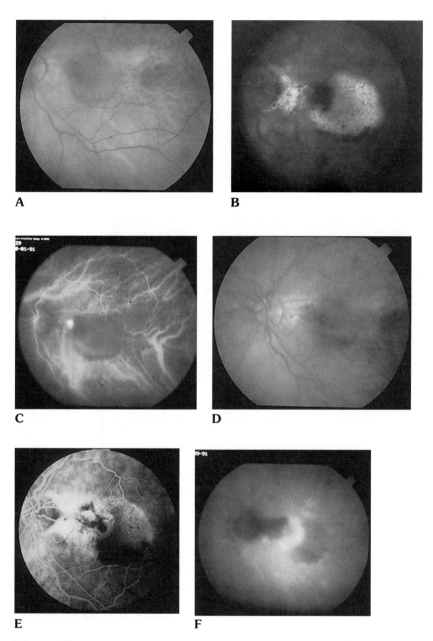

Figure 25 Occult recurrent CNV with serous PED. (A) Clinical photograph demonstrating a serosanguineous PED in the central macula. (B) Late-phase FA study demonstrating a serous PED. There is evidence of occult CNV in the papillomacular bundle. (C) Early-phase ICG study demonstrating a focal hot spot of CNV at the nasal margin of the PED. (D) Clinical photograph after treatment demonstrating a serosanguineous PED and exudative macular detachment. (E) Late-phase FA study demonstrating hyperfluorescence of the serous component of the PED and blocked fluorescence of the hemorrhagic component of the PED. There is also ill-defined hyperfluorescence around the treatment scar. (F) Late-phase ICG study demonstrating recurrence of the CNV at the temporal edge of the treatment scar in the papillomacular bundle. See also color insert, Fig. 7.25A, D.

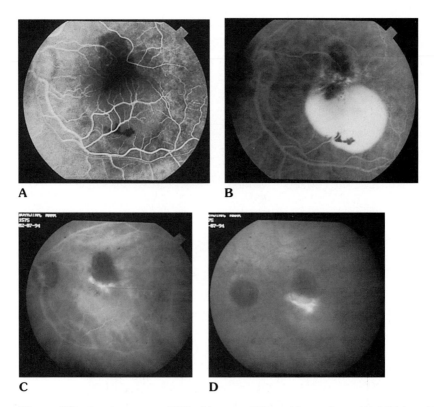

Figure 26 Occult recurrent CNV with serous PED and hemorrhage. (A) Midphase FA study in a patient with recurrent CNV demonstrating early filling of the serous component of a PED and blocked fluorescence by subretinal hemorrhage. (B) Late-phase FA study demonstrating intense hyperfluorescence of the serous PED. The previous treatment site appears hypofluorescent superiorly. No clear area of recurrent CNV is identified. (C) Midphase ICG study demonstrating a well-defined area of recurrent CNV at the inferior edge of the treatment scar. (D) Late-phase ICG study demonstrating leakage of the recurrent CNV in the serous PED.

ing in an aneurysmal bulge or outward projection, visible clinically as a reddish-orange, spheroid, polyp-like structure. The disorder is associated with multiple, recurrent serosanguineous detachments of the RPE and neurosensory retina, secondary to leakage and bleeding from the peculiar choroidal vascular abnormality (55–58).

ICG angiography has been used to detect and characterize the IPCV abnormality with enhanced sensitivity and specificity (Figs. 31, 32) (58–60). In the initial phases of the ICG study, a distinct network of vessels within the choroid becomes visible. In patients with juxtapapillary involvement, the vascular channels extend in a radial, arching pattern and are interconnected with smaller spanning branches that become more evident and numerous at the edge of the IPCV lesion.

Early in the course of the ICG study, the larger vessels of IPCV network start to fill before the retinal vessels, but the area within and surrounding the network is relatively hypofluorescent compared with the uninvolved choroid. The vessels of the network appear to fill more slowly than the retinal vessels. Shortly after the network can be identified on the ICG angiogram, small hyperfluorescent "polyps" become visible within the choroid.

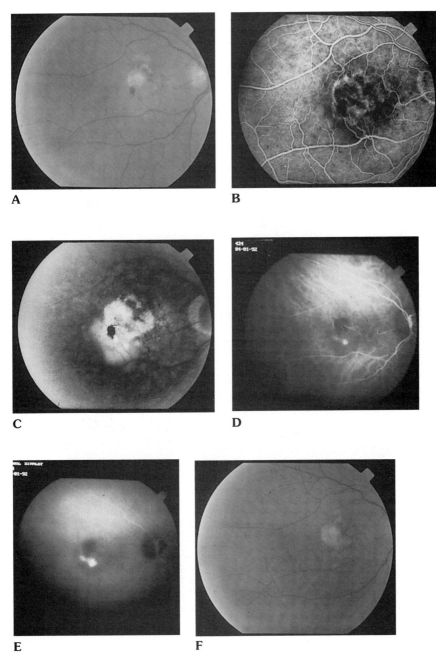

Figure 27 Treatment of recurrent occult CNV with hemorrhage. (A) Clinical photograph of a case of recurrent CNV 4 years after laser treatment. Note the presence of subretinal hemorrhage and neurosensory detachment. (B) Early-phase FA study demonstrating irregular hyperfluorescence surrounding the treatment scar. No classic CNV is seen. (C) Late-phase FA study demonstrating diffuse leakage in the neurosensory detachment. (D) Early-phase ICG study clearly demonstrating the recurrent CNV at the inferior edge of the treatment scar. (E) Midphase ICG study demonstrating leakage of the CNV. (F) Clinical photograph 6 weeks after ICG-guided laser treatment. There is complete resolution of the neurosensory detachment.

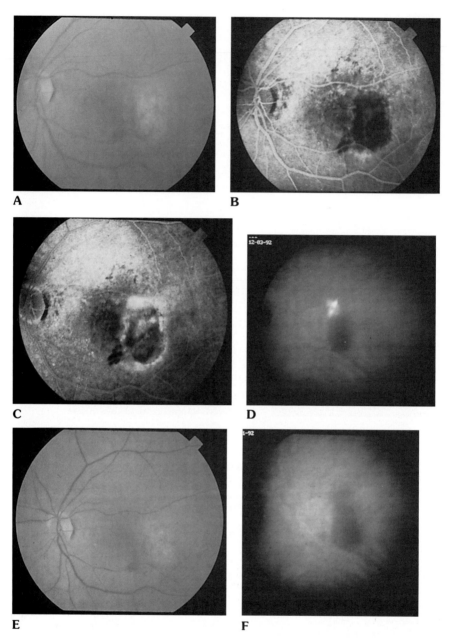

Figure 28 Treatment of recurrent occult CNV with hemorrhage. (A) Clinical photograph of recurrent CNV 6 months after laser treatment. There is a temporal chorioretinal scar and a recurrent serosanguineous retinal detachment. (B) Early-phase FA study demonstrating ill-defined hyperfluorescence around the laser scar. (C) Late-phase FA study demonstrating leakage and staining along the margin of the previous treatment site. No classic recurrent CNV is identified. (D) Late-phase IVG study demonstrating a hot spot of recurrent CNV at the superonasal edge of the treatment scar. An area of mild hyperfluorescence nasal to the chorioretinal scar may represent a plaque of occult CNV. (E) Clinical photograph 3 weeks after laser treatment demonstrating reduction of the neurosensory detachment. (F) Late-phase IVG study demonstrating complete obliteration of the recurrent CNV. The plaque of dormant CNV is unchanged. See also color insert, Fig. 7.28A, E.

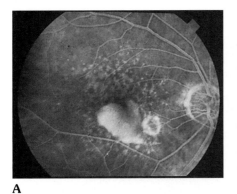

A

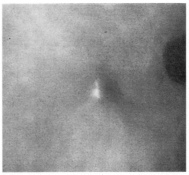

B

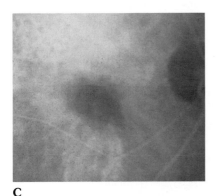

Figure 29 Treatment of recurrent occult CNV with serous PED. (A) Late-phase FA study of recurrent occult CNV 18 months after laser treatment. There is evidence of a serous PED. No well-defined recurrent CNV is noted. (B) Late-phase ICG study demonstrating hot spot of well-defined recurrent CNV nasal to the treatment scar. (C) Late-phase ICG study 6 weeks after laser treatment demonstrating resolution of the active CNV and of the serous PED after ICG-guide laser treatment.

C

These polypoidal structures correspond to the reddish-orange choroidal excrescence seen on clinical examination. They appear to leak slowly and the surrounding hypofluorescent area becomes increasingly hyperfluorescent. In the later phase of the angiogram there is a uniform disappearance of the dye ("washout") from the bulging polypoidal lesions. The late ICG staining characteristic of occult CNV is not seen in the IPCV vascular abnormality.

ICG angiography has also proven useful in recognizing cases of IPCV masquerading as CSR (61), and also in differentiating chronic cases of CSR from AMD (62–65). Spaide et al. demonstrated that in chronic CSR there is a characteristic hyperfluorescence of the choroidal vessels in the midphase of the ICG study, which disappear in the late phase of the study. This background hyperfluorescence in CSR has been attributed to hyperpermeability of the choroidal vasculature.

XIII. NEW TECHNIQUES IN ICG ANGIOGRAPHY

Recent advances in ICG angiography are real-time angiography (66), wide-angle angiography (66), digital subtraction ICG angiography (67), and dynamic ICG-guided feeder vessel laser treatment of CNV (68).

Real-time ICG angiography uses a modified Topcon 50IA camera with a diode laser illumination system that has an output at 805 nm (Topcon 501AL camera) that can produce images at 30 frames per second, and allows high-speed recording. The images can be acquired either as videotape, or as a single image at a frequency of 30 images per second. To

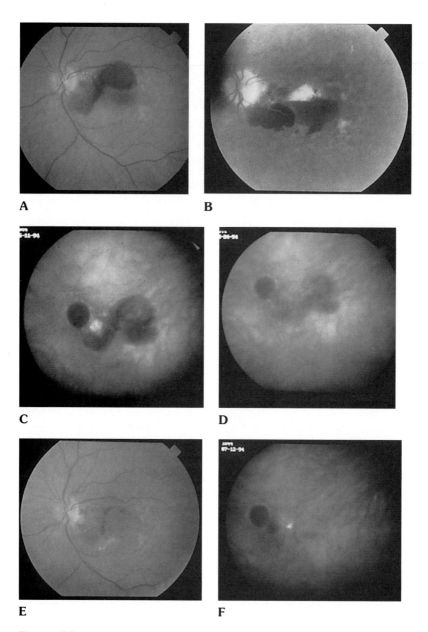

Figure 30 Treatment of recurrent occult CNV with serous PED. (A) Clinical photograph of a serosanguineous PED in a patient with AMD. (B) Late-phase FA study demonstrating blockage by the subretinal hemorrhage and leakage in the serous component of the PED. No well-defined CNV is identified. (C) Late-phase ICG study demonstrating a hot spot of well-defined CNV temporal to the optic disc. (D) Late-phase ICG study 2 weeks after laser treatment demonstrating hypofluorescence of the treatment site. (E) Clinical photograph 8 weeks after treatment demonstrating recurrence of the neurosensory macular detachment. (F) Late-phase ICG study demonstrating a hot spot of recurrent CNV just temporal to the previous laser treatment scar. See also color insert, Fig. 7.30A, E, G.

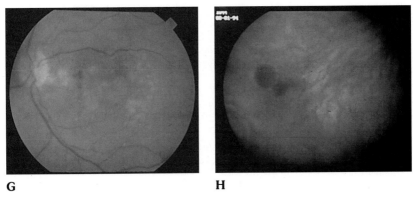

G   H

Figure 30 (cont.) (G) Clinical photograph 2 months after treatment of the recurrence demonstrating resolution of the neurosensory detachment. (H) Late-phase ICG study demonstrating complete elimination of the recurrent CNV.

make printed copies of these images, single frames are digitized, but the resolution is limited to 640 by 480 pixels.

Wide-angle images of the fundus can be obtained by performing ICG angiography with the aid of wide-angle contact lenses. The contact lenses used are the Volk SuperQuad 160, the Volk Quadraspheric, or the Volk Transequator (Volk, Mentor OH). Because the image formed by these lenses is located about 1 cm in front of the lens, the fundus camera is set on A or + so that the camera is focused on the image plane of the contact lens. This technique allows instantaneous imaging of a large area of the fundus. The combined usage of the contact lens and of the laser illumination system allows real-time imaging of a wide field of the choroidal circulation, up to 160 degrees of field of view (Figs. 33–36).

Digital subtraction ICG angiography (DS-ICGA) uses digital subtraction of sequentially acquired ICG angiographic frames to image the progression of the dye front in the choroidal circulation. A method of pseudocolor imaging of the choroid allows differentiation and identification of choroidal arteries and veins. DS-ICGA allows imaging of occult choroidal neovascularization (CNV) with greater detail and in a shorter period of time than with conventional ICG angiography.

Staurenghi et al. considered a series of 15 patients with subfoveal CNVM in whom feeder vessels (FVs) could be clearly detected by means of dynamic ICG angiography but not necessarily with FA. On the basis of the indications of the pilot study, the authors also studied a second series of 16 patients with FVs smaller than 85 microns. Treatment of FV using argon green laser was performed. The ICGA was performed immediately after treatment, after 2, 7, and 30 days, and then every 3 months, to assess FV closure. If a FV appeared to be still patent, it was immediately retreated and the follow-up was started again. The follow-up time ranged from 23 to 34 months for the pilot study and from 4 to 12 months for the second series. In the pilot study, the CNVM was obliterated after the first treatment in only one patient, five patients needed more than one treatment, and obliteration failed in nine patients (40% success rate). The rate of success was affected by the width and number of the FVs. The success rate in the second series of 16 patients was higher (75%). The authors concluded that dynamic ICGA may detect smaller FVs and makes it possible to control the laser effect and initiate immediate retreatment in the case of incomplete FV closure and should be considered mandatory for this type of treatment (68).

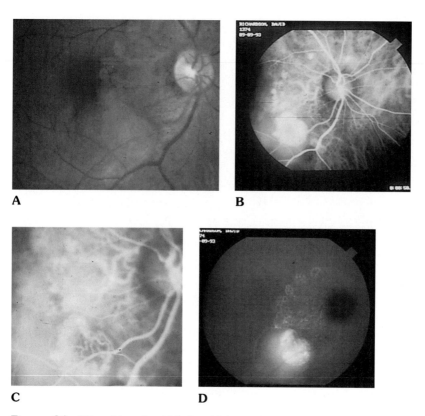

Figure 31 Idiopathic polypoidal choroidal vasculopathy. (A) Clinical photograph of a patient with idiopathic polypoidal choroidal vasculopathy demonstrating a pattern of polypoidal-like dilation of the choroidal vasculature in the peripapillary area. A larger, bulging dilation is present inferiorly. (B) Early-phase ICG study of a patient with idiopathic polypoidal choroidal vasculopathy demonstrating the vascular network in the papillomacular bundle at the level of the inner choroid with polypoidal lesions at its temporal border. Inferiorly an elevated network of tortuous vessels appears to fill from this vascular network and extend anteriorly. (C) High-magnification early-phase ICG study better reveals the network of vessels in the inferior lesion extending anteriorly. (D) Late-phase ICG study showing ring-like staining of the polypoidal structure temporally. The larger lesion inferiorly has intense staining with leakage into the subRPE space. (Courtesy of Richard F. Spaide, MD, New York. From Yannuzzi LA, Flower RW, Slakter JS. Indocyanine Green Angiography. St. Louis: CV Mosby, 1997:332–333.) See also color insert, Fig. 7.31A.

XIV. SUMMARY

ICG videoangiography is a useful adjunctive technique to FA for the diagnosis of AMD. This is especially true in the presence of occult CNV. Furthermore, ICG allows better recognition of subtypes of occult CNV such as vascularized PED, hot spots, plaques, and RCA Preliminary studies suggest that ICG-guided laser photocoagulation may be beneficial in the treatment of CNV. Further research is necessary to improve our understanding of all the information obtained by ICG angiography. Real-time ICG angiography, wide-angle ICG angiography, and digital subtraction ICG angiography may improve our diagnostic ability in AMD.

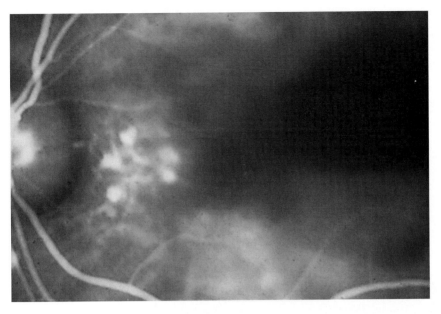

Figure 32 Idiopathic polypoidal choroidal vasculopathy. This patient presented with submacular hemorrhage. ICG angiography shows poly-like bulging of the inner choroidal circulation in the papillomacular bundle.

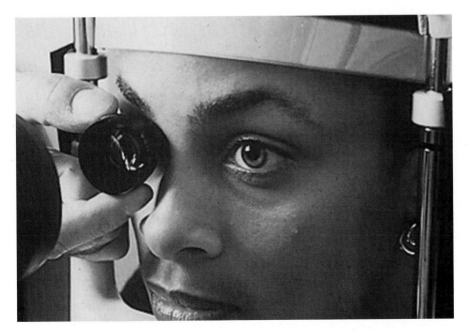

Figure 33 Wide-angle ICG angiography. A Volk SuperQuad 160-fundus lens is held in contact with the patient's eye to perform wide-angle ICG angiography of the fundus.

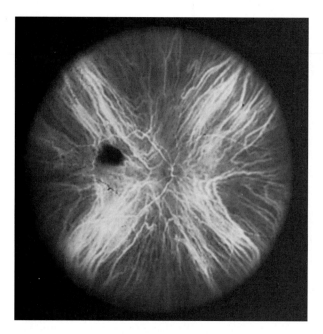

Figure 34 Wide-angle ICG angiography. Wide-angle ICG angiography picture of a patient with a choroidal nevus. Note the typical butterfly distribution of the choroidal circulation. (Courtesy of Richard F. Spaide, MD, New York. From Yannuzzi LA, Slakter JS, Flower RW. Indocyanine Green Angiography. St. Louis: CV Mosby, 1997.)

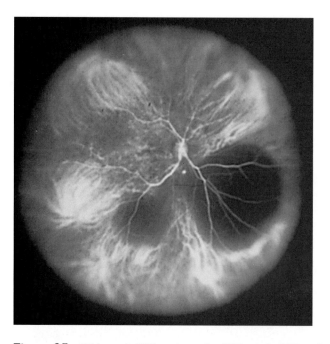

Figure 35 Wide-angle ICG angiography. Wide-angle ICG angiography picture of a patient with subretinal hemorrhage secondary to idiopathic polypoidal choroidal vasculopathy. The image shows 160 degrees of the fundus. (Courtesy of Richard F. Spaide, MD, New York, New York.)

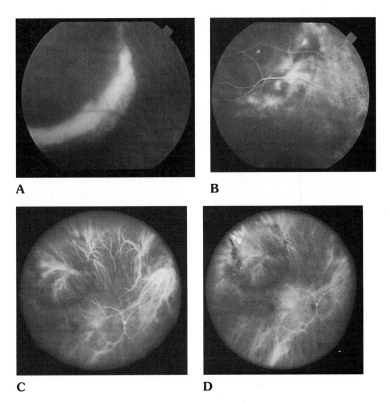

A   B

C   D

Figure 36 Wide-angle ICG angiography. Peripheral CNV. (A) Clinical photograph demonstrating a neurosensory detachment and subretinal exudates in the superotemporal fundus. (B) Late-phase FA study demonstrating ill-defined staining in the area of the subretinal exudates. (C) Early-phase wide-angle ICG study better demonstrating the area of exudative retinal detachment in the superotemporal fundus. The inferior edge of the detachment is hypofluorescent because of blockage by the exudates. (D) Late-phase ICG study demonstrating three focal hot spots of active CNV at the most peripheral margin of the neurosensory detachment. See also color insert, Fig. 7.36A.

ACKNOWLEDGMENT

This work was supported by the LuEsther T. Mertz Macula Foundation, New York, New York.

REFERENCES

1. Schatz HS, Burton T, Yannuzzi LA, Rabb MF. Interpretation of Fundus Fluorescein Angiography. St. Louis: Mosby-Year Book, 1978.
2. Yannuzzi LA, ed. Laser Photocoagulation of the Macula. Philadelphia: JB Lippincott, 1989.
3. Guyer DR, Puliafito CP, Mones JM, Friedman E, Chang W, Verdooner SR. Digital indocyanine green angiography in chorioretinal disorders. Ophthalmology 1992;99:287–290.
4. Yannuzzi LA, Slakter JS, Sorenso JS, Guyer DR, Orlock DA. Digital indocyanine green videoangiography and choroidal neovascularization, Retina 1992;12:191–223.
5. Geeraets WJ, Berry ER. Ocular spectral characteristics as related to hazards from lasers and other light sources. Am J Ophthalmol 1968;66:15–20.

6. Fox IJ, Wood EH. Application of dilution curves recorded from the right side of the heart or venous circulation with the aid of a new indicator dye. Proc Mayo Clin 1957;32:541.

7. Fox IJ, Wodd EH. Indocyanine green: physical and physiological properties Mayo Clin Proc 1960;35:732.

8. Kogure K, David NJ, Yamanouchi U, Choromokos E. Infrared absorption angiography of the fundus circulation. Arch Ophthalmol 1970;83:209–214.

9. David NJ. Infrared absorption fundus angiography. In: Proceedings of International Symposium on Fluorescein Angiography, Albi, France, 1969. Basel: Karger, 1971:189–192.

10. Hochheimer BF. Angiography of the retina with indocyanine green. Arch Ophthalmol 1971;86:564–565.

11. Flower RW. Infrared absorption angiography of the choroid and some observations on the effects of high intraocular pressures, Am J Ophthalmol 1972;74:600–614.

12. Flower, RW, Hochheimer BF. Clinical infrared absorption angiography of the choroid (letter). Am J Ophthalmol 1972;73:458–459.

13. Flower RW, Hochheimer BF. A clinical technique and apparatus for simultaneous angiography of the separate retinal and choroidal circulation. Invest Ophthalmol 1973;12:248–261.

14. Flower RW, Hochheimer BF. Indocyanine green dye fluorescence and infrared absorption choroidal angiography performed simultaneously with fluorescein angiography. Johns Hopkins Med J 1976;138:3–42.

15. Hyvarinen L, Flower RW. Indocyanine green fluorescent angiography. Arch Ophthalmol 1980;58:528–538.

16. Bischoff PM, Flower RW. Ten Years experience with choroidal angiography using indocyanine green dye: a new routine examination or an epilogue? Doc Ophthalmol 1985;60:235–291.

17. Hayashi K, DeLaey JJ. Indocyanine green angiography of neovascular membranes. Ophthalmologica 1985;190:30–39.

18. Hayashi K, Hasegawa Y, Tazawa Y, Delaey JJ. Clinical application of indocyanine angiography to choroidal neovascularization. Jpn J Clin Ophthalmol 1989;33:57–68.

19. Hayashi K, Hasegawa Y, Tokoro T. Indocyanine green angiography of central serous chorioretinopathy. Int Ophthalmol 1986;9:37–41.

20. Hayashi K, Hasegawa Y, Tokora T, Delaey JJ. Value of indocyanine green angiography in the diagnosis of occult choroidal neovascular membrane. Jpn J Clin Ophthalmol 1988;42:827–829.

21. Destro M, Puliafito CA. Indocyanine green videoangiography of choroidal neovascularization. Ophthalmology 1988;96:846–853.

22. Scheider A, Schroedel C. High resolution indocyanine green angiography with scanning laser ophthalmoscope. Am J Ophthalmol 1989;108:458–459.

23. Patz A, Flower RW, Klein ML, Orth DH, Fleishman JA, MacLeod D. Clinical applications of indocyanine green angiography. Doc Ophthalmol Proc Series 1976;9:245–251.

24. Cherrick GR, Stein SW, Leevy CM, et el. Indocyanine green: observations on its physical properties, plasma decay, and hepatic extraction. J Clin Invest 1960;39:592.

25. Baker KJ. Binding of sulfobromophthalein (BSP) sodium and indocyanine green (ICG) by plasma al-lipoproteins. Proc Soc Exp Biol Med 1966;122:957.

26. Goresky CA. Initial distribution and rate of uptake of sulfobromophthalein in the liver. Am J Physiol 1964;207:13.

27. Leevy CM, Bender J, Silverberg M, et al. Physiology of dye extraction by the liver: comparative studies of sulfobromophthalein and indocyanine green. Ann NY Acad Sci 1963;111:161.

28. Ketterer SG, Wiengand BD. The excretion of indocyanine green and its use in the estimation of hepatic blood flow. Clin Res 1959;7:71.

29. Ketterer SG, Wiengand BD. Hepatic clearance of indocyanine green. Clin Res 1959;7:289.

30. Probst P, Paumgartner G, Caucig H, Frauohlich H, Grabner G. Studies on clearance and placental transfer of indocyanine green during labotn. Clin Chim Acta 1970;29:157.

31. Leevy CM, Smith F, Kierman T. Liver function test. In: Bockus HL, ed. Gastroenterology, 3rd ed. Vol 3. Philadelphia: WB Saunders, 1976:68.

32. Shabetai R, Adolph RJ. Principles of cardiac catheterization. In: Fowler NO, ed. Cardiac Diagnosis and Treatment, 3rd ed. Hagerstown, MD: Harper & Row, 1980:117.

33. Hope Ross M., Yannuzzi LA, Gragoudas ES, et al. Adverse reactions due to indocyanine green. Ophthalmology 1994;101:529–533.

34. Olsen TW, Lim JI, Capone A, Myles RA, Gilman JP. Anaphylactic shock following indocyanine green angiography. Arch Ophthalmol 1996;114:97.

35. Macular Photocoagulation Study Group. Occult choroidal neovascularization: influence on visual outcome in patients with age-related macular degeneration. Arch Ophthalmol 1996;114:400–412.

36. Schwartz S,Guyer DR, Yannuzzi LA, et al. Indocyanine green videoangiography guided laser photocoagulation of primary occult choroidal neovascularization in age-related macular degeneration. Invest Ophthalmol Vis Sci 1995;36:186.

37. Slakter JS, Yannuzzi LA, Scheider U, Sorenson JA, Ciardella AP, Guyer DR, Spaide RF, Freund KB, Orlock DA. Retinal choroidal anastomosis and occult choroidal neovascularization. Ophthalmology 2000;107:742–753.

38. Kuhn D, Meunier I, Soubrane G, Coca G. Imaging of chorioretinal anastomoses in vascularized retinal pigment epithelium detachments. Arch Ophthalmol 1995;113:1392–1396.

39. Lafaut B A, Aisenbrey S, Vanden Broecke C, Bartz-Schmidt KU. Clinicopathological correlation of deep retinal vascular complex in age related macular degeneration. Br J Ophthalmol 2000;84:1269–1274.

40. Scheider A, Kaboth A, Neuhasuer L. Detection of subretinal neovascularization membranes with indocyanine green and infrared scanning laser ophthalmoscope, Am J Ophthalmol 1992;113:45–51.

41. Lim JI, Stenberg P, Capone A, Aaberg TM, Gilman JP. Selective use of indocyanine green angiography for occult choroidal neovascularization. Am J Ophthalmol 1995;120:75–82.

42. Yannuzzi LA, Hope-Ross M, Slakter JS, et al. Analysis of vascularized pigment epithelium detachments using indocyanine green videoangiography. Retina 1994;14:99–113.

43. Guyer DR, Yannuzzi LA, Slakter JS, et al. Digital indocyanine-green videoangiography of occult choroidal neovascularization. Ophthalmology 1994;101:1727–1737.

44. Guyer DR, Yannuzzi LA, Slakter JS, et al. Classification of choroidal neovascularization by digital indocyanine green videoangiography. Ophthalmology 1996;103:2054–2060.

45. Chang B, Yannuzzi LA, Ladas ID, et al. Choroidal neovascularization in second eyes of patients with unilateral exudative age-related macular degeneration. Ophthalmology 1995;102:1380–1386.

46. Lee BL, Lim JI, Grossniklaus HE. Clinicopathologic features of indocyanine green angiography-imaged, surgically excised choroidal neovascular membranes. Retina 1996;16:64–69.

47. Chang TS, Freund KB, de la Cruz Z, et al. Clinicopathologic correlation of choroidal neovascularization demonstrated by indocyanine green angiography in a patient with retention of good vision for almost four years. Retina 1994;14:114–24.

48. Guyer DR, Yannuzzi LA, Ladas I, et al. Indocyanine green guided laser photocoagulation of focal spots at the edge of plaques of choroidal neovascularization: a pilot study. Arch Ophthalmol 1996;114:693–697.

49. Slakter, JS, Yannuzzi, LA, Sorenson, JA, et al. A pilot study of indocyanine green videoangiography-guided laser photocoagulation of occult choroidal neovascularization in age-related macular degeneration. Arch Ophthalmol 1994;112:465–472.

50. Regillo SD, Benson WE, Maguire JI, et al. Indocyanine green angiography and occult choroidal neovascularization. Ophthalmology 1994;101:280–288.

51. Freund KB, Yannuzzi LA, Sorenson JA, et al. Age-related macular degeneration and choroidal neovascularization. Am J Ophthalmol 1993;115:786–791.

52. Mandava N, Guyer DR, Yannuzzi LA, et al. Indocyanine green videoangiography-guided laser photocoagulation of occult choroidal neovascularization. Ophthal Surg Lasers 1997;28:844–852.

53. Lim JI, Aaberg TM, Sr, Capone A, Jr, Stemberg P Jr. Indocyanine green angiography-guided photocoagulation of choroidal neovascularization associated with retinal pigment epithelial detachment. Am J Ophthalmol 1997;123:524–532.

54. Sorenson JA, Yannuzzi LA, Slakter JS, et al. A pilot study of digital indocyanine green videoangiography for recurrent occult choroidal neovascularization in age-related macular degeneration. Arch Ophthalmol 1994;112:473–479.

55. Kleiner RC, Brucker AJ, Johnston RL. The posterior uveal bleeding syndrome. Ophthalmology 1984;91 (Suppl 9):110.

56. Kleiner RC, Brucker AJ, Johnston RL. The posterior uveal bleeding syndrome. Retina 1990;10:9–17.

57. Yannuzzi LA, Sorenson JS, Spaide RF, et al. Idiopathic polypoidal choroidal vasculopathy. Retina 1990;10:1–8.

58. Yannuzzi LA, Ciardella AP, Spaide RF, et al. The expanding clinical spectrum of idiopathic polypoidal choroidal vasculopathy. Arch Ophthalmol 1999;115:478–485.

59. Ross RD, Gitter KA, Cohen G, et al. Idiopathic polypoidal choroidal vasculopathy associated with retinal arterial macroaneurysm and hypertensive retinopathy. Retina 1996;16:111.

60. Spaide RF, Yannuzzi LA, Slakter JS, et al. Indocyanine green videoangiography of idiopathic polypoidal choroidal vasculopathy. Retina 1995;15:100–110.

61. Yannuzzi LA, Freund KB, Goldbaum M, Scassellati-Sforzolini B, Guyer DR, Spaide RF, Maberley D, Wong DW, Slakter JS, Sorenson JA, Fisher YL, Orlock DA. Polypoidal choroidal vasculopathy masquerading as central serous chorioretinopathy. Ophthalmology 2000;107:767–777.

62. Spaide RF, Hall L, Haas A, et al. Indocyanine green videoangiography of older patients with central serous chorioretinopathy. Retina 1996;16:203–213.

63. Spaide RF, Campeas L, Haas A, et al. Central serous chorioretinopathy in younger and older adults. Ophthalmology 1996;103:2070–2080.

64. Guyer DR, Yannuzzi LA, Slakter JS, et al. Digital indocyanine green videoangiography of central serous chorioretinopathy. Arch Ophthalmol 1994;112:1057–1062.

65. Piccolino FC, Borgia L, Zinicola E, et al. Indocyanine green angiographic findings in central serous chorioretinopathy. Eye 1995;9:324–332.

66. Spaide RF, Orlork DA Herrmann-Delamazure B, et al. Wide-angle indocyanine green angiography. Retina 1998;18:44–49.

67. Spaide RF, Orlock DA, Yannuzzi LA, et al. Digital subtraction indocyanine green angiography of occult choroidal neovascularization. Ophthalmology 1998;105:680–688.

68. Staurenghi G, Orzalesi N, La Capria A, Aschero M. Laser treatment of feeder vessels in subfoveal choroidal neovascular membranes: a revisitation using dynamic indocyanine green angiography. Ophthalmology 1998;105:2297–2305.

8

Optical Coherence Tomography for Age-Related Macular Degeneration

Mark J. Rivellese and Elias Reichel
New England Eye Center, Tufts University School of Medicine, Boston, Massachusetts

Adam Martidis
Wills Eye Hospital, Thomas Jefferson University School of Medicine, Philadelphia, Pennsylvania

I. INTRODUCTION

Optical coherence tomography (OCT) is a noninvasive imaging modality capable of producing micron-resolution cross-sectional images of biological tissues. Developed less than a decade ago, it has demonstrated utility as both a research and clinical diagnostic tool for diseases of the retina and vitreoretinal interface (1–4). OCT accurately represents specific structural characteristics of the retina and can provide objective anatomical measurements. The diagnostic information complements conventional imaging techniques such as fluorescein and indocyanine green angiography.

II. OVERVIEW

The mechanism of OCT is analogous to ultrasound B-mode imaging with several distinct advantages. The use of light instead of acoustic waves allows for spatial resolution in the 10–20-micron range, approximately 10 times higher than B-mode ultrasound. Traditional B-mode ultrasound using a sound wave frequency of 10 MHz yields spatial resolutions of approximately 150 microns. In addition, the use of light allows an image to be obtained noninvasively, without direct contact to the globe. Cross-sectional images can be obtained rapidly in approximately 2.5 s.

III. APPLICATION

OCT has a wide range of applications in ophthalmology, particularly for diseases of the macula. The technology has been used to study patients with epiretinal membranes, macular holes, central serous chorioretinopathy, diabetic retinopathy, age-related macular degeneration, and other disorders. A particularly useful application of OCT is in the

171

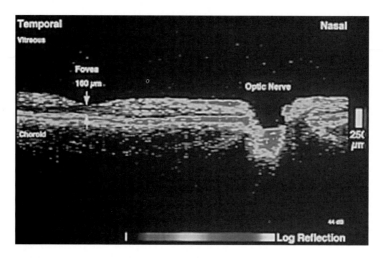

Figure 1   OCT of a normal eye through the optic nerve and fovea. See also color insert, Fig. 8.1.

localization, detection, and measurement of retinal fluid. A fluid collection is accurately depicted in its anatomical layer, may it be intraretinal, subretinal, or under the retinal pigment epithelium. OCT can provide clinically useful information about any retinal disease that manifests by changing macular thickness or accumulation of fluid in the macula. It also has utility in following response to treatments that alter macular structure.

IV.   OPTICAL COHERENCE TOMOGRAPHY INTERPRETATION

Interpretation of OCT images of ophthalmic disease such as age-related macular degeneration requires familiarity with the OCT representation of a normal posterior segment and knowledge of basic OCT principles.

The strength of the OCT signal at a particular tissue layer is dependent on several factors. Signal strength is defined by the following: the amount of incident light transmitted to a particular layer without being absorbed by intervening tissue, the amount of transmitted light that is backscattered, and the fraction of backscattered light that returns to the detector without being further attenuated. The reflectivity is the portion of incident light that is directly backscattered by a tissue. Therefore, the OCT signal from any particular tissue layer is a function of its reflectivity and the absorption and scattering properties of the overlying tissue layers (1). For example, a tissue with a high level of backscatter that lies deep to a tissue with low absorption and low backscatter will produce a high signal.

The signal strength can be represented in gray scale or as the false color representation used for the images that follow. Figure 1 shows an OCT image of a normal eye scanned through the optic nerve and fovea. The vitreoretinal interface is characterized by a demarcation in contrast from the nonreflective vitreous and the highly reflective nerve fiber layer (NFL). High backscatter is represented by red-orange color and low backscatter appears blue-black. False color is represented by the normal visible spectrum. The fovea has a characteristic depression with thinning of the retina corresponding to its normal anatomy.

A bright red-orange layer that delineates the posterior boundary of the retina corresponds to the retinal pigment epithelium (RPE) and choriocapillaris. Again, there is contrast between the less reflective photoreceptors and the highly backscattering RPE. The thin, dark layer anterior to the RPE layer represents the photoreceptor layer. Relatively weak backscatter returns from the choroid and appears green on the tomogram. The intermediate layers between the highly reflective NFL and RPE exhibit moderate backscatter and are represented on the false color scale as yellow-green.

V. NONEXUDATIVE MACULAR DEGENERATION

Cross-sectional imaging of eyes with nonexudative age-related macular degeneration (AMD) shows the characteristic appearance of drusen and geographic atrophy. Soft drusen cause a modulation in the highly reflective posterior boundary of the retina consistent with the accumulation of material within the RPE (Fig. 2). The small elevations of the RPE can appear similar to RPE detachments. Geographic atrophy shows thinning of the overlying retina and the hypopigmented RPE allows deeper penetration of the incident light into the choroid. The choroidal layer will have higher-than-normal backscatter owing to a decrease in signal absorption from the atrophic retina and RPE (Fig. 3).

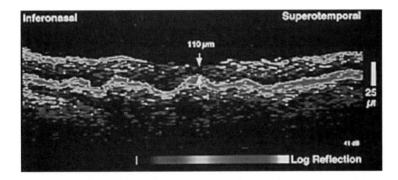

Figure 2 Soft drusen. See also color insert, Fig. 8.2.

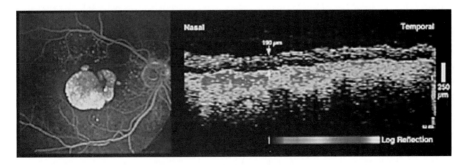

Figure 3 Geographic atrophy. See also color insert, Fig. 8.3.

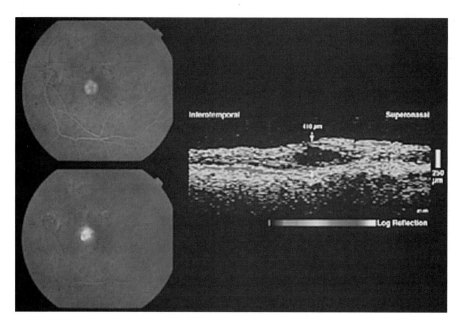

Figure 4   Retinal thickening. See also color insert, Fig. 8.4.

VI.   EXUDATIVE MACULAR DEGENERATION

Optical coherence tomograms of exudative macular degeneration may aid in the diagnosis and management of this condition. OCT is particularly valuable for detecting subretinal fluid and retinal pigment epithelial detachments, as well as changes in retinal thickness from intraretinal fluid. Measurements of retinal thickness provide an objective method of comparing retinal edema and subretinal fluid before and after intervention. There is some variability in the appearance of choroidal neovascularization on OCT. However, OCT may represent a new technique for visualizing angiographically occult choroidal neovascularization.

A.   Intraretinal and Subretinal Fluid

The presence of intraretinal fluid may be represented as retinal thickening or as the accumulation of fluid in well-defined spaces. (Fig. 4, 5). Intraretinal fluid in localized cysts (cystoid macular edema) appears as areas of discrete decreases in backscatter within the intermediate retinal layers, while diffuse edema will show an increase in thickness without definite spaces. Neurosensory detachments from the accumulation of subretinal, fluid appear in cross-section as elevations of the neurosensory retina above an optically clear space. The fluid space has well-defined boundaries at the fluid-retinal and fluid-RPE interfaces. In contrast to RPE detachments, the highly reflective RPE is imaged at the posterior border of the detachment (Fig. 6).

B.   Retinal Pigment Epithelial Detachments

It is possible to distinguish between serous and hemorrhagic retinal pigment epithelial detachments (PED) based on OCT images. Serous pigment epithelial detachments appear as

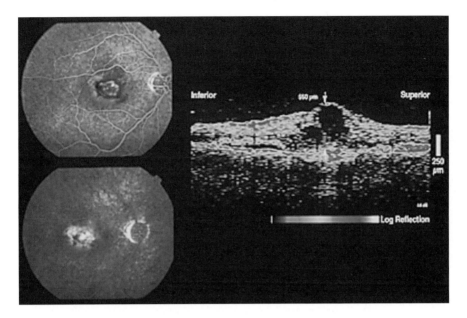

Figure 5 Cystoid macular edema secondary to choroidal neovascularization. See also color insert, Fig. 8.5.

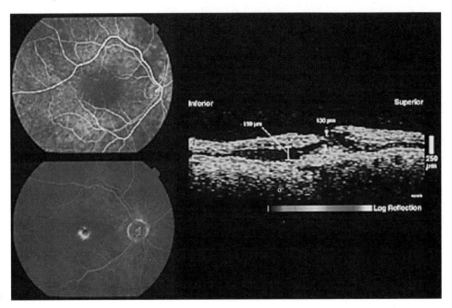

Figure 6 Neurosensory detachment secondary to subretinal fluid. See also color insert, Fig. 8.6.

dome-shaped elevations of the RPE with an elevated reflective band corresponding to the RPE. The intervening nonreflective layer is fluid in the sub-RPE space. The margins are sharp and there typically is shadowing of the reflections returning from the deeper choroid. This may be due to increased reflectivity and attenuation of the light through the decompensated RPE (Fig. 7). Hemorrhagic PEDs have a similar appearance. However, images of

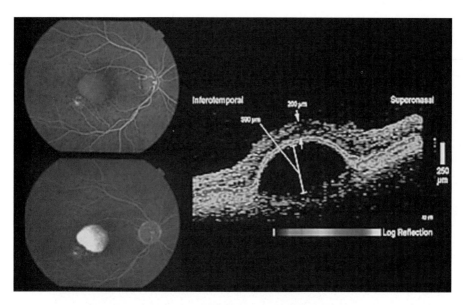

Figure 7   Serous retinal pigment epithelial detachment. See also color insert, Fig. 8.7.

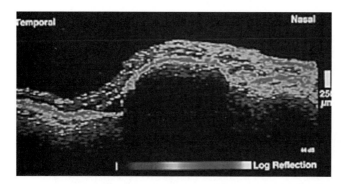

Figure 8   Hemorrhagic retinal pigment epithelial detachment. See also color insert, Fig. 8.8.

hemorrhagic detachments tend to show a band of high backscatter under the RPE band at the apex of the detachment (Fig. 8). This corresponds to the accumulated blood, decreasing light penetration, and attenuating choroidal reflection. Hemorrhagic PEDs and subretinal hemorrhages are sometimes difficult to distinguish on OCT because blood and the detached RPE have similar reflectivity.

C.   Choroidal Neovascularization

The presentation of choroidal neovascularization on OCT typically falls into one of three categories, but may show variability. Neovascular complexes that are angiographically well defined typically present as fusiform enlargement of the RPE/choriocapillaris reflective band with discrete borders (Fig. 9). Occasionally, the membrane may be imaged in the subretinal space (Fig. 10). Neovascular complexes that are poorly defined angiographically

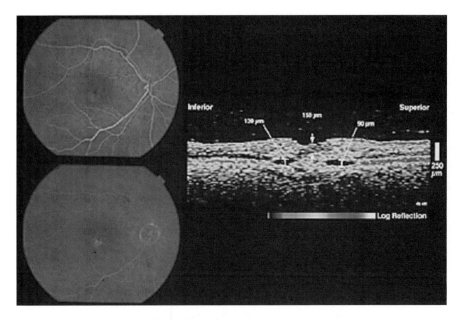

Figure 9 Well-defined choroidal neovascularization. See also color insert, Fig. 8.9.

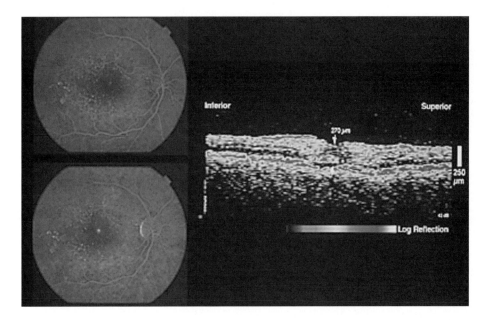

Figure 10 Choroidal neovascularization in the subretinal space. See also color insert, Fig. 8.10.

and fall into the category of occult fibrovascular PEDs display a well-defined elevation of the RPE reflective band with a mildly backscattering region below, corresponding to fibrous proliferation (Fig. 11). No shadowing of the choroidal reflection is present. Many choroidal neovascular complexes display enhanced choroidal reflection without a discrete

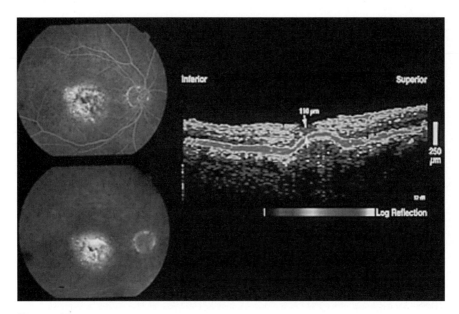

Figure 11   Fibrous pigment epithelial detachment. See also color insert, Fig. 8.11.

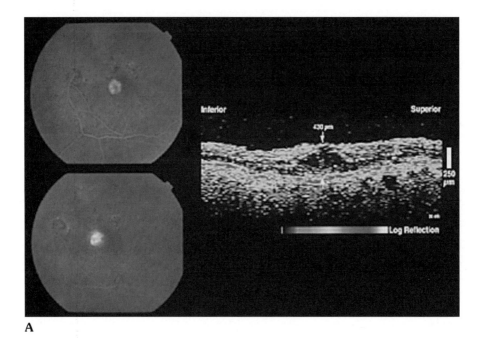

A

Figure 12   (A) Choroidal neovascularization before photodynamic therapy. (B) Same eye after photodynamic therapy. See also color insert, Fig. 8.12A, B.

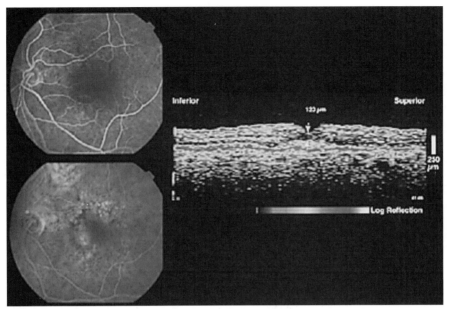

B

Figure 12 (cont.)

membrane. This may be due to increased optical penetration secondary to retinal pigment epithelial changes (1).

The ability to detect small changes in retinal thickness and the presence of fluid make OCT particularly useful for following patients after conventional laser treatment, photodynamic therapy, or transpupillary thermotherapy. Figure 12 shows a patient before and after treatment with verteporfin photodynamic therapy. Note the change in retinal thickness secondary to intraretinal fluid absorption.

VII. SUMMARY AND FUTURE DEVELOPMENT

OCT is a noninvasive imaging modality capable of providing accurate, reproducible images of the posterior segment. The retinal and RPE changes in age-related macular degeneration have a characteristic appearance on OCT. OCT is useful in detecting small changes in retinal thickness, subretinal and sub-RPE fluid, and choroidal neovascularization. It accurately localizes these processes and may provide an objective measurement. This is particularly useful in monitoring the response to therapeutic intervention in concert with conventional fluorescein and indocyanine green angiography.

REFERENCES

1.   Puliafito CA, Hee MR, Schuman JS, et al. Optical Coherence Tomography of Ocular Diseases. Thorofare, NJ: Slack, 1996.
2.   Hee MR, Puliafito CA, Duker JS, et al. Topography of diabetic macular edema with optical coherence tomography. Ophthalmology 1998;105:360–370.

3. Puliafito CA, Hee MR, Lin CP, et al. Imaging of macular diseases with optical coherence to-mography. Ophthalmology 1995;102:217–229.
4. Hee MR, Puliafito CA, Wong C, et al. Optical coherence tomography macular holes. Ophthal-mology 1995;102:748–756.
5. Hee MR, Baumal C, Puliafito CA, et al. Optical coherence tomography of age related macular degeneration and choroidal neovascularization. Ophthalmology 1996;103:1260–1270.

9

Laser Photocoagulation for Choroidal Neovascularization in Age-Related Macular Degeneration

Jonathan Yoken, Jacque L. Duncan, Jeffrey W. Berger, Joshua L. Dunaief, and Stuart L. Fine
Scheie Eye Institute, University of Pennsylvania Health System, Philadelphia, Pennsylvania

I. INTRODUCTION

Age-related macular degeneration (AMD) is the leading cause of blindness in developed countries (1), and choroidal neovascularization (CNV) is responsible for most of the severe visual loss (SVL) associated with AMD (2). Since the 1970s, laser photocoagulation had been recognized as a potentially beneficial treatment modality for CNV (3), and the initial report of the Macular Photocoagulation Study (MPS) Group (4) for the first time confirmed that argon laser photocoagulation of CNV guided by fluorescein angiography reduced the risk of SVL in AMD. In this chapter, the methodology and results of the MPS are reviewed and reinterpreted in light of the new data recently reported from the ongoing Photodynamic Therapy (PDT) trials (5). In addition, results generated from case series and trials of laser photocoagulation for CNV outside of the MPS are presented and discussed.

II. MACULAR PHOTOCOAGULATION STUDY

Prior to the MPS findings, "the prevailing notion was that nothing could be done to preserve the central vision once the exudative process was under way" (6). Patz and associates (3) first recommended that CNV > 125 microns from the foveal avascular zone (FAZ) edge be considered for laser treatment, based upon clinical experience and intuition, but no prospective, controlled trial had yet been performed nor was there a thorough understanding of treatment impact as a function of underlying disease process or size and location of CNV. The MPS, a prospective, randomized, multicenter clinical trial, initially set out to answer the question "does coagulating a leaking vessel (i.e., CNV) outside the fovea prevent significant loss of visual acuity?" (7). Subsequently, the MPS also addressed the visual outcomes of eyes receiving photocoagulation for new or recurrent juxtafoveal and subfoveal CNV.

A. MPS Eligibility Criteria, Methodology, and Outcome Measures

In the initial study of extrafoveal CNV (Fig. 1), patients in the AMD arm consented to have their study eye assigned to either observation or immediate argon laser treatment. Study eyes were required to have angiographic evidence of well-defined CNV 200–2500 microns from the center of FAZ, best-corrected visual acuity of 20/100 or better, CNV-related symptoms such as decreased acuity, metamorphopsia, or monocular diplopia, and drusen in either the study or the fellow eye (4,8). Also, the patient must have reached 50 years of age at the time of randomization. Exclusion criteria included a history of prior retinal photocoagulation, coexisting ocular disease potentially affecting visual acuity, and visual acuity worse than 20/400 (4,8). The subsequent studies evaluating treatment of juxtafoveal CNV required that the edge of the CNV be located 1–199 microns from the center of the FAZ or more than 200 microns from the FAZ if adjacent blood or pigment extended to within 200 microns. Eligible eyes were randomized to either observation or treatment with krypton red laser (9,10).

   The MPS also evaluated AMD patients with new and recurrent subfoveal CNV. Inclusion criteria for the New Subfoveal CNV Study required a fluorescein angiogram obtained less than 96 h before randomization, demonstrating CNV with well-demarcated borders, new vessels under the FAZ center, and a total lesion size < 3.5 MPS standard disk areas (1 MPS standard area = 1.77 mm²) with most of the lesion composed of classic or occult CNV. Best-corrected visual acuity at randomization was required to be in the range of 20/40–20/320 (11). In the Recurrent Subfoveal CNV Study, a fluorescein angiogram obtained < 96 h prior to randomization had to demonstrate either CNV under the FAZ center contiguous with a prior treatment scar or CNV within 150 microns of the FAZ center contiguous with a scar

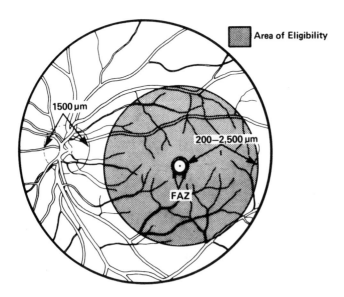

Figure 1   Eligibility for laser treatment in the extrafoveal studies. (Reproduced with permission from Macular Photocoagulation Study Group. Argon laser photocoagulation for neovascular maculopathy: three year results from randomized clinical trials. Arch Ophthalmol 1986;104: 694–701. Copyright 1986, American Medical Association.)

that had expanded under the FAZ center (12). Best-corrected visual acuity at randomization was required to be in the range of 20/40–20/320 (11). Additionally, following the proposed laser treatment, some portion of the retina within 1.5 mm from the center of FAZ would have to remain untreated. The total area occupied by prior and new treatment areas had to be < 6 MPS disk areas. Except for scar, most of the lesion had to be composed of CNV. Patients with prior treatment involving the center of the FAZ were excluded.

The primary outcome of the MPS comparing treated to observed eyes was SVL, defined as a loss of six or more lines of visual acuity (or a quadrupling of the visual angle). Visual acuity was measured in all studies. Critical reading print size was measured in the extrafoveal and juxtafoveal studies. Reading speed and contrast threshold were measured in the subfoveal studies. The rates of recurrent and persistent CNV in treated eyes and the incidence of new CNV in observed eyes were also reported. The standardized techniques utilized for measuring visual acuity, contrast threshold, and reading speed have been described previously (13).

B. MPS Laser Treatments, General Considerations

Photocoagulation of all neovascular lesions was performed according to a protocol standardized among the clinical centers depending on whether the lesion was extrafoveal, juxtafoveal, or subfoveal. The MPS protocol required retrobulbar anesthesia for all extrafoveal and juxtafoveal treatments. Retrobulbar anesthesia was recommended but not required for subfoveal treatments.

C. Extrafoveal Treatment

In the extrafoveal study, patients were treated with argon blue-green or green photocoagulation. The neovascular complex including contiguous blood was to be completely covered with laser burns sufficient to produce uniform retinal whitening. Noncontiguous 100-micron-diameter burns were used to outline the boundaries of the treatable lesion. Treatment for extrafoveal lesions was to extend 100–125 microns beyond the borders of the neovascular complex using overlapping 200- to 500-micron spots with 0.5-s exposures (Fig. 2). When treating within 350 microns of the FAZ center, 100-micron spots were used with 0.1- to 0.2-s-duration burns. Eyes with peripapillary CNV were also treated if treatment of the CNV would spare at least one and one-half clock hours of the peripapillary nerve-fiber layer, and no spots were delivered <200 microns from the edge of the optic nerve. Immediately following treatment, stereoscopic photographs were taken and compared to an intensity standard at the Fundus Photograph Reading Center (Fig. 3) (14). Angiograms taken at selected intervals following treatment were examined at the Reading Center for evidence of transit-phase hyperfluorescence that extended in later phases. This was considered either persistence (within 6 weeks of treatment) or recurrence (after 6 weeks) of CNV. Definite fluorescein leakage along the margins of the laser scar or at a second location mandated retreatment if the lesion remained extrafoveal, i.e., no closer than 200 microns from the center of the FAZ.

D. Juxtafoveal Treatment

When the initial MPS began, the wavelength most available to investigators was argon blue-green. However, since macular xanthophyll pigment absorbs blue light, it was be-

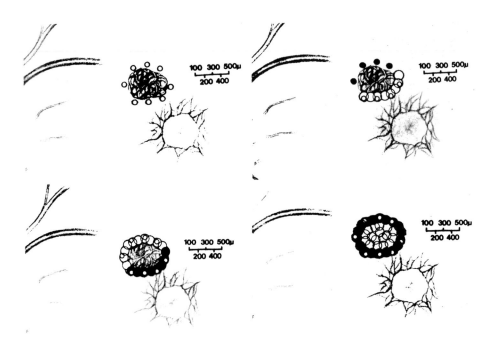

Figure 2   Schematic of protocol treatment. (A) Noncontiguous 100-micron burns are used to outline the choroidal neovascularization. (B) Foveal edge is treated with overlapping 200-micron 0.2-s burns. (C) Perimeter of the complex is treated with overlapping 200-micron 0.2-s burns. (D) Entire complex is treated with overlapping 200–500-micron 0.5-s burns. (Reproduced with permission from Macular Photocoagulation Study Group. Ocular histoplasmosis. Arch Ophthalmol 1983;101:1350. Copyright 1983, American Medical Association.)

lieved that this might contribute toward unintentional damage to the inner retina overlying an area of photocoagulation. When the MPS trials for treating juxtafoveal lesions were developed in 1981, investigators chose to use the krypton red laser to allow for better penetration through macular xanthophyll and thin layers of blood (15).

An angiogram less than 72 h old was required to guide the treatment of juxtafoveal lesions. The laser treatment was to extend for 100 microns beyond the border of the neo-vascular complex, except on the foveal side where treatment beyond the border of the lesion was not required unless the hyperfluorescence was greater than 100 microns from the center of the FAZ. Treatment of all areas of blood or blocked fluorescence associated with the CNV was not required (9).

E. Subfoveal Treatment

In this arm of the study, patients who were randomized to laser treatment were further randomized to either argon green or krypton red laser treatment. Intense photocoagulation burns had to extend for 100 microns beyond the borders of the lesion. For areas of the lesion covered by thick blood, the burns were to extend up to, but not beyond, the borders of the lesion. This part of the treatment protocol was applied to both the new and recurrent subfoveal CNV groups (11,12). Patients with recurrent subfoveal CNV required laser treatment to extend for 300 microns into the prior-treatment scar, and to obliterate any visible

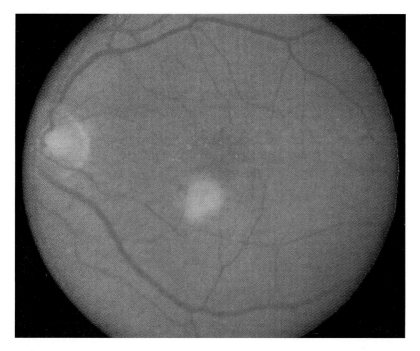

Figure 3 Treatment intensity standard. Posttreatment fundus photographs were compared with this photograph to determine compliance with treatment protocol. (Reproduced with permission from Macular Photocoagulation Study Group: Krypton laser photocoagulation for neovascular lesions of ocular histoplasmosis: results of a randomized clinical trial. Arch Ophthalmol 105:1499–1507, 1987. Copyright 1987, American Medical Association.) See also color insert, Fig. 9.3.

feeder vessel for 100 microns on either side of the vessel and for 300 microns beyond the vessel base (12).

III. SUMMARY OF MAJOR RESULTS OF THE MPS

A. Results of Extrafoveal CNV Treatment

Eighteen months into the study, enrollment of patients into the extrafoveal AMD arm of the MPS was terminated owing to an unequivocal treatment benefit: 60% of untreated eyes versus 25% of treated eyes developed SVL by 18 months (4). The treatment benefit persisted, and after 5 years of follow-up, 64% of untreated versus 46% of treated eyes had SVL (16). Recurrences of CNV were common, either independent or contiguous with the prior laser treatment, and were seen in 54% of treated eyes at 5 years (16). These recurrences were most common in the first year after treatment; 75% of all recurrences occurred in the first year. An association with smoking and likelihood of recurrence was noted in that 85% of patients who smoked more than 10 cigarettes per day versus 51% of nonsmokers suffered a recurrence (8). Patients who had recurrent CNV had a decreased average visual acuity, 20/250 as compared to 20/50 for those patients without recurrences (16) (Table 1).

Table 1   Outcome of CNV Treatment Secondary to AMD in the MPS, Risk of SVL

MPS AMD Study	1 year		2 year		3 year		5 year	
	Treated eyes	Control eyes	Treated eyes	Control eyes	Treated eyes	Control eyes	Treated eyes	Control eyes
Extrafoveal CNV(16)	24%	41%	33%[b]	51%[b]	45%	63%	46%	64%
Juxtafoveal CNV(10,18)	31%	45%	45%	54%	51%	61%	55% (54%)[c]	65% (72%)[c]
Subfoveal new CNV (20)	24% (20%)[a]	30% (11%)[a]	23%	39%	23%[d]	45%[d]		
Subfoveal recurrent CNV (20)	11%	29%	9%	28%	17%	39%		

[a] Three months
[b] Eighteen months (reflects 18-month data after 5 years of follow-up).
[c] Patients with classic CNV only.
[d] Four years.

B.   Results of Juxtafoveal CNV Treatment

For juxtafoveal CNV, at 3 years of follow-up 61% of untreated versus 51% of treated eyes had SVL. By 5 years of follow-up, 65% of untreated eyes versus 55% of treated eyes had developed SVL (10). The greatest treatment benefit was observed in treated patients without definite hypertension. Patients were defined as having definite hypertension if their systolic blood pressure was 160 mmHg or greater or their diastolic pressure was 95 mmHg or greater or they were currently taking antihypertensive medications. Seventy percent of untreated eyes versus 38% of treated eyes of patients without definite hypertension suffered SVL while no treatment benefit was observed in patients with definite hypertension (67% treated vs. 62% observed). Sixty-eight percent of eyes of untreated suspect hypertensive patients versus 55% of treated suspect hypertensive patients developed SVL. This outcome has not been observed in other MPS AMD studies, and therefore, it is still generally recommended to treat hypertensive patients otherwise meeting eligibility criteria. However, aspects of the MPS outcome data for hypertensives should be part of the informed consent process. Persistence and recurrence were again common, occurring 32% and 47% of the time 5 years, respectively (17). Not surprisingly, eyes without persistence or recurrence sustained better final visual acuity than those eyes that had persistence or recurrence (20/80–20/100 vs. 20/200–20/250). This relatively high level of persistence and recurrence was felt to be secondary to increased difficulty of treatment within the FAZ. Even though the investigators had a high level of proficiency in treating CNV with photocoagulation, reluctance to treat within the FAZ and decreased visibility of landmarks were thought to contribute to a 40% incomplete or inadequate treatment of lesions on the foveal side (17).

A subsequent publication from the MPS Fundus Photograph Reading Center outlined revised criteria for differentiating classic and occult CNV (18). This allowed for reevaluation of the juxtafoveal data previously reported (18). The greatest benefit at 5 years was observed in treated eyes with lesions composed purely of classic CNV. Fifty-four percent of treated eyes versus 72% of untreated eyes developed SVL, which was in part attributable to treatment adequacy. Classic-only and occult-only CNV lesions were completely covered by adequate photocoagulation in 89% and 35% of eyes, respectively. The classic CNV component of eyes with mixed CNV lesions was completely covered in 63% of these eyes as compared to less than 50% of the occult component being covered. No benefit was detected in treating the classic component of a combined lesion or part of an occult-only lesion (18).

C. Results of Subfoveal Treatment

The high rates of recurrent CNV that invovled the fovea seen in the juxtafoveal and extrafoveal studies motivated the MPS group to investigate the effects of laser treatment for subfoveal recurrent CNV (12). Eligible patients in this study had an average initial visual acuity of 20/125. By 3 and 24 months after enrollment, laser-treated eyes had maintained an average visual acuity of 20/250 while eyes assigned to observation had dropped to an average visual acuity of 20/200 by 3 months and 20/320 by 24 months. At 24 months of follow-up, 9% of treated eyes versus 28% of observed eyes had developed SVL. By 3 years, 17% of treated eyes versus 39% of observed eyes experienced SVL. Furthermore, treated eyes maintained a better average contrast threshold and average reading speed than observed eyes throughout the study period.

The MPS group also reported the results of laser treatment versus observation for new subfoveal CNV (19,20). In this arm, eyes that had well-defined subfoveal CNV no larger than 3.5 MPS disk areas were randomized to laser treatment with either argon green or krypton red wavelengths and compared to observation. At 3 months, the observed eyes fared better with only 11% experiencing SVL compared to 20% of treated eyes. However, by 24 months, 23% of treated eyes suffered SVL while the percentage of observed eyes with SVL had increased to 39%. Laser-treated eyes maintained contrast thresholds for large letters at or near baseline throughout the 3 years of follow-up while contrast sensitivity for observed eyes declined. After 5 years of follow-up, these treatment benefits persisted (20). Persistence or recurrence of CNV was seen in 51% of treated eyes by 24 months of follow-up, but interestingly this was not associated with a worse visual acuity (21). At 3 years of follow-up in the Subfoveal New CNV Study, eyes with persistence, eyes with recurrence, and eyes with neither persistence nor recurrence had mean visual acuities of 20/400, 20/250, and 20/320, respectively.

Throughout 5 years of follow-up, there was no significant difference in average loss of visual acuity or contrast sensitivity from baseline when comparing treatment with argon green or krypton red wavelengths (15). Also, there was no difference in the rates of recurrence or persistence of CNV. Small differences in average reading speed favored argon green treatment for recurrent subfoveal lesions, but since this parameter was markedly abnormal in both groups, its significance is uncertain.

The MPS investigators evaluated the influence of initial lesion size and visual acuity on visual outcome in the New Subfoveal CNV Study (22). Four patterns of clinical behavior were recognized and labeled A, B, C, and D (Fig. 4). All subgroups, except group D, that were treated suffered less SVL than observed eyes, but the treatment benefit was realized sooner for eyes with smaller lesions and worse initial visual acuity. Eyes with larger lesions but better initial visual acuity (group D) seemed to have no obvious treatment benefit (Fig. 5).

IV. LASER TREATMENT OUTSIDE THE MPS

Since most AMD lesions are not eligible for laser treatment guided by the MPS, and since treatment of subfoveal lesions results in immediate loss of central vision, recent efforts

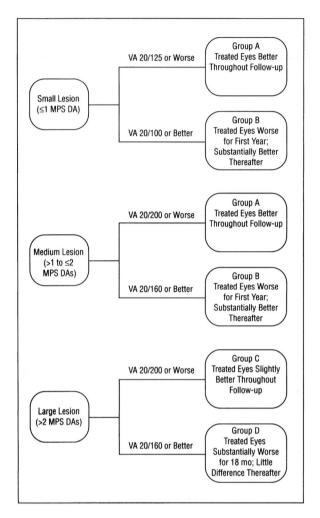

Figure 4 Schematic aid for determining the pattern of visual loss for eyes with subfoveal choroidal neovascularization. (Reproduced with permission from Macular Photocoagulation Study Group. Visual outcome after laser photocoagulation for subfoveal choroidal neovascularization secondary to age-related macular degeneration: the influence of initial lesion size and visual the acuity. Arch Ophthalmol 1994;112:480–488. Copyright 1994, American Medical Association.)

have been directed toward the development of prophylaxis strategies and more selective treatments for exudative AMD.

V. LASER TREATMENT OF OCCULT LESIONS

Initially, the MPS extrafoveal and juxtafoveal studies did not distinguish between occult and classic CNV. As discussed earlier, when a subsequent report from the MPS reading center was issued, reanalyzing all angiograms from the juxtafoveal study, it was determined that treated lesions composed of entirely classic CNV benefited most from laser

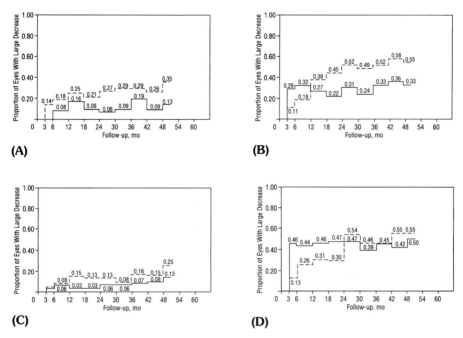

Figure 5   Proportion of eyes in groups (A), (B), (C), and (D) with a six- or more line decrease in visual acuity following subfoveal laser treatment. The solid and broken lines depict the treatment and no-treatment groups, respectively. (Reproduced with permission from Macular photocoagulation Study Group. Visual outcome after laser photocoagulation for subfoveal choroidal neovascularization secondary to age-related macular degeneration: the influence of initial lesion size and visual acuity. Arch Ophthalmol 1994;112:480–488. Copyright 1994, American Medical Association.)

treatment and had the lowest rates of SVL (18). Eyes that had both classic and occult components and received treatment only to the classic component or received variable coverage of the occult component fared no better than untreated eyes. The number of treated eyes with occult CNV only was too small to draw meaningful conclusions.

The natural history of occult CNV is variable, complicating interpretation of treatment studies, particularly those studies without controls (23). A retrospective study by Soubrane and co-workers (24) demonstrated no benefit for treatment of nonfoveal occult CNV. The study group consisted of 163 eyes, 77 treated and 79 observed, with initial visual acuity of 20/100 or better and angiographic evidence of occult CNV that spared the center of the FAZ by at least 100 microns. The treated patients received intense, confluent laser burns to the entire lesion as identified by fluorescein angiography plus an additional 100 microns sparing the center of the FAZ. At the end of follow-up (12– 84 months), SVL was demonstrated in 53% of treated eyes versus 40% of untreated eyes.

Some investigators have examined the use of laser treatment for AMD-associated pigment epithelial detachment (PED). These lesions were specifically excluded from the MPS because it was believed that the PED might limit the treating ophthalmologists' ability to treat the entire CNV complex, thereby increasing the chances for recurrence or persistence.

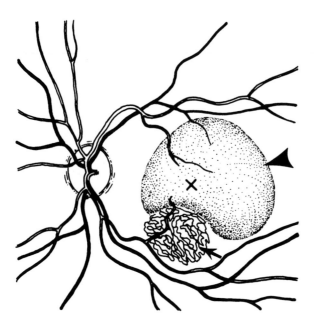

Figure 6 Choroidal neovascular membrane (arrow) with an adjacent subfoveal retinal pigment epithelial detachment (arrowhead). (Reprinted from Maguire JI, Benson WE, Brown GC. Treatment of foveal pigment epithelial detachments with contiguous extrafoveal choroidal neovascular membranes. Am J Ophthalmol 1990;109:523–529. Copyright 1990, with permission from Elsevier Science.)

The Moorfields Macular Study (25) demonstrated that argon blue-green grid photocoagulation to PEDs without clinical or angiographic evidence of CNV accelerated the loss of visual acuity. At 18 months, 73% of treated versus 41% of observed eyes had lost two lines of Snellen visual acuity. Geographic atrophy was also seen more frequently and earlier in treated eyes. The increased frequency of visual loss in the treated versus untreated eyes was sustained in a later report that included 4 years of follow-up (25).

Occasionally, PED is observed adjacent to CNV. Maguire et al. treated a small group of AMD patients (14 eyes) with foveal PEDs and adjacent extrafoveal CNV (Fig. 6) (26). These investigators treated only the adjacent extrafoveal CNV with laser photocoagulation. Closure of the CNV and subsequent collapse of the PED was observed in 8 of the 14 eyes treated (57%). Six of these eight eyes also had visual improvement at 6–64 months of follow-up. Although this was a small pilot study with no randomization or control group, the authors point to the poor natural history of these types of lesions as an incentive to consider treatment with photocoagulation (27–30). A prospective randomized study further evaluating this notion has not been performed.

VI. LASER TREATMENT OF SUBFOVEAL CNV, OUTSIDE MPS

Some investigators, in an effort to limit the immediate visually disturbing effects of photocoagulation of subfoveal lesions, have explored "foveal sparing" techniques. Coscas and

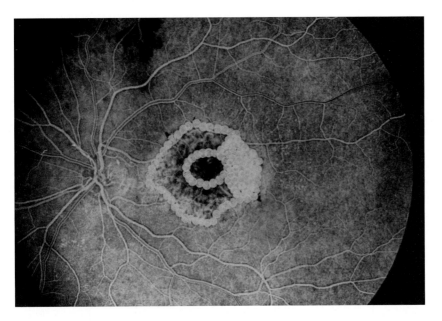

Figure 7 Treatment protocol for perifoveal laser treatment of subfoveal choroidal neovascular membrane. Protocol consists of confluent overlapping burns applied to the peripheral border of the neovascular membrane. Similar burns delineate the foveal avascular zone. The surface between these two limits is filled with laser photocoagulation. (Reproduced with permission from Coscas G, et al. Perifoveal laser treatment for subfoveal choroidal new vessels in age-related macular degeneration. Results of a randomized clinical trial. Arch Ophthalmol 1991;109:1258–1265. Copyright 1991, American Medical Association.)

associates (31) reported the largest series of patients treated with "annular" photocoagulation treatment for subfoveal CNV. In a prospective, randomized, controlled clinical trial, 160 patients with AMD and angiographic evidence of subfoveal CNV, either classic or occult, with or without a serous PED were randomized to either perifoveal laser treatment or observation. Visual acuity at presentation had to be in the range of 20/100–20/1000 without any prior history of laser treatment in the eligible eye. The treatment protocol required sparing of the central 400 microns of the FAZ and placement of confluent burns to the peripheral extent of the CNV lesion, or to the limits of any vascularized PED if present (Fig. 7). With more than 1 year of follow-up, visual acuity remained stable or improved in 41% of treated versus 20% of observed eyes. The authors further remarked that final results did not differ between those eyes that had well-defined versus occult CNV. Orth and co-workers (32) described a case series of three patients for whom this technique of annular photocoagulation provided dramatic visual improvement. The three patients described had the most favorable results of a larger group of 34 patients who were treated similarly. The three study patients varied from one another in that one had classic subfoveal CNV, one had recurrent subfoveal CNV, and one had a PED associated with subfoveal CNV. Their visual acuities improved from 20/100 to 20/40, 20/200 to 20/60, and 20/100 to 20/50 at 6 months, respectively. These three patients had complete resolution of exudation on fluorescein angiography as well. The authors of this report describe the other 31 patients treated with this technique typically as having visual acuity stabilization and a paracentral scotoma. This is a remarkable result when considering that typically patients who receive subfoveal photocoagulation develop a sudden decline in their visual acuity. Despite the potential promise of this technique, it has not gained widespread acceptance nor has it been studied with rigor.

Many small pilot studies and anecdotal reports initially indicated that there might be some benefit to the use of scatter ("grid") photocoagulation for subfoveal CNV (33–35). Tornambe et al. (33) conducted a small pilot study in which 40 eyes with well-demarcated subfoveal neovascularization secondary to AMD involving 100% of the FAZ were treated with either extrafoveal scatter alone (18 eyes) or scatter plus focal, confluent ablation of extrafoveal CNV (22 eyes). Scatter treatments were placed outside the area subtended by CNV. Fluorescein angiography and visual acuity were monitored at periodic intervals with average follow-up of 2.4 years (ranging from 1 to 4 years). The results indicated that 55% of all patients had persistent angiographic leakage, which included 56% of patients who received scatter alone and 55% of patients who received scatter plus focal ablation. At enrollment, 28% of eyes had a visual acuity of 20/80 or better and 80% had a visual acuity of 20/200 or better. At completion, 18% of eyes had 20/80 or better and 53% were 20/200 or better. Sixty percent of eyes attained the same or better visual acuity. There was no significant difference in final visual acuity between groups with or without persistent angiographic leakage, nor between groups treated with scatter alone versus scatter plus focal ablation. Importantly, there was no control group, which makes it difficult to draw definitive conclusions from this study.

Another small pilot study, conducted by Soubrane and Coscas (36), also investigated the use of macular scatter photocoagulation for ill-defined subfoveal CNV. These authors randomized eyes of patients 50 years or older with poorly defined subfoveal CNV and visual acuity of 20/100 or better to either treatment or observation. Treatment consisted of 300–500 nonconfluent 0.2-s-duration krypton laser burns of "minimal intensity" to the CNV complex. By 2 years of follow-up, no statistically significant differences were noted between groups (36).

Bressler et al. (37) reported the results of a randomized, prospective pilot trial of macular scatter photocoagulation for poorly demarcated subfoveal CNV related to AMD. A total of 103 eyes of patients with symptomatic occult CNV secondary to AMD, with or without a classic component, with poorly demarcated borders were randomized to either laser treatment or observation. Two subgroup treatments were developed using either direct grid treatment alone or grid plus focal ablation of classic CNV. The results of this study did not demonstrate any benefit from this type of treatment (Fig. 8). In fact, at 6 months treated eyes had two more lines of visual acuity loss as compared to observed eyes, suggesting that the treatment might even have been harmful at that point. However, by 24 months of follow-up, a crossover point was observed. There was no significant difference in visual function between groups such that 40% of each group had suffered severe visual loss at 2 years. The results of this trial have largely discouraged the use of scatter treatment for poorly demarcated subfoveal lesions, especially in light of the highly variable natural course of this type of CNV lesion (24,38).

VII. INDOCYANINE GREEN–GUIDED LASER TREATMENTS

Kogure and Choromokos reported the first use of indocyanine green (ICG) for fundus imaging in 1969 (39). However, owing to its low fluorescence (only 4% that of

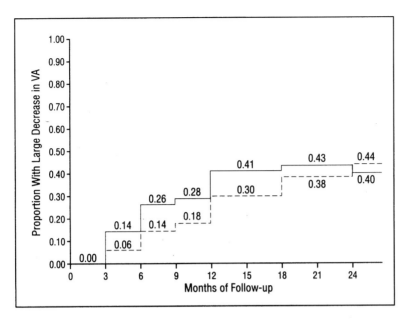

Figure 8 Percentages of eyes with severe visual loss for treated (solid line) and untreated (broken line) groups following macular scatter laser treatment for poorly demarcated subfoveal choroidal neovascularization. (Reproduced with permission from Bressler NM, et al. Macular scatter ("grid") laser treatment of poorly demarcated subfoveal choroidal neovascularization in age-related macular degeneration: results of a randomized pilot trial. Arch Opthalmol 1996;114:1456–1464. Copyright 1996, American Medical Association.)

fluorescein), it was difficult to detect ICG with the imaging systems of that day. More sensitive detectors have allowed for acquisition and rendering of high-quality angiograms with more readily discernible normal landmarks and pathological features.

ICG has two important differences from fluorescein. (1) ICG absorbs and emits in the near-infrared portion of the spectrum, which is less absorbed by the pigment epithelium, macular xanthophyll, media opacities, and blood when compared to visible light. (2) ICG is almost completely bound to plasma proteins (98%) and therefore is mostly confined to the intravascular space. This allows for better visualization of the choroidal vasculature as compared to fluorescein, which easily leaks from the small fenestrations of the choriocapillaris. In one study, Lim et al. noted that in 153 consecutive patients, imaged with both fluorescein and ICG angiography, 50% of patients with occult lesions on fluorescein angiography had hyperfluorescent lesions with "well-demarcated" margins on ICG (40).

Three basic patterns of ICG fluorescence of occult CNV have been described. These include small, focal "hot spots," plaques, and mixed lesions (41–43). The focal hot spot is a bright area of fluorescence smaller than one disk area that fluoresces early and is usually present by the midphase of the angiogram. It is thought to represent actively proliferating vessels with highly permeable areas of neovascularization. Plaque lesions are greater than one disk area in size, tend not to fluoresce early and fluoresce less intensely in the later stages of the angiogram, and can be either well defined or ill defined (60%). Mixed types of ICG fluorescence, which have both a plaque and a focal spot, include three important subtypes characterized by the location of the focal spot. The focal spot can be adjacent to, overlying, or remote from the plaque. In a review of 1000 consecutive eyes with occult CNV imaged with fluorescein and ICG, Guyer et al. reported that plaques, focal spots, and mixed lesions were observed in 61%, 29%, and 8% of the patients, respectively (43,44). Pilot studies using ICG-guided photocoagulation have primarily targeted the focal hot spot as a potential treatment site.

Although no large, randomized, controlled trials have been reported evaluating the use of ICG-guided photocoagulation, data exist from many pilot studies that have examined this issue (42,43,45–48). In one of the earliest reports, Regillo et al. (42) retrospectively reviewed all patients over a 5-month period who had undergone ICG angiography and who had exudative AMD with ill-defined CNV on fluorescein angiography. Of 19 patients who demonstrated well-defined, hyperfluorescent extrafoveal lesions on ICG and underwent subsequent ICG-guided photocoagulation, 63% experienced clinical resolution of exudation and stabilization (within one line) or improvement of Snellen acuity at 6 months. In one of the largest series reported to date, Slakter et al. (46) subsequently evaluated 347 consecutive patients with clinical and angiographic evidence of occult CNV. Of these, 79 (23%) were found to have focal hot-spot type lesions eccentric to the fovea with ICG. These lesions were treated as described by the MPS for extrafoveal, classic CNV (4). Two groups of potentially treatable patients were identified. Those in group 1, termed the vascularized pigment epithelial detachment group, included patients with a distinct detachment of the RPE on clinical examination greater than one disc diameter with minimal irregular hyperfluoresence on early fluorescein angiography that gradually increased in intensity and eventually stained the subpigment epithelial tissue late. Also, a serous PED in association with the occult CNV was seen filling in the late stages of the angiogram. Group 2 included patients with CNV beneath the RPE that appeared clinically as a shallow, solid thickening of the RPE without an associated serous PED. Forty-four patients (56%) had complete resolution of their exudative manifestations following treatment. Visual acuity improvement was noted in 10 eyes (13%) (two or more lines of Snellen acuity) and vision stabilization was noted in 42 eyes (53%). Follow-up ranged from 6 weeks to 16 months with a median of 23 weeks. The authors concluded, despite the lack of a contemporaneous control group, that this anatomical success rate was similar to that seen in the extrafoveal, classic CNV arm of the MPS (4,9,16). They also noted that 43% of eyes had one or more recurrences, again similar to MPS rates of recurrence (8,47). However, it is important to note the shorter follow-up time of this group compared to the MPS patients. The authors reported slightly less favorable anatomical, visual acuity, and recurrence outcomes in patients who presented with a serous PED (group 1), and offered three possibilities to explain these outcomes: (1) These patients may have had attenuated treatment secondary to turbid subretinal pigment epithelial fluid despite apparently satisfactory clinical "burns" noted at the time of treatment; (2) the turbid PED may still obscure the margins of the CNV despite the enhanced visualization capabilities of ICG, resulting in incomplete treatment; and (3) vascularized PEDs with a serous component may represent a naturally more aggressive form of exudative disease. Several retrospective analyses have demonstrated the poor natural course of eyes with serous and nonserous PEDs (28–30)

More recently, Weinberger et al. (48) reported a similar prospective pilot study, utilizing early ICG of occult CNV to guide treatment, with follow-up ranging from 12 months to 48 months (mean follow-up of 30 months). At 12 months, 13 of 21 eyes (62%) had obliteration of their lesions on fluorescein angiography and 66% of 21 eyes had stabilized or improved visual acuity. By 36 months, 6 of 10 eyes (60%) had obliteration of their lesions on fluorescein angiography, but only 30% of 10 eyes had stabilized or improved visual acuity, with 40% experiencing severe visual loss. Again, this study demonstrates the importance of long-term follow-up and careful comparison to control groups.

Guyer et al. (43) reported their success in treating only the focal hot spot adjacent to a plaque lesion. Of 23 eyes that were evaluated and treated, 19 eyes were available for follow-up at 1 year. Anatomical success was achieved in 13 eyes (68%) and stabilization or improvement of visual acuity was achieved in 9 (69%) of these 13 eyes. Again, longer follow-up and comparison to a control group are needed to assess fully this outcome.

ICG also has been examined for use in treating recurrent occult CNV. Sorenson et al. (47) consecutively evaluated 66 patients who presented with clinical signs and symptoms of recurrent occult CNV but had no well-defined or classic CNV on fluorescein angiography. Sixty-four (97%) were deemed to have recurrent CNV by ICG angiography. Of these, 29 (44%) were believed to have well-defined CNV lesions that were treated with ICG-guided photocoagulation. Twenty-three lesions were extrafoveal or juxtafoveal and six were subfoveal. At the end of follow-up, which averaged 6 months, 18 eyes (62%) had resolution of their exudative manifestations with stabilization or improvement of visual acuity.

In recent work presented in abstract form, Glaser and co-workers have observed "modulating" vessels that fill early and then fade quickly as seen on high-speed ICG videoangiography (49). It appears that selective treatment of these modulating vessels may be associated with a more widespread reduction in dye leakage. This modality is discussed more fully elsewhere in this book, and additional data are being accumulated, although no randomized, controlled clinical trial has yet been performed.

ICG remains a useful tool that allows for further classification and understanding of CNV lesions and may ultimately increase the number of patients eligible for standard photocoagulation. Definite recommendations await large, controlled clinical trials. As yet, none have been conducted.

VIII. LASER TREATMENT OF AMD USING PHOTODYNAMIC THERAPY

Novel treatments for AMD attempt to stop or prevent the growth of CNV without the concurrent damage to the retina and RPE caused by laser photocoagulation. One very promising approach is photodynamic therapy (PDT). In PDT, dye molecules are injected intravenously. Dye molecules preferentially localize to choroidal neovascularization-associated endothelial cells. Low-intensity, long-exposure irradiation promotes the photochemical production of reactive oxygen species including singlet oxygen, hydroxyl radicals, and superoxide anion, which promote thrombosis and vascular injury. The laser power is lower than that required for thermal retinal injury, conferring selectivity; CNV can be treated, while sparing overlying, potentially functional retina.

Although many different photosensitizing drugs exist (50), only benzoporphyrin derivative, also called verteporfin, has been evaluated, in Phase I, II and III clinical studies, and has recently been approved by the Food and Drug Administration (5,51,52). Encouraging 1- and 2 year reults have been reported for verteporfin. Subfoveal lesions composed of 50% or greater classic CNV (predominantly classic) had a significant improvement in outcome with verteporfin treatment: at 2 years 67% of eyes treated lost less than 15 letters, compared to 39% of eyes receiving placebo. Lesions in which some classic component was present, where the classic component subtended less than 50% of the lesion area, and patients with recurrent CNV had no improvement in outcome with verteporfin compared to placebo.

IX. IMPLICATIONS FOR CLINICAL PRACTICE

Patients at risk for the development of CNV should monitor central vision in each eye separately with alternate monocular cover testing on a daily basis. Any symptomatic change in reading vision, distance vision, or on Amsler grid testing should prompt examination to identify a potentially treatable lesion (13). AMD is a bilateral disease, and treatable pathology may be present in the fellow asymptomatic eye, so examination and imaging studies should be perfomed in both eyes.

Informed consent among patients who are eligible for thermal laser treatment should include discussion of potential risks and benefits of laser treatment. Patients should understand that many people report scotomata after treatment, and that persistence and recurrence are common. Even after initially successful laser treatment, progressive visual loss is the rule rather than the exception, owing to persistence, recurrence, or the development of new CNV.

Patients with CNV due to AMD that benefited from thermal laser photocoagulation in the MPS, were those with well-defined, classic CNV lesions. This type of lesion is present in not more than 13% of patients with neovascular AMD (53), and thus the vast majority of patients with neovascular AMD do not meet MPS eligibility criteria for laser treatment. However, thermal laser treatment has been shown to be effective in reducing the rates of severe vision loss among the patients eligible for treatment. In treated eyes that do not develop postlaser leakage, the mean visual acuity 3 years post treatment is 20/50. Unfortunately, over half of those treated have recurrent CNV with associated vision loss (10,16), and expansion of the laser scar may be associated with further decline in visual function for extrafoveal, juxtafoveal, and subfoveal lesions. In addition, thermal laser treatment of subfoveal CNV results in immediate iatrogenic loss of central vision from damage to retinal tissue overlying the CNV. These factors have prompted investigation into new treatment modalities, with the goal of developing a treatment that would benefit patients with larger, less well-defined CNV lesions, and would selectively obliterate CNV with minimal damage to the overlying retina.

PDT provides a new tool for the treatment of subfoveal lesions with minimal damage to overlying retina, and without immediate loss of vision as may be associated with photocoagulation of subfoveal lesions. Long-term outcome data comparing eyes treated with verteporfin to eyes that received placebo will yield better understanding of its role in the treatment of patients with CNV due to AMD. It is not possible at this time to determine the precise indications for thermal laser or PDT for patients with CNV due to AMD. The follow-up to date in clinical studies of PDT is limited to 12–24 months, and the natural course of CNV from AMD, as studied in the MPS, includes a high rate of recurrence and persistence with associated visual loss over time. Demonstration of long-term efficacy and safety, especially in an approach requiring retreatments as often as every 3 months, will require evaluation of longer-term follow-up data.

However, certain recommendations for treatments of CNV in patients with AMD can be made. Data support treatment of extrafoveal CNV lesions meeting MPS criteria with traditional laser. Five-year follow-up has shown a significant improvement in visual outcome with laser treatment compared to observation for this type of CNV (16), and treatment of extrafoveal CNV has not been evaluated with PDT. Second, MPS data support treatment of recurrent CNV that extends under the geometrical center of the fovea with thermal laser (20). The subgroup of 59 patients in TAP with recurrent subfoveal CNV who received PDT fared no better than the 23 patients who received placebo (5). However, the TAP study was not designed specifically to investigate patients with recurrent CNV, and likely did not have the power necessary to detect a treatment effect in this group of patients.

The results of the TAP study support treatment of subfoveal CNV from AMD that is predominantly classic with verteporfin (5). PDT is especially likely to benefit patients with subfoveal CNV that can be classified into groups B, C, and D of the MPS (small lesions with good initial visual acuity and large lesions), because at 12-month follow-up, patients treated with laser in each of these groups had worse visual outcomes than patients who were observed (22), while patients treated with verteporfin had better visual outcomes at this time compared to placebo (5). For patients with recurrent subfoveal CNV, and for patients with new subfoveal lesions, especially those characterized as MPS group A (small lesions with moderate or poor visual acuity, or medium-size lesions with poor visual acuity), thermal laser treatment should be considered. Patients were found to benefit from thermal laser by the MPS for up to 5 years after treatment (22), compared to the treatment benefit shown at only 24 months with PDT (5).

Currently, the data do not support strongly treatment of certain types of CNV with either thermal laser or PDT. The MPS demonstrated a treatment benefit from thermal laser in patients with juxtafoveal CNV, but this benefit was modest. The average visual acuity at 5 years was 20/200 in the treated group versus 20/250 in the untreated group, and 52% of treated versus 61% of untreated patients lost six or more lines of best-corrected visual acuity (10). Persistence and recurrence were frequent, occurring at a rate of 78% over 5 years (10). Patients with juxtafoveal CNV and hypertension were not shown to have a treatment benefit with thermal laser by the MPS (9,10). At this time, laser photocoagulation is recommended for well-defined juxtafoveal CNV; however, accumulating data, subgroup analysis, and future trials may shed additional light on the potential benefits of PDT for juxtafoveal CNV.

Patients with subfoveal CNV lesions that are less than 50% classic, without well-demarcated boundaries, do not meet MPS eligibility criteria, and additionally were found not to benefit from treatment with PDT. There remains no proven treatment for patients with predominantly occult CNV. This type of lesion is being investigated in a number of case series and prospective randomized trials with treatments such as external-beam radiation, transpupillary thermal therapy, submacular surgery, and pharmacological treatments (54).

The large majority of patients with visual loss due to CNV in AMD have subfoveal, occult CNV for which no treatment benefit with PDT has been demonstrated. An effective treatment or prophylactic intervention for the majority of patients with vision loss due to CNV has not yet been identified, and research is ongoing to find an effective modality to reduce rates of vision loss in these patients. Until an effective intervention is found, referral to a low-vision specialist may help to ensure that patients with vision loss due to AMD benefit from all visual aids and community resources available to them.

X. SUMMARY

Laser treatment, as described by the MPS Study Group, is beneficial for eligible eyes with extrafoveal, juxtafoveal, and subfoveal CNV. Subgroup analysis in the subfoveal new study revealed that treated eyes with worse initial visual acuity and smaller initial lesion size fared better than observed eyes. Group D eyes with larger lesions and good initial visual acuity sustained no treatment benefit. Recurrences of CNV were common, seen in 54% of treated eyes at (5) years in the extrafoveal study. No benefit was observed for treating the classic component of a lesion composed of both classic and occult components.

The natural history of occult CNV is variable, complicating interpretation of treatment studies, partcularly those studies without controls. Currently, no good data exist to guide the treatment of predominantly occult lesions. Patients at risk for the development of CNV should monitor central vision in each eye separately with alternate monocular cover testing on a daily basis. Any symptomatic change in reading vision, distance vision, or on Amsler grid testing should prompt examination to identify a potentially treatable lesion. Patients should be counseled that scotomata persistence and recurrence are common even after successful treatment.

REFERENCES

1. Fine SL, Berger JW, Maguire MG, Ho AC. Age-related macular degeneration. N Engl J Med 2000;342:483–92.
2. Ferris FL III, Fine SL, Hyman L. Age-related macular degeneration and blindness due to neovascular maculopathy. Arch Ophthalmol 1984;102:1640–1642.
3. Patz A, Fine SL, Finkelstein D, Yassur Y. Diseases of the macula: the diagnosis and management of choroidal neovascularization. Trans Am Acad Ophthalmol Otolaryngol 1977;83:468–475.
4. Macular Photocoagulation Study Group. Argon laser photocoagulation for senile macular degeneration. Results of a randomized clinical trial. Arch Ophthalmol 1982;100:912–918.
5. Treatment of Age Related Macular Degeneration with Photodynamic Therapy (TAP) Study Group. Photodynamic therapy of subfoveal choroidal neovascularization in age-related macular degeneration with verteporfin: one-year results of 2 randomized clinical trials-TAP report. Arch Ophthalmol 1999;117:1329–1345.
6. Fine SL. Further thoughts on the diagnosis and treatment of patients with macular degeneration. Arch Ophthalmol 1983;101:1189–1190.
7. Fine SL. Macular Photocoagulation Study. Arch Ophthalmol 1980;98:832.
8. Macular Photocoagulation Study Group. Recurrent choroidal neovascularization after argon laser photocoagulation for neovascular maculopathy. Arch Ophthalmol 1986;104:503–512.
9. Macular Photocoagulation Study Group. Krypton laser photocoagulation for neovascular lesions of age-related macular degeneration. Results of a randomized clinical trial. Arch ophthalmol 1990;108:816–824.
10. Macular Photocoagulation Study Group. Laser photocoagulation for juxtafoveal choroidal neovascularization. Five-year, results from randomized clinical trials. Arch Ophthalmol 1994;112:500–509.
11. Macular Photocoagulation Study Group. Subfoveal neovascular lesions in age-related macular degeneration. Guidelines for evaluation and treatment in the Macular Photocoagulation Study. Arch Ophthalmol 1991;109:1242–1257.
12. Macular Photocoagulation Study Group. Laser photocoagulation of subfoveal recurrent neovascular lesions in age-related macular degeneration. Results of a randomized clinical trial. Arch Ophthalmol 1991;109:1232–1241.
13. Berger JW, Fine SL. Laser treatment for choroidal neovascularization. In: Berger Fine SL, Maguire MG, eds. Age-Related Macular Degeneration. St. Louis: CV Mosby, 1999: 279–296.

14. Chamberlin JA, Bressler NM, Bressler SB, Elman SJ, Murphy RP, Flood TP, Hawkins BS, Maguire MG, Fine SL. The use of fundus photographs and fluorescein angiograms in the identification and treatment of choroidal neovascularization in the Macular Photocoagulation Study. The Macular Photocoagulation Study Group. Ophthalmology 1989;96:1526–1534.

15. Macular photocoagulation Study Group. Evaluation of argon green vs krypton red laser for photocoagulation of subfoveal choroidal neovascularization in the Macular Photocoagulation Study. Arch Ophthalmol 1994;112:1176–1784.

16. Macular photocoagulation Study Group. Argon laser photocoagulation for neovascular maculopathy. Five-year results from randomized clinical trials. Arch Ophthalmol 1991;109:1109–1114.

17. Macular photocoagulation Study Group. Persistent and recurrent neovascularization after krypton laser photocoagulation for neovascular lesions of age-related macular degeneration. Arch Ophthalmol 1990;108:825–831.

18. Macular Photocoagulation Study Group. Occult choroidal neovascularization. Influence on visual outcome in patients with age-related macular degeneration. Arch Ophthalmol 1996;114:400–412.

19. Macular Photocoagulation Study Group. Laser photocoagulation of subfoveal neovascular lesions in age-related macular degeneration. Results of randomized clinical trial. Arch Ophthalmol 1991;109:1220–1231.

20. Macular Photocoagulation Study Group. Laser photocoagulation of subfoveal neovascular lesions of age-related macular degeneration. Updated findings from two clinical trials. Arch Ophthalmol 1993;111:1200–1209.

21. Macular Photocoagulation Study Group. Persistent and recurrent neovascularization after laser photocoagulation for subfoveal choroidal neovascularization of age-related macular degeneration. Arch Ophthalmol 1994;112:489–499.

22. Macular Photocoagulation Study Group. Visual outcome after laser photocoagulation for subfoveal choroidal neovascularization secondary to age-related macular degeneration. The influence of initial lesion size and initial visual acuity. Arch Ophthalmol 1994;112:480–488.

23. Stevens TS, Bressler NM, Maguire MG, Bressler SB, Fine SL, Alexander J, Phillips DA, Margherio RR, Murphy PL, Schachat AP. Occult choroidal neovascularization in age-related macular degeneration. A natural history study. Arch Ophthalmol 1997;115:345–350.

24. Soubrane G, Coscas G, Francais C, Koenig F. Occult subretinal new vessels in age-related macular degeneration. Natural history and early laser treatment. Ophthalmology 1990;97:649–657.

25. Barondes MJ, Pagliarini S, Chisholm IH, Hamilton AM, Bird AC. Controlled trial of laser photocoagulation of pigment epithelial detachments in the elderly: 4 year review. Br J Ophthalmol 1992;76:5–7.

26. Maguire JI, Benson WE, Brown GC. Treatment of foveal pigment epithelial detachments with contiguous extrafoveal choroidal neovascular membranes. Am J Ophthalmol 1990;109:523–529.

27. Singerman LJ, Stockfish JH. Natural history of subfoveal pigment epithelial detachments associated with subfoveal or unidentifiable choroidal neovascularization complicating age-related macular degeneration. Graefes Arch Clin Exp Ophthalmol 1989;227:501–507.

28. Meredith TA, Braley RE, Aaberg TM. Natural history of serous detachments of the retinal pigment epithelium. Am J Ophthalmol 1979;88:643–651.

29. Poliner LS, Olk RJ, Burgess D, Gordon ME. Natural history of retinal pigment epithelial detachments in age-related macular degeneration. Ophthalmology 1986;93:543–551.

30. Elman MJ, Fine SL, Murphy RP, Patz A, Auer C. The natural history of serous retinal pigment epithelium detachment in patients with age-related macular degeneration. Ophthalmology 1986;93:224–230.

31. Coscas G, Soubrane G, Ramahefasolo C, Fardeau C. Perifoveal laser treatment for subfoveal choroidal new vessels in age-related macular degeneration. Results of a randomized clinical trial. Arch Ophthalmol 1991;109:1258–1265.

32. Orth DH, Rosculet JP, De Bustros S. Foveal sparing photocoagulation for exudative age-related macular degeneration. Retina 1994;14:153–159.
33. Tornambe PE, Poliner LS, Hovey LJ, Taren D. Scatter macular photocoagulation for subfoveal neovascular membranes in age-related macular degeneration. A pilot study. Retina 1992;12:305–314.
34. Buzney SM, Weiter JJ, Freilich BD. Scatter macular photocoagulation for age- related subfoveal neovascularization (ARVO abstract). Invest Ophthalmol Vis Sci 1995;36:S225.
35. Midena E, Valenti M, Piermarocchi S, Bertoja E, Degli-Angeli C, Segato T. Functional effects of scatter macular photocoagulation for age-related subfoveal neovascularization (ARVO abstract). Invest Ophthalmol Vis Sci 1996;37:S111.
36. Soubrane G, Coscas G. Photocoagulation of poorly defined choroidal neovascular membranes associated with age-related macular degeneration. In: Lewis H, Ryan SJ, eds. Medical and surgical retina: advances, controversies, and management. St. Louis: Mosby, 1994:48–53.
37. Bressler NM, Maguire MG, Murphy PL, Alexander J, Margherio R, Schachat AP, Fine SL, Stevens TS, Bressler SB. Macular scatter ("grid") laser treatment of poorly demarcated subfoveal choroidal neovascularization in age-related macular degeneration. Results of a randomized pilot trial. Arch Ophthalmol 1996;14:1456–1464.
38. Bressler NM, Bressler SB, Fine SL. Age-related macular degeneration. Surv Ophthalmol 1988;32:375–413.
39. Kogure K, Choromokos E. Infrared absorption angiography. J Appl Physiol 1969 26:154–157.
40. Lim JI, Sternberg P Jr, Capone A Jr, TM Sr, Gilman JP. Selective use of indocyanine green angiography for occult choroidal neovascularization. Am J Ophthalmol 1995;120:75–82.
41. Yannuzzi LA, Slakter JS, Sorenson JA, Guyer DR, Orlock DA. Digital indocyanine green videoangiography and choroidal neovascularization. Retina 1992;12:191–223.
42. Regillo CD, Benson WE, Maguire JI, Annesley WH Jr. Indocyanine green angiography and occult choroidal neovascularization. Ophthalmology 1994;101:280–288.
43. Guyer DR, Yannuzzi LA, Ladas I, Slakter JS, Sorenson JA, Orlock D. Indocyanine green-guided laser photocoagulation of focal spots at the edge of plaques of choroidal neovascularization. Arch Ophthalmol.1996;114:693–697.
44. Kwun RC, Guyer DR. Indocyanine green angiography. In: Berger JW, Fine SL, Maguire MG, eds. Age-Related Macular Degeneration. St. Louis: CV Mosby, 1999:237–247.
45. Lim JI, Aaberg TM, Capone A Jr, Sternberg P Jr. Indocyanine green angiography-guided photocoagulation of chroidal neovascularization associated with retinal pigment epithelial detachment. Am J Ophthalmol 1997;123:524–532.
46. Slakter JS, Yannuzzi LA, Sorenson JA, Guyer DR, Ho AC, Orlock DA. A pilot study of indocyanine green videoangiography-guided laser photocoagulation of occult choroidal neovascularization in age-related macular degeneration. Arch Ophthalmol 1994;112:465–472.
47. Sorenson JA, Yannuzzi LA, Slakter JS, Guyer DR, Ho AC, Orlock DA. A pilot study of digital indocyanine green videoangiography for recurrent occult choroidal neovascularization in age-related macular degeneration. Arch Ophthalmol 1994;112:473–479.
48. Weinberger AW, Knabben H, Solbach U, Wolf S. Indocyanine green guided laser photocoagulation in patients with occult choroidal neovascularisation. Br J Ophthalmol 1999;83:168–172.
49. Glaser BM, Murphy RP, Lakhanapal RR, Lin SB, Baudo TA. Identification and treatment of modulating choroidal vessels associated with occult choroidal neovascularization (ARVO abstract). Invest Opthalmol Vis Sci 2000;41:S320.
50. Husain D, Gragoudas ES, Miller JW. Photodynamic Therapy. In: Berger JW, Fine SL, Maguire MG, eds. Age-Related Macular Degeneration. St. Louis: CV Mosby, 1999: 297–307.
51. Miller JW, Schmidt-Erfurth U, Sickenberg M, Pournaras CJ, Lagua H, Barbazetto I, Zografos L, Piguet B, Donati G, Lane AM, Birngruber R, van den Berg H, Strong A, Manjuris U, Gray T, Fsadni M, Bressler NM, Gragoudas ES. Photodynamic therapy with verteporfin for choroidal

neovascularization caused by age-related macular degeneration: results of a single treatment in a phase 1 and 2 study. Arch Ophthalmol 1999;117:1161–1173.

52. Schmidt-Erfurth U, Miller JW, Sickenberg M, Lagua H, Barbazetto I, Gragoudas ES, Zografos L, Piguet B, Pournaras CJ, Donati G, Lane AM, Birngruber R, van den Borg H, Strong A, Manjuris U, Gray T, Fsedni M, Bressier NM. Photodynamic therapy with verteporfin for choroidal neovascularization caused by age-related macular degeneration: results of retreatments in a phase 1 and 2 study. Arch Ophthalmol 1999;117:1177–1187.

53. Freund KB, Yannuzzi LA, Sorenson JA. Age-related macular degeneration and choroidal neovascularization. Am J Ophthalmol 1993;115:786–791.

54. Schachat AP. Review of ongoing clinical trials for AMD. American Academy of Ophthalmology, Vitreoretinal Update, Orlando, Florida, 1999.

10
Photodynamic Therapy

Mark S. Blumenkranz
Stanford University School of Medicine, Stanford, California

Kathryn W. Woodburn
AP Pharma, Redwood City, California

I. INTRODUCTION

A. Historical Overview

Photodynamic therapy (PDT) is an emerging therapeutic modality that entails the administration of a photosensitizer, subsequent accumulation in the target tissue, and then activation by nonthermal monochromatic light corresponding to the sensitizer's absorption profile (1). Powerful oxidizing agents such as cytotoxic singlet oxygen and radicals are produced causing irreversible cellular damage. PDT has traditionally focused on the treatment of cancer (2), but the potential for selective destruction of diseased vessels, while sparing normal overlying tissues, coupled with promising clinical efficacy has spawned increasing nonclinical and clinical PDT research for the treatment of age-related macular degeneration (AMD), particularly subfoveal choroidal neovascularization (CNV). PDT is selective, both through photosensitizer retention in new vessels and through light application. Illumination is restricted to the diseased area and the limited depth of light penetration restricts damage to underlying tissues.

B. Vascular Targeting

PDT has been used successfully in the treatment of certain cancers owing to the remarkable selectivity of many photosensitizers for tumor tissue. PDT causes direct cellular injury in addition to microvascular damage or "shutdown" within the illuminated tumor. Uptake is considered to be due to the increased expression of low-density lipoprotein (LDL) receptors on tumor cells and neovascular endothelial cells. Porphyrin photosensitization in mammals was studied as early as 1910 when Hausmann investigated the effects of hematoporphyrin and light on mice (3). The results established the phototoxic propensity of porphyrins and Hausmann concluded that the peripheral vasculature was one of the primary PDT targets. In 1963, Castellani and co-workers demonstrated the microvasculature to be a crucial target (4). PDT-mediated neovascular damage has now become an emerging re-

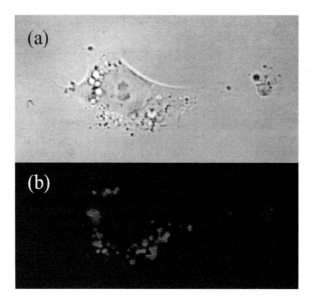

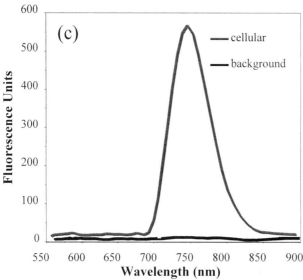

Figure 1 Photosensitizer accumulation in endothelial cells. Human umbilical vein endothelial cells, phase contrast micrograph shown in (a), were incubated with motexafin lutetium and fluorescence microscopy was performed revealing the subcellular localization sites (red in b). Fluorescence emission spectra taken from discrete cellular localization sites in (b) revealed the distinctive 750-nm-wavelength emission profile characteristic of the sensitizer (c). Background spectra were also obtained.

search area with many researchers showing differences in efficiency between photosensitizers in a number of vascular models (5,6).

Endothelial cells accumulate certain photosensitizers and are susceptible to PDT-induced destruction. The subcellular localization of motexafin lutetium (Lu-Tex) was deter-

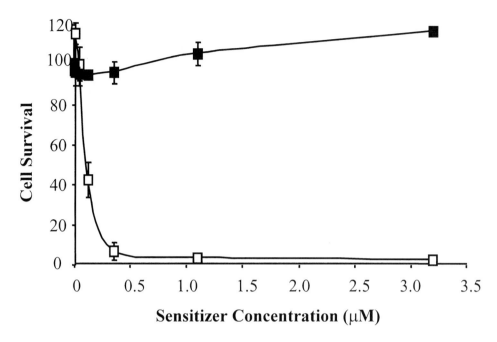

Figure 2 Cytotoxicity following photodynamic therapy. The effect of PDT with motexafin lutetium on the survival of human umbilical vein endothelial cells was assessed (open squares) and compared to sensitizer-only subsets (closed squares). Cells were incubated with varying sensitizer concentrations and then activated using 2 J/cm^2 of 732-nn-wvavelength light.

mined in human umbilical vein endothelial cells using fluorescence microscopy; a typical micrograph is displayed in Figure 1. Lu-Tex exhibits a fluorescence emission profile at 750 nm and this signature fluorescence marker is used to characterize and quantify sensitizer concentrations within tissues. Lu-Tex was found to localize within the lysosomes and endoplasmic reticulum as evidenced by costaining with organelle-specifie fluoroprobes. Following illumination some relocalization of the sensitizer occurred with partitioning being observed in the mitochondria, suggesting the primary subcellular localization site could not possibly fully account for all of the PDT-induced damage. Sensitizer-alone and light administration-alone treatment groups did not induce any changes in cell viability. Significant cell death due to Lu-Tex-mediated PDT was observed in endothelial cells producing a steep dose response (Fig. 2).

Vascular occlusion following PDT is marked by the release of vasoactive molecules, vasoconstriction, blood cell aggregation, endothelial cell damage, blood flow stasis, and hemorrhage. The response is dependent on sensitizer type, concentration, and the time interval between administration and treatment. Benzoporphyrin derivative monoacid ring A (BPD-MA)-induced PDT yielded selective destruction of tumor microvasculature, using a chrondosarcoma rodent model, compared to the surrounding normal microvasculature when illumination occurred within 30 min following sensitizer administration (7). However, no acute change in vascular status was observed when illumination occurred at 3 h. The vascular shutdown results correlated with the antitumor effect since tumor-bearing animals treated at 5 min responded more positively than those treated at 3 h.

C. Light Application

The light used for ophthalmic applications is nonthermal monochromatic laser light matched to the sensitizer's far-red absorbance profile. Far-red wavelength light possesses greater transmission through both blood and tissue than light at lower wavelengths, thereby enabling the treatment of pigmented or hemorrhagic lesions. The energy at which light is delivered is a product of the radiant power (expressed in milliwatts per square centimeter, mW/cm^2) and the time of illumination. The radiant energy, often termed fluence, is expressed as joules per square centimeter (J/cm^2). Therefore, to deliver a fluence of 50 J/cm^2 light at a power density of 600 mW/cm^2 an illumination time of 83 is required.

Upon illumination (Fig. 1), photons (hυ) interact with the ground singlet-state sensitizer (^{1}Sensitizer) causing it to undergo an electronic transition to an activated, short-lived, excited singlet state (^{1}Sensitizer*). The singlet state can then convert back to the ground state causing fluorescence or undergo intersystem crossing to generate the longer-lived excited triplet-state sensitizer (^{3}Sensitizer*). From the triplet state, a photon can be emitted causing phosphorescence with conversion to the ground state or the triplet state can interact with oxygen or biological substrates leading to microvascular damage (8,9). As schematically represented in Figure 3, two photo-oxidation processes can occur between the triplet state and molecular oxygen ($^3O_2$) causing irreversible damage to vascular components. The direct interaction of the excited triplet state with biomolecular substrates is termed the type I mode and is favored in areas with low oxygen concentrations. Biomolecular radicals are generated and react with oxygen forming cytotoxic oxidizing products. The type II mechanism entails interaction from the excited triplet-state sensitizer to ground-state oxygen producing singlet oxygen ($^1O_2$) with theoretical regeneration of the ground-state sensitizer. However, photobleaching and photo-product formation can deplete the ground-state sensitizer concentration.

Singlet oxygen is highly electrophilic, oxidizing biological substrates and initiating a cascade of radical chain reactions that damage cellular components. Singlet oxygen production is thought to be responsible for most of the damage induced by PDT. Singlet oxygen possesses a reactive pathlength of less than 0.02 micron so any effect has a limited potency (2). The photochemical processes involved are complex and are different for each sensitizer and are also subject to the microenvironment. Intersystem crossing is kinetically important for the formation of the excited triplet state and for PDT potency. Molecules with high fluorescence quantum yields will generate lower triplet quantum yields and are more likely to be used as diagnostic agents. Conversely, molecules with low fluorescence quantum yields will generate high triplet quantum yields and therefore should produce a high yield of cytotoxic species.

D. PDT Candidates

The ideal photosensitizer should be chemically pure and possess the appropriate physical and biological properties that make it inherently nontoxic until activated by light. The agent should possess strong absorption properties in the far-red spectral region (660–780 nm) where light has greatest penetration into blood and tissue and possess efficient photophysical properties for destroying neovascular endothelial cells. The sensitizer should also localize selectively in the neovasculature while being rapidly cleared from the blood and overlying photoreceptors. In addition, rapid cutaneous clearance would limit cutaneous photosensitivity. Several photosensitizers are currently being explored and are in different stages of preclinical and clinical development.

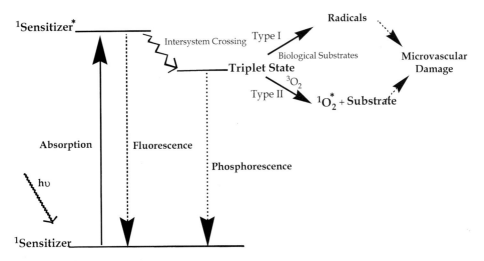

Figure 3 Photochemical processes involved in photodynamic therapy.

Photosensitizing candidate molecules are generally related to porphyrins (Fig. 4, 5). Porphyrins are fused tetrapyrrolic macrocycles that are omnipresent in nature as major biological pigments. Protoporphyrin IX, a typical porphyrin molecule, forms the nonprotein portion of hemoglobin. Reduction, oxidation, or expansion of the macrocyclic ring leads to different molecular subclasses. A reduction at one of the four pyrrole rings in the porphyrin macrocycle yields a chlorin molecule. The electronic conjugation system is altered causing further absorption into the far-red wavelength region, from 630 to approximately 660–690 nm. Increasing the macrocycle conjugation system further, by the formation of a pentadentate metallophotosensitizer, yields a texaphyrin molecule and results in even further absorption in the far-red spectral region (700–760 nm). Phthalocyanines are tetrapyrrolic structures fused together by nitrogen atoms instead of carbon bridges; absorption is exhibited in the 650- to 700-nm-wavelength region. Purpurins possess a reduced pyrrole ring and also an extended ring conjugation system; the absorption maxima is between 650 and 690 nm. The chemical structures of the main photosensitizers now being evaluated clinically are shown in Figure 4 while those in preclinical development are in Figure 5. The singlet oxygen quantum yield ($^1O_2 \ \phi_\delta$) and the extinction coefficient (ϵ) at the wavelength used for photoactivation are also shown.

E. Benzoporphyrin Derivative Monoacid (Verteporfin, Visudyne, BPD-MA)

BPD-MA (benzoporphyrin derivative monoacid ring A) consists of equal amounts of two regioisomers that differ in the location of the carboxylic acid and methyl ester on the lower pyrrole rings of the chlorin macrocycle (see Fig. 2). BPD-MA, owing to its hydrophobicity, is formulated with liposomes. The monoacid analogs were developed because they produced greater PDT responses compared to the diacids (10). The monoacid regioisomers are converted, in the liver, to the diacids. The regioisomers responded similarly in experimental efficacy settings; however, the pharmacokinetic properties were different in the rat, dog,

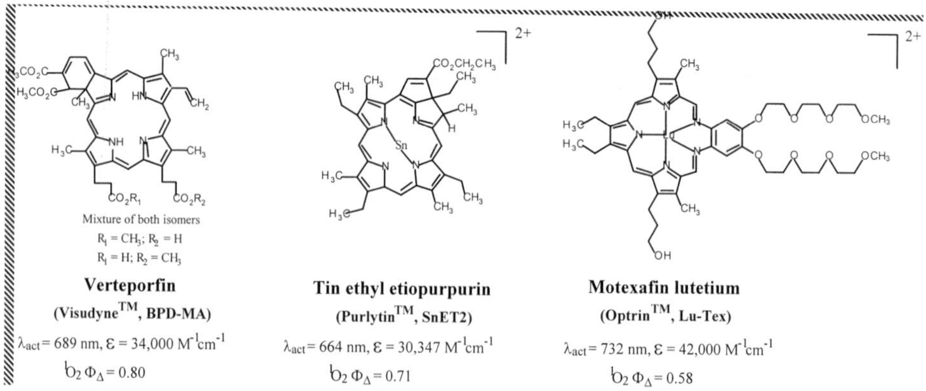

Figure 4 Chemical structures and photophysical properties of photodynamic therapy agents now in clinical trials.

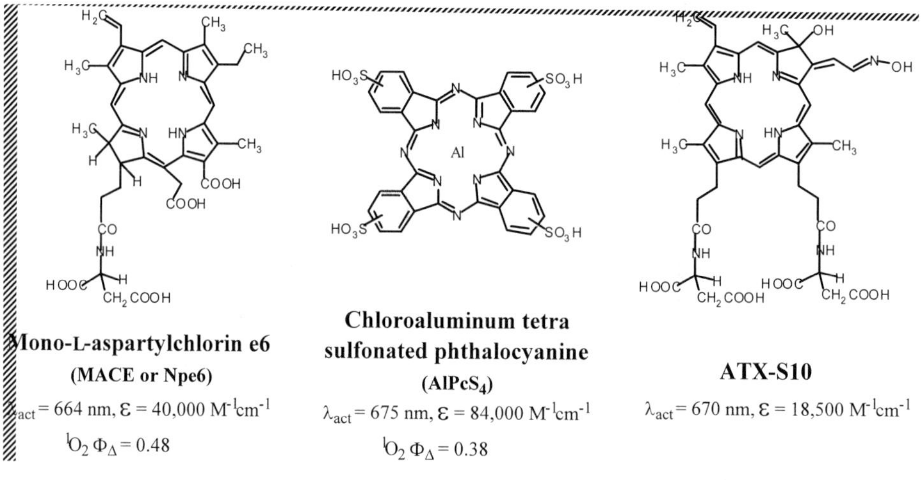

Figure 5 Chemical structures and photophysical properties of photodynamic therapy agents now undergoing preclinical development.

and monkey but not in humans, where the plasma half-life was 5–6 h (11,12). It is thought the latter may be due to differences in plasma esterases or lipoprotein profiles.

PDT studies undertaken using experimentally induced CNV in primates resulted in closure of the neovasculature and choriocapillaris, but not the retinal vasculature.

Liposomal BPD-MA was infused at a dose of 0.375 mg/kg over 10–32 min; illumination with a fluence of 150 J/cm^2 (689–692 nm laser light at 600 mW/cm^2) occurred 30–55 min following infusion initiation (9). When the same treatment parameters were performed on normal primate eyes, some retinal pigment epithelium (RPE) damage and choriocapillaris closure occurred; however, little harm was observed in contiguous tissues. When light was delivered within 30–45 min following sensitizer delivery, sensitizer administration rates had little effect on vascular occlusion rates. BPD-MA localization in the choroid and RPE was confirmed using fluorescence microscopy in rabbits. Retention occurred within 5 min with progression to the outer segments within 20 min. No BPD-MA was detected within the choroid or photoreceptors at 2 h; however, a small trace was detected in the RPE at 24 h (13). A similar pharmacokinetic pattern was observed in monkeys using in vivo fluorescence imaging (14).

The long-term effects on the retina and choroid were evaluated in cynomolgus monkeys with experimental CNV (15). Fundus photography and angiography analyses were performed at 24 h and then weekly for 4–7 weeks following a treatment of 0.375 mg BPD-MA/kg and a fluence of 150 J/cm^2. Eyes were examined histologically at the end of the follow-up period. CNV closure also resulted in closure of the choriocapillaris with damage occurring to RPE cells. However, these areas appeared to regenerate somewhat in the 4–7-week study period. Of 28 CNV lesions followed for 4 weeks 72% remained closed.

Lesion retreatment was determined to be needed to sustain vessel closure. The effect of three treatments was evaluated in disease-free primate eyes (16). Treatments, using sensitizer doses of 6, 12, or 18 mg/m^2 20 min after drug infusion and a fluence of 100 J/cm^2, were performed every 2 weeks. A cumulative dose response was observed; damage to the retina, choroid, and optic nerve was limited in the 6 mg/m^2 sensitizer subgroup while the higher-dose groups exhibited severe choriocapillaris and photoreceptor damage at 6 weeks.

F. Tin Ethyl Etiopurpurin (Purlytin, SnET2)

The purpurin SnET2 has been clinically evaluated for the palliation of symptoms associated with recurrent cutaneous metastatic breast cancer (17). The sensitizer possesses a large extinction coefficient at 660 nm and since it is hydrophobic it is formulated in a lipid emulsion. SnET2-mediated PDT was found to occlude CNV experimentally induced in rats (18). SnET2 was intravenously administered at a dose of 1 mg/kg; the eyes were then exposed at 10 min with 10, 15, or 25 J/cm^2 of 664-nm light using an irradiance of 150 mW/cm^2.

All vessels were occluded in the 25 J/cm^2 subset at the 28-day follow-up with no evidence of damage to contiguous tissues.

G. Motexafin Lutetium (Optrin, Lutetium Texaphyrin, Lu-Tex)

Motexafin lutetium is a water-soluble pentadentate metallophotosensitizer that absorbs strongly in the far-red wavelength region. Subsequent activation at this wavelength enables greater light transmission through blood, lipids, and other endogenous pigments thereby maximizing the induction of cytotoxic species at the diseased site. Lu-Tex possesses a strong, broad fluorescence emission profile centered at 750 nm that is not hindered by endogenous chromophores, thereby exhibiting potential advantages over conventional angiographic dyes (19). The sensitizer is presently in oncological and atherosclerotic clinical trials (20, 21). Rapid clearance is exhibited in humans with plasma half-lives of 0.25 and 8.8 h, thereby reducing cutaneous phototoxicity and limiting systemic toxicity (21).

Studies in rabbits confirmed the potential utility of Lu-Tex as both a photodynamic and angiographic agent (22). Rapid clearance of the sensitizer from retinal vessels, detected using fluorescence angiography was observed in primates. The fluorescence signal peaked in the CNV region at 10–45 min with minimal leakage occurring at 5 h (22). CNV primate closure, with limited damage to retinal and choroidal tissues, was obtained using 1- and 2-mg/kg sensitizer doses and fluences of 50–100 J/cm^2 (23).

H. Light Considerations

Generally any light source that is matched to the photosensitizer's absorption profile can be used for PDT. For ophthalmology fiberoptic delivery of a laser source is required to permit focusing on the retina with a slit lamp system. Lasers are needed because high-energy monochromatic collimated light can be coupled efficiently to fiberoptics allowing delivery within an acceptable time frame. Diode lasers that are stable, compact, and relatively inexpensive in the 630- to 730-nm-wavelength range are now available.

II. CLINICAL OUTCOMES

PDT is now thought to be a superior alternative to laser photocoagulation, when CNV lies beneath the geometrical center of the fovea, since the overlying retina can be spared. Using preclinical CNV models, the neovascularization and normal choriocapillaris can be closed while the outer and inner retina is preserved. In contrast, during the process of destroying neovascularization lying beneath the RPE and sensory retina with photocoagulation, thermal conductance to the retina results in acute necrosis of all layers of the retina, which can later atrophy leading to loss in vision. However, with PDT visual acuity generally remains stable immediately following treatment and has been shown, in a minority of patients, to immediately improve, suggesting the relative preservation of photoreceptors and inner retinal elements (25).

A. Verteporfin Human Trials

The safety and efficacy of verteporfin (BPD-MA, Visudyne) have been confirmed in Phase I, II, and a recently completed pivotal Phase III trial in humans (24,25,29). The photosensitizer is being developed jointly by QLT Phototherapeutics, Vancouver, Canada, and CIBA Vision AG, Bülach, Switzerland. The Phase I and II study proved that a single treatment of verteporfin PDT could occlude CNV vessels, as measured by fluorescein angiography, for 1–4 weeks following administration (24). The maximal tolerated light dose, defined by retinal closure, was 150 J/cm^2. A light dose of 25 J/cm^2 was needed to achieve minimal closure of the vessels. Fluorescein leakage recurred by 4–12 weeks after PDT. CNV progression was noted at 3 months in 51% of eyes with classic CNV.

Since fluorescein leakage recurred by 12 weeks after a single PDT treatment, the investigators believed the neovascular vessels would regrow causing a further subsequent loss in vision. Therefore, the trial was extended to analyze the safety and efficacy of repeat treatments to an eye with subfoveal CNV (29). It should be noted that the reperfusion area was smaller than the pretreatment area. Verteporfin was infused at a dose of 6 mg/m^2 over a period of 10 min and then two different light-dosing regimens were used. In the first regimen patients received 100 J/cm^2 of light 20 min after infusion initiation while in the second regimen 50, 75, or 100 J/cm^2 of light was applied 15 min after commencement of the infusion. Patients received up to two retreatments at 2 or 4 weeks after the initial PDT procedure. The visual acuity change in the first regimen was 0.2 line and in the second regimen was −1.0 line at follow-up times of 16–20 weeks after the initial treatment. Fluorescein leakage recurred in almost all patients by 4–12 weeks. The leakage was, however,

Table 1 Baseline Demographics and Follow-Up Results

	Verteporfin ($n = 402$)	Placebo ($n = 207$)
1. Completion of follow-up		
a. 12 months	94%	94%
b. 24 months	87%	86%
2. Cumulative treatments		
24 months	5.6	6.5

$n = 609$ patients.
Source: Modified and reprinted with permission from the Arch Ophthalmol 1999; 117: 1329–1345.

reduced with multiple treatments. Ocular and systemic side effects were not increased following multiple PDT treatments.

The TAP study (Treatment of Age-Related Macular Degeneration with Photodynamic Therapy) evaluated 609 patients with subfoveal choroidal neovascularization (CNV) who were randomized to treatment with either verteporfin or placebo in a ratio of 2:1. Patients were required to have CNV beneath the geometrical center of the fovea, as one component of a lesion that also contained some component of classic new vessels. Lesions were classified on the basis of baseline color photographs and fluorescein angiography as being either predominantly classic or minimally classic depending on whether the area of CNV occupied greater or less than 50% of the total lesion, respectively, for purposes of statistical analysis. Greatest linear dimension (GLD) was limited to 5400 microns or less.

Patients received either verteporfin at a dose of 6 mg/m² over 10 min in 30 mL of D5w or placebo intravenous injection and were then irradiated 15 min after the start of the infusion for 83 s with 689 nm light from a diode laser at a power setting of 600 mW/cm² for a total fluence of 50 J/cm². The diameter of the treatment zone was set to exceed the GLD of the total lesion including CNV, as well as other lesion components such as blood, or blocked fluorescence if applicable by a total of 1000 microns or approximately 500 microns beyond the furthest edge on all sides if possible. Patients were instructed to avoid direct sunlight and wear sunglasses for at least 48 h following treatment and to return for follow-up at 3-month intervals. At each follow-up visit, the patient underwent visual acuity screening with both ETDRS charts and contrast sensitivity charts by an examiner masked with respect to their treatment category, followed by fluorescein angiography. If the lesion was judged to be actively leaking on fluorescein angiography, retreatment was performed by an identical method to the first session, except that the margins of the lesion and consequent retreatment spot size were calculated on the basis of the most recent angiogram.

The first published report indicated that visual acuity, contrast sensitivity, and fluorescein angiographic outcomes were more favorable in the verteporfin-treated eyes than in the placebo-treated eyes. Twelve months following initial treatment, 246 (61%) of 402 eyes assigned to verteporfin compared with 96 (46%) of 207 eyes assigned to placebo had lost fewer than 15 letters of visual acuity from baseline p < 0.001). In subgroup analyses, the visual acuity benefit (<15 letters lost) of verteporfin therapy was clearly demonstrated (67% vs. 39%; p <0.001) when the area of classic CNV occupied 50% or more of the area of the entire lesion. These results remained significant with longer follow-up of 24 months. Over that time period, verteporfin patients received on average 5.6 treatments compared with 6.5 treatments for patients receiving placebo (Table 1). The percentage of patients with predominantly classic CNV losing less than 15 letters remained relatively constant at

Table 2 Primary Vision Endpoints at 12 and 24 months

	Verteporfin	Placebo
<15 letter loss (12 months)		
Predominantly classic	67%	39%
Minimally classic	56%	55%
No classic	63%	30%
<15 letter loss (24 months)		
Predominantly classic	59%	31%
Minimally classic	47%	44%
No classic	56%	30%

Source: Modified and reprinted with permission from the Arch Ophthalmol 1999; 117:1329–1345.

Table 3 Adverse Events (cumulative 24 months)

	Vertiporfin	Placebo
Any visual disturbance	22.1%	15.5%
Vision decreased	10.2%	6.3%
Acute loss (>20 letters within 7 days)	<1.0%	0.0%
Infusion-related back-pain	2.5%	
Injection site trauma	15.9%	
Photosensitivity reaction	3.5%	

Source: Modified and reprinted with permission from the Arch Ophthalmol 1999; 117: 1329–1345.

59% compared with 31% who lost less than 15 letters in the placebo group (39). In contrast, in the minimally classic group at 24 months, 47% of verteporfin-treated patients lost less than 15 letters compared with 44% of the placebo group, a difference that is neither statistically nor clinically significant. Interestingly, at both 12 and 24 months, a small subset of patients who were judged by the reading center to not have any classic component of CNV (86 patients) also had less vision loss in the verteporfin arm than the placebo arm (Table 2).

Adverse events including vision disturbance, infusion-related back pain, injection site trauma, and photosensitivity reaction were rare, although statistically significantly different between the two groups (24,25) (Table 3). These results were a significant landmark in the treatment of this disease since other therapies have not been shown to be successful in reducing loss of visual acuity over time compared with placebo. With laser photocoagulation there exists the serious complication of immediate vision loss as a result of thermal damage to the surrounding normal retina (26–28). In contrast, although PDT when successful generally results in the temporary closure of choroidal new vessels for a period of approximately 1–4 weeks, by 12 weeks most patients have reperfusion or reproliferation of choroidal new vessels resulting in the need for retreatment to achieve continued closure and visual stabilization. However, the risk of adverse events such as acute vision loss does not increase with PDT retreatment, unlike that associated with conventional thermal photocoagulation.

Owing to the strong evidence from the TAP trial supporting the use of verteporfin in reducing vision loss, the sensitizer was recently approved by the regulatory agencies of 22

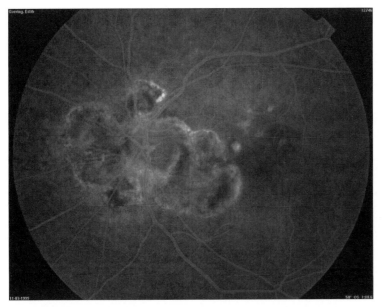

Figure 6 Ninety-year-old female with prior successful treatment of peripapillary choroidal neovascular (CNV) membrane. Visual acuity is 20/60.

countries, including the United States, European Union, Canada, and Australia, for the treatment of age-related macular degeneration (AMD) in patients with predominantly classic subfoveal choroidal neovascularization.

B. Case Example

A 90-year-old woman with a history of AMD, and a diskiform scar in the fellow right eye underwent successful treatment of a peripapillary choroidal neovascular membrane in the left eye with retention of 20/60 vision (Fig. 6). She subsequently developed a recurrence of predominantly classic CNV into the center of the fovea in her left eye. The early and late phases of the pretreatment angiogram are seen in Figures 7 and 8, respectively.

Visual acuity was reduced from 20/60 to 20/200. The patient underwent photodynamic therapy with Visudyne to the left eye according to the methods described in the TAP study on December 16, 1999. Early and late-phase fluorescein angiographic images taken 1 week later (Figs. 9 and 10, respectively) demonstrated hypofluorescence in the area of prior hyperfluorescence confirming temporary closure of the active classic CNV. However, by 3 months following initial treatment, the CNV had become reperfused, as demonstrated in Figures 11 and 12, necessitating retreatment. Visual acuity was stabilized at the 20/200 level, permitting reading with low-vision aids.

PDT with Visudyne is only suited for patients with predominantly classic subfoveal CNV. There was no visual acuity difference between placebo-treated and Visudyne-treated eyes when the lesion had less than 50% classic CNV composition (39). The Verteporfin In Photodynamic Therapy Trial (VIP) evaluated the use of Visudyne for occult CNV. The VIP Trial found no significant difference between placebo-treated and Visudyne-treated eyes with occult CNV at 1 year (40). Further studies will investigate the use of different treatment parameters in the treatment of occult CNV with PDT.

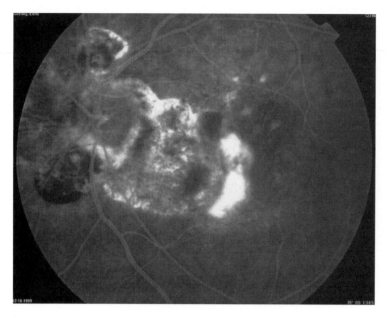

Figure 7   Early frame angiogram from same patient 1 month later with reduction in visual acuity to 20/200 with recurrence of classic CNV from temporal edge of prior treatment scar into center of fovea.

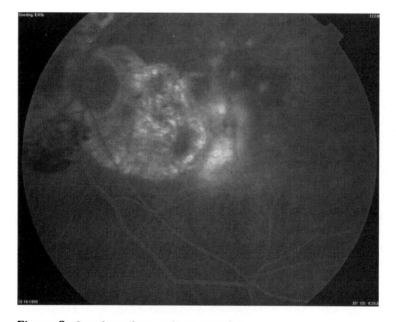

Figure 8   Late frame from study on same date.

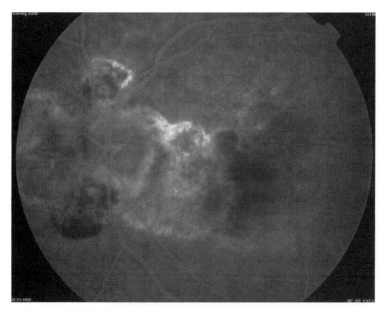

Figure 9 Early frame angiogram of same patient one week following photodynamic therapy with verteporfin. Note absence of hyperfluorescence in foveal region, previously seen in Figure 8.

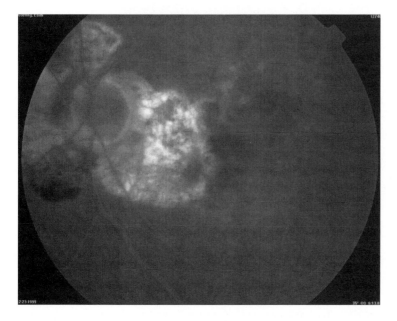

Figure 10 Late frame angiogram 1 week following photodynamic therapy. Note persistence of hyperfluorescence indicating absence of leakage from and presumed closure of subfoveal choroidal neovascularization.

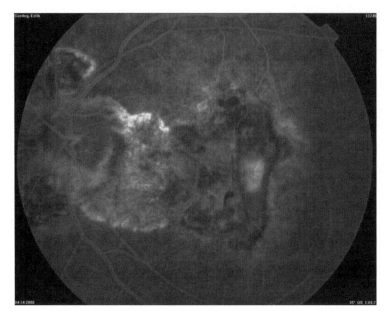

Figure 11   Same patient seen in Figure 6, seen 3 months following initially successful photodynamic therapy. The midframe angiogram demonstrates regrowth of subfoveal choroidal neuvascularization with slight enlargement compared with Figure 7.

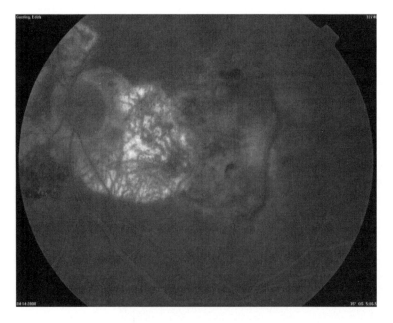

Figure 12   Late frame angiogram of same patient confirming staining of lesion.

III. OTHER AGENTS

Differences exist, however, in the quantum yield, clinical efficiency, and light and sensitizer dose requirements between different classes of agents. While Verteporfin (Visudyne) is the first photosensitizing agent to be approved, other photodynamic therapy agents, such as tin ethyl etiopurpurin (Purlytin) and motexafin lutetium (Optrin), are currently undergoing Phase III and Phase II trials, respectively, and may also prove useful in the area of photodynamic therapy.

A. Tin Ethyl Etiopurpurin Human Trials

Phase I/II tin ethyl etiopurpurin (Purlytin, SnET2) studies have confirmed the preclinical studies prediction of efficacy in the treatment of subfoveal choroidal neovascularization in humans (30). The trials are cosponsored by Miravant Medical Technologies, Santa Barbara, California, and Pharmacia Upjohn, Kalamazoo, Michigan. Forty eyes with subfoveal CNV were treated in an open-label dose-escalation study in which they received between 0.25 and 1.0 mg/kg of tin ethyl etiopurpurin and 664-nm light ranges from fluences of 36–126 J/cm^2 at a rate of 600 mW/cm^2. Twenty-three of 40 eyes (58%) remained at baseline or improved. At the preferred drug light combination of 0.5–0.75 mg/kg and 36 J/cm^2, visual acuity changes from baseline ranged from +1.9 to +3.5 lines 12 weeks after treatment. Retreatment was frequently required. Fourteen eyes were evaluated at 6 months and were found to have a decline of −1.1 line in visual acuity. Based on these results, a pivotal Phase III trial is currently underway for patients 50 years or older who have subfoveal CNV of less than 3000 microns with at least some classic component secondary to AMD and a best corrected visual acuity score of 20/63–20/500. Eyes with prior laser treatment, recent intraocular surgery, high myopia, or large amounts of submacular damage were excluded.

B. Motexafin Lutetium Human Trials

Human studies performed in Europe (sponsored by Pharmacyclics, Sunnyvale, CA, and Alcon Laboratories, Fort Worth, TX) confirmed the utility of using motexafin lutetium (Optrin, lutetium texaphyrin, Lu-Tex) as a PDT agent for the treatment of subfoveal CNV in humans at selected drug doses and light fluences. In patients receiving 2.5–3.0 mg/kg of drug and fluences ranging from 50 to 125 J/cm^2 (732 nm) complete or partial closure of CNV was achieved in nine of 13 patients. Twenty of 26 patients receiving at least 4 mg/kg of drug had partial or complete closure. Higher light doses were associated with higher closure rates; only three of 18 patients closed with 50–75 J/cm^2 while eight of nine closed with 125–150 J/cm^2. Changes in visual acuity were strongly correlated with angiographic closure with an improvement of 0.5 line in patients with complete or partial closure compared with a mean decrease of 0.33 line in patients without closure ($p < 0.03$). Patients treated with 4.0 mg/kg were more likely to experience paresthesias, which were thought to represent a mild photosensitizing effect. There was one case of obvious facial photosensitization. Based upon these studies, a Phase I/II study was begun in the United States with sites in the San Francisco Bay area, New York, Los Angeles, and Boston to further evaluate the safety and efficacy of Lu-Tex (2.0–3.0 mg/kg and 50–125 J/cm^2) for both angiography and PDT in 45 patients.

C. Complications

To date, verteporfin has had the longest follow-up, so most of the adverse events are known for this sensitizer. Recurrence of CNV and vision disturbances has occurred in some patients. For verteporfin, injection site reactions (13.4%), infusion-related back pain (2%), and cutaneous photosensitivity reactions (3%) have been reported. Transient visual disturbances occurred in 18% of PDT patients compared to 12% of placebo patients. The long-term effects of treatment, in terms of both safety and vision stabilization, are largely unknown as follow-up, thus far, has been limited to 2 years. The use of fluorescein angiography as a surrogate clinical endpoint is questionable. In subgroup analyses of many of the photosensitizers it seems that this is not the ultimate predictor for vision improvement, so in the absence of visual acuity data, caution must be used when designing retreatment regimens.

IV. FUTURE DEVELOPMENTS

A. Photodynamic Angiography

One area of current investigation and potential utility is photodynamic angiography. As indicated earlier, upon illumination of the sensitizer with a paired laser light source, it undergoes an electronic transition to an activated short-lived excited singlet state, which may either intrasystem crossing to generate the longer-lived excited triplet state or convert back to the ground state with consequent fluorescence (Fig. 3). Even when the conversion to a triplet occurs, photons are still generated during reversion to the ground state producing fluorescence. The quantum yield for emitted fluorescence varies from compound to compound much as does the quantum yield for free radicals. One potentially useful side effect of this emitted fluorescence is the ability to image the photosensitzer in vivo employing sensitive detectors matched to the emission wavelength of the photosensitizer. In the case of Motexafin Lutetium, maximal absorbance occurs in two regions, 470 nm, and 732 nm, and emission at 750 nm (Fig. 1) When specialized filters centered around 75 nm are used, a florescein angiogram demonstrating the biodistribution of this photosensitizer can be displayed (Fig. 13). The information available from this type of real-time analysis, may permit the development of more refined treatment regimens based upon the differential pharmacokinetics of different sensitizers, individualized for type of CNV and specific patient pharmacokinetic factors, as a supplement to conventional fluorescein angiography (19,22).

B. Mono-L-Aspartyl Chlorin e6 (NPe6 or MACE)

Preclinical studies in pigmented rabbits and monkeys confirm the utility of NPe6 in the closure of experimental choroidal neovasculature and the normal choriocapillaris while sparing the retina (31). Effective occlusion of normal vessels was achieved at 2 mg/kg with a fluence of 2.3–7.5 J/cm^2 or 10 mg/kg using 0.46–0.75 J/cm^2, using relatively short pulses of 1–10 s (450–750 mW/cm^2 and 664 nm) 5 min after injection. The combination of higher doses of drug and higher fluences was highly toxic to the retina. NPe6 could also be imaged in the retinal and choroidal circulation using specialized digital capture equipment and matched filters.

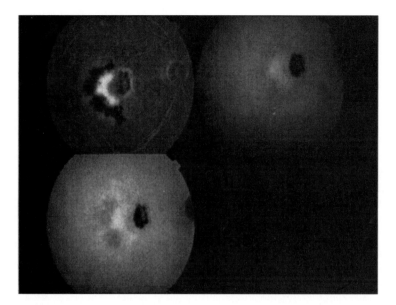

Figure 13 Composite photograph demonstrating different angiographic views of patient with classic recurrent CNV emanating from temporal edge of previously treated CNV. The image at top left is a late frame fluorescein angiogram with the temporal margin obscured by blood. The image at top right is an ICG angiogram taken on the same day. The image at bottom left is an angiographic image taken with an excitation and barrier filters of approximately 730 and 750 nm, respectively, optimized to demonstrate the biodistribution of motexafin lutetium. Note the relative similarity between the ICG and Lu-Tex images related to their capture in the infrared spectrum, and relatively greater molecular weight and protein binding than fluorescein.

C. Chloroaluminum Sulfonated Phthalocyanine (A1PcS4)

A1PcS4-mediated PDT produced closure of retinal medullary ray vessels and choroidal vessels in normal nonpigmented and pigmented rabbits. Histological evaluation revealed marked thrombosis of medullary ray and choroidal vessels with minimal changes to surrounding tissues including the neurosensory retina. In pigmented rabbits higher sensitizer doses were needed for complete closure compared to the nonpigmented rabbits. Kliman and colleagues undertook a diagnostic and therapeutic study using A1PcS4 in monkeys that had photothermal-induced choroidal neovascularization (32,33). A1PcS4 is highly fluorescent. Excitation at 600 nm induces fluorescence around 680 nm. Angiographic monitoring of the monkey eyes using 3 mg A1PcS4/kg displayed localization of the dye in the neovascular vessels for up to 24 h. Light dose and time interval dependencies for vascular occlusion were observed. Illumination 30 min following sensitizer administration with a fluence of 34 J/cm^2 at a rate of 283 mW/cm^2 produced complete CNV closure as seen at 48 h. Using the same illumination parameters at 24 h did not produce vessel closure. Increasing the fluence to 85 J/cm^2 at 24 h elicited partial vessel closure.

To increase the targeting ability of A1PcS4 heat-sensitive liposomes have been used as a delivery vehicle. This method of laser-targeted delivery has been described by Asrani and Zeimer (34). Albino rats were administered 7.5 mg A1PcS4/kg and then were irradiated within 5 min of administration. A dye laser at 577 nm was used so that significant blood absorption would take place thereby heating the liposomes and subsequently releasing the A1PcS4 that was then activated by the sensitizer. Activation at this wavelength of A1PcS4 is not ideal, as it is 14 times less than the peak at 675 nm, but it is still feasible. Vessel occlusion was achieved, suggesting that laser-targeted delivery may be feasible in humans.

D. ATX-S10

ATX-S10 [13,17-bis (1-carboxypropionyl) carbamoylethyl-8-ethenyl-2-hydroxy-3-hydroxyimino-ethylidene-2, 7,12,18-tetramethyl 6 porphyrin sodium] is a hydrophilic chlorin photosensitizer that has been shown to close CNV in the rat (35,36). Fluorescence microscopy using ATX-S10 as its own fluorophore confirmed the presence of the drug in the lumen of the retinal and choroidal vessels within 5 h. The sensitizer cleared rapidly from the normal retina. Laser illumination applied immediately and 2–4 h following sensitizer injection at fluences of 7.4 J/cm^2 and 22 J/cm^2, respectively, caused CNV occlusion without significant damage to the normal retinal and larger choroidal vessels.

ATX-S10-mediated PDT was found to induce selective occlusion of experimental CNV in primate eyes (37). Optimal treatment regimens included dosing regimens of 30–40 J/cm^2 with illumination 30–74 min after administration of 8 mg ATX-S10/kg, and 1–10 J/cm^2 illumination at 30–74 min or 30–74 J/cm^2 illumination 75–150 min after administration of 12 mg ATX-S10/kg.

V. FUTURE PDT DIRECTIONS

Microvasculature damage occurs soon after PDT causing blood flow stasis leading to hypoxia. Hypoxia induces angiogenesis marking disease continuation. Antiangiogenic treatment has recently been shown to increase the antitumor effectiveness of PDT using experimental tumor models (38). It therefore envisioned combining antiangiogenic treatments with clinical PDT for AMD patients for both acute and sustained vessel closures. The fluorescent properties of the photo sensitizers can be taken advantage of to allow diagnostic localization.

VI. CONCLUSION

Subfoveal CNV associated with AMD has a poor prognosis. The potential for selective destruction of the CNV by PDT is being realized with the recent evaluation of randomized clinical trials. Visudyne (BPD-MA) has shown clinical benefits in treated patients catalyzing the exploration of other photodynamic agents. Further evaluation of light-dosing parameters, pharmacokinetics, plasma protein binding, subcellular localization, sensitizer absorption, degradation, and metabolism is currently underway which will help to discern the differences between the various sensitizers. It is anticipated that further refinements will be made in protocol and treatment design enabling this technique to become a widely practiced, beneficial treatment modality.

VII. ADDENDUM

The 2-year results for the occult CNV with no classic group showed a statistically significant difference between the verteporfin and the placebo groups (40). Verteporfin therapy reduced the risk of moderate and severe vision loss in the AMD patients. The benefit was greater for patients presenting with either smaller lesion size (4 disk areas or less)—regardless of initial acuity—or lower levels of visual acuity (letter score less than 65 letters, 20/50-1 or less equivalent) regardless of initial lesion size.

There is at present no proven benefit of verteporfin for treatment of minimally classic lesions at this time. The Verteporfin in Minimally Lesion Study is ongoing and will address this application.

REFERENCES

1. Henderson BW, Dougherty TJ. How does photodynamic therapy work? Photochem Photobiol 1992;55:145–157.
2. Dougherty TJ, Gomer CJ, Henderson BW, Jori G, Kessel D, Korbelik M, Moan J, Peng Q. Photodynamic therapy. J Natl Cancer Inst 1998;90:889–905.
3. Hausmann WH. Die sensibilisierende Wirkung des Hamatoporphyrins. Biochem Z 1911;30:276–316.
4. Castellani A, Page GP, Concioli M. Photodynamic effect of haematoporphyrin on blood microcirculation. J Pathol Bacteriol 1963;86:99–102.
5. Selman SH, Kreimer-Birnbaum M, Klaunig JE, Goldblatt PJ, Keck RW, Britton SL. Blood flow in transplantable bladder tumors treated with hematoporphyrin derivative and light. Cancer Res 1984;44:1924–1927.
6. Star WM, Marijnissen HP, van den Berg-Blok AE, Versteeg JA, Franken KA, Reinhold HS. Destruction of rat mammary tumor and normal tissue microcirculation by hematoporphyrin derivative photoradiation observed in vivo in sandwich observation chambers. Cancer Res 1986;46:2532–2540.
7. Fingar VH, Kik PK, Haydon PS, Cerrito PB, Tseung M, Abang E, Wieman TJ. Analysis of acute vascular damage after photodynamic therapy using benzoporphyrin derivative (BPD). Br J Cancer 1999;79:1702–1708.
8. Fingar VH. Vascular effects of photodynamic therapy. J Clin Laser Med Surg 1996; 14:323–328.
9. Husain D, Miller JW, Kenney AG, Michaud N, Flotte TJ, Gragoudas ES. Photodynamic therapy and digitial angiography of experimental iris neovascularization using liposomal benzoporphyin derivative. Ophthalmology 1997;104:1242–1250.
10. Richter AM, Waterfield E, Jain AK, Allison B, Sternberg ED, Dolphin D, Levy JG. Photosensitising potency of structural analogues of benzoporphyrin derivative (BPD) in a mouse tumor model. Br J Cancer 1991;63:87–93.
11. Richter AM, Jain AK, Canaan AJ, Waterfield E, Sternberg ED, Levy JG. Photosensitizing efficiency of two regioisomers of the benzoporphyrin derivative monoacid ring A (BPD-MA). Biochem Pharmacol 1992;43:2349–2358.
12. Levy JG, Chan A, Strong A. Clinical status of benzoporphyrin derivative. Proc SPIE 1995;2625:86–95.
13. Haimovici R, Kramer M, Miller J, Hasan T, Flotte TJ, Schomacker KT, Gragoudas ES. Localization of lipoprotein-delivered benzoporphyrin derivative in the rabbit eye. Curr Eye Res 1997;16:83–90.
14. Husain D, Miller JW. Photodynamic therapy of exudative age-related macular degeneration. Semin Ophthalmol 1997;12:14–25.
15. Husain D, Kramer M, Kenny AG, Michaud N, Flotte TJ, Gragoudas ES, Miller JW. Effects of photodynamic therapy using vertepofin on experimental choroidal neovascularization and normal retina and choroid up to 7 weeks after treatment. Invest Ophthalmol Vis Sci 1999;40:2322–2331.
16. Reinke MH, Canakis C, Husain D, Michaud N, Flotte TJ, Gragoudas ES, Miller JW.

Verteporfin photodynamic therapy retreatment of normal retina and choroid in the cynomolgous monkey. Ophthalmology 1999;106:1915–1923.

17. Mang TS, Allison R, Hewson G, Snyder W, Moskowitz R. A phase II/III clinical study of tin ethyl etiopurpurin (Purlytin)-induced photodynamic therapy for the treatment of recurrent cutaneous metastatic breast cancer. Cancer J Sci Am 1998;4:378–384.

18. Primbs GB, Casey R, Wamser K, Snydner WJ, Crean DH. Photodynamic therapy for corneal neovascularization. Ophthal Surg Lasers 1998;29:832–838.

19. Blumenkranz MS, Woodburn KW, Qing F, Verdooner S, Kessel D, Miller R. Lutetium texaphyrin (Lu-Tex): a potential new agent for ocular fundus angiography and photodynamic therapy. Am J Ophthalmol 2000;129:353–362.

20. Rockson SG, Lorenz DP, Cheong WF, Woodburn KW. Photoangioplasty: an emerging clinical cardiovascular role for photodynamic therapy. Circulation. 2000: 102;591–596.

21. Renschler MF, Yuen AR, Panella TJ, Wieman TJ, Dougherty S, Esserman L, Panjehpour M, Taber SW, Fingar VH, Lowe E, Engel JS, Lum B, Woodburn KW, Cheong W, Miller RA. Photodynamic therapy trials with lutetium texaphyrin (Lu-Tex) in patients with locally recurrent breast cancer. Proc SPIE 1998;3247:35–39.

22. Graham KB, Arbour JD, Connolly EJ, Delori F, Carson D, Gragoudas ES, Miller JW. Digital angiography using lutetium texaphyrin in a monkey model of choroidal neovascularization (abstract). Invest Ophthalmol Vis Sci 1999;40 (Suppl):S402.

23. Arbour JD, Connolly EJ, Graham K, Carson D, Michaud N, Flotte T, Gragoudas ES, Miller JW. Photodynamic therapy of experimental choroidal neovascularization in a monkey model using intravenous infusion of lutetium texaphyrin (abstract). Invest Ophthalmol Vis Sci 1999;40 (Suppl):S401.

24. Miller JW, Schmidt-Erfurth U, Sickenberg M, Pournaras CJ, Laqua H, Barbazetto I, Zografos L, Piguet B, Donati G, Lane AM, Birngruber R, van den Berg H, Strong A, Manjuris U, Gray T, Fsadni M, Bressler NM, Gragoudas ES. Photodynamic therapy with verteporfin for choroidal neovascularization caused by age-related macular degeneration: results of a single treatment in a Phase 1 and 2 study. Arch Ophthalmol 1999;117:1161–1173.

25. Photodynamic therapy of subfoveal choroidal nsovascularization in age-related macular degeneration with verteporfin: one-year results of 2 randomized clinical trials—TAP report 1. Treatment of Age-Related Macular Degeneration with Photodynamic Therapy (TAP) Study Group. Arch Ophthalmol 1999;117:1329–1345.

26. Dastgheib K, Bressler SB, Green WR. Clinicopathologic correlation of laser lesion expansion after treatment of choroidal neovascularization. Retina 1993;13:345–352.

27. Visual outcome after laser photocoagulation for subfoveal choroidal neovascularization secondary to age-related macular degeneration. The influence of initial lesion size and visual acuity. Macular Photocoagulation Study Group. Arch Ophthalmol 1994;112:480–488.

28. Laser photocoagulation for juxtafoveal choroidal neovascularization: five-year results from randomized clinical trials Macular Photocoagulation Study Group. Arch Ophthalmol 1994;112:500–509.

29. Schmidt-Erfurth U, Miller JW, Sickenberg M, Laqua H, Barbazetto I, Gragoudas ES, Zografos L, Piguet B, Pournaras CJ, Donati G, Lane AM, Bimgruber R, van den Berg H, Strong HA, Manjuris U, Gray T, Fsadni M, Bressler NM, Photodynamic therapy with verteporfin for choroidal neovascularization caused by age-related macular degeneration: results of retreatments in a Phase 1 and 2 study. Arch Ophthalmol 1999;117:1177–1187.

30. Thomas EL, Rosen R, Murphy R, Puliafitto C, Jonsson P. Visual acuity stabilizes after a single treatment with SnET2 photodynamic therapy in patients with subfoveal choroidal neovascularization (abstract). Invest Ophthalmol Vis Sci 1999;40(Suppl):S401.

31. Mori K, Yoneya S, Ohta M, Sano A, Anzai K, Peyman GA, Moshfeghi DM. Angiographic and histologic effects of fundus photodynamic therapy with a hydrophilic sensitizer (mono-L-aspartyl chlorin e6). Ophthalmology 1999;106:1384–1391.

32. Kliman GH, Puliafito CA, Stern D, Borirakchanyavat S, Gregory WA. Phthalocyanine photo-

dynamic therapy: new strategy for closure of choroidal neovasculariaztion. Lasers Surg Med 1994;15:2–10.

33. Kliman GH, Puliafito CA, Grossman GA, Gregory WA. Retinal and choroidal vessel closure using phthalocyanine photodynamic therapy. Lasers Surg Med 1994;15:11–18.

34. Asrani S, Zeimer R. Feasibility of laser targeted photo-occlusion of ocular vessels. Br J Ophthalmol 1995;79:766–770.

35. Gohto Y, Obana A, Kaneda K, Miki T. Photodynamic effect of a new photosensitizer ATX-S10 on corneal neovascularization. Exp Eye Res 1998;67:313–322.

36. Obana A, Gohto Y, Kanede K, Nakajima S, Takemura T, Miki T. Selective occlusion of choroidal neovasculariazation by photodynamic therapy with a water-soluble photosensitizer, ATX-S10. Lasers Surg Med 1999;24:209–222.

37. Obana A, Gohto Y, Kanai M, Nakajima S, Kaneda K, Miki T. Selective photodynamic effects of the new photosensitizer ATX-S10(Na) on choroidal neovascularization in monkeys. Arch Ophthalmol 2000;118:650–658.

38. Ferrario A, von Tiehl KF, Rucker N, Schwarz MA, Gill PS, Gomer CJ. Antiangiogenic treatment enhances photodynamic therapy responsiveness in a mouse mammary carcinoma. Cancer Res 2000;60:4066–4069.

39. Therapy (TAP) Study Group. Photodynamic therapy of subfoveal choroidal neovascularization in age-related macular degeneration with verteporfin: two-year results of 2 randomized clinical trials—TAP Report 2. Arch Ophthalmol 2001;119:198–207.

40. Tap Study Group Verteporfin therapy of subfoveal choroidal neovascularization in age-related macular degeneration: two-year results of a randomized clinical trial including lesions with occult with no classic choroidal neovascularization—Verteporfin in photodynamic therapy report 2. Am J Ophthalmol 2001:131:541–559.

11

Radiation Treatment in Age-Related Macular Degeneration

Christina J. Flaxel

Doheny Retina Institute of the Doheny Eye Institute, University of Southern California Keck School of Medicine, Los Angeles, California

Paul Finger

New York AMDRT Center, New York, New York

I. INTRODUCTION

Age-related macular degeneration (AMD) is a leading cause of severe visual loss and legal blindness in developed countries (1,2). Ten million Americans are visually disabled due to AMD and 10% of patients aged 66–74 years have signs of AMD (3,4). Estimates of prevalence range from 7 to 30% in persons aged 75–85 years (4–6). The wet form of AMD is responsible for the most severe and rapid vision loss. In North America, 200,000– 400,000 people will develop the most severe, or wet, form of AMD each year. This wet form accounts for 12% of cases overall but 90% of cases of legal blindness (4).

Macular degeneration is likely to reach epidemic proportions. It is estimated that the U.S. population over the age of 85 years is currently 5 million, a number expected to triple by the middle of this century (2). Because of increasing life expectancies in developed countries, more and more people will live long enough to develop vision loss from AMD.

Vision loss due to neovascular (wet) AMD involves the growth of abnormal "new" vessels through breaks in Bruch's membrane from the choroid and under the retinal pigment epithelium (RPE). This neovascular process is felt to be due to age-related degeneration of the RPE. In the normal eye by-products of retinal metabolism, specifically of the photoreceptors, are usually removed by cells of the RPE layer. These materials build up and are seen clinically as drusen in the macula. It is felt that aging slows down the RPE cell metabolism and is associated with RPE cell death, so that this layer is no longer able to remove these waste products, which in turn accumulate and are seen clinically as drusen. It is also unclear why in the dry form of AMD this accumulation leads to cell loss and atrophy, while in wet macular degeneration drusen appear to be a stimulus for blood vessels to grow from the choroid. It has been postulated that neovascularization is an attempt to clear the waste. Unfortunately, these new vessels, called choroidal neovascular membranes (CNV), cause many of the problems related to the wet form of the disease.

A. Laser Treatment for AMD

Neovascular membranes due to AMD are identified as either classic or occult or present as a combination of the two forms: classic CNV are characterized by discrete areas of hyperfluorescence in the early phase of the fluorescein angiogram (FA) that expand in the later phase while occult CNV lack the typical features of classic CNV and show areas of stippled hyperfluorescence in the early phase, often associated with elevation of the RPE, associated with dye leakage in the later phase. Typically, classic CNV have well-demarcated borders on FA and result in significant vision loss within the first year of onset while occult CNV have poorly defined borders and cause gradual decline in vision over an extended period of time. Though patients selected for the Macular Photocoagulation Study (MPS) were to have classic CNV, the MPS investigators undertook a rereview of baseline FAs with attention to degree of occult CNV and determined that half the patients had classic only and half had some degree of occult CNV (11). More than half of the patients with classic CNV only developed recurrent CNV within 1 year of treatment but the treatment was still beneficial. In the patients with occult CNV there was no difference in outcome between treated and untreated eyes and no benefit was found in treating only the classic component in these cases (11).

B. Rationale for Laser

Until recently, the only treatment for AMD proven by randomized clinical trial was laser photocoagulation of the abnormal and leaking blood vessels. In these studies, the location of the CNV along with the fluorescein angiographic characteristics determined whether the lesion was treatable.

The MPS series demonstrated the benefit of treating extrafoveal, juxtafoveal, and subfoveal CNV due to AMD (7–9). Unfortunately, laser photocoagulation of subfoveal lesions induces an immediate central scotoma that is poorly tolerated by most patients, in all groups, only 10–15% of eyes with neovascular AMD meet the criteria for laser treatment, recurrent CNV is very common, and the majority of patients with neovascular AMD become legally blind despite laser treatment (10).

The MPS group found that most treated eyes had an average visual acuity of 20/200–20/320 at 3 years, which is better than untreated eyes, and that treated eyes maintained better contrast sensitivity than untreated eyes (12). Within 5 years of treatment, more than half of patients required retreatment and most eyes became legally blind (visual acuity $\geq$ 20/200). Recurrent CNV is the major reason for additional vision loss after argon laser treatment for juxta- and extrafoveal CNV because these recurrences are often subfoveal (10). Laser treatment of subfoveal CNV has been shown to be beneficial in eyes with classic, well-demarcated lesions of relatively small size with relatively good vision (13). Many eyes with subfoveal lesions are not good candidates for laser because the CNV is too big, the vision is too good, or the lesion cannot be clearly demarcated using standard FA techniques (14).

C. New Approaches in Treatment of AMD

Alternative newly developed therapeutic approaches for subfoveal CNV include surgical removal of the neovascular membrane with or without transplantation of pigment epithelial cells (15–18). This approach is currently undergoing clinical trials in the United States as the Subfoveal Surgery Trial (sponsored by the National Institutes of Health). Other methods, such as macular translocation surgery, involve rotation of the retina and CNV away from the macula thus allowing the CNV to be lasered in an extrafoveal location (19–22). Photodynamic therapy (PDT) is a new treatment option that has been shown to temporarily close CNV due to AMD and high myopia (23–29). A number of antiangiogenic drug trials for AMD are also underway (30–34).

Of these new methods, only PDT (using the photoactive drug Visudyne) has been proven to slow down visual loss in treated eyes in a randomized placebo-controlled clinical trial (29). The TAP study showed that 54% of sham-treated eyes versus 39% of treated eyes lost three or more lines of vision after 1 year and that PDT is indicated only when the CNV is greater than 50% classic in composition (29). However, the treatment does have some shortcomings including the need for repeated treatment at 3-month intervals. Recent 2-year results from the VIP Study do show efficacy of PDT in subfoveal occult membrane in slowing visual loss (34a).

Other methods currently undergoing evaluation include plasmapheresis, which is undergoing pilot studies (35,36), low-dose transpupillary thermal therapy (TTT) (37), and drug therapy including the use of intraocular administration of antiangiogenic agents.

II. RADIATION THERAPY FOR AMD

When compared with these other experimental treatment methods, theoretical advantages of radiation therapy include absence of iatrogenic mechanical or laser damage or systemic side effects (38). An additional advantage to radiation treatment is that eyes with primarily occult CNVs are potentially eligible for treatment (38) and, unlike PDT, only one treatment would be necessary. The scientific rationale for using radiation therapy for a benign disease characterized by neovascular growth is based on experimental and clinical evidence. Radiation is known to potentially destroy vascular tissue (39–42). Specifically, low-dose radiation has been shown to inhibit neovascularization (43–46). An example is seen in plaque-irradiated choroidal melanomas where a ring of chorioretinal atrophy is commonly found around the tumor's base and decreased or absent blood flow is demonstrated by FA. These findings demonstrate the ability of radiation to destroy normal and neovascular blood vessels, but the resultant chorioretinal atrophy is an unacceptable endpoint when treating macular degeneration (46,47).

In contrast, if relatively low-dose radiotherapy could inhibit CNVs and secondary disciform scars, then patients should have better visual outcomes (Fig 1–3). The main question persists: is there a therapeutic window in which the dose of radiation used is high enough to induce regression of CNV but low enough to spare the normal retina and choroid? Radiation specialists believe this is possible: proliferating endothelium is more susceptible to radiation damage than are nonproliferating capillary endothelial cells and larger vessels; thus neovascular endothelial cells as well as inflammatory cells are particularly radiosensitive (48). There is also the potential for radiotherapy to inhibit further neovascular growth and induce neovascular regression by induction of programmed cell death and by modifications of growth factor profiles of the neovascular complexes (41,49). In addition, it is also thought that inflammation may play a role in neovascularization and, as noted, radiation inhibits the inflammatory response (41,50). Benign intracerebral arteriovenous malformations as well as choroidal hemangiomas have been shown to regress using ionizing beams (51–53).

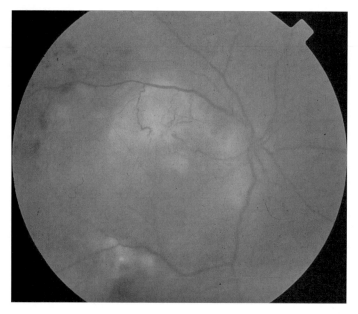

Figure 1 Right eye of 72-year-old patient with diskiform scar. See also color insert, Fig. 11.1.

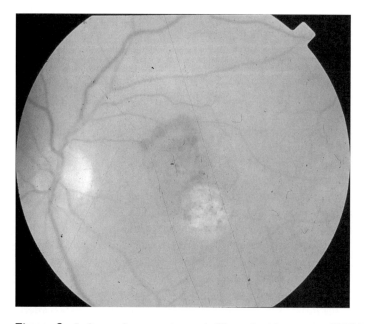

Figure 2 Left eye of same patient as in Figure 1 with recurrent CNV following laser treatment. See also color insert, Fig. 11.2.

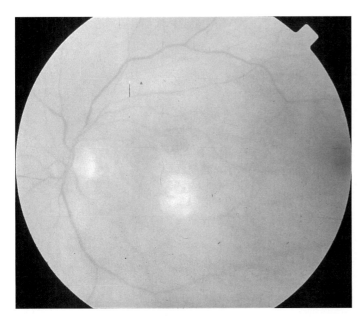

Figure 3 Same eye as in Figure 2, 6 months status post–proton radiation left eye for recurrent CNV. See also color insert, Fig. 11.3.

A. Radiation Toxicity

The potential toxicity of radiation is well known. (42,44,54–59). Studies have shown that the normal neural retina and choroid are relatively radioresistant (57,58). It is also known that factors influencing development of radiation retinopathy include total dose delivered, daily fraction size, preexisting microangiopathy, diabetes, or prior chemotherapy (47,48).

Radiation-induced retinopathy has been reported at doses of 30–35 Gy, but is more commonly associated with doses of 45–60 Gy (Fig. 4). Radiation optic neuropathy is rare at doses below 50 Gy (47,48,54–56) (Fig. 5, A and B) Fraction sizes greater than 2.5 Gy may predispose to toxicity especially with total doses greater than 45 Gy (55,56). However, there is increasing evidence that fractionated doses with larger daily fraction size in lower than standard overall doses can be delivered safely and effectively to small regions. Lens dose of 15 Gy or more will induce cataract and transient dry eye; keratitis and epiphoria are expected complications (54–56,60). Other concerns are exposure to brain and contralateral eye (50,54–56).

III. PRIOR STUDIES

Initial reports regarding radiation for AMD began to appear in the literature in 1993 (61). Chakravarthy's preliminary results included 19 patients with subfoveal CNV due to AMD treated with radiation therapy and seven matched controls. At 1 year 63% of treated patients showed stabilization of vision, while there was deterioration of acuity in eyes of all controls over the same period. This study also showed significant neovascular membrane re-

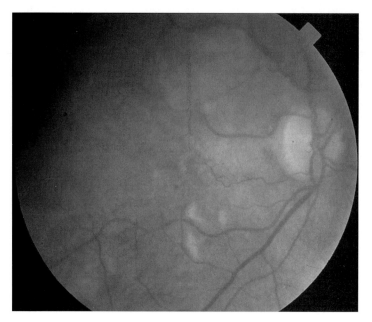

Figure 4   Radiation retinopathy 1 year following proton beam radiation using 14 GE. See also color insert, Fig. 11.4.

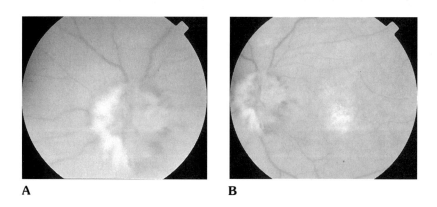

A   B

Figure 5   (A) Postradiation optic neuropathy after 14 GE proton beam treatment, 1 year post-treatment. (B) In this view the CNV appears dry. See also color insert, Fig. 11.5A, B.

gression in 77% of treated patients at 1 year by image analysis with concurrent progressive enlargement of the neovascular membranes in all controls over the same time period (61). These results and the results from other centers led to an ongoing prospective-randomized British and European Trial of radiation therapy (62). Multiple subsequent reports involving both external-beam radiotherapy (EBR) and plaque radiotherapy showed promising but variable results.

In 1996, Finger and colleagues reported their results with low-dose external-beam radiation of 12–15 Gy and plaque radiotherapy with equivalent dosage in 137 patients and showed decreased subretinal hemorrhages, exudates, and leakage of neovascular membranes with maintenance of visual acuity (63). Subsequently, Stalmans et al. from Belgium reported failure of control of CNV with radiation dosage of 20 Gy in 2-Gy fractions in 111 patients (64). A similar finding was noted by Spaide and his group in 1998 when they reported a dose of 10 Gy in 5-Gy fractions failed to control neovascular growth in AMD. This study never disclosed what percentage of irradiated patients were "recurrent CNVs" (previously treated by laser photocoagulation) (65). Several further reports in 1998 and 1999 reported possible beneficial effects of radiation—the Radiotherapy Study from the French group reported a potential beneficial effect of using 16 Gy in four sessions of 4 Gy each with mean follow-up of 6.4 months (66). A second group from France reported stabilization of visual acuity and anatomical outcome, also in occult CNV in eyes with AMD, in 1999 (67). However, this group also reported a significant complication rate including radiation retinopathy, optic neuropathy, choroidal vasculopathy, and branch retinal vein occlusion using either 20 Gy in 5 fractions via lateral beam (giving an effective dose of 30 Gy) or 16–20 Gy in 4–5 fractions delivered via lateral arc (67). This study did not include a control group and follow-up ranged from 12 to 24 months (67).

In another report from Finger and his group, plaque radiotherapy was employed in eyes with neovascular AMD with no adverse effects (68). This group concluded that plaque radiotherapy was unilateral treatment as opposed to external beam allowing a higher radiation dose to be delivered to the macula with less irradiation delivery to the surrounding tissues. They found no sight-limiting complications in their phase I clinical trial in which they treated 23 eyes with palladium-103 plaques (68). Berginks group from the Netherlands reported good results with relatively high radiation doses of 24 Gy and concluded that there was a dose-response effect with a more favorable effect at higher dosages (69,70).

In June 2000, Flaxel et al. published their report in EYE, discussing the use of proton beam irradiation for subfoveal CNV in AMD along with their data from the phase I/II planned dose-escalation clinical trial (71). Proton beam is another method for the delivery of radiation that allows a higher dose (at a high dose rate) to be delivered to a specific area. Like most forms of EBR, proton beam therapy requires an entry site and irradiates within its path; the dose volume is limited to a section of the eye, decreasing irradiation of normal tissues outside the beam and the contralateral eye. Flaxel et al. used proton beam irradiation in a single-dose, light-field patient orientation with temporal beam entry initially with 8 GE (Grey equivalent) beginning in March 1994, then increasing to 14 GE in March 1995 when no adverse effects relating to the radiation were noted. Twenty-one eyes were treated with 8 GE. Flaxel et al. noted an initial stabilization of subretinal leakage on FA in 50% of eyes at 12 months' follow-up but with regrowth in all but three eyes at 15 months' follow-up. However, in the 14 GE-treated eyes, 83% showed no leakage at 12 months of follow-up and 78% of eyes had unchanged or improved vision. Additionally, for those eyes with more than 9 months of follow-up in the 14-GE-treated patients, 83% of eyes that had 20/100 or better vision prior to proton beam treatment showed improvement in vision. Also, severe visual loss increased up to 37% at 2 years with 8-GE-treated eyes, while with 14 GE, the incidence of severe visual loss was essentially none through the follow-up period. However, in regard to complications related to the radiation treatment, there were no cases of cataract, dry eye, lash loss, or optic neuropathy in any of the study eyes and there was no case of radiation retinopathy in the 8-GE-treated eyes, but these complications were found in 50% of eyes treated with 14 GE. There was one case outside of the study of severe proliferative radiation retinopathy and optic neuropathy within 1 year of treatment with se-

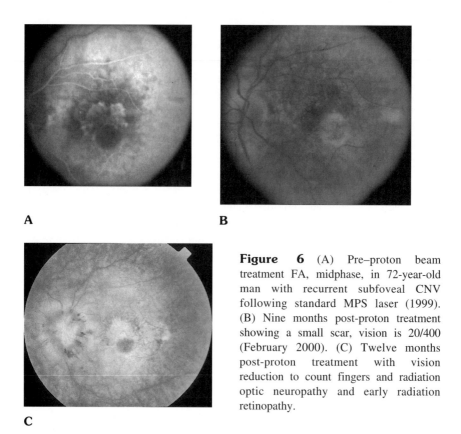

A   **B**

Figure 6 (A) Pre–proton beam treatment FA, midphase, in 72-year-old man with recurrent subfoveal CNV following standard MPS laser (1999). (B) Nine months post-proton treatment showing a small scar, vision is 20/400 (February 2000). (C) Twelve months post-proton treatment with vision reduction to count fingers and radiation optic neuropathy and early radiation retinopathy.

C

vere visual loss (Fig. 6, A, B, and C). The authors concluded that their preliminary data suggest that proton beam irradiation correlates with CNV regression, maintains visual function, is more effective at 14 GE, is less beneficial in larger lesions, and that radiation complications are more common with longer follow-up but only in the 14-GE-treated group (71). Because of the significant risk of complications, proton beam treatment is currently not being recommended until further studies can be done regarding dose delivery with consideration of fractionization of the dosage.

IV. CURRENT STUDIES

There are now several ongoing studies of the use of radiation in AMD. Two recent reports are from Holz's RAD Study Group in Germany (72) and Kobayashi and Kobayashi in Japan (73). The RAD Study is a randomized, prospective, double-blind, placebo-controlled trial, performed at nine centers throughout Germany (72). This study enrolled 205 patients treated with either 8 fractions of 2 Gy, (101 eyes) or 8 fractions of 0 Gy (104 eyes). At 1-year follow-up, no benefit was seen in either classic or occult subfoveal CNV due to AMD; approximately one-half of treated eyes were occult-only CNV while the other half were mixed classic plus occult CNV. No serious complications relating to the radiation treatment have occured to date (72). The Japanese study is also a randomized, prospective, placebo-controlled trial carried out at one center in Japan (73). This study enrolled 101 patients and followed them for 2 years. They also reported no significant treatment-related side-effects and they used a total dose of 20 Gy delivered in 10 divided doses over 14 days with irradiation through a single lateral port. They concluded that radiotherapy showed a beneficial effect compared with untreated eyes with favorable factors being smaller area of CNV, higher degree of occult CNV, and better initial visual acuity (73). Both groups are continuing follow-up on all patients.

Several studies are currently in progress including a set of prospective, double-masked, randomized studies at the Medical College of Georgia evaluating the efficacy of low-dose EBR using 14 Gy in 2-Gy fractions for new subfoveal CNV in AMD and in a trial using EBR as an adjunct for laser treatment to prevent recurrence; thus far no results have been reported. However, in their uncontrolled series of EBR for patients presenting with recurrent CNV after laser treatment, this group has reported a better response to treatment in the patients treated with 3-Gy fractions than in those treated with 2-Gy fractions, at least by clinical impression. In the United Kingdom, Chakravarthy and co-workers have been performing a prospective, single-masked, multicenter clinical trial evaluating EBR using 12 Gy in 2-Gy fractions in the treatment of subfoveal CNV with a classic component since 1995 (62). The clinical impression is that there is no difference between the treated and control groups. Finger, Berson, and colleagues have verbally reported a small randomized pilot study of EBR utilizing 18 Gy in 2-Gy fractions. With 8 months' follow-up, best-corrected visual acuities in treated patients were not significantly different from those of observed controls (personal communication).

Conflicting data from multiple studies led the NEI to sponsor a prospective randomized pilot study in the United States (38). This nonfunded, multicenter, pilot study includes two groups, with randomization to either treatment or observation, and is called the Age-Related Macular Degeneration Radiation Trial (AMDRT) (74). Eligibility criteria for the new subfoveal CNV Study include lesions not amenable to MPS laser treatment; classic, mixed, or occult CNV by FA; blood obscures less than 50% of the lesion; VA > 20/320; and no contraindication to EBR (i.e., prior chemotherapy, diabetes, history of periorbital or ocular radiation). Randomization is to either EBR (5 daily sessions of 4 Gy for a total dose of 20 Gy) or observation. The primary outcome measure is a 3-line or greater loss of visual acuity over the 5-year follow-up period. There is also a recurrent CNV study arm with similar criteria (74). Twelve centers are involved; many have completed initial enrollment of 10 eyes but there are no available data. No serious adverse effects of EBR have been reported to date.

V. CONCLUSIONS

The only well-organized, multicenter, masked study that has shown no benefit of EBR is Holz's German RAD study with 18 Gy in 2-Gy fractions (72). It is possible that either a higher total dose or larger fractions would be beneficial and other trials are currently evaluating this theory (including the AMDRT in the United States) (74). It is also possible that radiation in conjunction with another treatment modality might be of benefit such as combined with PDT or antiangiogenic agents: for example, allowing complete closure of the neovascular complex with PDT, followed by radiation to extend the affect of treatment. Other groups are looking at this possibility as well as the benefit of combining low-dose

EBR with conventional laser treatment to decrease the recurrence rate. Similarly, other groups are studying the use of low-dose proton beam combined with PDT in the hope that this will limit CNV recurrence. This approach might avoid the complications seen with higher doses of radiation using the proton beam.

The current AMDRT protocol should demonstrate whether there is any effect at a higher dose and dose rate. Any higher levels of radiation would be expected to demonstrate significant radiation-related side effects.

Although past studies have found that radiation halts the growth of choroidal neovascularization, the studies reported to date do not provide enough evidence to support widespread treatment of patients. Clearly, further prospective randomized studies are needed to actually show whether higher radiation doses would stabilize or improve vision in patients affected by exudative macular degeneration (38). Hopefully, studies such as the AMDRT will help to sort out this very difficult question.

VI. SUMMARY

Neovascular AMD is responsible for rapid and severe visual loss in developed countries. Discussed in this chapter are

> Mechanism of visual loss in wet AMD
> Classic versus occult CNV and laser photocoagulation
> The MPS
> Rationale for using laser in AMD and the results of the MPS
> New approaches in AMD treatment including surgical removal macular translocation surgery, photodynamic therapy, antiangiogenic drugs, steroid injections, plasmapheresis, and transpupillary thermal therapy
> Advantages of radiation therapy in AMD including inhibition of diskiform scar formation
> Toxicity of radiation including retinopathy and optic neuropathy
> Studies in the past using radiation therapy for AMD including external-beam and plaque radiotherapy
> Current studies including AMDRT, proton beam, RAD Study group from Germany, British EBR trial, and the Japanese study

REFERENCES

1. Ferris FL, Fine SL, Hyman L. Age-related macular degeneration and blindness due to neovascular maculopathy. Arch Ophthalmol 1984;102:1640–1642.
2. American Academy of Ophthalmology. Age-Related Macular Degeneration, Preferred Practice Pattern. San Francisco: American Academy of Ophthalmology, 1998.
3. Leibowitz HM, Krueger DE, Maunder LR, Milton RC, Kini MM, Kahn HA, Nickerson RJ, Pool J, Colton TL, Ganley JP, Loewenstein JI, Dawber TR. The Framingham Eye Study monograph: an ophthalmological and epidemiological study of cataract, glaucoma, diabetic retinopathy, macular degeneration, and visual acuity in a general population of 2631 adults, 1973–1975. Surv Ophthalmol 1980;24(Suppl):335–610.
4. Kahn HA, Leibowitz HM, Ganley JP, Kini MM, Colton T, Nickerson RS, Dawber TR. The Framingham eye study. II. Association of ophthalmic pathology with single variables previously measured in the Framingham heart study. Am J Epidemiol 1977;106:33–41.

5. Klein BE, Klein R. Cataracts and macular degeneration in older Americans. Arch Ophthalmol 1982;100:571–573.

6. Vinding T. Age related macular degeneration, macular changes, prevalence and sex ratio. An epidemiological study of 1000 aged individuals. Acta Ophthalmol 1989;67:609–616.

7. Macular Photocoagulation Study Group. Argon laser photocoagulation for AMD: results of a randomized clinical trial. Arch Ophthalmol 1982;100:912–918.

8. Macular Photocoagulation Study Group. Juxtafoveal CNVM. Arch Ophthalmol 1990; 108:1442.

9. Macular Photocoagulation Study Group. Subfoveal neovascular lesions in AMD: guidelines for evaluation and treatment in the Macular Photocoagulation Study. Arch Ophthalmol 1991; 109:1242–1257.

10. Macular Photocoagulation Study Group. Recurrent CNV after argon laser treatment for neovascular maculopathy. Arch Ophthalmol 1986;104:503–512.

11. Macular Photocoagulation Study Group. Occult choroidal neovascularization. Influence on visual outcome in patients with age-related macular degeneration. Arch Ophthalmol 1996; 114:400–412.

12. Macular Photocoagulation Study Group. Laser photocoagulation of subfoveal neovascular lesions in AMD: results of a randomized clinical trial. Arch Ophthalmol 1991;109:1220–1231.

13. Macular Photocoagulation Study Group. Visual outcome after laser photocoagulation for subfoveal CNV secondary to AMD: the influence of initial lesion size and initial visual acuity. Arch Ophthalmol 1994;112:480–488.

14. Freund KB, Yanuzzi LA, Sorenson JA. Age-related macular degeneration and choroidal neovascularization. Am J Ophthalmol 1993;115:786–791.

15. Algvere PV, Berglin L, Gouras P, Sheng Y. Transplantation of fetal retinal pigment epithelium in age-related macular degeneration with subfoveal neovascularization. Graefe's Arch Clin Exp Ophthalmol 1994;232:707–716.

16. Rezai KA, Kohen L, Wiedermann P, Heimann K. Iris pigment epithelium transplantation. Graefe's Arch Clin Exp Ophthalmol 1997;235:558–562.

17. Thomas MA, Grand MG, Williams DF, Lowe MA. Surgical management of subfoveal choroidal neovascularization. Ophthalmology 1992;99:952–968.

18. Scheider A, Gundisch O, Kampik A. Surgical extraction of subfoveal choroidal new vessels and submacular haemorrhage in age-related macular degeneration; results of a prospective study. Graefe's Arch Clin Exp Ophthalmol 1999;237:10–15.

19. Machemer R, Steinhorst UH. Retinal separation, retinotomy, and macular relocation. II. A surgical approach for age-related macular degeneration? Graefe's Arch Clin Exp Ophthalmol 1993;231:635–641.

20. Ninomiya Y, Lewis JM, Hasegawa T, Tana Y. Retinotomy and foveal translocation for surgical management of subfoveal choroidal neovascular membranes. Am J Ophthalmol 1996; 122:613–621.

21. Eckardt C, Eckardt U, Conrad HG. Macular rotation with and without counterrotation of the globe in patients with age-related macular degeneration. Graefe's Arch Clin Exp Ophthalmol 1999;37:313–325.

22. Lewis H, Kaiser PK, Lewis S, Estafanous M. Macular translocation for subfoveal choroidal neovascularization in age-related macular degeneration: A prospective study. Am J Ophthalmol 1999;128:135–146.

23. Husain D, Miller JW, Michaud N, Connolly E, Flotte TJ, Gragoudas ES. Intravenous infusion of liposomal benzoporphyrin derivative for photodynamic therapy of experimental choroidal neovascularization. Arch Ophthalmol 1996;114:978–985.

24. Kliman GH, Puliafito CA, Stern D, Borirakchanyavat S, Gregory WA. Phthalocyanine photodynamic therapy: new strategy for closure of choroidal neovascularization. Lasers Surg Med 1994;15:2–10.

25. Lin SC, Lin CP, Feld JR, Duker JS, Puliafito CA. The photodynamic occlusion of choroidal vessels using benzoporphyrin derivative. Curr Eye Res 1994;13:513–522.

26. Miller JW, Walsh AW, Kramer M, Hasan T, Michaud N, Flotte TJ, Haimovici R, Gragoudas ES. Photodynamic therapy of experimental choroidal neovascularization using lipoprotein-delivered benzoporphyrin. Arch Ophthalmol 1995;113:810–818.

27. Peyman GA, Moshfeghi DM, Moshfeghi A, Khoobehi B, Doiron DR, Primbs GB, Crean DH. Photodynamic therapy for choroicapillaris using tin ethyl etiopurpurin (SnET2). Ophthalmic Surg Lasers 1997;28:409–417.

28. Schmidt-Erfurth U, Miller J, Sickenberg M, Bunse A, Laqua H, Gragoudas E, Zografos L, Birngruber R, van den Bergh H, Strong A, Manjuris U, Fsadni M, Lane AM, Piguet B, Bressler NM Photodynamic therapy of subfoveal choroidal neovascularization: clinical and angiographic examples. Graefe's Arch Clin Exp Ophthalmol 1998;236:365– 374.

29. Treatment of age-related macular degeneration with photodynamic therapy (TAP) Study Group. Photodynamic therapy of subfoveal choroidal neovascularization in age-related macular degeneration with verteporfin: one-year results of 2 randomized clinical trials— TAP report. Arch Ophthalmol 1999;117:1329–1345.

30. Challa JK, Gillies MC, Penfold PL, Gyory JF, Hunyor AB, Billson FA. Exudative degeneration and intravitreal triamcinolone: 18 month follow up. Aust NZ J Ophthalmol 1998;26:277–281.

31. D'Amato RJ, Loughan MS, Flynn E, Folkman J. Thalidomide is an inhibitor of angiogenesis. Proc Natl Acad Sci USA 1994;91:4082–4085.

32. Pharmacological Therapy for Macular Degeneration Study Group. Interferon-2a is ineffective for patients with choroidal neovascularization secondary to age-related macular degeneration. Results of a prospective randomized placebo-controlled clinical trial. Arch Ophthalmol 1997;115:865–872.

33. Thomas MA, Ibanez HE. Interferon alfa-2a in the treatment of subfoveal choroidal neovascularization. Am J Ophthalmol 1993;115:563–568.

34. Ciulla TA, Danis RP, Harris A. Age-related macular degeneration: review of experimental treatments. Surv Ophthalmol 1998;32:134–146.

34a. Verteporfin in Photodynamic Therapy [VIP] Study Group. Photodynamic therapy of subfoveal choroidal neovascularization in age-related macular degeneration with Verteporfin: two year results of a randomized clinical trial including lesions with occult but not classic neovascularization—VIP Report #2. Am J Ophthalmol 2001; in press.

35. Brunner R, Widder RA, Walter P, Luke C, Godehardt E, Bartz-Schmidt KU, Heimann K, Borberg H. Influence of membrane differential filtration on the natural course of age-related macular degeneration, a randomized trial. Retina 2000;20:483–491.

36. Inhoffen W, Nussgens Z. Rheological studies on patients with posterior subretinal neovascularization in age-related macular degeneration. Graefe's Arch Clin Exp Ophthalmol 1990;228:316–320.

37. Mainster MA, Reichel E. Transpupillary thermotherapy for age-related macular degeneration: long-pulse photocoagulation, apoptosis and heat-shock proteins. Ophthalmic Surg Lasers 2000;313:359–373.

38. Finger PT and Augsberger JJ. Controversies, radiotherapy and the treatment of age-related macular degeneration. Arch Ophthalmol 1998;116:1507–1511.

39. Baker DG, Krochak RJ. The response of the microvascular system to radiation: a review. Cancer Invest 1989;37:287–294.

40. Krishnan L, Krishnan EC, Jewell WR. Immediate effect of irradiation on microvasculature. J Rad Oncol Biol Phys 1988;15:147–150.

41. Finger PT, Immonen I, Freire J, Brown G. Brachytherapy for macular degeneration associated with subretinal neovascularization. In: Alberti WE, Richard G, Sagerman RH, eds. Age-Related Macular Degeneration. Berlin: Springer-Verlag, 2001:167–172.

42. Chakravarthy U, Gardiner TA, Archer DB, Maguire CJF. A light microscopic and autoradiographic study of non-irradiated and irradiated ocular wounds. Curr Eye Res 1989;8:337–348.

43. Archambeau JO, Mao XW, Yonemoto LT, Slater JD, Friedrichsen E, Teichman S, Preston W, Slater JM. What is the role of radiation in the treatment of subfoveal membranes? Review of ra-

diobiologic, pathologic, and other considerations to initiate a multimodality discussion. Int J Radiat Oncol Biol Phys 1998;40:1125–1136.

44. De Gowin RL, Lewis JL, Hoak JC, Mueller AL, Gibson DP. Radiosensitivity of human endothelial cells in culture. J Lab Clin Med 1974;84:42–48.

45. Hosoi Y, Yamamoto M, Ono T, Sakamoto K. Prostacyclin production in cultured endothelial cells is highly sensitive to low doses of ionizing radiation. Int J Radiat Biol 1993;63:631–638.

46. Johnson LK, Longenecker JP, Fajardo LF. Differential radiation response of cultured endothelial cells and smooth myocytes. Anal Quant Cytol 1982;4:188–198.

47. Finger PT. Radiation therapy for choroidal melanoma. Surv Ophthalmol 1997;42:215–232.

48. Sagerman RH, Chung CT, Alberti WE: Radiosensitivity of ocular and orbital structures. In: WE Alberti,RH Sagerman, eds. Radiotherapy of Intraocular and Orbital Tumors. Berlin: Springer-Verlag, 1993.

49. Langley RE, Bune EA, Quartuccio SG, Medeiras D, Braunhut SJ. Radiation induced apoptosis in microvascular endothelial cells. Br J Cancer 1997;75:666–672.

50. Finger PT, Chakravarthy Y. External beam radiation therapy is effective in the treatment of age-related macular degeneration. Arch Ophthalmol 1998;116:1507–1509.

51. Perez CA, Brady LW: Principles and Practice of Radiation Oncology, 2nd ed. Philadelphia: JB Lippincott, 1992.

52. Schilling H, Sauerwein W, Lommatzsch A, Friedrichs W, Brylak S, Bornfeld N, Wessing A. Long-term results after low dose ocular irradiation for choroidal haemangiomas. Br J Ophthalmol 1997;81:267–273.

53. Engenhart R, Wowra B, Debus J, Kimmig BN, Hover KH, Lorenz W, Wannenmacher M. The role of high-dose, single-fraction irradiation in small and large intracranial arteriovenous malformations. Int J Radiat Oncol Biol Phys 1994;30:521–529.

54. Scott TA, Augsburger JJ, Brady LW, Hernandez C, Woodleigh R. Low dose ocular irradiation for diffuse choroidal hemangiomas assoicated with bullous nonrhegmatogenous retinal detachment. Retina 1991;11:389–393.

55. Brown GC, Shields JA, Sanborn G, Augsburger JJ, Savino PJ, Schatz NJ. Radiation retinopathy. Ophthalmology 1982;1494–1501.

56. Chan RC, Shukovsky LJ. Effects of irradiation on the eye. Radiology 1976;120:673–675.

57. Parsons JT, Fitzgerald CR, Hood CI, Ellingwood KE, Bova FJ, Million RR. The effects of irradiation on the eye and optic nerve. Int J Radiat Oncol Biol Phys 1983;9:609–622.

58. Johnson LK, Longenecker JP, Fajardo LF. Differential radiation response of cultured endothelial cells and smooth myocytes. Anal Quant Cytol 1982;4:188–198.

59. Archer DB, Amoaku SMK, Gardinier TA. Radiation retinopathy, clinical, histological and ultrastructural correlations. Eye 1991;5:239–251.

60. Plowman PN, Harnett AN. Radiotherapy in benign orbital disease. I: Complicated ocular angiomas. Br J Ophthalmol 1988;72:286–288.

61. Chakravarthy U, Houston RF, Acher DB. Treatment of age-related subfoveal neovascular membranes by teletherapy: a pilot study. Br J Ophthalmol 1993;77:265–273.

62. Study Protocol. Radiotherapy in the Management of Subfoveal Choroidal Neovascular Membranes of Age-Related Macular Degeneration. Belfast: 1995.

63. Finger PT, Berson A, Sherr D, Riley R, Balkin RA, Bosworth JL. Radiation therapy for subretinal neovascularization. Ophthalmology 1996;103:878–889.

64. Stalmans P, Leys A, Van Limbergen E. External beam radiation therapy (20 Gy, 2 Gy fractions) fails to control the growth of choroidal neovascularization in age-related macular degeneration: a review of 111 cases. Retina 1997;17:481–492.

65. Spaide RF, Guyer DR, McCormick B, Yanuzzi LA, Burke K, Mendelsohn M, Haas A, Slakter JS, Sorenson JA, Fisher YL, Abramson D. External beam radiation therapy for choroidal neovascularization. Ophthalmology 1998;105:24–30.

66. Donati G, Soubrane D, Quaranta M, Coscas G, Soubrane G. Radiotherapy for isolated occult subfoveal neovascularisation in age-related macular degeneration: a pilot study. Br J Ophthalmol 1999;83:646–651.

67. Mauget-Faysse M, Chiquet C, Milea D, Romestaing P, Gerard JP, Martin P, Koenig F. Long term results of radiotherapy for subfoveal choroidal neovascularisation in age related macular dgeneration. Br J Ophthalmol 1999;83:923–928.

68. Finger PT, Berson A, Ng T, Szechter A. Ophthalmic plaque radiotherapy for age-related macular degeneration associated with subretinal neovascularization. Am J Ophthalmol 1999;127:170–177.

69. Bergink GJ, Deutman AF, van den Broek JFCM, van Daal WA, van der Maazen RW. Radiation therapy for age-related subfoveal choroidal neovascular membranes, a pilot study. Doc Ophthalmol 1995;90:67–74.

70. Bergink GJ, Hoyng CB, van der Maazen RWM. A randomized controlled trial on efficacy of radiation therapy in the control of subfoveal choroidal neovascularization in age-related macular degeneration: radiation versus observation. Graefe's Arch Clin Exp Ophthalmol 1998;236:321–325.

71. Flaxel CJ, Friedrichsen EJ, Smith JO, Oeinck SC, Blacharski PA, Garcia CA, Chu HH. Proton beam irradiation of subfoveal choroidal neovascularization in age-related macular degeneration. Eye 2000;14:155–164.

72. The Radiation Therapy for Age-related Macular Degeneration (RAD) Study Group, A prospective, randomized, double-masked trial on radiation therapy for neovascular age-related macular degeneration (RAD Study). Ophthalmology 1999;106:2239–2247.

73. Kobayashi H and Kobayashi K. Age-related macular degeneration: Long-term results of radiotherapy for subfoveal neovascular membranes. Am J Ophthalmol 2000;130:617-635.

74. Study Protocol. The Age-Related Macular Degeneration Radiation Trial (AMDRT), United States, 1999.

12
Photocoagulation of AMD-Associated CNV Feeder Vessels

Robert W. Flower

New York University School of Medicine, New York, New York, and University of Maryland School of Medicine, Baltimore, Maryland

I. INTRODUCTION

Treatment of age-related macular degeneration (AMD)-associated choroidal neovascularization (CNV) by photocoagulation of the vessel—or vessels—supplying blood to the CNV has long been considered an attractive approach, particularly when the neovascularization is very near or underlies the fovea. Although elegantly simple as a concept, successfully implementing this treatment approach has proven to be a protracted process. The history of its development spans a period of nearly 30 years, and the case can be made its development has been coupled to the evolution of fundus angiography technology, especially choroidal angiography.

A. Origins of the Concept

Perhaps the earliest description of feeder vessel treatment in ophthalmology was in 1972 by Behrendt, who discussed argon laser photocoagulation of intraretinal and vitreous feeder vessels of neovascular membranes associated with diabetic retinopathy (1). The then-recent availability of visible-light-wavelength lasers led to numerous such novel approaches aimed at controlling ocular neovascularization. Understandably, all of those were related to retinal and anterior segment neovascularizations, since they could be directly visualized by means of readily available optical devices. The choroidal vasculature, on the other hand, was not a popular target of interest, since direct visualization of it was obscured by retinal and choroidal pigments, and in sodium fluorescein angiography images it appeared mostly only as a diffuse "choriocapillaris flush." The deeper-lying vascular layers remained obscured so far as routine clinical observations were concerned.

At about that same time, in the early 1970s, the concept of routine clinical angiography of the choroidal circulation using indocyanine green (ICG) dye was being developed. ICG fluorescence angiography initially had been explored as an investigative tool for studying choroidal blood flow in animal experiments. However, since ICG dye already had

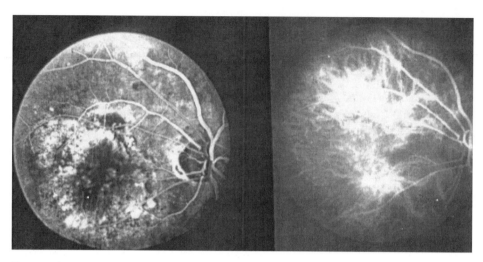

Figure 1 Simultaneously acquired fluorescein (left frame) and ICG (right frame) angiogram images of the first patient with CNV studied by use of ICG fluorescence angiography.

a long-documented history of biocompatibility, exploring its use in human subjects as well was compelling. Since up to that time relatively little attention had been paid to the choroidal circulation compared to the retina, there was no well-defined clinical goal at first in visualizing human choroidal blood flow beyond academic curiosity, so a rudimentary survey of both normal and diseased eyes was undertaken (2). One of the first groups of patients considered in the survey were those with macular degeneration.

Figure 1 shows simultaneously acquired fluorescein and ICG angiogram images of the first patient successfully studied by that methodology. The greatly improved ability to visualize the angioarchitecture of AMD-associated CNV lesions afforded by ICG angiography, coupled with the concept of feeder vessel photocoagulation, led to the first attempts at ICG-guided photocoagulation of CNV feeder vessels. Unfortunately, the results of those first attempts were not encouraging: Clear differentiation between CNV afferent and efferent vessels was not easy—or in most cases not possible—since both spatial and temporal resolution of the early ICG fluorescence angiogram images was limited, the spot size and aiming precision of the first visible light laser photocoagulation delivery systems also was limited, and, perhaps most important, the laser light wavelengths available were not ideally suited to the task.

For some time thereafter the concept of feeder vessel photocoagulation was not seriously pursued as a clinical tool. Instead, the dominant treatment approach for AMD-associated CNV came to be based on Macular Photocoagulation Study (MPS) recommendations (3). These included destruction of the entire CNV membrane—as delineated by fluorescein angiography—along with an additional margin around the CNV, even when the procedure resulted in an immediate, nonrecoverable additional loss of visual acuity. The results of the MPS suggested that despite an immediate vision loss, 3 years later a patient so treated statistically would have better visual acuity than if untreated. Those results not withstanding, few ophthalmologists remained comfortable with the notion of having to destroy the retina to save it, preferring for the most part to avoid photocoagulation near the fovea.

B. Revisiting the Concept

The first notable clinical application of ICG fluorescence angiography was its use in guiding laser photocoagulation of CNV. This method was applied to patients whose clinical and fluorescein angiographic features did not meet the eligibility criteria for laser therapy defined by the MPS recommendations; generally it was applied to cases of poorly defined, or occult, CNV. In this application, use of ICG angiography resulted in improved localization of abnormal choroidal vessels, thereby making treatment by photocoagulation possible (4,5). Whereas this clinical use of ICG undoubtedly contributed to sustaining interest in ICG angiography, arguably it was the commercial availability of the scanning laser ophthalmoscope (SLO) that contributed to increasing interest in ICG angiography. Compared to the predominantly available commercial ICG angiography systems based on fundus camera optics—capable of acquiring images at a rate of about one per second—the SLO afforded the ability to perform high-speed imaging. Ready access to high-speed ICG image acquisition systems was an important component of renewed interest in feeder vessel photocoagulation treatment.

The concept of feeder vessel photocoagulaton currently is being revisited as a treatment for AMD-associated CNV. In February 1998 Shiraga et al., reported the results of a pilot trial to assess the feasibility of extrafoveal photocoagulation of subfoveal CNV secondary to AMD (6). Their results included finding feeder vessels in 37 of 170 consecutive patients (22%), using SLO ICG angiography. In 70% of those 37 cases (26 cases) extrafoveal photocoagulation of the feeder vessels, using 575- to 630-mn-wavelength light, resulted in resolution of the exudative manifestations and improved or stabilized visual acuity. The following December, Straurenghi et al. (7), also using SLO ICG angiography, reported finding treatable feeder vessels in 15 of 22 patients having subfoveal CNV not amenable to the treatment suggested by the MPS (3). They successfully obliterated the feeder vessels in 40% of the cases, resulting in improved or stabilized visual acuity after more than 2 years. In a second group of 16 patients they reported a much higher success rate of 75%, attributed to the smaller feeder vessel diameters (<85 μm) found in this group. In December 1997, yet another series of feeder vessel treatments was begun using a high-speed, pulsed-laser (HSPL) fundus camera system for feeder vessel identification (Flower RW, Glaser BM, Murphy RP, Macula Society. Presentation, 1999.) The HSPL used in this study consisted of a Zeiss fundus camera modified to include a pulsed 805-nm-wavelength diode laser for excitation of ICG dye fluorescence in the choroidal circulation; images were acquired at a rate of 30/s (8). In this latter study, a higher incidence (about 66%) of feeder vessel identification was achieved, apparently owing to use of the HSPL system and different angiogram analysis techniques. Nevertheless, treatment success of the latter study appears to be equivalent to that of the other groups, even though the follow-up period was shorter and it focused on occult CNV, whereas the other studies appear to have focused on classic CNV.

The common experience of all these studies was that feeder vessel photocoagulation appeared to be a viable treatment approach and worthy of continued pursuit, even though the exact nature of the vessels being treated and the most efficacious application of laser energy remain to be determined. Clearly, there is a "catch 22" associated with this methodology: There are no histological data on treated CNV feeder vessels, per se, and the only proof currently available of the accuracy of angiographic CNV feeder vessel identification is improvement or stabilization of the patient's visual acuity following treatment. But this standard of proof is biased toward failure, since conventional laser photocoagulation of

CNV feeder vessels already has proven to be difficult or incomplete in some cases. Therefore, if the full potential of feeder vessel treatment is to be accurately assessed and eventually realized, a more consistently successful approach to laser photocoagulation must be devised. And at the same time, a much better understanding of the hemodynamic consequences of feeder vessel photocoagulation must be developed to facilitate rational analysis of treatment successes and failures.

II. WHAT IS A FEEDER VESSEL?

Properly characterizing CNV feeder vessels in terms of their locations within the choroid, their vessel wall structure, and their blood flow is a necessary step in developing the most efficacious photocoagulation method. In that regard, however, histological data about CNV angioarchitecture appear to be at odds with the angiographic appearance of the so-called feeder vessels being treated.

A. Histological Appearance of CNV Feeder Vessels

The vessels passing through breaks in Bruch's membrane and connecting a CNV to the choroidal blood supply can be capillaries, arteries, or veins, as determined by the vessel wall structure. In general, CNV complexes up to 300 μm diameter have only one break containing a capillary-like vessel (9,10). Complexes on the order of 500 μm have two to four breaks, and at least one or two contain a capillary-like vessel; the other transmit only cells. CNV complexes of these dimensions consist of a single layer of capillary vessels on the inner surface of Bruch's membrane, and they arise from a layer of vessels that lies just beneath, instead of between, the intercapillary pillars, so it is assumed these are new vessels replacing the choroidal capillaries. Because many tissue sections must be cut to find and track these vessels, there are only a few examples in which the vessels can actually be tracked in the choroid, and even then it is not always clear whether they lead to an artery or a vein (Sarks JP, Sarks SH, written communication, March 14, 1999).

Complexes on the order of 200 μm have more than four breaks, and the vessels passing through are of medium size. These complexes usually are two layers thick, but still beneath the retinal pigment exithelium (RPE), and they can be served by well formed arterial and venous vessels. Complexes from patients with diskiform scars have breaks containing larger arteries and veins; these disrupt the RPE and invaded the retina, (Sarks JP, Sarks SH, written communication, March 14, 1999).

It has been suggested that on average, there are 2.3 vessels passing through Bruch's membrane and connecting each CNV to the underlying choroidal vasculature (11). The frequency with which these vessels are capillaries, arteries, or veins has not yet been reported, but it is clear that the majority of penetrating vessels encountered are relatively short capillary-like vessels. It is clear also that such small vessels are not likely to be recognized in ICG angiogram images.

B. Angiographic Appearance of CNV Feeder Vessels

The most frequently identified and treated feeder vessels reported in studies to date appear to be on the order of one to several millimeters long, a dimension quite large with respect to the penetrating vessels most frequently found in histological preparations. Figure 2 shows examples of feeder vessels, identified using the HSPL fundus camera system, that have been successfully photocoagulated, resulting in improved or stabilized vision. In using that system, identification of feeder vessels is made by first carefully examining the area surrounding the location of a known or suspected CNV complex in high-speed ICG angiogram images, since the most obvious characteristic of a feeder vessel is proximity to CNV. Some feeder vessels are easily identified, as in Figure 2A and D, when they are prominent and easily distinguishable from adjacent choroidal vessels. Often, however, feeder vessels are less prominent, as in Figure 2B and C, and identification requires use of an analytical technique such as phi-motion angiography,* which helps differentiate a feeder vessel from its surroundings by enhancing visualization of blood flow through it, toward the CNV. Determining direction of flow is essential to correctly identifying CNV feeder vessels—as opposed to their draining vessels—even when their angioarchitecture seems obvious.

C. Reconciling Histological and Angiographic Data

Clearly, the vessels identified in histological specimens as the conduits of blood from the choriocapillaris (CC) to CNVs appear to be different from the so-called feeder vessels identified in angiograms. Typically "feeder vessel" refers to an afferent vessel supplying blood to a particular vascular complex, one directly connected to the complex. To be precise, in the case of CNV that definition should apply to the short capillary-like vessels that penetrate Bruch's membrane and form a CNV/CC connection. The vessels in ICG angiograms dubbed "feeder vessels"in the recently reported studies of CNV feeder vessel photocoagulation— especially in the case of occult CNV— meet the criterion of being afferent, but they appear to be much larger than the capillary-like vessels seen in the histological specimens. Strictly speaking, therefore, the term "CNV feeder vessel,"as applied in angiographic descriptions, appears to be a misnomer for some other choroidal vessels—most likely Sattler's layer arterioles.

The so-called feeder vessels (FVs) seen in angiograms very much resemble vessels of the choroidal middle layer, or Sattler's layer, which lies just beneath the CC. Comparison of the ICG angiogram images of the feeder vessels in Figure 2 to the scanning electron micrographs of corrosion casts of the anterior aspect of the CC in Figure 3 demonstrates this similarity. Therefore, it seems a reasonable assumption that the feeder vessels identified in ICG angiograms and reported to have been successfully treated by photocoagulation are Sattler's layer arteriolar vessels.

---

* Phi-motion is a phenomenon first identified by Wertheimer in 1912 (12): it refers to visual perception of motion where none exists. In a situation where there is a gap in visual information, the brain fills in what is missing. An example of the case in point is the appearance of two spatially separated points of light wherein first one is illuminated and, a finite time later, the second one is illuminated. The perception is that of a single point *moving* from the location of the first point to that of the second. By repeatedly viewing an appropriate segment of a high-speed angiogram image sequence in continuous-loop fashion and at an appropriate speed, the phi-motion phenomenon accentuates perception of the movement of dye through vessels.

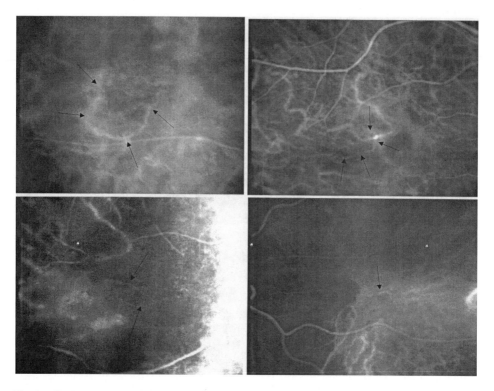

Figure 2 Examples of CNV feeder vessels, identified using the HSPL (high-speed, pulsed-laser) fundus camera system, that were successfully photocoagulated, resulting in improved or stabilized vision. In each case, arrows inidcate the course of the feeder vessel. (Reprinted from Flower RW. Experimental studies of indocynine green dye-enhanced photocoagulation of choroidal neovascularization feeder vessels. Am J Ophthalmol 2000; 129: 506, Fig 3. Copyright 2000, with permission from Elsevier Science.)

There is additional evidence to support the notion that the angiographically defined CNV feeder vessels are Sattler's layer vessels: A commonly observed characteristic of successfully treated FVs is their 'beaded" appearance in ICG angiograms (RP Murphy, symposium presentation, Chicago, June 3, 2000); an example of that appearance is shown in Figure 4A. The most likely explanation for the beaded appearance is that the dye-filled FV is crossed throughout its length by smaller choroidal vessels. This same phenomenon is more pronounced in high-speed ICG angiograms of rhesus monkey eyes following carotid arterial dye injection, as demonstrated in Figure 4B, wherein carotid dye injection improved dye wave front definition, enhancing observation of the temporal filling differences between various layers of choroidal vessels. When crossed by small non-dye-filled vessels, the crossings result in dark segments along the feeder vessel; when crossed by small dye-filled vessels, the crossings result in hyperfluorescence, due to additivity of fluorescence from the overlapping vessels. The presence of small vessels between the FV and the CC fixes the FV location well below the CC, consistent with the notion that CNV-FVs are Sattler's layer vessels.

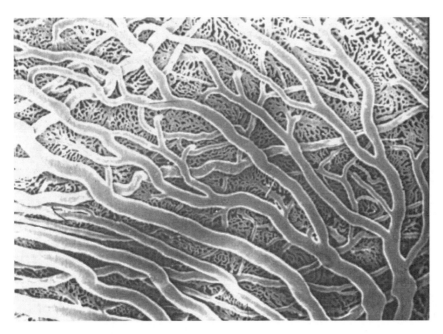

Figure 3 A scanning electron micrograph of a corrosion cast of the posterior (Sattler's) layer of small-diameter choroidal arteries and veins that feed and drain the choriocapillaris, which can be seen in the background. For the most part, the veins are oriented from the upper left-hand corner of the image toward the lower right-hand corner; they overlie the arteries. (Courtesy of Dr. Andrzej W. Fryczkowski.) (Reprinted from Flower RW. Experimental studies of indocyanine green dye-enhanced photocoagulation of choroidal neovascularization feeder vessels. Am J Ophthalmol 2000; 129:507, Fig 4. Copyright 2000, with permission from Elsevier Science.)

Additionally, Arnold et al. (13) have shown the choroids of AMD eyes to be as little as half the thickness of those in age-matched normal eyes (e.g., 90 μm compared to 180 μm), primarily owing to a significant decrease in the number of vessels that normally occupy the middle choroidal layers (Sattler's layer). So it is possible that the relatively high contrast of some FVs see (Fig. 2) is a result of there being fewer-than-normal adjacent vessels in the same layer, and in the absence of the normal number of adjacent vessels, the FVs may have become preferential channels for blood flow through a diminished Sattler's layer. Therefore, the assumption that many of the FV investigators have identified and photocoagulated are Sattler's layer arteriolar vessels is at least consistent with the evidence at hand.

III. THE RELATIONSHIP BETWEEN SATTLER'S LAYER VESSELS AND CNVs

The explanation for apparently successful photocoagulation treatment of so-called CNV FVs (i.e., Sattler's layer vessels) lies in the hemodynamic relationship between the Sattler's layer vessels and the capillary-like vessels that form the CC/CNV communication.

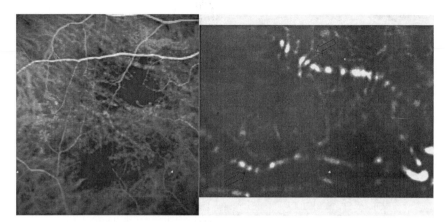

Figure 4 (A) ICG angiogram demonstrating the commonly observed "beaded" appearance of CNV feeder vessels. (B) The same "beaded" appearance seen more prominently in the high-speed ICG angiograms of rhesus monkey eye following carotid arterial dye injection. When crossed by small non-dye-filled vessels, the intersections appear as dark segments along the feeder vessel (vessel indicated by the lower arrow); when crossed by small dye-filled vessels, the intersections appear hyperfluorescent owing to additivity of fluorescence from the overlapping vessels (vessel indicated by the upper arrow). (Reprinted from Flower RW, von Kerczek C, Zhu L, Ernest A, Eggleton C, Topoleski LDT. A theoretical investigation of the role of choriocapillaris blood flow in treatment of sub-foveal choroidal neovascularization associated with age-related macular degeneration. Am J Ophthalmol 2001;132:85–93.)

A. An Anthropomorphic Model of the CC/CNV Connection

The relationship proposed to exist between these two types of vessels is modeled in Figure 5, wherein there is no anatomical continuity between them, although functionally they be-have as if there were. The figure also demonstrates how blood could move in a function-ally contiguous manner from a Sattler's layer FV, into the CC, and then through a nearby capillary vessel leading from the CNV during the systolic phase of the intraocular pressure pulse.

By comparison to the sinusoid-like structure of the CC vascular plexus, it is likely that resistance to blood flow would be higher through a parallel CNV complex, connected to the CC by the capillary-like vessels that penetrate Bruch's membrane. In this model, blood flow through the CNV would occur, but it would not be as great as through the un-derlying CC. In keeping with the pulsatile nature of CC blood flow shown to exist as the result of the perpendicular interface of arterioles and the wide, flat choriocapillaries (8,14), a high hydrostatic pressure-head must exist at the interface early during systole, relative to the surrounding CC (as indicated by the collapsed state of the choriocapillaries and the CNV vessels in Figure 5A and B). In addition to pushing blood into the choriocapillaries, the pressure-head would be partially dissipated in forcing some blood into the adjacent pen-etrating vessel. Thus, a small, pulsatile pressure gradient would be established through the CNV, even though the majority of flow would be through the CC. In this model, closure of the FVs, or even significant partial closure, would have the effect of reducing the pressure head available at the penetrating vessel to a level so low that resistance to flow through the CNV could not be overcome, thereby effectively closing the CNV as well.

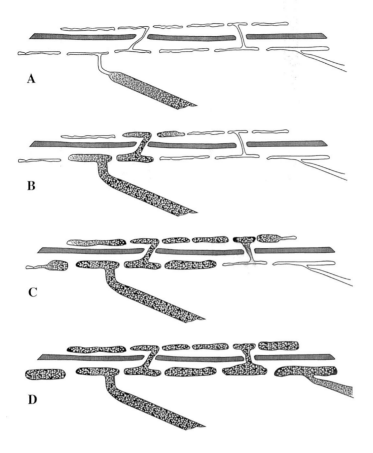

Figure 5 Schematic representation of the presumed relationship between a vessel penetrating Bruch's membrane (penetrating vessel) and connecting a CNV membrane to the choriocapillaris. The posterior margin of Bruch's membrane is represented by the dark horizontal line. A Sattler's layer choroidal arteriole (presumably a feeder vessel) is shown entering the choriocapillaris (CC) from beneath. The four frames of the figure indicate how blood would move in a functionally contiguous manner from a Sattler's layer feeder vessel, into the CC, and then through another nearby penetrating vessel during the systolic phase of the intraocular pressure pulse even though the penetrating and feeder vessels are not anatomically contiguous. (A) At the onset of the blood pressure pulse, a high hydrostatic pressure-head of blood (represented by the black dots) would develop at the perpendicular interface of arteriole and the wide, flat CC (as indicated by the collapsed state of the choriocapillaries and the CNV membrane). (B) Slightly later during the pulse, in addition to pushing blood into the choriocapillaries, part of the pressure-head would be dissipated in forcing some blood into the adjacent penetrating vessel. Thus, a small pressure gradient would be established through the CNV. (C) Still later, blood flow through the CNV would occur, but it would not be as great as through the underlying CC, because by comparison to the sinusoid-like structure of the CC vascular plexus, it is likely that resistance to blood flow through a parallel CNV complex, connected to the CC by capillary-like penetrating vessels, would be higher. (D) Eventually, flow through the CNV would be complete. (Reprinted from Flower RW. Experimental studies of indocyanine green dye-enhanced photocoagulation of choroidal neovascularization feeder vessels. Am J Ophthalmol 2000;129:507, Fig 5. Copyright 2000, with permission from Elsevier Science.)

Thus, there is considerable evidence to support the hypothesis that ultimately the source of blood supplying a CNV is a Sattler's layer arteriole whose entry into the CC is situated near one of the capillary-like vessels that penetrate Bruch's membrane, forming a CC/CNV communication. That is, the FVs identified for focal photocoagulation treatment of CNV appear to be Sattler's layer arterioles that are functionally—but not directly physically—connected to the CNV. Throughout the rest of this discussion, the term "CNV feeder vessel" is intended to imply a Sattler's layer vessel that is functionally contiguous with a CNV. This leads to the possibility that in some cases direct, anatomically contiguous connection between a Sattler's layer vessel and a CNV eventually could evolve, obviating any CC involvement at all; indeed, such an evolution might be the path leading from occult to classic CNV.

B. A Model of the FV/CC/CNV Hemodynamic Relationship

The simple anthropomorphic model of FV/CNV blood flow described above was conceived to account for the clinically observed resolution of retinal edema following FV photocoagulation, even when only partial FV vessel closure is achieved (15). However, since the submacular CC is a true vascular plexus—fed and drained by multiple interspersed arteries and veins— a much more sophisticated model is needed to describe the changes in CC blood flow beneath the CNV following FV photocoagulation. Therefore, a theoretical model for the human CC, based on available histological and hemodynamic data, was developed to simulate the CC blood flow field before and after FV photocoagulation.*

Known angioarchitectural and hemodynamic parameters for the CC and CNV from the literature were used to construct the theoretical model of a section of submacular CC and a small overlying CNV membrane shown in Figure 6. The CC plexus consists of two parallel sheets separated by 7.5 microns between which 10-micron-diameter columns are placed at regular intervals, leaving 15-micron-wide channels in between to simulate the CC plexus. Isolated, but well-separated, precapillary arterioles and venules communicate with the CC plexus and perfuse it with blood. The cross-sectional dimensions of the arterioles and venules are of the same order as the CC thickness, h. The center-to-center spacing between adjacent arterioles and venules is much larger than h. Therefore, the CC was modeled as a planar porous medium containing a widely dispersed set of fluid inflows and fluid outflows, simulating the feeding and draining vessels of Sattler's layer. Feeding arteriolar and draining venous vessels consist of, respectively 7.5 and 15-micron-diameter tubes entering the CC from beneath.

An overlying CNV membrane was modeled as a parallel miniature version of the CC, but with smaller dimensions that will result in a significantly higher resistance to fluid flow. The communication between the CNV and the CC is by way of two capillary-dimensioned vessels that penetrate Bruch's membrane. In the model, the position of the CNV could be changed to achieve various spatial relationships between the penetrating vessels and the Sattler's layer vessels that feed and drain the CC.

---

* This model was developed in collaboration with C. von Kerczek, L. Zhu, A. Ernest, C. Eggleton, and L. D. T. Topoleski from the Department of Mechanical Engineering University of Maryland, Baltimore, MD.

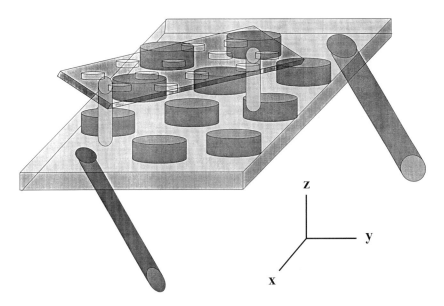

Figure 6 Schematic representation of the computer-simulated model of the choriocapillaris (CC) and an overlying choroidal neovascular (CNV) membrane. The CC segment is represented by the thin green rectangular box; the red disks within the volume of the box represent the interstitial spaces surrounded by the network of choriocapillaries. One Sattler's layer arteriolar (red cylinder) and one venous (blue cylinder) vessel are shown connected to the posterior CC. A CNV membrane is. represented by the very thin purple rectangular box. Two capillary-like vessels (green cylinders) penetrate Bruch's membrane (not depicted) and form the CC/CNV connection (penetrating vessels) as shown; in the text, these are referred to as penetrating vessels. In the simulation, the position of the penetrating vessels with respect the Sattler's layer vessels was varied. (Reprinted from Flower RW, von Kerczek C, Zhu L, Ernest A, Eggleton C, Topoleski LDT. A theoretical investigation of the role of choriocapillaris blood flow in treatment of sub-foveal choroidal neovascularization associated with age-related macular degeneration. Am J Ophthalmol 2001;132:85–93.)

This theoretical model became the basis for computer simulation of blood flow distribution in a segment of human subfoveal CC approximately 1300 × 1000 microns in area. The actual placement of the multiple Sattler's layer vessels to feed and drain blood from the simulated CC plexus segment was made according to the histologically determined locations of those vessels in one normal human eye (16). Figure 7 shows the anterior aspect of the computer-simulated segment of that human submacular CC, marked with the actual locations of arteriolar and venous vessels Sattler's layer vessels connected to its posterior aspect; the figure also shows the simulated CNV in two different locations. Blood flow rates in the feeding arterioles and venules were then estimated by matching the predicted precapillary arteriole and venule pressure difference to experimentally measured data; the experimentally measured maximum pressure difference between a feeding arteriole and venule was found to be 4.5 mmHg (17). Experimentally measured pressures and pressure differences were applied across the feeding and draining vessels to generate maps of blood flow through the computer-simulated model CC segment. Figure 8 shows the normal isobar and iso-blood-speed distributions in the computer simulated segment of CC from

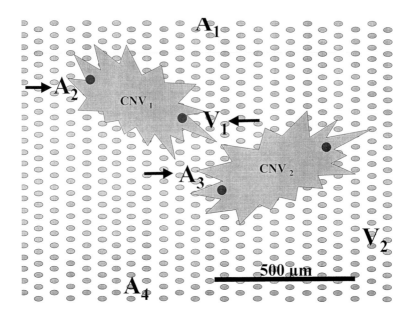

Figure 7 The anterior aspect of the computer-simulated segment of a human submacular CC, marked with the actual locations of arteriolar and venous vessels. Sattler's layer vessels connected to its posterior aspect; the figure also shows the simulated CNV in two different locations. (Reprinted from Flower RW, von Kerczek C, Zhu L, Ernest A, Eggleton C, Topoleski LDT. A theoretical investigation of the role of choriocapillaris blood flow in treatment of sub-foveal choroidal neovascularization associated with age-related macular degeneration. Am J Ophthalmol 2001;132:85–93.

Figure 7; it also shows how those distributions are altered when one of the Sattler's layer feeding arterioles is completely occluded.

A significant reduction in the local CC pressure probably results in significant changes in the blood flow through an overlying CNV network, since the driving force for CNV blood flow is the pressure difference between the capillary-like vessels that penetrate Bruch's membrane, forming the CC/CNV communication. Clinical observations indicate that partial—as well as complete—photocoagulation of the (presumed Sattler's layer) FV adjacent to a CNV's penetrating vessel(s) is an effective means of decreasing the blood flow in the CNV (BM Glaser, RP Murphy, G Staurenghi, personal communications, 1999). Therefore, the model also was used to simulate blood flow through a CNV before and after FV laser photocoagulation; the simulation was performed for the CNV membrane situated in two different locations, as indicated in Figure 7. The first location, CNV #1, was between arteriole #2 and venule #1, while the second, CNV #2, was between arteriole #3 and a point in the venous pressure, equidistant from venules #1 and #2. Photocoagulation of arteriole #2 and of venule #1 resulted in significant reduction of CNV #1 blood flow (71% and 79%, respectively), with similar results in CNV #2 when arteriole #3 was photocoagulated (84% reduction). On the other hand, even the complete closure of venules #1 or #2 produced less than 30% decrease in blood velocity through CNV #2.

CC Blood Pressure Field (mm Hg)

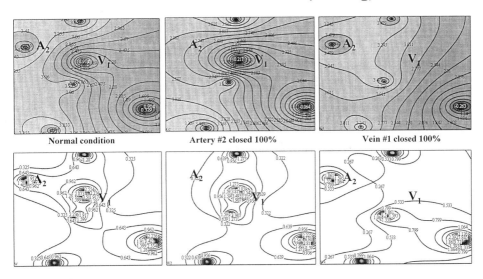

CC Blood Speed Field (mm/s)

Figure 8 Isogramic maps of the blood pressure and blood speed fields of the choriocapillaris segment shown in Figure 7 under normal and simulated vascular photocoagulation conditions. The isogramic lines in the left-hand two frames identify locations of constant pressure (upper frame) and flow (lower frame) throughout the CC segment under normal conditions. The pattern of these lines change, as shown in the other pairs of frames, when either the underlying Sattler's layer arteries (middle frames) or veins (right-hand frames) are occluded. The particular vessels occluded in these examples are aretriole A_1 and venule V_1, identified in Figure 7. (Reprinted from Flower RW, von Kerczek C, Zhu L, Ernest A, Eggleton C, Topoleski LDT. A theoretical investigation of the role of choriocapillaris blood flow in treatment of sub-foveal choroidal neovascularization associated with age-related macular degeneration. Am J Ophthalmol 2001;132:85–93.)

C. Implications of the FV/CC/CNV Hemodynamic Relationship

This model predicts that even 50% closure of a blood vessel entering the posterior aspect of the CC in the vicinity of a capillary-like vessel leading to a CNV can be effective in reducing or possibly stopping CNV blood flow, regardless of whether that vessel is a feeding arteriole or a draining venule. In other words, the important hemodynamic event with respect to reducing or stopping CNV blood flow is significant reduction of the blood pressure—hence, blood flow as well—in the local underlying CC. Thus, the predictions of the present computer-simulated model support the novel approach to CNV management made previously, namely that (1) rather than total obliteration of a CNV (which frequently results in recurrence), the endpoint of laser photocoagulation treatment can be reduction of CNV blood flow to the extent that undesirable manifestations of the CNV—most notably retinal edema—are halted or reversed, and (2) CNV blood flow reduction can be mediated by reduction of blood flow through the underlying CC (15).

There are two important implications to that novel approach, one related to F V treatment and the other related to the mechanics of successful CNV treatments in general. Regarding FV photocoagulation treatment of CNV, the selection criterion for targeted FVs might be extended to include venous as well as arteriolar vessels entering the posterior CC in the vicinity of a CNV membrane. If indeed reduction of the underlying CC blood flow is the important treatment goal, then depending upon the orientation of the CNV's penetrating vessels with respect to the field of vessels feeding and draining the CC, targeting veins or veins in conjunction with arteries may yield the best results. After all, the ramifications of occluding a venous drainage channel to a true vascular plexus, like the posterior-pole CC, is not the same as occlusion of the drainage vein of a true end-arteriolar vascular complex. In the former case, blood is diverted to adjacent venous channels, without excessive increase in capillary transmural pressure, whereas in the latter case, venous occlusion likely results in blood flow stasis and elevation of capillary transmural pressure to a level near that across the feeding arterial vessel wall.

Since the predicted relationship between CC and CNV blood flows actually is independent of the specific means by which CC blood flow is reduced, the second implication of the results is that reduction of CC blood flow underlying a CNV membrane may be a component mechanism common to all successful CNV treatments, including photocoagulation, photodynamic therapy (PDT), transpupillary thermal therapy (TTT), and drusen photocoagulation. It is well established that post-PDT angiograms routinely evidence reduced CC fluorescence (18), and that appears also to be the case following TTT (19). In the case of TTT, reduced CC blood flow may be due to increased resistance to plexus blood flow resulting from heat-induced interstitial tissue swelling and concomitant reduction of CC luminal space. Angiographic data specifically related to submacular blood flow following photocoagulation destruction of macular drusen have not been presented anywhere; however, it has been demonstrated that CC obliteration occurs with application of moderate to heavy laser burns and that loss of choriocapillaries can add significant resistance to blood flow through the CC plexus (8).

If reduced CC blood flow is a component mechanism of successful CNV treatment, regardless of the modality used, then FV photocoagulation arguably might be viewed as the most effective method. The difference between FV photocoagulation and the other methods is analogous to removing a weed from a lawn by pulling out its roots (FV) versus just cutting off the weed's leaves. It can be argued that FV photocoagulation is the most precise of the various methods in terms of manipulating CC blood flow, and it minimizes the area of tissue/laser interaction. Moreover, since blood flow through a particular CC area apparently can be manipulated by modulation of adjacent venous or arteriolar vessels connected to the plexus's anterior side, it may be that the most precise manipulation of CC blood flow—and, hence, treatment of CNV—will be by controlled, partial photocoagulation of carefully selected combinations of arterioles and venules in Sattler's layer vessels.

IV. DEVELOPMENT OF A MORE EFFICACIOUS METHOD OF FV TREATMENT

The models of CNV FVs are consistent with the clinical observation that often, even incomplete closure of a FV produces reduction of CNV dye filling, resolution of associated edema, and improved visual acuity. Of course, partial closure of targeted FVs at present is an unintended endpoint of argon and krypton laser photocoagulation application. In such cases, failure to completely close the relatively deep-lying targeted vessels may be attributable to generation of an insufficiently high temperature gradient, emanating from the RPE, where laser light-to-heat transduction occurs. The temperature gradient that is produced does extend into the sensory retina and can produce significant damage there, so the location for FV photocoagulation must be chosen so as not to involve the fovea. It would be desirable, therefore, to avoid the concomitant retinal damage and to make FV photocoagulation more efficient and predictable. This would have the additional potential benefit of allowing such treatment to be applied much closer to the fovea than is presently possible, thereby increasing the number of patients who might benefit from CNV FV treatment.

A. The Concept of ICG-Dye–Enhanced Photocoagulation

An example of a successfully treated FV is shown in Figure 9, and it also shows an undesirable side effect as well: damage to the nerve fiber layer overlying the site of FV photocoagulation. Since CNV FVs apparently lie below the plane of the CC, a method of photocoagulation that moves the epicenter of the laser-generated heat closer to those vessels and away from the sensory retina would be an improvement over the presently available method. The concept of ICG-dye–enhanced photocoagulation has that potential and, therefore, should be revisited for this application, bearing in mind that its use must be optimized to accommodate characteristics of the targeted choroidal vasculature. The main premise of dye-enhanced photocoagulation is that application of laser light energy with a wavelength matched to the primary wavelength absorbed by a bolus of dye passing through the target blood vessel produces the most efficient photocoagulation burn in terms of vessel closure with minimum damage to surrounding tissue. Figure 10 demonstrates the main aspects of ICG-dye-enhanced photocoagulation and compares it to FV photocoagulation by conventional laser light photocoagulation.

The concept of improving the efficiency of the photocoagulation process by ICG-dye enhancement is not new to treatment of AMD-related CNV, as Reichel and co-workers utilized it for treating poorly defined subfoveal CNV. Eventually they reported their initial clinical investigation in 10 patients (20), but in terms of visual outcome, their results, were equivocal, and the technique did not achieve widespread use. The particular dye-enhancement technique they used, however, relied on absorption of infrared laser light energy by *dye-stained* choroidal blood vessel walls minutes following dye injection. That apparently is a very inefficient process, compared to one in which the same laser energy is absorbed by *dye molecules within* the target vessels during transit of a high-concentration dye bolus (15).

B. A Combined ICG Angiography/Dye-Enhanced Photocoagulation System

Performance of ICG-dye-enhanced photocoagulation requires use of a laser delivery system that permits visualization of intervenously injected ICG dye as it traverses the vasculature. Such a system was constructed from a Zeiss fundus camera (Carl Zeiss, Oberkochen, Germany) modified to include a pulsed diode laser light source and a synchronized, gated CCD camera for performing high-speed ICG angiography, as previously described (8,21). The fundus camera was further modified so that the output tip of the fiberoptic of an 810-nm diode laser photocoagulator (Oculight SLX, Iris Medical Instru-

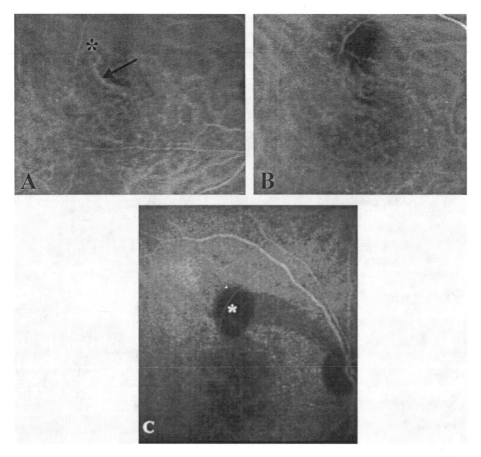

Figure 9 ICG angiogram images of a successfully treated FV. (A) Pretreatment; the FV is indicated by an arrow, and the site of the laser beam is indicated by *. (B) Post-treatment; note lack of CNV dye-filling. (C) Image shows an undesirable side effect: damage to the nerve fiber layer overlying the site of FV photocoagulation. (Reprinted from Flower RW. Experimental studies of indocyanine green dye-enhanced photocoagulation of choroidal neovascularization feeder vessels. Am J Ophthalmol 2000;129:502, Fig 1. Copyright 2000, with permission form Elsevier Science.)

ments, Mountain View, CA) can be positioned in the plane of the fundus illumination optics pathway normally occupied by the internal fixation-pointer; that plane is conjugate to the fundus of the subject's eye. The He-Ne aiming beam emitted by the photocoagulator appears as a sharply focused spot when viewed through the fundus camera's video system, and the position of the fiberoptic with respect to the subject's fundus can be controlled by the micromanipulator's X and Y adjustments. With this configuration, it is possible to deliver 810-nm photocoagulation light pulses to precisely located areas of the fundus while observing the fundus with visible light through the fundus camera eyepiece, making it possible to synchronize photocoagulation laser pulse delivery with arrival of a dye bolus at a targeted vessel site. The fundus camera system is shown in Figure 11.

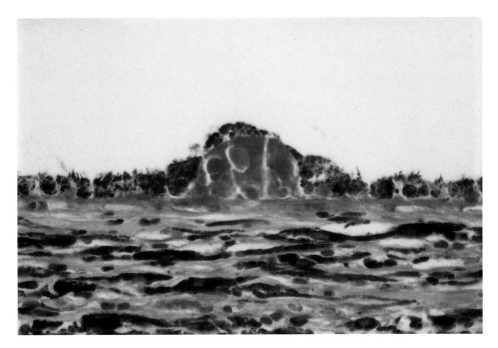

Figure 2.1 A hard druse. A globular hyaline deposit with overlying RPE atrophy. The retina is artifactually detached, thus not shown in this picture (H&E).

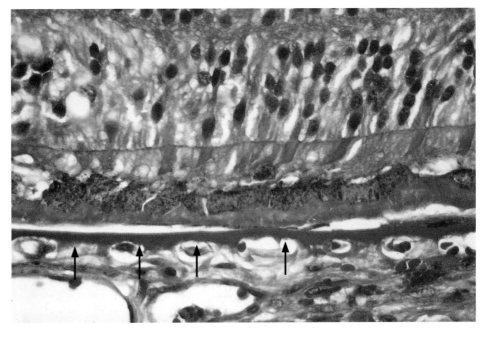

Figure 2.4 Basal deposits ("diffuse drusen"). There is a marked sub-RPE thickening of the Bruchs' membrane (arrows) (PAS).

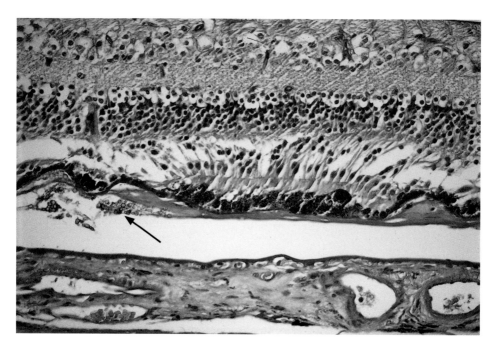

Figure 2.5 Diskiform scarring, low magnification. Notice dystrophic calcification. Calcium crystals are seen within the substance of the sub-RPE fibrous plaque (arrow).

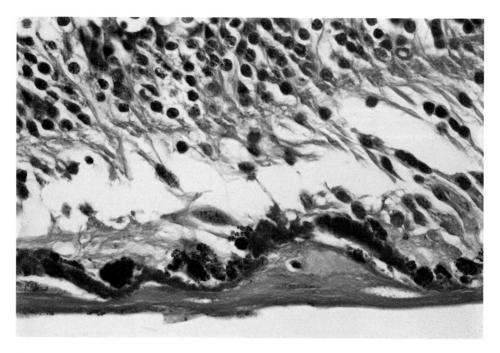

Figure 2.6 Same case as in Figure 2.5, higher magnification. Notice degenerated outer segments of photoreceptors and atrophic RPE. There is a sub-RPE fibrous sheet.

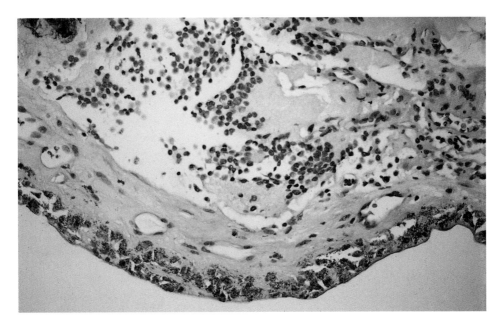

Figure 2.9 Surgically excised subfoveal choroidal neovascular membrane specimen from an 82-year-old man with AMD. Outer retinal elements were included in the excised specimen. Notice a dense fibrovascular membrane above the RPE and underneath the photoreceptor nuclei. This is a type II, or subretinal, membrane, which, according to Gass' theory, is more typical of non-AMD membranes (21).

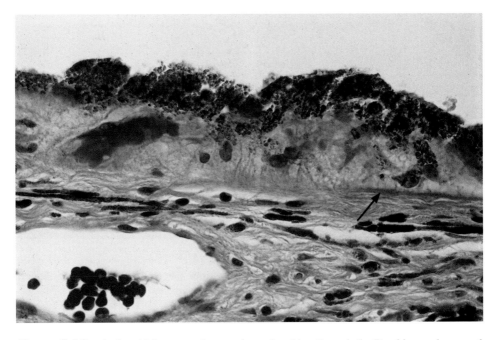

Figure 2.10 A choroidal neovascular membrane breaking through the Bruch's membrane and into the sub-RPE plane ("type II" membrane). Notice intact Bruch's membrane at the right side of the picture (arrow). Elements seen in the membrane include a capillary, a few mononuclear leukocytes, endothelial cells, RPE cells, and collagen (PAS).

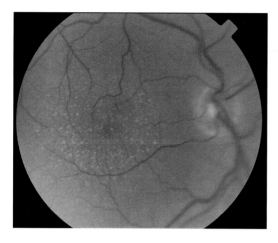

Figure 4.1 Color photograph of hard drusen in a 65-year-old asymptomatic man.

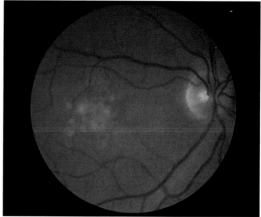

Figure 4.6 Color photograph showing soft drusen in a mildly symptomatic 70-year-old patient (mild distortion on Amsler grid testing).

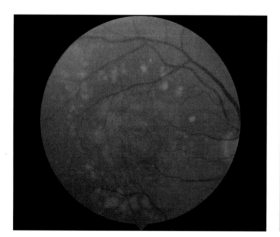

Figure 4.7 Color photograph of geographic atrophy and drusen.

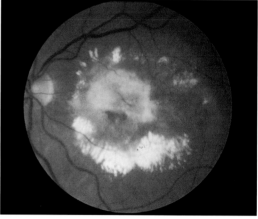

Figure 4.8 Color photograph showing the end-stage appearance of the fellow eye of the patient in Figure 4.6 with high-risk drusen.

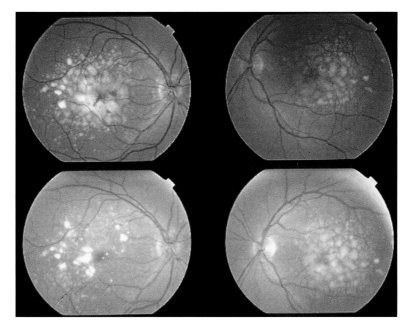

Figure 4.9 Example of pre- (upper left and upper right) and post- (lower left and lower right) subthreshold diode laser showing drusen disappearance in a 45-year-old man with a hereditary form of AMD.

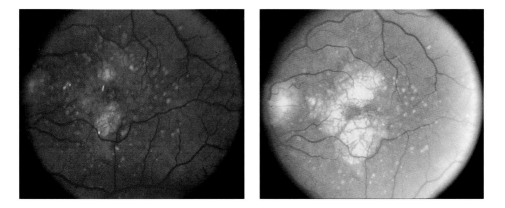

Figure 5.1 Four-year progression in geographic atrophy. (Left) There are multifocal areas of geographic atrophy, along with drusen and pigmentary alteration. (Right) Four years later, the areas of geographic atrophy have enlarged and coalesced, forming a horseshoe of atrophy surrounding the fovea.

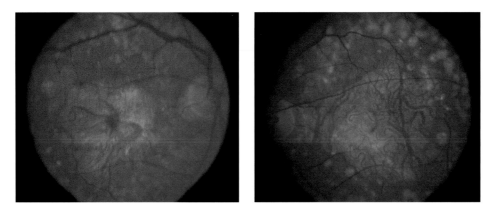

Figure 5.2 Bilateral geographic atrophy. (Left) This eye had 20/30 visual acuity, and the patient was able to read 80 words per minute, using the spared central area. (Right) The fellow eye did not have a useable spared region and had 20/400 visual acuity.

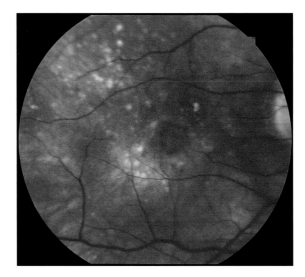

Figure 6.1 Subfoveal gray pigmented CNV. Soft large drusen surround CNV.

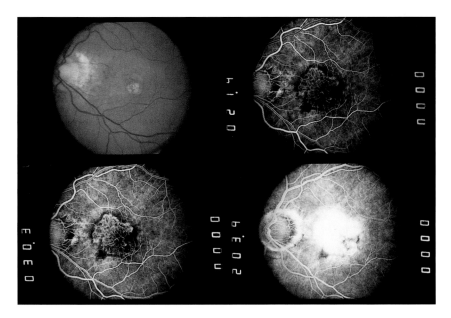

Figure 6.2 (A) Upper left: Color photo of the left eye shows an atrophic extrafoveal laser scar surrounded by a grayish subretinal lesion. There is overlying subretinal fluid. (B) Upper right: Fluorescein angiogram shows early lacy hyperfluorescence in the subfoveal area surrounding the laser scar. Note the ring of blocked fluorescence around the lacy CNV. There is some extrafoveal occult CNV beyond the blocked fluorescence. (C) Lower left: Occult CNV is present and surrounds the blocked fluorescence around the classic CNV. (D) Lower right: The occult and the classic components show late leakage.

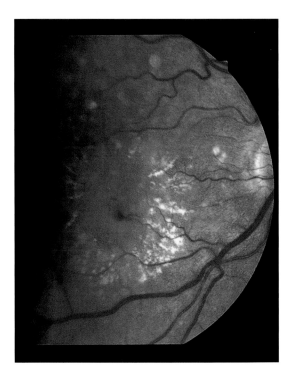

Figure 6.3 Ring of hard exudates surround an area of turbid fluid with a few spots of intraretinal hemorrhage overlying the central lesion.

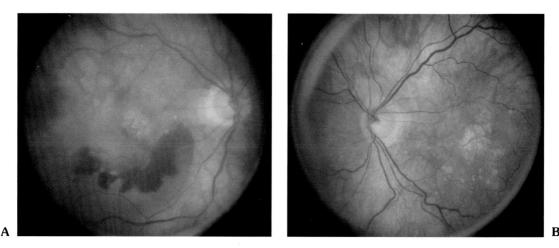

Figure 6.4 (A) Right eye shows subretinal blood (red) and sub-RPE blood (grey-green) is seen adjacent to an area of geographic atrophy. There is another area of subretinal blood temporal to the macula. There is overlying subretinal fluid. Visual acuity is 6/200. (B) Left eye showing more advanced geographic atrophy is found in the subfoveal area; visual acuity is 20/200.

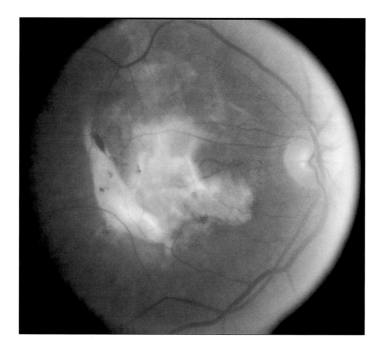

Figure 6.5 Color photo shows subretinal fibrosis. Note the sharp margins and the whitish color of the scar.

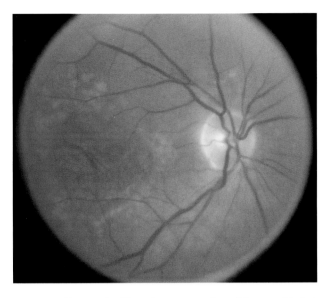

Figure 6.6 Early geographic atrophy. Note the orange color of the atrophic lesion and the visibility of the deep choroidal blood vessels within the area. There are no drusen in the atrophic area but soft drusen in the area adjacent to the lesion.

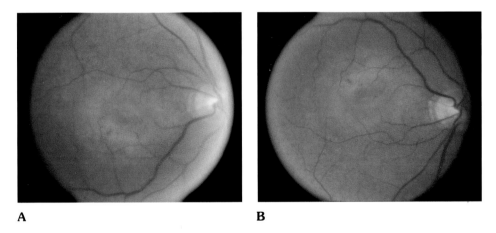

A   B

Figure 6.8 (A) Left stereo pair. (B) Right stereo pair. Stereoscopic photographs show a pigment epithelial detachment with overlying subretinal fluid and spots of subretinal blood. Visual acuity was 20/300. Three weeks later, the amount of subretinal blood increased and the CNV was more clearly seen as a greenish lesion in the subfoveal area.

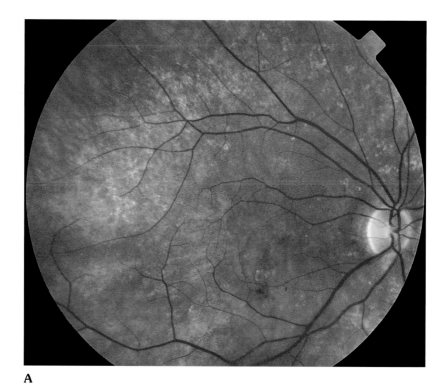

A

Figure 6.9 (A) Color fundus photo shows subretinal blood and a subretinal pigmented lesion.

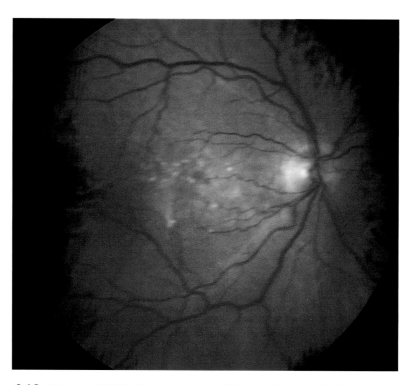

Figure 6.12 Pigmented CNV with some subretinal blood and surrounding large, soft, confluent drusen.

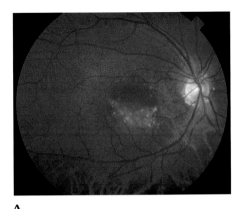

A

Figure 7.2 Classic CNV. (A) Clinical photograph demonstrating radial basal laminar drusen and RPE disturbances. There is an overlying neurosensory macular detachment.

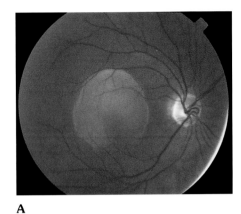

A

Figure 7.3 Occult CNV with PED (V-PED). (A) Clinical photograph demonstrating an irregularly shaped PED with turbid yellowish sub-RPE fluid.

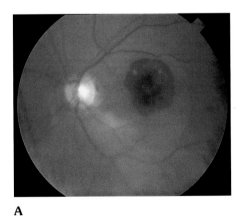

A

Figure 7.5 Occult CNV with sub-RPE hemorrhage and focal spot. (A) Clinical photograph demonstrating a subretinal hemorrhage in the central macula in a patient with AMD.

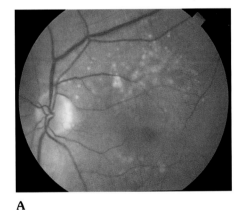

A

Figure 7.6 Active occult CNV. (A) Clinical photograph demonstrating a serous PED in the central macula.

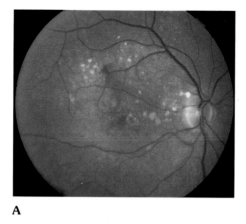

A

Figure 7.7 Inactive occult CNV. (A) Clinical photograph demonstrating thickening of the RPE and chronic exudative changes in the central macula.

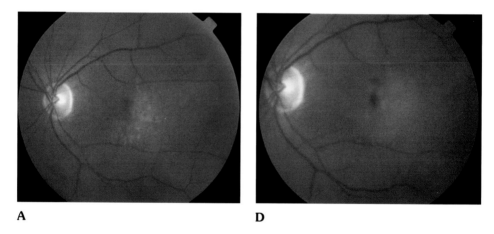

A   **D**

Figure 7.9 Occult CNV with serous PED and RCA. (A) Clinical photograph demonstrating exudation in the central macula with subretinal hemorrhage, lipid, and a serous PED. (D) Clinical photograph 3 months following treatment demonstrating persistent turbid detachment of the PED and subretinal hemorrhage.

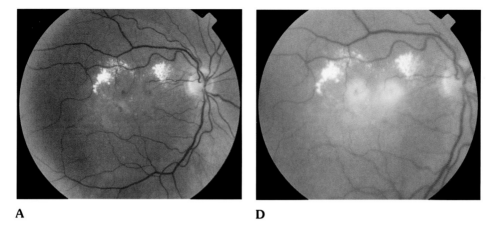

A   **D**

Figure 7.12 Occult CNV with serous PED and RCA. (A) Clinical photograph demonstrating hemorrhage, subretinal lipid exudates, and a PED in the macula. (D) Clinical photograph obtained immediately following laser treatment of the two sites of CNV. The reddish lesion now highlighted within the treatment site represents a network of vessels rather than hemorrhage.

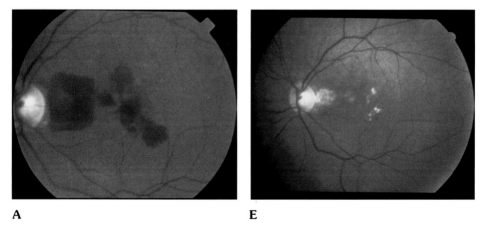

A   **E**

Figure 7.13 Polypoidal-type occult CNV with subretinal hemorrhage. (A) Clinical photograph demonstrating subretinal hemorrhage secondary to CNV. (E) Clinical photograph 3 months after laser treatment demonstrating resolution of the subretinal hemorrhage.

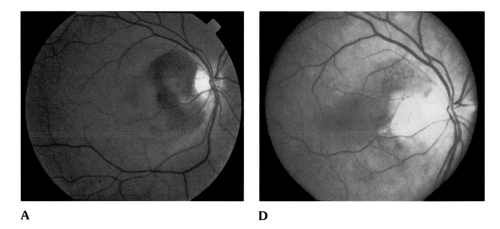

A   D

Figure 7.14 Polypoidal-type occult CNV with subretinal hemorrhage. (A) Color photograph demonstrating hemorrhagic detachment of the macula. Note the absence of drusen at the posterior pole. (D) Clinical photograph 1 year after ICG-guided laser treatment demonstrating resolution of the subretinal hemorrhage. Visual acuity improved from 20/200 to 20/25.

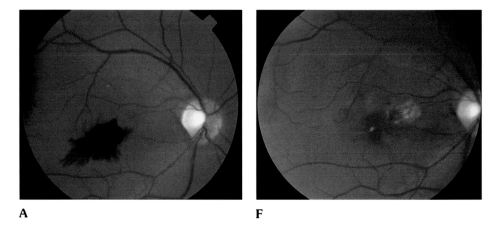

A   F

Figure 7.15 Occult CNV treatment technique. (A) Clinical photograph demonstrating a subretinal hemorrhage in the macular area. (F) Clinical photograph obtained 6 months after treatment demonstrating mottling of the RPE at the site of laser treatment and complete resolution of the subretinal hemorrhage.

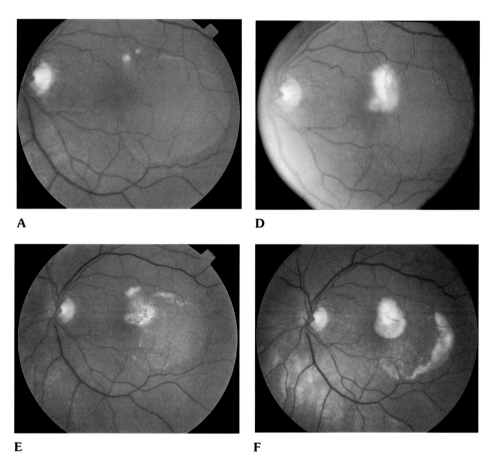

A

D

E

F

Figure 7.16 ICG-guided laser treatment of occult CNV with serous PED. (A) Clinical photograph demonstrating a large, lobular serous PED in the temporal macula. (D) Clinical photograph immediately after ICG-guided laser treatment of the CNV. (E) Clinical photograph 1 month later demonstrating partial resolution of the PED and a chorioretinal scar at the site of the treatment. (F) Four years later there is flattening of the PED. Fibrous metaplasia is seen temporally at the site of prior exudation.

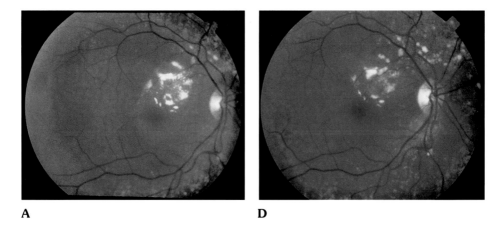

A   D

Figure 7.17 ICG-guided laser treatment of occult CNV. (A) Clinical photograph revealing an exudative macula detachment, with multiple confluent drusen beneath the neurosensory elevation. (D) Clinical photograph 1 month after ICG-guided laser photocoagulation of the hot spot of focal CNV. There is complete resolution of the neurosensory detachment of the macula.

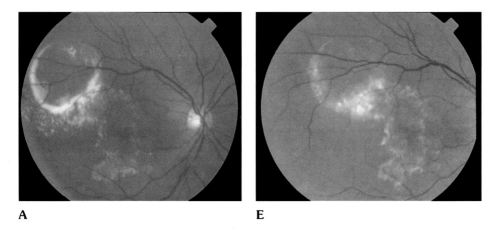

A   E

Figure 7.19 Hot spot at the margin of a plaque. (A) Clinical photograph demonstrating a turbid PED with lipid exudates in the temporal macula. Central RPE mottling and thickening is noted. (E) Three months following treatment there is complete flattening of the PED and resolution of the lipids. No change is noted in the central lesion.

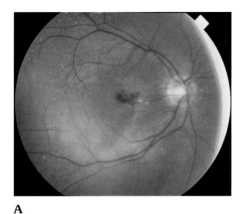

A

Figure 7.22 Occult recurrent CNV. (A) Clinical photograph demonstrating a serosanguineous PED at the temporal margin of a laser photocoagulation scar. A choroidal nevus is partially visible superotemporally.

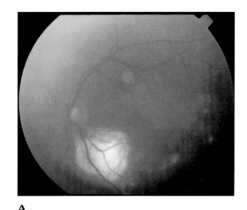

A

Figure 7.24 Occult recurrent CNV. (A) Clinical photograph demonstrating an exudative macular detachment following two previous laser treatments for CNV—one inferonasally and one inferotemporally to the fovea.

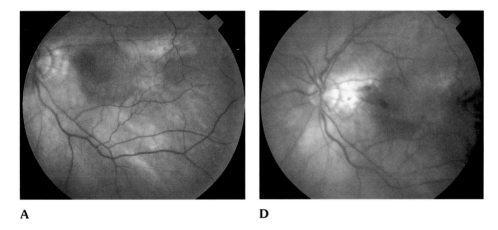

A   D

Figure 7.25 Occult recurrent CNV with serous PED. (A) Clinical photograph demonstrating a serosanguineous PED in the central macula. (D) Clinical photograph after treatment demonstrating a serosanguineous PED and exudative macular detachment.

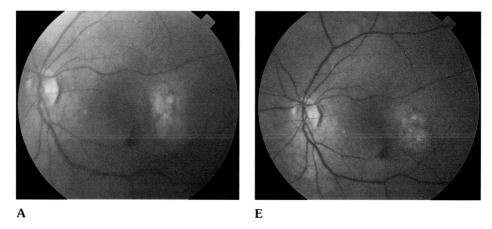

A   E

Figure 7.28 Treatment of recurrent occult CNV with hemorrhage. (A) Clinical photograph of recurrent CNV 6 months after laser treatment. There is a temporal chorioretinal scar and a recurrent serosanguineous retinal detachment. (E) Clinical photograph 3 weeks after laser treatment demonstrating reduction of the neurosensory detachment.

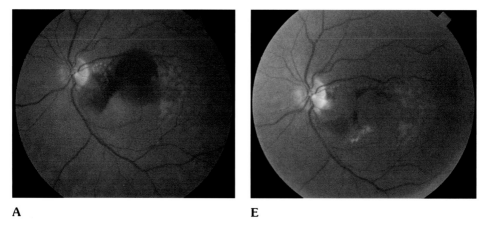

A   E

Figure 7.30 Treatment of recurrent occult CNV with serous PED. (A) Clinical photograph of a serosanguineous PED in a patient with AMD. (E) Clinical photograph 8 weeks after treatment demonstrating recurrence of the neurosensory macular detachment.

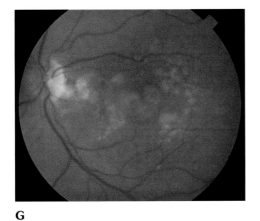

G

Figure 7.30 *(continued)* (G) Clinical photograph 2 months after treatment of the recurrence demonstrating resolution of the neurosensory detachment.

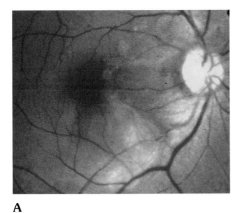

A

Figure 7.31 Idiopathic polypoidal choroidal vasculopathy. (A) Clinical photograph of a patient with idiopathic polypoidal choroidal vasculopathy emonstrating a pattern of polypoidal-like dilation of the choroidal vasculature in the peripapillary area. A larger, bulging dilation is present inferiorly.

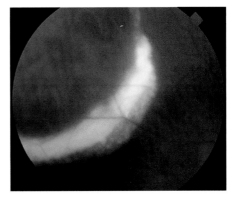

A

Figure 7.36 Wide-angle ICG angiography. Peripheral CNV. (A) Clinical photograph demonstrating a neurosensory detachment and subretinal exudates in the superotemporal fundus.

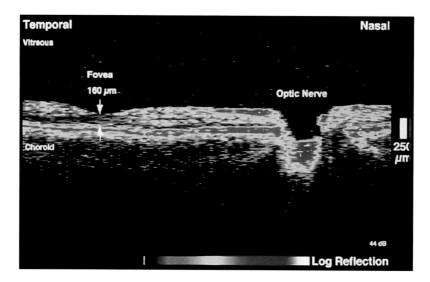

Figure 8.1 OCT of a normal eye through the optic nerve and fovea.

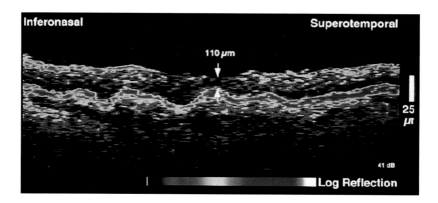

Figure 8.2 Soft drusen.

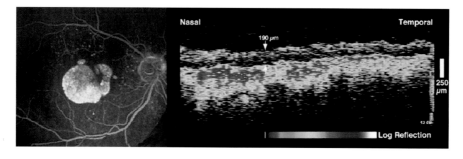

Figure 8.3 Geographic atrophy.

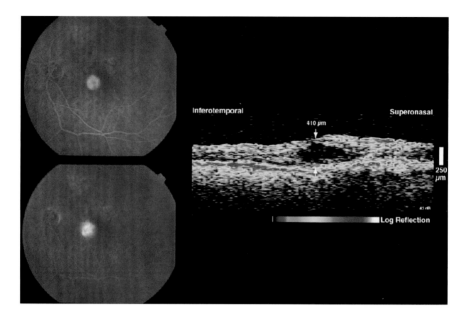

Figure 8.4 Retinal thickening.

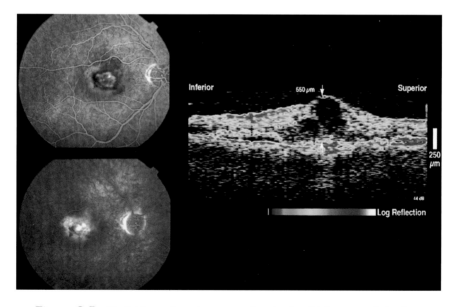

Figure 8.5 Cystoid macular edema secondary to choroidal neovascularization.

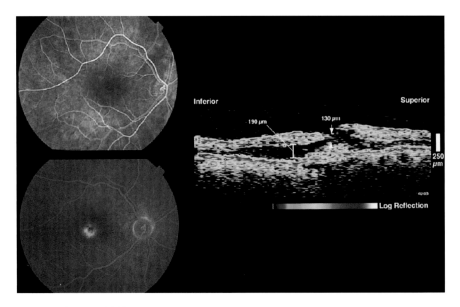

Figure 8.6 Neurosensory detachment secondary to subretinal fluid.

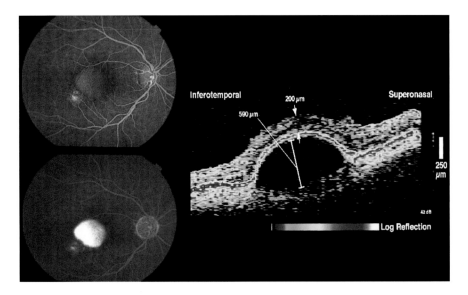

Figure 8.7 Serous retinal pigment epithelial detachment.

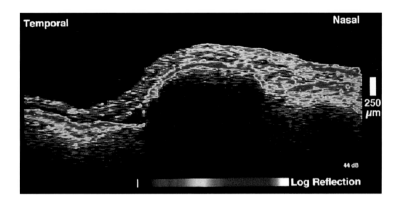

Figure 8.8 Hemorrhagic retinal pigment epithelial detachment.

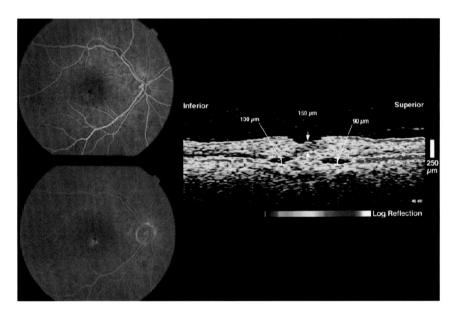

Figure 8.9 Well-defined choroidal neovascularization.

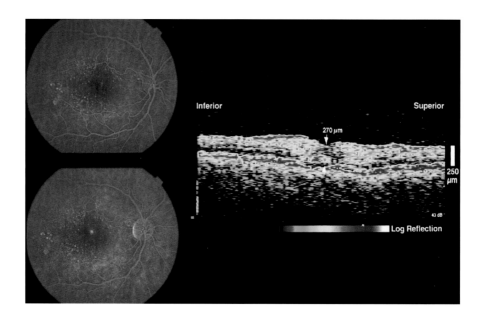

Figure 8.10 Choroidal neovascularization in the subretinal space.

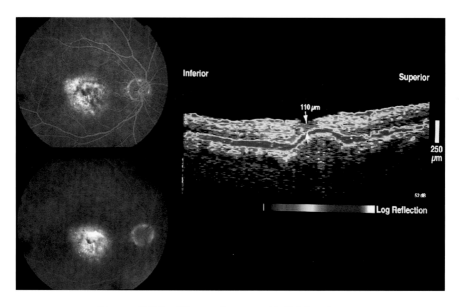

Figure 8.11 Fibrous pigment epithelial detachment.

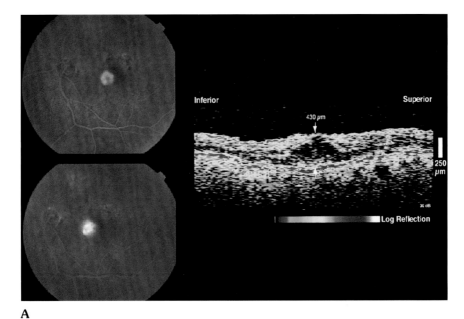

Figure 8.12 (A) Choroidal neovascularization before photodynamic therapy. (B) Same eye after photodynamic therapy.

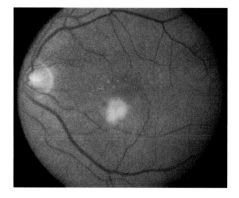

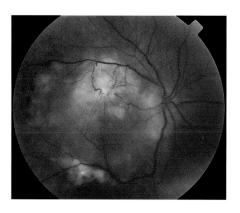

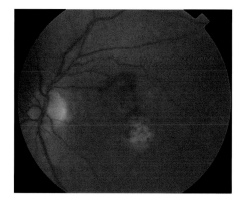

Figure 9.3 Treatment intensity standard. Post-treatment fundus photographs were compared with this photograph to determine compliance with treatment protocol. (Reproduced with permission from Macular Photocoagulation Study Group: Krypton laser photocoagulation for neovascular lesions of ocular histoplasmosis: results of a randomized clinical trial. Arch Ophthalmol 105:1499–1507, 1987. Copyrighted 1987, American Medical Association.)

Figure 11.1 Right eye of 72-year-old patient with diskiform scar.

Figure 11.2 Left eye of same patient as in Figure 1 with recurrent CNVM following laser treatment.

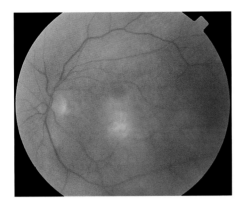

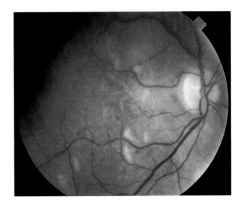

Figure 11.3 Same eye as in Figure 11.2, 6 months status post proton radiation left eye for recurrent CNVM.

Figure 11.4 Radiation retinopathy 1 year following proton beam radiation using 14 CGE.

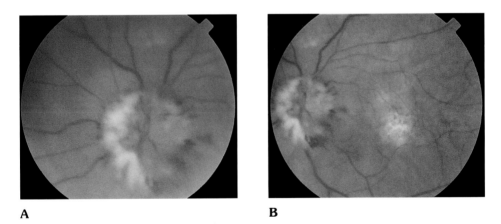

A   B

Figure 11.5 (A) Postradiation optic neuropathy after 14 CGE proton beam treatment, 1 year posttreatment. (B) In this view the CNVM appears dry.

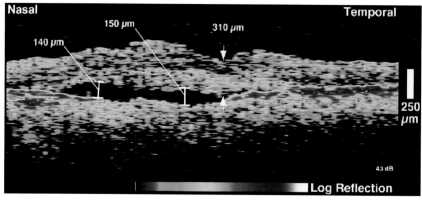

B

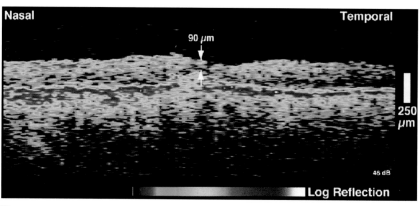

D

Figure 13.2 (B) OCT demonstrated subretinal fluid and TTT was performed. One year following treatment the visual acuity remained 20/50. Examination demonstrated mild retinal pigmentary changes. (D) Subretinal fluid had resolved on OCT.

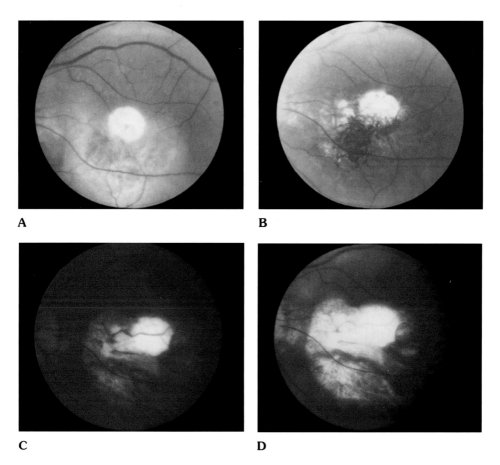

Figure 15.6 (A) Color photograph of a patient with geographic atrophy and a subretinal neovascular membrane due to age-related macular degeneration. Visual acuity is 20/300. There was no previous laser therapy. (B) Photograph taken 1 month following submacular surgery, revealing some residual subretinal blood at the excision site. (C) Photograph taken 3 years following surgery, revealing RPE and choriocapillary atrophy in the area of preexisting subretinal neovascular membrane. Visual acuity is 20/200. (D) Photograph taken 7 years following surgery, demonstrating that the area of atrophy has increased in size. Visual acuity is 20/200.

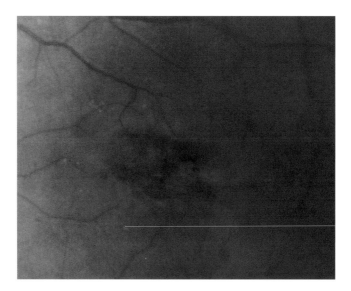

Figure 16.20 Fundus photograph at presentation demonstrates a subfoveal choroidal neovascular membrane approximately one MPS disk area in size under the geometrical center of the foveal avascular zone in the left eye. Visual acuity is 20/200-1.

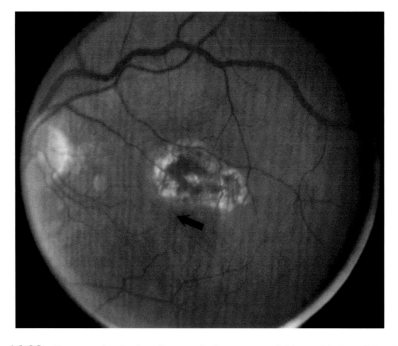

Figure 16.22 Postoperative fundus photograph shows successful laser ablation of the choroidal neovascular membrane with no evidence of recurrence. The geometrical center of the foveal avascular zone (arrow) is preserved. Visual acuity is 20/40.

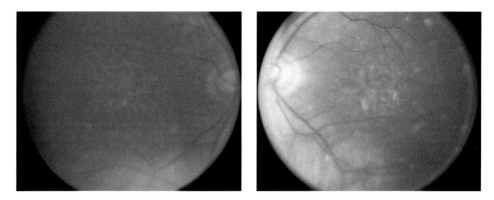

Figure 18.1 Baseline color fundus photographs of a patient with age-related macular degeneration, and bilateral drusen. Visual acuity is 20/30 OU. Multiple, soft, confluent drusen are noted.

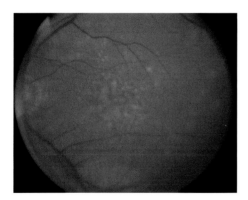

Figure 18.3 The left eye is randomized to low-intensity laser treatment. Twenty gray-white laser spots are placed in temporal arc in the macula. The laser spots are subtle.

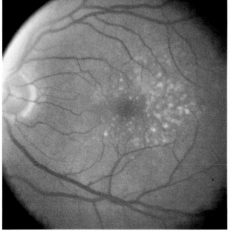
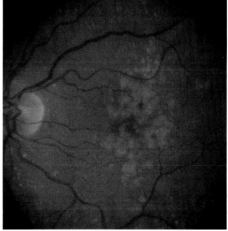

Figure 19.2 (Left) Fundus of an eye with many macular drusen of a variety of sizes. (Right) Fundus of another eye showing very large confluent drusen.

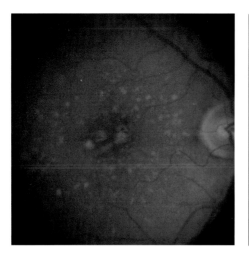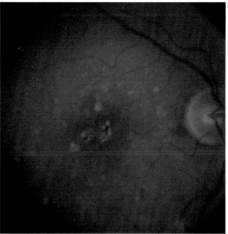

Figure 19.6 (Left) The right fundus of a patient with multiple, large macular drusen. (Right) Twelve months after treatment with subthreshold laser lesions, drusen resorption has been dramatic.

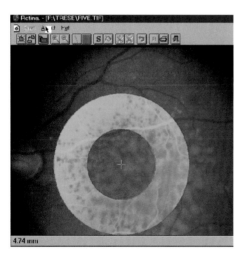

Figure 19.7 Using a drusen analysis software program, drusen located within the large circle (alzer 1 ring) are selected for analysis and the area of regard is displayed. A drusen detection algorithm identifies and displays the drusen it found in false color.

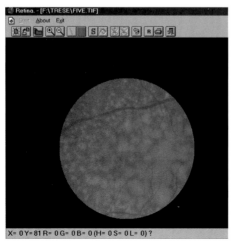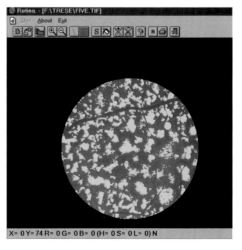

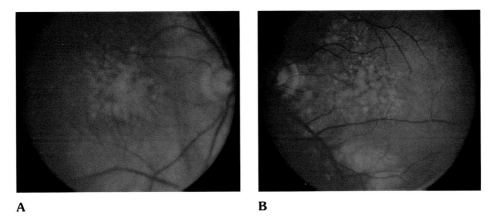

A   **B**

Figure 20.4   Six-month color fundus photographs show no significant change in drusen in either eye. Visual acuity remains 20/30 OU.

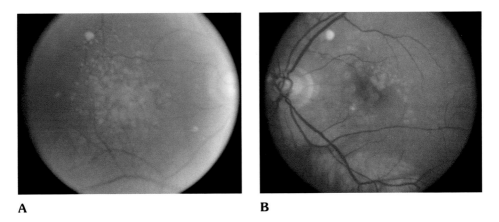

A   **B**

Figure 20.5   Twelve-month color fundus photographs show marked resolution of drusen in the treated left eye. The right eye remains stable with no significant change in dursen. Visual acuity is 20/30 OD and 20/20 OS.

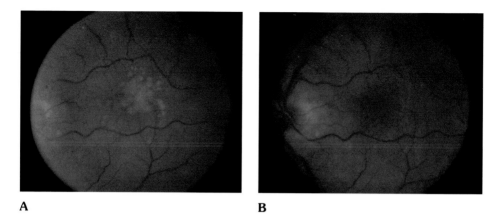

A   B

Figure 20.6 (A) Baseline fundus photograph demonstrating multiple, large drusen. The eye was treated with 20 laser spots in the temporal macula per the CNVPT protocol. (B) Six months later there is significant drusen reduction and the vision has changed from 20/32 to 20/25.

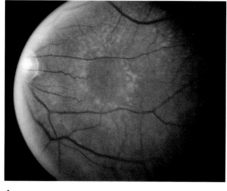

Figure 20.7 (A) Color fundus photograph 6 months after CNVPT laser treatment showing submacular fluid and the visual acuity has dropped from 20/20 to 20/60.

A

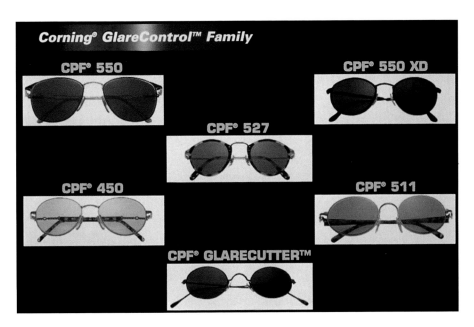

Figure 22.15 Corning family of filters.

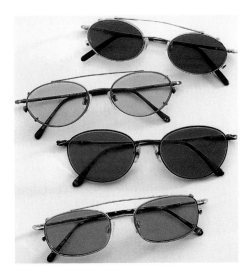

Figure 22.16 Corning's X series, which are slightly darker than their corresponding filters.

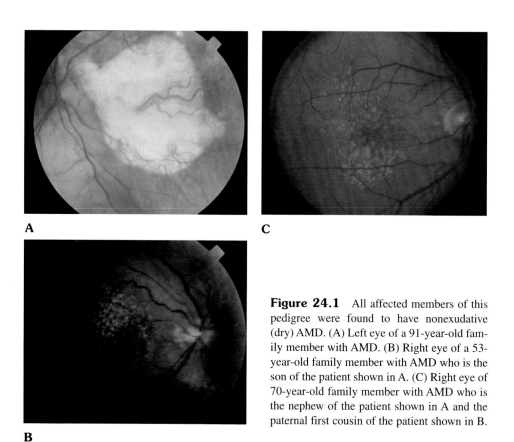

Figure 24.1 All affected members of this pedigree were found to have nonexudative (dry) AMD. (A) Left eye of a 91-year-old family member with AMD. (B) Right eye of a 53-year-old family member with AMD who is the son of the patient shown in A. (C) Right eye of 70-year-old family member with AMD who is the nephew of the patient shown in A and the paternal first cousin of the patient shown in B.

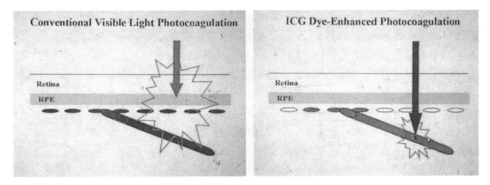

Figure 10 Schematic comparison of choroidal vessel photocoagulation by conventional laser and ICG–dye-enhanced laser. (Reprinted from Flower RW. Experimental studies of indocyanine green dye-enhanced photocoagulation of choroidal neovascularization feeder vessels. Am J Ophthalmol 2000;129:503, Fig 2. Copyright 2000, with permission from Elsevier Science.)

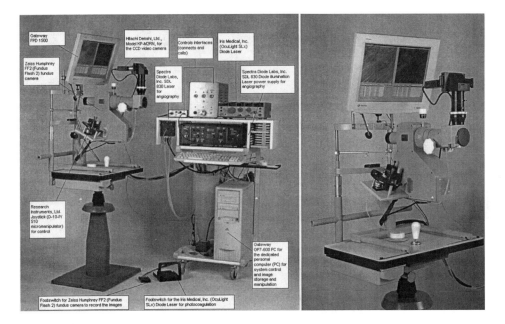

Figure 11 The fundus camera/photocoagulation system.

C. Demonstration of ICG Dye–Enhanced Photocoagulation

No animal model exists of CNV FVs, but the choroidal vasculature of pigmented rabbit eyes can serve as a model system in which to demonstrate principles that may pertain to the human eye. For example, the rabbit CC is a reasonable equivalent of its human counterpart, and being a vascular plexus, it also can serve as a model of CNV, in that CNV also is a vascular plexus—albeit one with high resistance to flow compared to the CC.

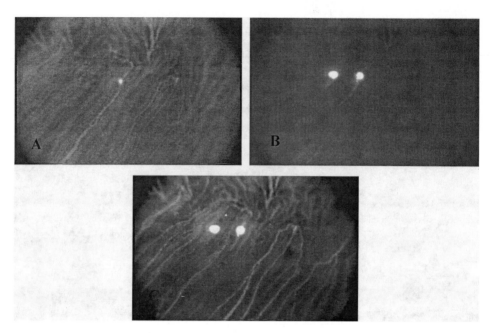

Figure 12   Demonstration of use of the ICG dye–enhanced camera system. (A) Application of laser energy during transit of a high-concentration dye bolus. (B) Incarceration of ICG dye distal to the burn site. (C) Validation of vessel closure by injection of another dye bolus.

Likewise, the arterioles feeding the rabbit eye CC can serve as a model for FVs, so the pigmented eyes of Dutch belted rabbits were used to demonstrate ICG-dye-enhanced photocoagulation.

Use of the ICG dye–enhanced camera system is demonstrated in the three frames of Figure 12, which show application of laser energy during transit of a high concentration dye bolus (A), incarceration of ICG dye distal to the burn site (B), and validation of vessel closure by injection of another dye bolus (C). Incarceration of ICG dye immediately following laser photocoagulation (B) not only provides immediate feedback as to the success of the procedure, but the incarcerated dye constitutes a strongly absorbing target for further laser application without the need to inject additional dye boluses. The reduction in retinal tissue damage concomitant to FV laser photocoagulation using ICG dye–enhancement is demonstrated in Figure 13, which compares the extent of RPE damage resulting from application of identical laser burns to identical choroidal arteries, one with and one without presence of a transiting high-concentration dye bolus.

V.   THE FUTURE OF CNV FEEDER-VESSEL TREATMENT

Aggressive CNV behavior—rapid membrane growth, edema formation, etc.—has been viewed as a destructive event, and conventional treatment aims to remedy such behavior by complete CNV obliteration. But the frequent recurrence of CNV following such treatment

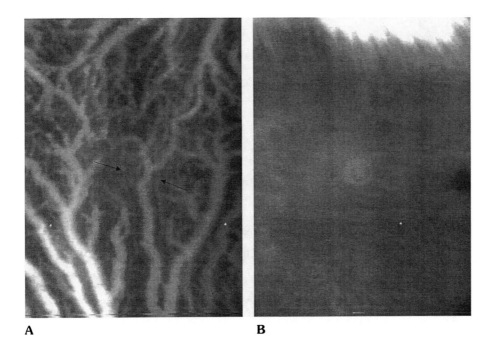

A   B

Figure 13 Demonstration of the reduction in retinal tissue damage concomitant to FV laser photocoagulation using ICG dye enhancement, using identical choroidal arteries arising from a common origin in a pigmented rabbit eye as a model. (A) Arrows indicate locations of laser burns of identical energy on the two identical choroidal arterioles. The left-hand burn was applied without use of ICG dye enhancement, and the right-hand burn was placed during transit of a high-concentration bolus of ICG dye. (B) Comparison of the extent of RPE damage resulting from application of the identical laser burns inferior to the medullary rays.

could be nature's continuing effort to compensate for the original—and perhaps now exac-erbated—defect. Instead, such aggressive CNV behavior could be viewed as an overcom-pensation for some metabolic or other blood-flow-related defect. And if laser treatment were to be applied in such a way as to just reduce the blood flow to aggressive CNV by an appropriate amount—perhaps until the CNV vasculature matures—then further aggressive behavior might be avoided; those cases of inadvertent incomplete FV closure resulting in improved vision would be examples.

Photocoagulating the FVs supplying CNV associated with AMD can be a successful treatment method (6,7)—especially for occult CNV. Indeed, there may be an important dif-ference between the response of CNV evoked by direct application of laser energy, as in conventional treatment, and that evoked by reducing blood flow through the otherwise undisturbed membrane. If ultimately FV photocoagulation treatment were to be refined along these lines, the laser would become more a precision instrument to modulate blood flow than a weapon for destruction of the very retinal tissue whose function we are trying to conserve. Additionally, because of the pre- and post-treatment high-speed ICG an-giograms the method requires, information about choroidal hemodynamics is being ac-crued that otherwise probably would not be available.

REFERENCES

1. Behrendt T. Therapeutic vascular occlusions in diabetic retinopathy. Arch Ophthal Mol 1972;87:629–633.
2. Patz A, Flower RW, Klien ML, Orth DH, Fleischman JA, McLeod DS. Clinical application of indocyanine green angiography. In: Delay JJ, ed. International Symposium on Fluorescein Angiography. Documenta Ophthalmologica Proceedings Series, Vol 9. The Hague: Dr. W. Junk bv, 1976, p 245.
3. Macular Photocoagulation Study Group. Subfoveal neovascular lesions in age-related macular degeneration: guidelines for evaluation and treatment in the macular photocoagulation study. Arch Ophthalmol 1991;109:1242–1257.
4. Slakter JS, Yannuzzi LA, Sorensen JS, et al. A pilot study of indocyanine green videoangiography-guided laser treatment of primary occult choroidal neovascularizaton. Arch Ophthalmol 1994;112:465–472.
5. Schwartz S, Guyer DR, Yannuzzi LA, et al. Indocyanine green videoangiography guided laser photocoagulation of primary occult choroidal neovascularizaton in age-related macular degeneration. Invest Ophthalmol Vis Sci 1995;36:S244.
6. Shiraga F, Ojima Y, Matsuo T, Takasu I, Matsuo N. Feeder vessel photocoagulation of subfoveal choroidal neovascularization secondary to age-related macular degeneration. Ophthalmology 1998;105:662–669.
7. Staurenghi G, Orzalesi N, La Capria A, Aschero M. Laser treatment of feeder vessels in subfoveal choroidal neovascular membranes: a revisitation using dynamic indocyanine green angiography. Ophthalmology 1998;105:2297–2305.
8. Flower RW. Extraction of choriocapillaris hemodynamic data from ICG fluorescence angiograms. Invest Ophthalmol Vis Sci 1993;34:2720–2729.
9. Sarks SH. Aging and degeneration in the macular region: a clinicopathological study. Br J Ophthalmol 1976;60:324–341.
10. Schneider S, Greven CM, Green WR. Photocoagulation of well-defined choroidal neovascularization in age-related macular degeneration. Retina 1998;18:242–250.
11. Green WR, Enger C. Age-related macular degeneration: histopathologic studies. The 1992 Lorenz E Zimmerman lecture. Ophthalmology 1993;100:1519–1535.
12. Wertheimer M. Experimentelle Studien ueber das Sehen von Bewegung. Z Psychol 1912;61:161–265.
13. Arnold JJ, Sarks SH, Killingsworth, Sarks JP. Reticular pseudodrusen: a risk factor in age-related maculopathy. Retina 1995;15:183–191.
14. Flower RW. High-speed ICG angiography. In: Yannuzzi LA, Flower RW, Slakter JS, ed. Indocyanine Green Angiography. St. Louis: Mosby, 1997, pp 86–94.
15. Flower RW. Experimental studies of indocyanine green dye-enhanced photocoagulation of choroidal neovascularization feeder vessels. Am J Ophthalmol 2000;129:501–512.
16. Fryczkowski AW, Sherman MD. Scanning electron microscopy of human ocular vascular casts: the submacular choriocapillaris. Acta Anat 1988;132:265–269.
17. Maepea O. Pressures in the anterior ciliary arteries, choroidal veins and choriocapillaris. Exp Eye Res 1992;54:731–736.
18. Flower RW, Snyder WA, Expanded hypothesis on the mechanism of photodynamic therapy action on choroidal neovascularization. Retina 1999;19:365–369.
19. Reichel E, Berrocal AM, Ip M. Kroll AJ, Desai V, Duker JS, Puliafito CA. Transpupillary thermotherapy (TTT) of occult subfoveal choroidal neovascularization in patients with age-related macular degeneration. Ophthalmology 1999;106:1908–1914.
20. Reichel E, Puliafito CA, Duker JS, Guyer DR. Indocyanine green dye-enhanced diode laser photocoagulation of poorly defined subfoveal choroidal neovascularization. Ophthal Surg 1994;25:195–201.
21. Flower RW. Variability in choriocapillaris blood flow distribution. Invest Ophthalmol Vis Sci 1995;36:1247–1258.

13

Transpupillary Thermotherapy of Subfoveal Occult Choroidal Neovascularization

Adam H. Rogers and Elias Reichel
New England Eye Center, Tufts University School of Medicine, Boston, Massachusetts

Adam Martidis
Wills Eye Hospital, Thomas Jefferson University School of Medicine, Philadelphia, Pennsylvania

Audina M. Berrocal
Bascom Palmer Eye Institute, Miami, Florida

I. INTRODUCTION

Age-related macular degeneration (AMD) is a leading cause of central vision loss in patients older than 65 years of age. Despite a lower prevalence of neovascular AMD compared with nonneovascular AMD, an estimated 80% of severe vision loss occurs secondary to the formation of choroidal neovascularization (CNV) (1,2). Left untreated, most patients with subfoveal CNV have a poor visual outcome with only a small percentage maintaining visual acuity greater than 20/100 (3–5). Qualifying lesions, high recurrence rates, and an immediate decline in visual acuity have restricted treatment and prompted a search for alternative treatments.

II. TREATMENT OF CLASSIC SUBFOVEAL CHOROIDAL NEOVASCULARIZATION

Laser treatment of subfoveal CNV is one the only proven treatment modality, but it has been limited by both lesion size and characteristics based on fluorescein angiography. Laser photocoagulation of subfoveal CNV in the Macular Photocoagulation Study (MPS) required a small, well-defined lesion of 3.5 MPS disk areas or less. Treatment was complicated by an immediate loss of approximately three lines of visual acuity from thermal photocoagulation of the neurosensory retina. The MPS further failed to demonstrate a treatment benefit in visual acuity until 2 years after randomization (3–5). The Treatment of Age-Related Macular Degeneration with Photodynamic Therapy (TAP) Study Group (6) reported that the use of verteporfin, an intravenously injected photosensitizing agent activated with a 690-nm light source, statistically reduced vision loss. While this nonthermal

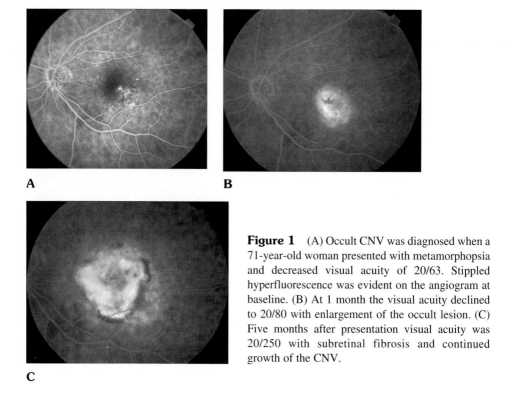

A   B

Figure 1 (A) Occult CNV was diagnosed when a 71-year-old woman presented with metamorphopsia and decreased visual acuity of 20/63. Stippled hyperfluorescence was evident on the angiogram at baseline. (B) At 1 month the visual acuity declined to 20/80 with enlargement of the occult lesion. (C) Five months after presentation visual acuity was 20/250 with subretinal fibrosis and continued growth of the CNV.

C

laser induced less injury to the surrounding neurosensory retina, a treatment benefit occurred only when the classic component of the CNV occupied greater than 50% of the entire lesion. Other treatments of CNV including interferon alfa-2a (7), submacular surgery (8), and irradiation (9) have proven unsuccessful.

III. NATURAL HISTORY OF OCCULT SUBFOVEAL CHOROIDAL NEOVASCULARIZATION

While the MPS and TAP studies treated predominantly well-demarcated, classic CNV, most patients present with occult CNV and are ineligible for treatment (10). Natural history studies of occult CNV demonstrate that significant visual loss occurs with these lesions (Fig. 1). Bressler et al. (11) retrospectively reviewed 84 eyes with occult CNV and reported that 63% lost three or more lines of vision with an average of 28 months of follow-up. The average visual acuity declined from an initial measurement of 20/80 to 20/250 during the same time period. Stevens et al. (12) prospectively followed 21 eyes with occult CNV over a 12-month period and reported that 29% lost six or more lines of vision. The Macular Photocoagulation Study (13) observed 26 eyes with occult CNV. Severe visual loss, consisting of a decrease in visual acuity of six or more lines of acuity, occurred in 41% of eyes at 12 months and 64% at 36 months. The median visual acuity at the 36-month point declined to 20/200 in the untreated eyes with occult CNV from an initial acuity of 20/50. Fifty-nine patients with occult CNV were followed as a control group in the Radiation Therapy for Age-related Macular Degeneration (RAD) Study Group. A mean of 3.4 lines of visual acuity were lost at 1 year (8).

Treatment options for occult CNV have been limited. Recently, both radiation and submacular surgery have been utilized as treatment options. In the RAD Study Group (8), eligible patients had subfoveal classic or occult CNV with a lesion size of six disk areas or less, visual acuity of 20/320 or better, visual symptoms of 6 months or less, and absence of foveal hemorrhage. A total of 101 patients were randomized to receive eight fractions of 2 Gy external-beam irradiation, while 104 patients received eight fractions of a sham treatment. Of the 88 patients receiving radiation treatment examined at 1 year, the mean decrease in visual acuity was 3.5 lines compared with a 3.7-line drop experienced by the 95 patients in the control group. No statistically significant difference existed whether classic or occult CNV was present in either the treatment or control group. Three or more lines of visual acuity were lost in 51.1% of the treated and 52.6% of the controls at 1 year. In general, external-beam radiation administered at a dose of 16 Gy applied in eight fractions of 2 Gy provided no statistically significant benefit for the treatment of subfoveal classic or occult CNV secondary to AMD.

The Submacular Surgery Trial (8) evaluated the surgical excision of a recurrent subfoveal CNV originating from the edge of a prior laser scar from previous photocoagulation of extrafoveal or juxtafoveal CNV secondary to AMD. The total lesion size could not exceed nine MPS disk areas, which included the prior laser scar, recurrent CNV, and any lesion components that block fluorescence. While classic CNV was required, the subfoveal portion of the lesion could be occult or classic. Seventy patients were enrolled in the Submacular Surgery Trial with 36 randomized to laser and 34 to submacular surgery when the study was closed in 1997. At the 24-month examination, 26% of the laser treated eyes and 14% of the surgically treated eyes improved by two or more lines of visual acuity. Of all patients, the surgical group on average lost two lines of visual acuity, while the laser group remained stable. The Submacular Surgery Trial concluded that surgical removal of recurrent subfoveal CNV provided no benefit over laser photocoagulation.

Macular translocation has gained popularity as an alternative treatment. The advantage of this surgical treatment is that it can treat both classic and occult CNV with poorly defined margins. Owing to the unpredictable nature of the procedure and potential surgical complications, further refinement of the surgical technique has been recommended (20).

IV. TRANSPUPILLARY THERMOTHERAPY

Transpupillary thermotherapy (TTT) has emerged as a recent advancement for the treatment of occult subfoveal choroidal neovascularization in patients with AMD (Fig. 2). TTT was initially used in the treatment of choroidal melanomas (14,15), and a recent pilot study of 16 eyes in 15 patients with occult subfoveal CNV treated with TTT demonstrated the effectiveness of this form of treatment in stabilizing visual acuity (16). With a mean follow-up of 12 months, three of 16 eyes (19%) improved by two or more lines of Snellen visual acuity. Nine eyes (56%) had no change in visual acuity, and four eyes (25%) declined by two or more lines. Fifteen of the 16 eyes treated with TTT demonstrated improvement in the amount of exudation. Diminished exudation was also present in three of four eyes that experienced a decline in visual acuity.

Miller-Rivero and Kaplan treated 30 eyes with TTT of which 22 were predominantly occult and eight were predominantly classic. Pretreatment visual acuity ranged from 20/40

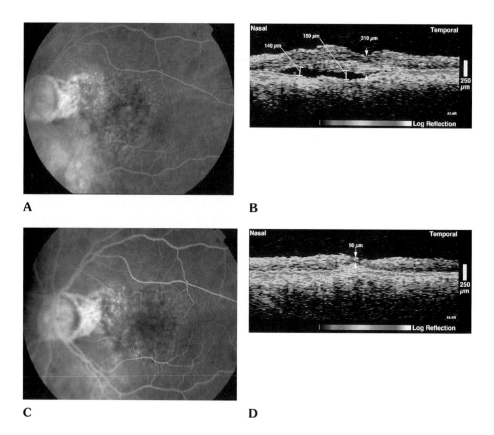

Figure 2 A 76-year-old woman presented with decreased visual acuity in the left eye measuring 20/50. (A) Stippled hyperfluorescence consistent with occult choroidal neovascularization was present on fluorescein angiography. (B) OCT demonstrated subretinal fluid and TTT was performed. One year following treatment the visual acuity remained 20/50. Examination demonstrated mild retinal pigmentary changes. (C) Fluorescein angiography was unchanged, and (D) subretinal fluid had resolved on OCT. See also color insert, Fig. 13.2B, D.

to count fingers. Eight eyes (26.7%) improved two lines or more, 13 eyes (43.3%) remained within one line of pretreatment visual acuity, and nine eyes (30.0%) declined two or more lines. Twenty-six eyes demonstrated a decrease in exudation after treatment, and seven eyes were retreated (17).

Newsome and associates (18) further evaluated the efficacy of TTT for the treatment of both classic and occult CNV. In a nonrandomized fashion 44 eyes of 42 patients with symptomatic visual loss and angiographic evidence of CNV secondary to AMD were enrolled for treatment. Twelve of the lesions were predominantly classic and 32 predominantly occult. The study population also included 11 eyes with serous pigment epithelial detachments. In the predominantly occult group, 78% of the lesions were closed with an average of 0.66 Snellen lines lost over 7.2 months of follow-up. Predominantly classic lesions were closed in 75% of eyes with an average of 0.75 Snellen lines lost. Stabilization or improvement in visual acuity occurred in 71% of eyes with occult lesions and 67% of eyes with classic lesions.

Reported complications from TTT are rare. Severe loss of vision has been estimated to occur in less than 1% of patients from several large series of cases. In the initial pilot study of 16 eyes with occult CNV (13), there was no evidence of damage to the neurosensory retina. Significant posttreatment hemorrhage was reported in two of 44 patients reported in the series by Newsome and associates (18). Shields et al. (15) treated 100 consecutive patients with choroidal melanoma using TTT. There were no reported lenticular or corneal complications. Branch retinal vein occlusion occurred in 23 patients with an associated branch retinal artery occlusion in 12 patients. However, the treatment of choroidal melanoma differs from the treatment of CNV in that it is considerably more intense with a desired endpoint of whitening of the tumor and overlying retina.

Transpupillary thermotherapy is administered through a slit-lamp-mounted delivery system attached to a modified infrared diode laser at 810 nm (Iris Medical Instruments, Mountain View, CA). The beam has an adjustable width of 1.2 mm, 2.0 mm, and 3.0 mm, and is transmitted to the retina via a diode-coated contact lens. The beam width may be further enlarged through contact lens magnification. In the study by Newsome and associates, several spot sizes were successfully used in a confluent, overlapping fashion to treat larger lesions during one treatment session (18). Treatment is initiated when the entire spot envelops the visible retinal lesion. The typical power settings range between 360 and 1000 mW based on the diameter of the spot size, fundus pigmentation, choroidal blood flow, and media clarity (19). The power to produce a given rise in temperature is dependent on the diameter of the laser spot, not the area. A doubling of the spot size requires a doubling in power, with the reverse being true if the spot size is halved. A typical setting with a 3-mm spot size consists of an initial power level between 650 and 800 mW for 60s. A thin, white slit beam is focused in the center of the red aiming beam on the lesion to view any retinal changes that occur during treatment. If any retinal whitening is observed the treatment is stopped, as the goal of treatment is to observe no retinal change in color. During treatment, only gentle pressure form the lens should be placed on the globe. This avoids compression of the choroidal vasculature, which may lead to thermal-induced damage of the retina and choroid from retained heat generated by the laser.

TTT treats occult CNV in a subthreshold manner with long exposure and large retinal spot sizes. At 810 nm, the energy transmitted to the eye penetrates to the choroid and retinal pigment epithelium (RPE) while minimizing absorption in the neurosensory retina. The choroidal vasculature further acts to dissipate generated heat. In contrast to threshold treatment from conventional short-pulsed photocoagulation where an estimated rise in retinal temperature of 42 °C occurs, the estimated retinal temperature elevation with TTT at standard settings (800 mW, 60 s, 3.0-mm spot size) is approximately 10 °C (19). Through this delivery of thermal energy to the choroid, the mechanism of treatment of CNV by TTT may occur through vascular thrombosis, apoptosis, thermal inhibition of angiogenesis (19), or the release of cytotoxic free radicals from irradiated tissue (18).

V. CONCLUSION

TTT offers patients with subfoveal occult CNV a treatment option for a disease that is inadequately treated by conventional laser (13), and whose natural history has a uniformly poor outcome. By penetrating deep in the choroid with infrared light at 810 nm, TTT causes heat-induced damage to the neovascular tissue while limiting injury to the neurosensory retina. Through a small pilot study of 16 eyes, TTT has been shown to stabilize visual acuity in 75% of patients over a follow-up period from 6 to 24 months. Other authors have confirmed the findings of the initial pilot study by Reichel and associates, and have further identified that TTT is useful in the stabilization of visual acuity in eyes with classic CNV (17,18). The use of TTT to treat occult subfoveal CNV secondary to age-related macular degeneration is further being evaluated in the ongoing Transpupillary Thermotherapy for Occult Choroidal Neovascularization (TTT4CNV) trial. This randomized, 2-year, multicenter study is currently recruiting patients with occult CNV and visual acuity ranging from 20/50 to 20/400. The TTT4CNV clinical trial will compare the effectiveness of TTT for occult CNV with the natural course of the disease. This study should help to define the role of TTT for the treatment of occult choroidal neovascularization.

VI. SUMMARY

TTT is emerging as a treatment for occult choroidal neovascularization. By penetrating deep in the choroid with infrared light at 810 mm, TTT causes heat-induced damage to the neovascular tissue while limiting injury to the neurosensory retina.

Multiple pilot studies have confirmed that TTT is useful in stabilizing the visual acuity in eyes with occult CNV. Recent pilot studies have identified that TTT stabilizes visual acuity in eyes treated with classic CNV. The use of TTT to treat occult CNV is currently under investigation in the TTT4CNV trial.

REFERENCES

1. Klein R, Klein BE, Linton KL. Prevalence of age-related maculopathy: the Beaver Dam Eye Study. Ophthalmology 1992;99:933–943.
2. Leibowitz HM, Krueger DE, Maunder LR, et al. The Framingham Eye Study Monograph. VI. Macular Degeneration. Surv Ophthalmol 1980;24(Suppl):428– 457.
3. Macular Photocoagulation Study Group. Laser photocoagulation of subfoveal neovascular lesions in age-related macular degeneration: results of a randomized clinical trial. Arch Ophthalmol 1991;109:1220–1231.
4. Macular Photocoagulation Study Group. Laser photocoagulation of subfoveal recurrent neovascular lesions in age-related macular degeneration: results of a randomized clinical trial. Arch Ophthalmol 1991;109:1232–1241.
5. Macular Photocoagulation Study Group. Subfoveal neovascular lesions in age-related macular degeneration: guidelines for evaluation of and treatment in the Macular Photocoagulation Study. Arch Ophthalmol 1991;109:1242–1257.
6. Treatment of Age-Related Macular Degeneration with Photodynamic Therapy (TAP) Study Group. Photodynamic therapy of subfoveal choroidal neovascularization in age-related macular degeneration with verteporfin. Arch Ophthalmol 1999;117:1329–1345.
7. Pharmacologic Therapy for Macular Degeneration Study Group. Interferon alfa-2a is ineffective for patients with choroidal neovascularization secondary to age-related macular degeneration. Arch Ophthalmol 1997;115:865–872.
8. Submacular Surgery Trials Pilot Study Investigators. Submacular surgery trials randomized pilot trial of laser photocoagulation versus surgery for recurrent choroidal neovascularization secondary to age-related macular degeneration. I. Ophthalmic outcomes. Submacular Surgery Trials Pilot Study report number 1. Am J Ophthalmol 2000;130:387–407.

9. The Radiation Therapy for Age-Related Macular Degeneration (RAD) Study Group. A prospective, randomized, double-masked trial on radiation therapy for neovascular age-related macular degeneration (RAD Study). Ophthalmology 1999;106:2239–2247.
10. Freund KB, Yannuzzi LA, Sorenson JA. Age-related macular degeneration and choroidal neovascularization. Am J Ophthalmol 1993;115:786–791.
11. Bressler MM, Frost, LA, Bressler SB, et al. Natural course of poorly defined choroidal neovascularization associated with macular degeneration. Arch Ophthalmol 1988;106:1537–1542.
12. Stevens TS, Bressler NM, Maguire MG, et al., Occult choroidal neovascularization in age-related macular degeneration; a natural history study. Arch Ophthalmol 1997;115:345–350.
13. Macular Photocoagulation Study Group. Occult choroidal neovascularization influence on visual outcome in patients with age-related macular degeneration. Arch Ophthalmol 1996;114:400–412.
14. Shields CL, Shields JA, DePotter P, Kheterpal S. Transpupillary thermotherapy in the management of choroidal melanoma. Ophthalmology 1996;103:1642–1650.
15. Shields CL, Shields JA, Cater J, et al. Transpupillary thermotherapy for choroidal melanoma: tumor control and visual results in 100 consecutive cases. Ophthalmology 1998;105:581–590.
16. Reichel E, Berrocal AM, Ip M, et al. Transpupillary thermotherapy of occult subfoveal choroidal neovascularization in patients with age-related macular degeneration. Ophthalmology 1999;106:1908–1914.
17. Miller-Rivero NE, Kaplan HJ. Transpupillary thermotherapy in the treatment of occult choroidal neovascularization. Invest Ophthalmol Vis Sci 2000;41:S179.
18. Newsome RSB, McAlister JC, Saeed M, McHugh JDA. Transpupillary thermotherapy (TTT) for the treatment of choroidal neovascularisation. Br J Ophthalmol 2001;85:173–178.
19. Mainster MA, Reichel E. Transpupillary thermotherapy for age-related macular degeneration: long-pulse photocoagulation, apoptosis, and heat shock proteins. Ophthalmic Surg Lasers 2000;31:359–373.
20. Lewis H, Kaiser P, Lewis S, Estafanous M. Macular translocation for subfoveal choroidal neovascularization in age-related macular degeneration: a prospective study. Am J Ophthalmol 1999;128:135–146.

14
Choroidal Neovascularization

Peter A. Campochiaro
Wilmer Eye Institute, Johns Hopkins University School of Medicine, Baltimore, Maryland

Frances E. Kane
Novartis Ophthalmics, Inc., Duluth, Georgia

I. INTRODUCTION

Choroidal neovascularization (CNV) is one of the most challenging problems faced by retina specialists. It is a common cause of severe visual loss in patients with age-related macular degeneration (AMD) and younger patients with one of many diseases that affect the choroid–Bruch's membrane–retinal pigmented epithelium (RPE) complex, including but not limited to ocular histoplasmosis, myopic degeneration, angioid streaks, and multifocal choroiditis. Current treatments are aimed at destroying CNV. However, even when ablative treatments are initially successful, they are plagued by high rates of recurrences, because they do not address underlying angiogenic stimuli (1). Understanding of the molecular signals involved in the occurrence of CNV could provide the basis for the development of new effective treatments.

II. INFERENCES FROM NEOVASCULARIZATION ELSEWHERE IN THE BODY

Angiogenesis is a critical process during embryonic development and wound repair and occurs in almost all tissues of the body. It is well tolerated in most tissues, but not in the eye where normal functioning depends upon maintenance of blood-ocular barriers. Angiogenesis varies somewhat in different tissues because endothelial cells differ in different parts of the body and surrounding cells participate in the neovascular response resulting in tissue-specific aspects. However, some common themes are shared among tissues.

In most tissues, angiogenesis is controlled by a balance between proangiogenic and antiangiogenic factors. Based upon in vitro assays and in vivo effects in some tissues, vascular endothelial growth factors (VEGFs) (2), fibroblast growth factors (FGFs) (3), tumor necrosis factor-α (TNF-α) (4), insulin-like growth factor-1 (IGF-1) (5,6), and hepatocyte growth factor (HGF) (7) are generally considered proangiogenic factors. Transforming growth factor-β (TGF-β) and related family members inhibit endothelial cell migration and proliferation in vitro, but have been suggested to be proangiogenic or antiangiogenic in vivo, depending on the context (8–10). Several purported endogenous inhibitors of angiogenesis have been described including angiostatin (11), endostatin (12), antithrombin III (13), platelet factor 4 (14), thrombospondin (15), and pigment epithelium-derived factor (PEDF) (16).

Along with soluble proangiogenic and antiangiogenic factors, extracellular matrix (ECM) molecules also participate in several ways in the regulation of neovascularization. They may bind and sequester soluble factors, preventing them from activating receptors on endothelial cells until they are released from the ECM by proteolysis (17–19). Acting through integrins on the surface of endothelial cells, ECM molecules may directly stimulate or inhibit endothelial cell processes involved in angiogenesis (20). Soluble angiogenic factors exert some of their effects through ECM molecules by altering expression of integrins on endothelial cells (21). Endothelial cells of dermal vessels have increased expression of αvβ3 integrin when participating in angiogenesis and αvβ3 antagonists block angiogenesis (22).

Angiogenesis in all tissues is likely to involve certain processes in endothelial cells, including proteolytic activity, migration, proliferation, and tube formation (23,24), but the molecular signals that mediate or modulate these processes might vary from tissue to tissue. For instance, two proteolytic systems have been implicated in the breakdown of ECM during angiogenesis, one involving the urokinase type of plasminogen activator (uPA) (25) and one involving matrix metalloproteinases (MMPs) (26,27) and the relative importance of these systems could vary in different types of angiogenesis. Tissue inhibitor of metalloproteinases-1 (TIMP-1) has been touted as an inhibitor of neovascularization (28), but it stimulates VEGF-induced neovascularization in the retina (29). Interferon α2a causes dramatic involution of hemangiomas (30) and inhibits iris neovascularization in a model of ischemic retinopathy (31), which led to the prediction that it would inhibit CNV. However, a multicenter, randomized, placebo-controlled trial demonstrated that patients with CNV who received interferon α2a did not have any involution of CNV and ended up with worse vision than those treated with placebo (32). Therefore, testing in relevant animal models is necessary to predict the effect of proteins or drugs on ocular neovascularization.

III. INFERENCES FROM RETINAL NEOVASCULARIZATION

It would be nice if information regarding retinal neovascularization could be applied to CNV, because more is known about the pathogenesis of retinal neovascularization. The clinical observation that retinal neovascularization almost always occurs in association with retinal capillary nonperfusion led to the hypothesis that retinal ischemia is the driving force (33–35). This hypothesis is supported by experimental models in which damage to retinal vessels leads to retinal neovascularization (31,36–39). Advances in the understanding of hypoxia-mediated gene regulation have suggested potential molecular signals such as hypoxia-inducible factor-1, involvement of which has been confirmed by experimental studies (40). As a result, many of the molecular signals involved in retinal neovascularization have been defined (for review, see Ref. 41).

Hypoxia has not been definitely implicated in the occurrence of CNV. While there is evidence that choroidal blood flow is decreased in patients with AMD, it is not clear whether the decrease is sufficient to cause hypoxia of photoreceptors and RPE (42, 43).

Furthermore, hypoxia cannot be invoked in patients with ocular histoplasmosis, myopic degeneration, angioid streaks, or many other diseases in which young people get CNV. Another difference between CNV and retinal neovascularization is the contribution of the RPE to CNV. Although the contribution of the RPE to CNV on a molecular level has not yet been clearly defined, it is clear that the RPE is intimately involved. Therefore, it is hazardous to use our knowledge of retinal neovascularization to draw inferences regarding CNV, unless they are confirmed experimentally.

IV. THE PATHOGENESIS OF CNV

One thing that patients with CNV share is that they all have abnormalities of Bruch's membrane and the RPE. In patients with AMD, pathological studies have demonstrated that diffuse thickening of Bruch's membrane is highly associated with the occurrence of CNV (44). Large soft drusen and pigmentary abnormalities are clinical risk factors for CNV (45); soft drusen indicate the presence of diffuse sub-RPE deposits and pigmentary changes suggest compromise of the RPE. Therefore, there is disordered metabolism of ECM in patients with AMD that may compromise RPE cells leading to cell dropout and proliferation, and CNV. Breaks in Bruch's membrane and/or other abnormalities of the ECM of RPE cell occur in other diseases in which CNV occurs. Patients with Sorsby's fundus dystrophy have a mutation in the tissue inhibitor of metalloproteinase-3 (TIMP-3) gene that results in abnormal processing of the protein so that it is deposited along Bruch's membrane (46). This collection of an ectopic protein along Bruch's membrane is associated with RPE and photoreceptor degeneration and a high incidence of CNV (47,48).

Why would abnormal ECM along the basal surface of RPE cells result in cell compromise and CNV? Like most epithelial cells, the phenotype and behavior of RPE cells is regulated in part by interaction with its ECM. Cultured RPE cells display alterations in morphology and gene expression when grown on different ECMs (49). Presentation of some ECM molecules such as vitronectin or thrombospondin to the apical or basal surface of RPE cells results in small increases in fibroblast growth factor-2 (FGF-2) and large increases in VEGF in the media of the cells (50). Therefore, alterations in the ECM of RPE cells can cause them to increase production of proteins with angiogenic activity.

Is increased production of angiogenic proteins in the retina sufficient to cause CNV? To address this question, bovine rhodopsin promoter was coupled to a full-length cDNA coding for $VEGF_{165}$ and transgenic mice (rho/VEGF mice) were generated (51). Three founder mice were obtained and crossed with C57BL/6 mice to generate transgenic lines. One of the lines (V6) had sustained increased expression of VEGF in photoreceptors starting on postnatal day (P) 7 and developed neovascularization that originated from the deep capillary bed of the retina and grew into the subretinal space. In contrast, transgenic mice with increased expression of FGF-2 in photoreceptors (rho/FGF2 mice) do not develop any neovascularization (52).

There are several possible explanations for why mice from the V6 line of rho/VEGF trangenics develop neovascularization that develops from deep retinal vessels, but not from choroidal vessels. One possibility is that the outer blood-retinal barrier constituted by the RPE prevents VEGF produced by photoreceptors access to choroidal vessels. Another possibility is that choroidal vessels cannot respond to VEGF. A third possibility is that Bruch's membrane provides a biochemical as well as a mechanical barrier to the growth of CNV.

The first possibility was addressed by Schwesinger et al. (53), who coupled the promoter for RPE-65 to a cDNA for VEGF 165 and generated transgenic mice with expression of VEGF in RPE cells. These mice failed to show any CNV, although they did show increased numbers of choroidal blood vessels indicating that the choroidal vessels had some response to the excess VEGF. In wild-type mice, laser-induced rupture of Bruch's membrane results in CNV (54). In rho/VEGF or rho/FGF2 transgenic mice, rupture of Bruch's membrane resulted in very large areas of CNV, much larger than those in wild-type mice (55). Low-intensity laser, which ruptured photoreceptor cells but did not rupture Bruch's membrane, resulted in CNV in rho/FGF2 mice, but not rho/VEGF or wild-type mice. These experiments demonstrate that choroidal vessels are capable of responding to excess VEGF or extracellular FGF2 when there is a concomitant rupture of Bruch's membrane. This suggests that Bruch's membrane constitutes a mechanical and biochemical barrier to CNV. Increased expression of VEGF or FGF2 is unable to cause a breech in the barrier. In the case of FGF2, sequestration is likely to be an important control mechanism, because low-intensity laser that ruptures photoreceptor cells and releases FGF2, but does not rupture Bruch's membrane, results in CNV. This is not the case for VEGF, which stimulates CNV only when the Bruch's membrane barrier has been disrupted by another means.

The importance of the Bruch's membrane barrier for prevention of CNV may help to explain difficulties in modeling CNV. Laser-induced rupture of Bruch's membrane, first established in primates and later adapted to rodents, has been widely used (54,56,57). All other models of CNV, whether they involve implantation of sustained-release polymers or gene transfer, have a component of surgical damage to Bruch's membrane (58,59). Therefore, as noted in genetic experiments mentioned above, some sort of compromise of Bruch's membrane must accompany increased levels of angiogenic factors to generate CNV.

Laser-induced rupture of CNV in mice (54) has provided a particularly valuable tool, because it can be used in genetically engineered mice to explore the role of individual gene products. Using this strategy, Ozaki et al. (52) demonstrated that mice with targeted deletion of FGF2 develop CNV similar to that in wild-type mice indicating that FGF2 is not necessary for the development of CNV after rupture of Bruch's membrane. This approach was also used to demonstrate that nitric oxide (NO) is proangiogenic in both the retina and the choroid, but different isoforms of nitric oxide synthetase play a role (60). For retinal neovascularization, eNOS plays an important role, while for CNV, nNOS is important. This suggests that NOS inhibitors may be useful in patients at risk for CNV.

V. PROSPECTS FOR PHARMACOLOGICAL TREATMENTS FOR CNV

Since hypoxia has not been definitely implicated in the development of CNV, unlike the situation for retinal neovascularization, there is no strong rationale for suspecting that VEGF, as opposed to the many other angiogenic factors that have been identified, plays a central role in CNV. Therefore, we were somewhat surprised to find that oral administration of drugs that inhibit VEGF receptor kinases dramatically inhibit CNV as well as retinal neovascularization (61,62). Antagonizing VEGF by other means could also be beneficial. Intravitreous injection of a fragment of an anti-VEGF antibody inhibits CNV after laser-induced rupture of Bruch's membrane in primates (63). Intravitreous injection of the same anti-VEGF antibody fragment (64) or an aptamer that binds VEGF (65) have been tested in phase 1 trials in patients with subfoveal CNV and are currently in phase 2 trials.

Another approach for treatment is to use an endogenous inhibitor of angiogenesis. Endostatin is a cleavage product of collagen XVIII that inhibits tumor angiogenesis resulting in dramatic tumor regression (12). However, proteins can be difficult to work with and some studies using the protein have suggested against a strong antiangiogenic effect. Gene transfer provides a strategy to achieve sustained release of endostatin and can circumvent difficulties arising from handling the protein. We performed intravascular injections of adnenoviral vectors containing a transgene consisting of murine Ig κ-chain leader sequence coupled to sequence coding for murine endostatin (66). Mice injected with a construct in which endostatin expression was driven by the Rous sarcoma virus promoter had moderately high serum levels of endostatin and significantly smaller CNV lesions at sites of laser-induced rupture of Bruch's membrane than mice injected with null virus. Mice injected with a construct in which endostatin expression was driven by the cytomegalovirus promoter had roughly 10-fold higher endostatin serum levels and had significantly less CNV with nearly complete inhibition. There was a strong inverse correlation between endostatin serum level and area of CNV. This study provides proof of the principle that gene therapy to increase levels of endostatin can inhibit the development of CNV.

A potential advantage of gene therapy is that intraocular injection of a vector containing an expression construct provides a potential means of sustained local delivery. We investigated the effect of adenoviral-mediated intraocular transfer of the *PEDF* gene. Intravitreous injection of an adenoviral vector encoding PEDF resulted in expression of *PEDF* mRNA in the eye measured by RT-PCR and increased immunohistochemical staining for PEDF protein throughout the retina. In mice with laser-induced rupture of Bruch's membrane, choroidal neovascularization was significantly reduced after intravitreous injection of PEDF vector compared to injection of null vector or no injection. Subretinal injection of the PEDF vector resulted in prominent staining for PEDF in retinal pigmented epithelial cells and strong inhibition of choroidal neovascularization. In two models of retinal neovascularization [transgenic mice with increased expression of vascular endothelial growth factor (VEGF) in photoreceptors and mice with oxygen-induced ischemic retinopathy], intravitreous injection of null vector resulted in decreased neovascularization compared to no injection, but intravitreous injection of PEDF vector resulted in further inhibition of neovascularization that was statistically significant. Several studies have suggested that PEDF has neuroprotective activity (67–72) and it might contribute to the trophic support of photoreceptors provided by RPE cells, because in an in vitro model of photoreceptor degeneration in which the RPE is removed from *Xenopus* eyecups, PEDF protected photoreceptors from degeneration and loss of opsin immunoreactivity (73). Therefore, intraocular PEDF gene transfer may provide a good approach in patients with AMD, because it could possibly benefit both neovascular and nonneovascular AMD.

Recently, it has been demonstrated that intraocular injection of an adenoassociated viral vector containing a cDNA for angiostatin inhibits laser-induced CNV. Therefore, three different proteins have been found to inhibit CNV (74).

VI. CONCLUSIONS

Current treatments for neovascular AMD do not address the underlying stimuli for abnormal blood vessel growth and are basically palliative treatments. As our understanding of the molecular signals that lead to AMD improves, opportunities for more effective pharmacological treatments will increase. Several agents, including VEGF receptor kinase inhibitors, anti-VEGF antibodies, PEDF, and angiostatin, that effectively prevent CNV in animal models have been identified. Over the next several years many clinical trials will be performed and it is highly likely that one or more beneficial drugs and/or transgenes will be identified.

ACKNOWLEDGMENTS

This work was supported by grants EY05951, EY12609, and P30EY1765 from the National Eye Institute, the Foundation Fighting Blindness, Lew R. Wasserman Merit Awards (SV and PAC), and unrestricted funds from Research to Prevent Blindness. PAC is the George S. and Dolores Dore Eccles Professor of Ophthalmology and Neuroscience.

REFERENCES

1. Macular Photocoagulation Study Group. Argon laser photocoagulation for neovascular maculopathy: five year results from randomized clinical trials. Arch Ophthalmol 1991; 109:1109–1114.
2. Connolly DT, Heuvelman DM, Nelson R, Olander JV, Eppley BL, Delfino JJ, Siegal NR, Leimgruber RM, Feder J. Tumor vascular permeability factor stimulates endothelial cell growth and angiogenesis. J Clin Invest 1989; 84:1470–1478.
3. Abraham JA, Whang JL, Tumolo A, Mergia A, Freidman J, Gospodarowicz D, Fiddes JC. Human basic fibroblast growth factor: nucleotide sequence and genomic organization. EMBO J 1986; 5:2523–2528.
4. Leibovich SJ, Polverini PJ, Shepard HM, Wiseman DM, Shively V, Nuseir N. Macrophage-induced angiogenesis is mediated by tumor necrosis factor-alpha. Nature 1987; 329:630–632.
5. Grant MB, Mames RN, Fitzgerald C, et al. Insulin-like growth factor I as an angiogenic agent. In vivo and in vitro studies. Ann NY Acad Sci 1993; 692:230–242.
6. Smith LEH, Kopchick JJ, Chen W, Knapp J, Kinose F, Daley D, Foley E, G. SR, Schaeffer JM. Essential role of growth hormone in ischemia-induced retinal neovascularization. Science 1997; 276:1706–1709.
7. Laterra J, Nam M, Rosen E, Rao JS, Lamszus K, Goldberg ID, Johnston P. Scatter factor/hepatocyte growth factor gene transfer enhances glioms growth and angiogenesis in vivo. Lab Invest 1997;76:565–577.
8. Madri J, Reidy M, Kocher O, Bell L. Endothelial cell behavior following denudation injury is modulated by TGF-beta and fibronectin. Lab Invest 1989;60:755–765.
9. Hayasaka K, Oikawa S, Hashizume E, Kotake H, Midorikawa H, Sekikawa A, Hoshi K, Hara S, Ishigaki Y, Toyota T. Anti-angiogenic effect of TGFbeta in aqeous humor. Life Sci 1998; 63:1089–1096.
10. Hasegawa Y, Takanashi S, Kanehira Y, Tsushima T, Imai T, Okumura K. Transforming growth factor-beta 1 level correlates with angiogenesis, tumor progression, and prognosis in patients with nonsmall cell lung carcinoma. Cancer 2001;91:964–971.
11. O'Reilly MS, Holmgren S, Shing Y, Chen C, Rosenthal RA, Moses M, Lane WS, Cao Y, Sage HE, Folkman J. Angiostatin: a novel angiogenesis inhibitor that mediates the suppression of metastases by a Lewis lung carcinoma. Cell 1994;79:315–328.
12. O'Reilly MS, Boehm T, Shing Y, Fukai N, Vasios G, Lane WS, Flynn E, Birknead JR, Olsen BR, Folkman J. Endostatin: an endogenous inhibitor of angiogenesis and tumor growth. Cell 1997;88:277–285.

13. O'Reilly MS, Pirie-Sheherd S, Lane WS, Folkman J. Antiangiogenic activity of the cleaved conformation of the serpin antithrombin. Science 1999; 285:1926–1928.

14. Maione TE, Gray GS, Petro J, Hunt AJ, Donner AL, Bauer SI, Carson HF, Sharpe RJ. Inhibition of angiogenesis by recombinant human platelet factor-4 and related peptides. Science 1990; 247:77–79.

15. Good DJ, Polverini PJ, Rastinejad F, et al. A tumor supressor-dependent inhibitor of angiogenesis is immunologically and functionally indistinguishable from a fragment of thrombospondin. Proc Natl Acad Sci USA 1990; 87:6624–6628.

16. Dawson DW, Volpert OV, Gillis P, Crawford SE, Xu H-J, Benedict W, Bouck NP. Pigment epithelium-derived factor: a potent inhibitor of angiogenesis. Science 1999; 285:245–248.

17. Vlodavsky I, Folkman J, Sullivan R, Fridman R, Rivka I-M, Sasse J, Klagsbrun M. Endothelial cell-derived basic fibroblast growth factor: synthesis and deposition into subendothelial extracellular matrix. Proc Natl Acad Sci USA 1987; 84:2292–2296.

18. Vlodavsky I, Korner G, Ishai-Michaeli R, Bashkin P, Bar-Shavit R, Fuks Z. Extracellular matrix-resident growth factors and enzymes: possible involvement in tumor metastasis and angiogenesis. Cancer Metast Rev 1990; 9:203–226.

19. Park JE, Keller G-A, Ferrara N. The vascular endothelial growth factor (VEGF) isoforms: differential deposition into the subepithelial extracellular matrix. Mol Biol Cell 1993; 4:1317–1326.

20. Dike LE, Ingber DE. Integrin-dependent induction of early growth response genes in capillary endothelial cells. J Cell Sci 1996; 109:2855–2863.

21. Friedlander M, Brooks PC, Shaffer RW, Kincaid CM, Varner JA, Cheresh DA. Definition of two angiogenic pathways by distinct alpha-v integrins. Science 1995; 270:1500–1502.

22. Brooks P, Clark R, Cheresh D. Requirement of vascular integrin alpha-v beta-3 for angiogenesis. Science 1994; 264:569–571.

23. Gross JL, Moscatelli D, Rifkin DB. Increased capillary endothelial cell protease activity in response to angiogenic stimuli in vitro. Proc Natl Acad Sci USA 1983; 80:2623–2627.

24. Sato Y, Rifkin DB. Autocrine activities of basic fibroblast growth factor: regulation of endothelial cell movement, plasminogen activator synthesis, and DNA synthesis. J Cell Biol 1988; 107:1199–1205.

25. Pepper MS, Vassalli J-D, Montesano R, Orci L. Urokinase-type plasminogen activator is induced in migrating capillary endothelial cells. J Cell Biol 1987; 105:2535–2541.

26. Moscatelli DA, Rifkin DB, Jaffe EA. Production of latent collagenase by human umbilical vein endothelial cells in response to angiogenic preparations. Exp Cell Res 1985; 156:379–390.

27. Cornelius LA, Nehring LC, Roby JD, Parks WC, Welgus HG. Human dermal microvascular endothelial cells produce matrix metalloproteinases in response to angiogenic factors and migration. J Invest Dermatol 1995;105:170–176.

28. Johnson MD, Kim H-RC, Chesler L, Tsao-Wu G, Bouck N, Polverini PJ. Inhibition of angiogenesis by tissue inhibitor of metalloproteinase. J Cell Physiol 1994; 160:194–202.

29. Yamada E, Tobe T, Yamada H, Okamoto N, Zack DJ, Werb Z, Soloway P, Campochiaro PA. TIMP-1 promotes VEGF-induced neovascularization in the retina. Histol Histopathol 2001; 16:87–97.

30. Ezekowitz RAB, Mulliken JB, Folkman J. Interferon alpha-2a therapy for life-threatening hemangioma of infancy. N Engl J Med 1992; 326:1456–1463.

31. Miller JW, Stinson W, Folkman J. Regression of experimental iris neovascularization with systemic alpha-interferon. Ophthalmology 1993;100:9–14.

32. Group PTfMDS. Interferon alfa-2a is ineffective for patients with choroidal neovascularization secondary to age-related macular degeneration. Results of a prospective randomized placebo-controlled clinical trial. Arch Ophthalmol 1997;115:865–872.

33. Michaelson I. The mode of development of the vascular system of the retina with some observations on its significance for certain retinal diseases. Trans Ophthalmol Soc UK 1948; 68:137–180.

34. Ashton N. Retinal vascularization in health and disease. Am J Ophthalmol 1957; 44(4):7–17.
35. Shimizu K, Kobayashi Y, Muraoka K. Midperipheral fundus involvement in diabetic retinopathy. Ophthalmology 1981; 88:601–612.
36. Virdi P, Hayreh S. Ocular neovascularization with retinal vascular occlusion. I. Association with retinal vein occlusion. Arch Ophthalmol 1980; 100:331–341.
37. Pournaras C, Tsacopoulos M, Strommer K, Gilodi N, Leuenberger PM. Experimental retinal branch vein occlusion in miniature pigs induces local tissue hypoxia and vasoproliferative microangiopathy. Ophthalmology 1990; 97:1321–1328.
38. Penn JS, Tolman BL, Lowery LA. Variable oxygen exposure causes preretinal neovascularization in the newborn rat. Invest Ophthalmol Vis Sci 1993; 34:576–585.
39. Smith LEH, Wesolowski E, McLellan A, Kostyk SK, D'Amato R, Sullivan R, D'Amore PA. Oxygen-induced retinopathy in the mouse. Invest Ophthalmol Vis Sci 1994; 35:101–111.
40. Ozaki H, Yu A, Della N, Ozaki K, Luna JD, Yamada H, Hackett SF, Okamoto N, Zack DJ, Semenza GL, Campochiaro PA. Hypoxia inducible factor-1a is increased in ischemic retina: temporal and spatial correlation with VEGF expression. Invest Ophthalmol Vis Sci 1999; 40:182–189.
41. Campochiaro PA. Retinal and choroidal neovascularization. J Cell Physiol 2000;184:301–310.
42. Grunwald J, Hariprasad S, DuPont J, Maguire M, Fine S, Brucker A, Maguire A, Ho A. Foveolar choroidal blood flow in age-related macular degeneration. Invest Ophthalmol Vis Sci 1998; 39:385–390.
43. Ross RD, Barofsky JM, Cohen G, Baber WB, Palao SW, Gitter KA. Presumed macular choroidal watershed vascular filling, choroidal neovascularization, and systemic vascular disease in patients with age-related macular degeneration. Am J Ophthalmol 1998; 125:71–80.
44. Green WR, Enger C. Age-related macular degeneration histopathologic studies. Ophthalmology 1993; 100:1519–1535.
45. Bressler SB, Maguire MG, Bressler NM, Fine SL, Group atMPS. Relationship of drusen and abnormalities of the retinal pigment epithelium to the prognosis of neovascular macular degeneration. Arch Ophthalmol 1990; 108:1442–1447.
46. Weber BHF, Vogt G, Pruett RC, Stohr H, Felbor U. Mutations in the tissue inhibitor of metalloproteinases-3 (TIMP3) in patients with Sorsby's fundus dystrophy. Nat Genet 1994; 8:352–356.
47. Sorsby A, Mason MEJ, Gardener N. A fundus dystrophy with unusual features. Br J Ophthalmol 1949; 33:67–97.
48. Hoskin A, Sehmi K, Bird AC. Sorsby's pseudoinflammatory macular dystrophy. Br J Ophthalmol 1981; 65:859–865.
49. Carapochiaro PA, Hackett SF. Corneal endothelial cell matrix promotes expression of differentiated features of retinal pigmented epithelial cells: implication of laminin and basic fibroblast growth factor as active components. Exp Eye Res 1993; 57:539–537.
50. Mousa SA, Lorelli W, Campochiaro PA. Extracellular matrix-integrin binding modulates secretion of angiogenic growth factors by retinal pigmented epithelial cells. J Cell Biochem 1999; 74:135–143.
51. Okamoto N, Tobe T, Hackett SF, Ozaki H, Vinores MA, LaRochelle W, Zack DJ, Campochiaro PA. Transgenic mice with increased expression of vascular endothelial growth factor in the retina: a new model of intraretinal and subretinal neovascularization. Am J Pathol 1997; 151(1):281–91.
52. Ozaki H, Okamoto N, Ortega S, Chang M, Ozaki K, Sadda S, Vinores MA, Derevjanik N, Zack DJ, Basilico C, Campochiaro PA. Basic fibroblast growth factor is neither necessary nor sufficient for the development of retinal neovascularization. Am J Pathol 1998; 153:757–765.
53. Schwesinger C, Yee C, Rohan RM, Joussen AM, Fernandez A, Meyer TN, Poulaki V, Ma JJK, Redmond TM, Liu S, Adamis AP, D'Amato RJ. Intrachoroidal neovascularization in transgenic mice overexpressing vascular endothelial growth factor in the retinal pigment epithelium. Am J Pathol 2001;158:1161–1172.

54. Tobe T, Ortega S, Luna L, Ozaki H, Okamoto N, Derevjanik NL, Vinores SA, Basilico C, Campochiaro PA. Targeted disruption of the *FGF2* gene does not prevent choroidal neovascularization in a murine model. Am J Pathol 1998; 153:1641–1646.

55. Yamada H, Yamada E, Ando A, Esumi N, Bora N, Saikia J, Sung C-H, Zack DJ, Campochiaro PA. FGF2 decreases hyperoxia-induced cell death in mice. Am J Pathol 2001;159:1113–1120.

56. Miller H, Miller B, Ryan SJ. The role of the retinal pigmented epithelium in the involution of subretinal neovascularization. Invest Ophthalmol Vis Sci 1986; 27:1644–1652.

57. Dobi ET, Puliafito CA, Destro M. A new model of choroidal neovascularization in the rat. Arch Ophthalmol 1989; 107:264–269.

58. Spilsbury K, Garrett KS, Shen WY, Constable IJ, Rakoczy PE. Overexpression of vascular endothelial growth factor (VEGF) in the retinal pigment epithelium leads to the development of choroidal neovascularization. Am J Pathol 2000; 157:135–144.

59. Baffi J, Byrnes G, Chan C-C, Csaky KG. Choroidal neovascularization in the rat induced by adenovirus mediated expression of vascular endothelial growth factor. Invest Ophthalmol Vis Sci 2000;41:3582–3589.

60. Ando A, Mori K, Yamada H, Yamada E, Takahashi K, Saikia J, Yang A, Kim M, Campochiaro PA. Nitric oxide plays an important role in both retinal and choroidal neovascularization. Invest Ophthalmol Vis Sci 2001; 42:S88.

61. Seo M-S, Kwak N, Ozaki H, Yamada H, Okamoto N, Fabbro D, Hofmann F, Wood JM, Campochiaro PA. Dramatic inhibition of retinal and choroidal neovascularization by oral administration of a kinase inhibitor. Am J Pathol 1999; 154:1743–1753.

62. Ozaki H, Seo M-S, Ozaki K, Yamada H, Yamada E, Hofmann F, Wood J, Campochiaro PA. Blockade of vascular endothelial cell growth factor receptor signaling is sufficient to completely prevent retinal neovascularization. Am J Pathol 2000; 156:679–707.

63. Afshari MA, Krzystolik MG, Adamis AP, O'Neill CA, Gragoudas ES, Michaud NA, Li W, Connolly E, Hartmangruber ML, Miller JW. Therapeutic and prophylactic effects of a recombinant human binding fragment of a monoclonal antibody directed to vascular endothelial growth factor (rhuFab VEGF) in a monkey model of laser-induced choroidal neovascularization. Invest Ophthalmol Vis Sci 2001; 42:5001.

64. Schwartz SD, Blumenkranz M, Rosenfeld PJ, Miller JW, Haller J, Fish G, Lobes L, Singerman L, Green WL, Reimann J. Safety of rhuFab V2, an anti-VEGF antibody fragment, as a single intravitreal injection in subjects with neovascular age-related macular degeneration. Invest Ophthalmol Vis Sci 2001; 42(suppl):S522.

65. Guyer DR, Martin DM, Klein M, Haller J, Group TE-TS. Anti-VEGF therapy in patients with exudative age-related macular degeneration. Invest Ophthalmol Vis Sci 2001; 42(suppl):S522.

66. Mori K, Ando A, Gehlbach P, Nesbitt D, Takahashi K, Goldsteen D, Penn M, Chen T, Mori K, Melia M, Phipps S, Moffat D, Brazzell K, Liau G, Dixon KH, Campochiaro PA. Inhibition of choroidal neovascularization by intravenous injection of adenoviral vectors expressing secretable endostatin. Am J Pathol 2001; 159:313–320.

67. Taniwaki T, Becerra SP, Chader GJ, Schwartz JP. Pigment epithelium-derived factor is a survival factor for cerebellar granule cells in culture. J Neurochem 1995; 64:2509–2517.

68. Araki T, Taniwaki T, Becerra SP, Chader GJ, Schwartz JP. Pigment epithelium-derived factor (PEDF) differentially protects immature but not mature cerebellar granule cells against apoptotic cell death. J Neurosci Res 1998; 53:7–15.

69. DeCoster MA, Schabelman E, Tombran-Tink J, Bazan NG. Neuroprotection by pigment epithelial-derived factor against glutamte toxicity in developing primary hippocampal neurons. J Neurosci Res 1999; 56:604–610.

70. Bilak MM, Corse AM, Bilak SR, Lehar M, Tombran-Tink J, Kuncl RW. Pigment epithelium-derived factor (PEDF) protects motor neurons from chronic glutamate-mediated neurodegeneration. J Neuropathol Exp Neurol 1999; 58:719–728.

71. Cao W, Tombrin-Tink J, Chen W, Mrazek D, Elias R, McGinnis JF. Pigment epithelium-derived factor protects cultured retinal neurons against hydrogen peroxide-induced cell death. J Neurosci Res 1999; 57:789–800.

72. Houenou LJ, D'Costa AP, Li L, Tugeon VL, Enyadike C, Alberdi E, Becerra SP. Pigment epithelium derived factor promotes the survival and differentiation of developing spinal motor neurons. J Comp Neurol 1999;412:506–514

73. Jablonski MM, Tombran-Tink J, Mrazek DA, Iannoaccone A. Pigment epithelium-derived factor supports normal development of photoreceptor neurons and opsin expression after retinal pigment epithelium removal. J Neurosci 2000; 20:7149–7157.

74. Lai C-C, Wu W-C, Chen S-L, Xiao X, Tsai T-C, Huan S-J, Chen T-L, Tsai RJ-F, Tsao Y-P. Suppression of choroidal neovascularization by adeno-associated virus vector expressing angiostatin. Invest Ophthalmol Vis Sci 2001; 42:2401–2407.

15

Submacular Surgery for Patients with Age-Related Macular Degeneration

P. Kumar Rao and Matthew A. Thomas
Barnes Retina Institute, Washington University, St. Louis, Missouri

I. INTRODUCTION

A. Historical Overview

In the late 1980s initial attempts at surgical removal of choroidal neovasacular membranes (CNVMs) were reported. De Juan and Machemer pioneered a technique that involved performing a vitrectomy followed by a large retinotomy around the macula (1). A retinal flap was reflected, the membrane was removed, the retina was repositioned, and endophotocoagulation was used to create adhesions to hold the retina in place. Unfortunately, poor visual results and the development of proliferative vitreoretinopathy with retinal detachment occurred. In an attempt to limit this complication, Blinder et al. performed scatter photocoagulation outside the vascular arcades prior to surgery (2). Vitrectomy was followed by endodiathermy to the retina just inside the arcades. Again a large flap retinotomy was created, the retina was folded back, the membrane was removed, the retina was once again repositioned, endophotocoagulation was applied to the retinotomy, and silicone oil was injected for prolonged tamponade. Oil removal was performed later, without the development of retinal detachments. These eyes had extensive macular pathology with poor preoperative vision, and visual results remained poor despite the lack of retinal detachments. More recent techniques have enhanced the safety and simplified the procedure.

B. Clinical Relevance/Importance

Vitrectomy techniques may be an appropriate management option for some patients with choroidal neovascularization (CNV) . Current techniques allow safe extraction of most subretinal membranes regardless of etiology but not all patients respond favorably to such an approach. Certain clinical and angiographic characteristics as well as underlying disease processes may allow favorable outcomes. However, no randomized prospective data are yet available to prove the role of these procedures. The National Institutes of Health–sponsored Submacular Surgery Trials will determine whether surgery or observation is better for eyes with subfoveal CNV in presumed ocular histoplasmosis syndrome or age-related macular degeneration and in eyes with age-related macular degeneration (AMD)-associated subretinal hemorrhage.

Laser photocoagulation and photodynamic therapy have both been shown to be advantageous over observation in the management of some eyes with AMD-associated subfoveal CNV (3–5). Although the Macular Photocoagulation Study (MPS) demonstrated effective laser treatment for some choroidal neovascular membranes (CNVM) in AMD, 2–5 years after treatment the visual outcome was poor, ranging from 20/100 to 20/400. The rate of persistent or recurrent CNV ranged from 50% to 70% (4,5). Additionally, MPS guidelines exclude many patients from laser treatment (6,7). These limitations have stimulated the search for other therapies.

Surgical excision of subretinal membranes is an alternative to laser treatment, and techniques for surgical removal have become quite safe. Currently there are no randomized prospective clinical trial data available to guide decisions regarding subretinal surgery for CNV. Fortunately the Submacular Surgery Trials (SST) are currently underway and will yield important data regarding this therapy. While recognizing the essential role of the SST, it is of value to review the current state of knowledge of subretinal surgery. This review represents information from retrospective studies, small series, case reports, and personal experience.

C. Patients or Settings Appropriate for Surgery

The best surgical candidates are those patients with type 2 CNV [membranes between the retinal pigment epithelium (RPE) and neurosensory retina] and with extrafoveal ingrowth sites (8–10). Clinically, the appearance of well-defined borders, a thin layer of blood between the membrane and the RPE, pigmented edges, patient age less than 50, and absence of biomicroscopic and stereoscopic fluorescein evidence of elevation of the RPE beyond a well-defined CNVM all suggest that the CNVM is between the RPE and retina (9,11). An anterior location can be determined by finding a rim of blocked fluorescence and absent late staining of surrounding tissues with fluorescein angiography (11). In addition, ocular coherence tomography can help reveal the position of the CNVM and thus help predict which eyes will do well with surgery (12).

Excision of CNVM may be accompanied by loss of underlying RPE. Angiography is often useful in predicting the size of this postoperative defect. This defect is generally greater for patients with AMD than those with multifocal choroidopathies or idiopathic CNVM (13). In AMD the area of the CNVM and the hyperfluorescent halo seen in the late phase of the angiogram before surgery is approximately 80% the size of the postoperative defect.

In many non-AMD eyes, the initial site of presumed ingrowth by the choroidal vessels can be detected preoperatively. The best surgical outcomes are seen with eccentric ingrowth sites (10). Eyes with an unidentifiable ingrowth site probably have more diffuse RPE involvement and may have worse outcomes following surgery. A light colored spot noted during fundus examination may indicate the ingrowth site. Fluorescein angiography may reveal a stalk in the earliest frames or a focal area of hyperfluorescence from which the membrane arises. Such characteristics may allow a preoperative indication for better postoperative outcomes.

D. Goals of the Procedure

The goal of subretinal membrane removal is to remove the pathological tissue and leave as much RPE and choroid as possible. Prevention of retinal detachment and hemorrhage is also important. Careful selection of the retinotomy site, gentle dissection of the membrane from overlying retina and underlying RPE, and control of intraocular pressure are essential to achieving these goals.

II. DESCRIPTION OF CURRENT TECHNIQUE

In the early 1990s Thomas and Kaplan described the use of a small retinotomy to accomplish CNVM removal (14). The current technique is as follows: complete vitrectomy is followed by removal of the posterior hyaloid (Fig. 1), and a 36-gauge pick is used to pierce the neurosensory retina (Fig. 2). A localized retinal detachment over the CNVM is created by infusing balanced salt solution through the retinotomy using a 33-gauge angled cannula (Fig. 3). The subretinal pick is then reinserted through the retinotomy to separate the neo-vascular complex from overlying retina and surrounding tissues . Subretinal forceps are then passed through the retinotomy, and the membrane is grasped and removed very slowly, to minimize RPE loss and to allow the retinotomy to stretch around the CNVM (Figs. 4 and 5). Great care is taken to achieve hemeostasis by elevating the intraocular pressure before the membrane is disconnected from the choroid. A gradual return to normal pressure while directly visualizing the excision site allows for immediate recognition of any subretinal bleeding. If any bleeding is seen, the pressure is promptly raised until hemostasis is verified. Once hemostasis is achieved and the intraocular pressure has been returned to normal, the membrane can be removed from the eye.

The intraocular fluid is exchanged for air and residual fluid is removed from the retinotomy site by aspirating just anterior to the retinotomy with a 33-gauge extrusion

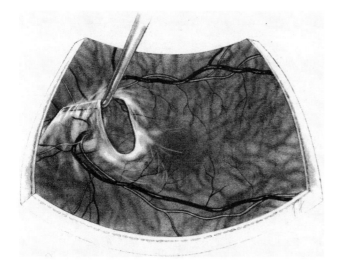

Figure 1   The 33-gauge pick (hyaloid lifter) is used to engage posterior cortical vitreous. (From Ryan SJ, ed. Surgical Removal of Subretinal Choroidal Neovascular Membranes in Retina, 3rd ed. St. Louis: Mosby, 2001:2562–2572, Fig. 153-1.)

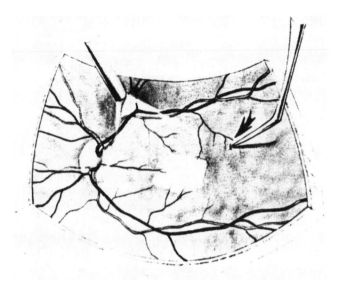

Figure 2 The 36-gauge pointed subretinal pick is used to perforate neurosensory retina. One may encounter a slight amount of hemorrhage as the retina is transected. Diathermy is not used. (From Ryan SJ, ed. Surgical Removal of Subretinal Choroidal Neovascular Membranes in Retina, 3rd ed. St. Louis: Mosby, 2001:2562–2572, Fig. 153-2.)

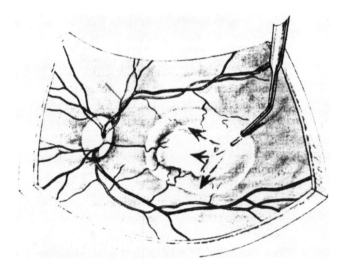

Figure 3 The angled 33-gauge subretinal infusion needle is used to gently infuse balanced salt solution beneath the neurosensory retina. Care is taken not to tear retina at previous laser scars or other adhesions to the underlying membrane. (From Ryan SJ, ed. Surgical Removal of Subretinal Choroidal Neovascular Membranes in Retina, 3rd ed. St. Louis: Mosby, 2001:2562–2572, Fig. 153-3.)

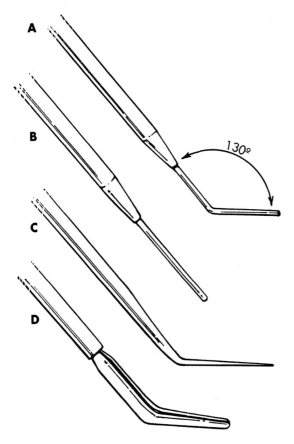

Figure 4 Current subretinal instruments include (A) a 33-gauge angled infusion needle, (B) an occasionally useful 33-gauge straight cannula, (C) sharpened subretinal picks (for engaging hyaloid, perforating retina, and subretinal work), 33 and 36 gauge, and (D) horizontal subretinal forceps. Additional instruments include subretinal vertical forceps, subretinal horizontal scissors, and subretinal vertical scissors. These latter instruments are only occasionally required. (From Ryan SJ, ed. Surgical Removal of Subretinal Choroidal Neovascular Membranes in Retina, 3rd ed. St. Louis: Mosby, 2001:2562–2572, Fig. 153-4.)

needle. If the retinotomy has not enlarged, fluid is infused until a 10–15% air bubble is left. Face-down postoperative positioning facilitates air tamponade of the retinotomy and prevents cataract formation. These techniques result in a low rate of complications (15,16).

III. CLINICAL OUTCOMES

A. Published Results

1. AMD
Many studies have examined the role of submacular surgery in patients suffering from AMD-related CNVMs. The results are mixed and may reflect the aspect of visual

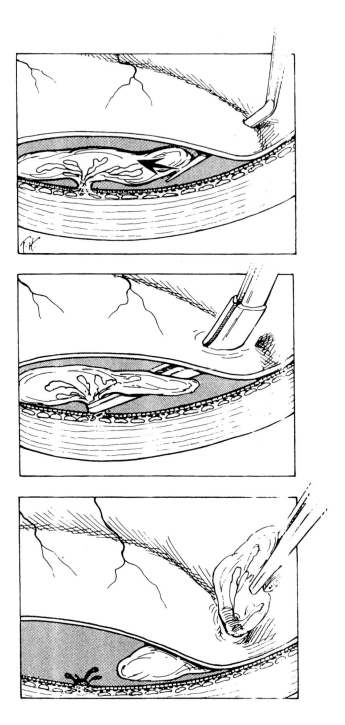

Figure 5   The pointed tip of the subretinal pick is used to engage and lift up the neovascular complex, which is subsequently grasped with horizontal forceps. Hemorrhage is prevented by raising the intraocular infusion pressure. (From Ryan SJ, ed. Surgical Removal of Subretinal Choroidal Neovascular Membranes in Retina, 3rd ed. St. Louis: Mosby, 2001:2562–2572, Fig. 153-5.)

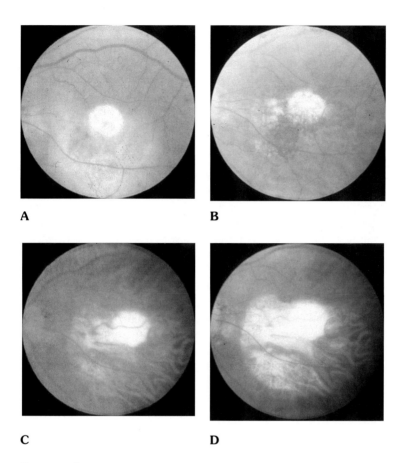

Figures 6 (A) Color photograph of a patient with geographic atrophy and a subretinal neovascular membrane due to age-related macular degeneration. Visual acuity is 20/300. There was no previous laser therapy. (B) Photograph taken 1 month following submacular surgery, revealing some residual subretinal blood at the excision site. (C) Photograph taken 3 years following surgery, revealing RPE and choriocapillary atrophy in the area of preexisting sub retinal neovascular membrane. Visual acuity is 20/200. (D) Photograph taken 7 years following surgery, demonstrating that the area of atrophy has increased in size. Visual acuity is 20/200. See also color insert, Fig. 15.6.

function that is measured. For example, after subretinal membrane removal, patients with AMD may occasionally have residual retinal function in the surgical site when tested with the scanning laser ophthalmoscope (17). Additionally, a recent retrospective case series of surgical removal of subfoveal membranes from patients suffering from AMD demonstrated vision improvement (gained three lines) in 30% or stabilized vision in 42% of surgically treated eyes. Unfortunately, 28% of patients also lost three or more lines of vision. The authors concluded that vision improved or stabilized in the majority of patients. While 72% of patients improved or remained stable, one could also argue that 70% of these patients remained stable or worsened (18).

Previous reports suggest that most patients with AMD do not improve in visual function following surgery (16). Additionally one recent report demonstrates possible worsening of visual acuity following surgery and the authors recommend not operating on AMD-associated subfoveal CNVMs (19). Patients with AMD generally do not achieve good vision after surgical excision of subretinal membranes because of the widespread nature of the disease (8,20–24). Another cause for visual decline following surgical treatment may be the loss of perfusion to the underlying choriocapillaris. Preserved perfusion of the choriocapillaris is associated with better postoperative results (25). Unfortunately, the choriocapillaris may continue to atrophy after surgery in patients with macular degeneration. This progressive atrophy may be due to the RPE loss that usually accompanies surgery for subretinal membranes in AMD (26) (Fig. 6).

Many patients with CNVM present with subretinal hemorrhage. Subretinal blood in patients with macular degeneration is often associated with decreased vision if left untreated (27–29). Numerous studies have documented either stabilization or improvement of vision after surgical removal of subretinal hemorrhage (30–34). In addition, evacuation of this blood may result in a smaller scotoma for patients with AMD (35). However, the best candidates for removal of subretinal blood are those who are young and have thick hemorrhages due to causes other than AMD (27,30).

Most of the previously mentioned studies are small series or retrospective reviews. The Submacular Surgery Trials (SST) are a prospective randomized series of studies that are currently enrolling patients and seek to illuminate the potential role this surgical approach may play in managing patients with CNV. The SST pilot study number 1 enrolled 70 patients who had previously received extrafoveal laser photocoagulation for an AMD-associated CNV and then developed subfoveal recurrent neovascularization. This trial was created to test methods and attain an estimate of the number of patients necessary for the larger multicenter trial. The recently published results from this pilot study suggest no reason to prefer surgery over photocoagulation for eyes with recurrent subfoveal CNV associated with AMD. There were few perioperative complications and the size of the surgically affected area was not significantly larger 2 years following surgery than the area of the neovascualar lesion at baseline (36). The SST pilot study number 2 examined quality-of-life outcomes following surgery and laser treatment of recurrent subfoveal CNVM associated with AMD. Of the 70 patients in SST pilot study number 1, 54 were interviewed with the 36-item Short Form Health Survey prior to randomization. At the conclusion of the study, there were no significant differences in quality-of-life outcome scores between the two treatment arms (37).

2. Other Diseases

Surgical treatment of CNVM is most successful in patients with focal abnormalities of the RPE. Patients with presumed ocular histoplasmosis syndrome (POHS), punctate inner choroidopathy, and CNVM formation following focal laser treatment presumably have only focal disturbances of the RPE. Those with myopia and angioid streaks have more diffuse disease, while those with AMD are thought to have widespread RPE disease. Surgery for CNVM in these disorders has variable reported success rates (19,38–42). CNV from idiopathic juxtafoveolar retinal telangiectasis probably should not be approached with our current surgical techniques. The membranes seen in this disease probably arise within the neurosensory retina and only secondarily do they connect to the choroid. Attempted removal has resulted in retinal defects and poor outcomes (43). Children may also develop CNVM from various causes. Our data and a recent report by Sears et al. describe good surgical outcomes for children who develop CNV (44,45). Declining vision, a protracted neurosensory detachment with the development of cystoid macular edema, or subfoveal bleeding may be indications for surgery (44).

3. Juxtafoveal Membranes

Patients with juxtafoveal membranes may also benefit from surgery. In a study of 35 patients followed for more than 6 months after surgical excision of juxtafoveal membranes of various etiologies, vision improved by three or more lines in 57% of cases. By definition these membranes do not have ingrowth sites beneath the fovea and therefore are likely to have better surgical outcomes (46).

4. Extrafoveal Membranes

Some extrafoveal membranes can be treated with laser according to MPS guidelines. Preservation of overlying retina is probably not as critical with these lesions and laser provides a presumed lower risk alternative to surgery in these cases.

5. Peripapillary Membranes

MPS guidelines do not recommend photocoagulation for membranes larger than 4.5 clock-hours adjacent to the temporal half of the optic nerve. In a small series of eyes with peripapillary membranes associated with POHS, 50% of those membranes with subfoveal extension achieved 20/40 vision or better following surgery. Additionally, three peripapillary membranes were strictly extrafoveal and ineligible for laser according to MPS criteria. All three cases achieved 20/20 vision with surgical excision (47). These are encouraging results for surgical treatment of large peripapillary membranes.

B. Complications

Complications can occur both during and after surgery. Intraoperative complications include those potentially associated with any pars plana vitrectomy, such as retinal tears or detachment, and bleeding. Intraoperative complications unique to this surgery include enlarged retinotomy sites with persistent subretial fluid or detachment, extensive subretinal hemorrhage, and large RPE defects. Delayed complications may include cataract formation, retinal detachment, and recurrent membrane formation. Recurrence of CNV after surgical removal of subretinal membranes has been reported to occur in 23–52% of cases (15,48). Melberg et al. found that when CNV recurred following surgery, the best visual outcomes were achieved for patients who underwent laser treatment for an extrafoveal recurrence (49). Benson et al. have noted that repeat surgery was not associated with worse visual outcome (48). Photodynamic therapy may also play a role in controlling recurrences. Recurrent membranes should be treated with laser if extrafoveal and with either laser photocoagulation or repeat surgery if juxtafoveal and with either repeat surgery, photodynamic therapy, or observation if the regrowth is central.

IV. FUTURE DEVELOPMENTS

The current surgical technique will undoubtedly evolve and improve, aided by further refinements in instrumentation (50). Photodynamic therapy offers another treatment option for some patients suffering from subretinal membranes. This therapy may prove especially useful for those patients who have recurrent CNV after subretinal surgery. The ongoing Submacular Surgery Trials will further define which patients, if any, will benefit from subretinal surgery. Ultimately, pharmacological agents will help prevent and/or inhibit CNV.

V. SUMMARY

Choroidal neovascularization can cause severe visual disturbances. Current management options include observation, laser photocoagulation, photodynamic therapy, and surgical excision. Current guidelines for laser therapy have been well established but exclude many patients. Photodynamic therapy may hold some promise but its value is limited by the need for repeated treatments. An alternative therapy for patients with subretinal membranes may be surgical removal.

The Submacular Surgery Trials seek to clarify the role of vitreous surgery in the management of CNV and are currently enrolling patients in all three arms: SST-H (subfoveal CNV associated with POHS and/or idiopathic cause), SST-N (AMD-associated CNV with at least some classic component and no prior laser therapy), and SST-B (large hematomas). The trials will determine whether patients with AMD and large subfoveal membranes that do not fit MPS guidelines or subfoveal hemorrhage have better outcomes following surgical excision or observation. Additionally, they will compare surgical outcomes to observation for patients with CNV from the presumed ocular histoplasmosis syndrome and idiopathic causes.

Excision of choroidal neovascular membranes is technically possible and safe. The best candidates are those with membranes between the RPE and retina (type 2 membranes). A small retinotomy, gentle dissection, and pressure tamponade are critical to the technique. The Submacular Surgery Trials will help determine which patients will benefit from surgery.

REFERENCES

1. De Juan E, Machemer R. Vitreous surgery for hemorrhagic and fibrous complications of age-related macular degeneration. Am J Ophthalmol 1988;105:25–29.
2. Blinder KJ, Peyman GA, Paris CL, Gremillion CM. Submacular scar excision in age-related macular degeneration. Int Ophthalmol 1991;15:215–222.
3. Treatment of Age-related Macular Degeneration with Photodynamic Therapy (TAP) Study Group. Photodynamic therapy of subfoveal choroidal neovascularization in age-related macular degeneration with verteporfin: one-year results of 2 randomized clinical trials—TAP Report 1. Arch Ophthalmol 1999;117:1329–1345.
4. Macular Photocoagulation Study Group. Persistent and recurrent neovascularization after krypton laser photocoagulation for neovascular lesions of age-related macular degeneration. Arch Ophthalmol 1990;108:825–831.
5. Macular Photocoagulation Study Group. Laser photocoagulation of subfoveal recurrent neovascular lesions in age-related macular degeneration: results of a randomized clinical trial. Arch Ophthalmol 1991;109:1232–1241.
6. Freund KB, Yannuzzi LA, Sorenson JA. Age-related macular degeneration and choroidal neovascularization. Am J Ophthalmol 1993;115:786–791.
7. Moisseiev JA, Masuri R, Treister G. The impact of the Macular Photocoagulation Study results on the treatment of exudative age-related macular degeneration. Arch Ophthalmol 1995;113:185–189.
8. Gass JD. Biomicroscopic and histopathologic considerations regarding the feasibility of surgical excision of subfoveal neovascular membranes. Am J Ophthalmol 1994; 118:285–298.
9. Grossniklaus HE, Gass JD. Clinicopathologic correlations of surgically excised type 1 and 2 type submacular choroidal neovascular membranes. Am J Ophthalmol 1998;126 (1) :59–69.

10. Melberg NS, Thomas MA, Burgess DB. The surgical removal of subfoveal choroidal neovascularization: ingrowth site as a predictor of visual outcome. Retina 1996;16:190–195.

11. Ibanez HE, Thomas MA. Surgical approach to subfoveal neovascularization and submacular hemorrhage. Semin Ophthalmol 1994;9:56–64.

12. Giovannini A, Amato GP, Mariotti C, Scassellati-Sforzolini B. OCT Imaging of choroidal neovascularisation and its role in the determination of patients' eligibility for surgery. Br J Ophthalmol 1999;83:438–442.

13. Giovannini A, Mariotti C, Scassellati-Sforzolini B, D'Altobrando E. Usefulness of fluorescein angiography in predicting the size of the atrophic area after surgical excision of choroidal neovascularization. Ophthalmologica 1999;213:139–144.

14. Thomas MA, Kaplan HJ. Surgical removal of subfoveal neovascularization in the presumed ocular histoplasmosis syndrome. Am J Ophthalmol 1991;111:1–7.

15. Holekamp NM, Thomas MA, Dickinson JD, Valluri S. Surgical removal of subfoveal choroidal neovascularization in presumed ocular histoplasmosis: stability of early visual results. Ophthalmology 1997;104:22–26.

16. Thomas MA, Dickinson JD, Melberg NS, Ibanez HE, Dhaliwal RS. Visual results after surgical removal of subfoveal choroidal neovascular membranes. Ophthalmology 1994;101:1384–1396.

17. Loewenstein A, Sunness JS, Bressler NM, Marsh MJ, De Juan E. Scanning laser ophthalmoscope fundus perimetry after surgery for choroidal neovascularization. Am J Ophthalmol 1998;125(5):657– 665.

18. Merrill PT, LoRusso FJ, Lomeo MD, Saxe SJ, Khan MM, Lambert HM. Surgical removal of subfoveal choroidal neovascularization in age-related macular degeneration. Ophthalmology 1999;106:782– 789.

19. Roth DB, Downie AA, Charles ST. Visual results after submacular surgery for neovascularization in age-related macular degeneration. Ophthalm Surg Lasers 1997;28(11):920–925.

20. Thomas MA, Grand MG, Williams DF, Lee CF, Pesin SR, Lowe MA. Surgical management of subfoveal choroidal neovascularization. Ophthalmology 1992;99:952–968.

21. Berger AS, Kaplan HJ. Clinical experience with the surgical removal of subfoveal neovascular membranes. Ophthalmology 1992; 99:969–976.

22. Lambert HM, Capone A, Aaberg T, Sternberg P, Mandell BA, Lopez PF. Surgical excision of subfoveal neovascular membranes in age-related macular degeneration. Am J Ophthalmol 1991;113:257–262.

23. Green WR, Enger C. Age-related macular degeneration histopathologic studies: the 1992 Lorenz E. Zimmerman Lecture. Ophthalmology 1993;100:1519–1535.

24. Ormerod LD, Puklin JE, Frank RN. Long-term outcomes after the surgical removal of advanced subfoveal neovascular membranes in age-related macular degeration. Ophthalmology 1994;101:1201–1210.

25. Akduman L, Del Priore LV, Desai VN, Olk RJ, Kaplan HJ. Perfusion of the subfoveal choriocapillaris affects visual recovery after submacular surgery in presumed ocular histoplasmosis syndrome. Am J Ophthalmol 1997;123(1):90–96.

26. Castellarin AA, Nasir M, Sugino IK, Zarbin MA. Progressive presumed choriocapillaris atrophy after surgery for age-related macular degeneration. Retina 1998;18(2):143–149.

27. Bennett SR, Folk JC, Blodi CF, Klugman M. Factors prognostic of visual outcome in patients with subretinal hemorrhage. Am J Ophthalmol 1990;109:33–37.

28. Berrocal MH, Lewis ML, Flynn HW. Variations in the clinical course of submacular hemorrhage. Am J Ophthalmol 1996;122:486– 493.

29. Avery RL, Fekrat S, Hawkins BS, Bressler NM. Natural history of subfoveal hemorrhage in age-related macular degeneration. Retina 1996;16:183–189.

30. Ibanez HE, Williams DF, Thomas MA, Ruby AJ, Meredith TA, Boniuk I, et al. Surgical management of submacular hemorrhage: a series of 47 consecutive cases. Arch Ophthalmol 1995;113:62–69.

31. Lewis H. Intraoperative fibriolysis of submacular hemorrhage with tissue plasminogen activator and surgical drainage. Am J Ophthalmol 1999;118:559–568.

32. Lim JI, Drews-Botsch C, Sternberg P Jr, Capone A, Aaberg TM. Submacular hemorrhage removal. Ophthalmology 1995;102:1393– 1399.

33. Kamei M, Tano Y, Maeno T, Mitsuda H, Yuasa T. Surgical removal of submacular hemorrhage using tissue plasminogen activator and perfluorocarbon liquid. Am J Ophthalmol 1996;121:267–275.

34. Hochman MA, Seery CM, Zarbin MA. Pathophysiology and management of subretinal hemorrhage. Surv Ophthalmol 1997;42:195–213.

35. Petersen J, Meyer-Riemann W, Ritzau-Tondrow U, Bahlmann D. Visual fields after removal of subretinal hemorrhages and neovascular membranes in age-related macular degeneration. Graefes Arch Clin Exp Ophthalmol 1998;236:241–247.

36. Submacular Surgery Trials Pilot Study Investigators. Submacular surgery trials randomized pilot trial of laser photocoagulation versus surgery for recurrent choroidal neovascularization secondary to age-related macular degeneration. I. Ophthalmic outcomes, Submacular Surgery Trials Pilot Study report number 1. Am J Ophthalmol 2000;130(4):387–407.

37. Submacular Surgery Trials Pilot Study Investigators. Submacular surgery trials randomized pilot trial of laser photocoagulation versus surgery for recurrent choroidal neovascularization secondary to age-related macular degeneration. II. Quality of life outcomes, Submacular Surgery Trials Pilot Study report number 2. Am J Ophthalmol 2000;130(4): 408–418.

38. Oslen TW, Capone A, Sternberg P, Grossniklaus H, Martin DF, Aaberg TM. Subfoveal choroidal neovascularization in punctate inner choroidopathy: surgical management and pathologic findings. Ophthalmology 1996;103:2061–2069.

39. Adelberg DA, Del Priore LV, Kaplan HJ. Surgery for subfoveal membranes in myopia, angioid streaks and other disorders. Retina 1995;15:198–205.

40. Bottoni F, Perego E, Airaghi P, Cigada M, Ortolina S, Carlevaro G, et al. Surgical removal of subfoveal choroidal neovascular membranes in high myopia. Graefes Arch Clin Exp Ophthalmol 1999; 237(7):573–582.

41. Chen CJ, Urban LL, Nelson NC, Fratkin JD. Surgical removal of subfoveal iatrogenic choroidal neovascular membranes. Ophthalmology 1998;105(9):1606–1611.

42. Berger AS, Conway M, Del Priore LV, Walker RS., Pollack JS, Kaplan HJ. Submacular surgery for subfoveal choroidal neovascular membranes in patients with presumed ocular histoplasmosis. Arch Ophthalmol 1997;115:991–996.

43. Berger AS, McCuen BW, Brown GC, Brownlow RL. Surgical removal of subfoveal neovascularization in idiopathic juxtafoveolar retinal telangiectasis. Retina 1997;17 (2): 94–98.

44. Sears J, Capone A, Aaberg T, Lewis H, Grossniklaus H, Sternberg P, et al. Surgical management of subfoveal neovascularization in children. Ophthalmology 1999;106(5):920–924.

45. Uemura A, Thomas MA. Visual outcome after surgical removal of choroidal neovascularizaion in pediatric patients. Arch Ophthalmol 2000;118:1373–1378.

46. Joseph DP, Thomas MA. Surgical treatment of juxtafoveal choroidal neovascularization. Invest Ophthalmol Vis Res 1997;38 (Suppl):457.

47. Atebara NH, Thomas MA, Holekamp NM, Mandell BA, Del Priore LV. Surgical removal of extensive peripapillary choroidal neovascularization associated with presumed ocular histoplasmosis syndrome. Ophthalmology 1998;105(6):1598–1605.

48. Benson MT, Callear A, Tsaloumas M, Chhina J, Beatty S. Surgical excision of subfoveal neovascular membranes. Eye 1998; 12:768–774.

49. Melberg NS, Thomas MA, Dickinson JD, Valluri S. Managing recurrent neovascularization after subfoveal surgery in presumed ocular histoplasmosis syndrome. Ophthalmology 1996;103:1064– 1068.

50. Loewenstein A, Rader RS, Shelley TH, De Juan E. A flexible infusion micro-cannula for subretinal surgery. Ophthalm Surg Lasers 1997;28(9):774–775.

16
Limited Macular Translocation

Kah-Guan Au Eong
*Wilmer Eye Institute, Johns Hopkins University School of Medicine,
Baltimore, Maryland*

Dante J. Pieramici
*California Retina Research Foundation, Santa Barbara, California, and Wilmer Eye Institute,
Johns Hopkins University School of Medicine, Baltimore, Maryland*

Gildo Y. Fujii and Eugene de Juan, Jr.
*Doheny Retina Institute of the Doheny Eye Institute, University of Southern California Keck
School of Medicine, Los Angeles, California*

I. INTRODUCTION

Age-related macular degeneration (AMD) is the leading cause of blindness in many developed countries (1,2). Hemorrhage and fibrovascular scarring from choroidal neovascularization (CNV) accounts for 80–90% of blindness from AMD, the remainder being attributable to atrophic changes in the macula. No therapy is currently available for the atrophic form, and few treatment options are available for the neovascular form.

The Macular Photocoagulation Study documented that laser photocoagulation of subfoveal CNV confers a statistically significant benefit with regard to long-term visual acuity when compared to the natural history of the condition (3–5). However, treatment of subfoveal CNV was associated with an immediate average reduction of three Bailey-Lovie lines and the benefits of treatment over no treatment only became apparent 6 months after the treatment. In addition, retention or recovery of good vision rarely occurred in patients treated with laser photocoagulation.

In a recent survey of all consultant ophthalmologists in the United Kingdom and the Republic of Ireland by Beatty and associates, only 13.6% of 339 ophthalmologists whose practice includes laser photocoagulation of CNV secondary to AMD stated that they ablate subfoveal CNV with laser photocoagulation (6). The main reason (73.6%) the ophthalmologists gave for withholding treatment was that they were not prepared to accept the likelihood of an immediate drop in visual acuity following laser ablation. This survey demonstrates that although laser photocoagulation has been shown to be effective in the management of subfoveal CNV secondary to AMD by a well-designed randomized clinical trial, at least in the United Kingdom and Ireland, many practicing ophthalmologists do not treat subfoveal CNV with laser photocoagulation.

Because of the limited therapy available for subfoveal CNV, many investigators have pursued alternative therapy such as interferon alpha-2a (7–10), radiation (11,12), subreti-

Table 1 Classification of Macular Translocation Surgery

Type of surgery	Other name	Authors (year)
Macular translocation with 360-degree peripheral circumferential retinotomy	Full macular translocation	Machemer and Steinhorst (1993) (27)
Macular translocation with large (but less than 360-degree) circumferential retinotomy		Ninomiya and associates (1996) (36)
Macular translocation with small (self-sealing) or no retinotomy/retinotomies, with or without scleral imbrication	Limited macular translocation	de Juan and associates (1998) (25)

nal endophotocoagulation (13), and submacular surgery (14–19) with no or limited success. More recently, photodynamic therapy with verteporfin (Visudyne, CIBA Vision Corp. Duluth, GA) showed some modest benefits but the therapy does not benefit all patients with subfoveal CNV and multiple retreatments are necessary (20–22). Six percent of eyes with subfoveal CNV treated with verteporfin therapy experienced three or more lines of improvement in visual acuity compared to 2.4% in eyes given placebo at 12 months following initiation of treatment (22). In recent years, several investigators have approached the management of subfoveal CNV with a totally new treatment paradigm. This new treatment is known by several names including retinal relocation (23), retinal translocation (24,25), macular relocation (26–28), macular translocation (29–34), macular rotation (35), and foveal translocation (36–40). The term macular translocation surgery is currently the most widely used in the United States.

Several different techniques are currently in use by investigators worldwide for macular translocation surgery. These techniques produce different degrees of postoperative foveal displacement. The various forms of macular translocation surgery may be broadly classified into three categories depending on the size of the retinotomy/retinotomies used: (1) macular translocation with 360-degree peripheral circumferential retinotomy, (26,27,29,31,41); (2) macular translocation with large (but less than 360-degree) circumferential retinotomy (34,36–40); and (3) macular translocation with either small (self-sealing) or no retinotomy/retinotomies, with or without scleral imbrication (Table 1) (24,25,28,33,42). Macular translocation with 360-degree peripheral circumferential retinotomy is also known as *full* macular translocation while another name for macular translocation with either small or no retinotomy/retinotomies is *limited* macular translocation. This chapter reviews the current state of knowledge and the technique of limited macular translocation for the management of subfoveal CNV secondary to AMD.

II. RATIONALE

Although the exact pathogenesis of CNV secondary to AMD is not known, the natural history of this condition is progressive loss of central vision over time. The initial retinal dysfunction responsible for impaired vision in eyes with subfoveal CNV may be attributable to factors such as subretinal fluid, subretinal hemorrhage, and impaired nutrition/waste exchange across the retinal pigment epithelium (RPE) and Bruch's membrane, and visual function may recover, at least partially, if these factors are removed. When fibrous proliferation and degeneration of the overlying photoreceptors occur during the later stages of the disease, the visual loss becomes irreversible.

The rationale of macular translocation surgery is that moving the neurosensory retina of the fovea in an eye with recent-onset subfoveal CNV to a new location before permanent retinal damage occurs may allow it to recover or maintain its visual function over a healthier bed of RPE–Bruch's membrane–choriocapillaris complex. In effect, macular translocation surgery attempts to achieve a more normal subretinal space beneath the fovea. The concept is attractive, but how well extrafoveal or extramacular RPE and choriocapillaris can support good foveal function is relatively unknown. The density and pigmentation of RPE cells and the pattern of choroidal circulation are not uniform throughout the ocular fundus. The macular area has the greatest density of RPE melanin pigmentation (43) and a lobular choroidal angioarchitecture that allows for extremely fast circulation (44). An 18-year-old man who had his fovea rotated 43 degrees superiorly following an open-globe injury retained good visual acuity despite foveal relocation to an area of extramacular RPE and choroid (45). Assuming comparatively good extramacular RPE and choroidal function in patients with subfoveal CNV secondary to AMD, macular translocation surgery may therefore be a viable treatment option. In addition to relocating the fovea to a comparatively healthier RPE-Bruch's membrane–choriocapillaris bed to support foveal function, relocating the fovea to an area outside the border of the CNV allows ablation of the CNV by laser photocoagulation without destroying the fovea, thereby arresting the progression of the CNV and preserving central vision.

Macular translocation surgery has also been combined with submacular surgery by some surgeons. Thomas and associates have shown that removal of subfoveal CNV secondary to AMD is frequently accompanied by removal of native RPE, accounting for the relatively poorer visual outcome of submacular surgery for AMD when compared to that for other etiologies such as ocular histoplasmosis syndromes (17). This is because the CNV in AMD typically lies in the sub-RPE space between the RPE and Bruch's membrane (type 1 CNV), as opposed to that found anterior to the native RPE in the subneurosensory retinal space (type 2 CNV) in eyes with ocular histoplasmosis, multifocal choroiditis, and idiopathic neovascular membranes (46). When combined with removal of CNV, macular translocation surgery allows the fovea to be relocated to an area outside the RPE defect created.

III. HISTORICAL BACKGROUND

Lindsey and associates were the first to report their experiment with retinal relocation in 1983, but their aim was to study the anatomical dependency of the foveal retina on foveal RPE and choroid (23). Their techniques included creation of a retinal detachment and relaxing retinal incisions, shifting of the neurosensory retina, and retinal reattachment. Their techniques were expanded in 1985 by Tiedeman and co-workers, who conceived the idea of rotating the macula of eyes with subfoveal CNV secondary to AMD to a new area of underlying RPE–Bruch's membrane–choriocapillaris complex as a treatment for the condition (47). They showed it was feasible to rotate the macula approximately 45 degrees around the optic disk with reattachment of the fovea in animal eyes.

After developing their surgical techniques in rabbit eyes (26), Machemer and Steinhorst in 1993 became the first surgeons to demonstrate in humans the feasibility of macular translocation surgery (27). Their technique involves lensectomy, complete vitrectomy, planned total retinal detachment by transscleral infusion of fluid under the retina, 360-degree peripheral circumferential retinotomy, rotation of the retina around the optic disk, and reattachment of the retina with silicone oil tamponade. Besides allowing retinal rotation to occur, the retinotomy also provided access to the subretinal space for removal of blood and choroidal neovascular membranes. A number of investigators have subsequently modified this technique, but many of them still require large or 360-degree peripheral circumferential retinotomy to allow rotation of the retina (31,35,36,41).

The early reports of proliferative vitreoretinopathy (PVR) complicating macular translocation with large retinotomy prompted Imai and de Juan to develop a new technique of macular translocation without the need for any retinotomy in 1996 (28). Their technique involves transscleral subretinal hydrodissection, anterior-posterior scleral shortening near the equator, and retinal reattachment. Using this technique, they were able to achieve a predictable macular relocation of greater than 500 microns in rabbit eyes. Because no retinal break was created, the likelihood of developing PVR was thought to be lower than with earlier techniques. As more experience is gained with the surgery, de Juan and associates have made several modifications to their original technique (24,25,33,42). They currently use a 41-gauge retinal hydrodissection cannula to make several tiny self-sealing retinotomies for subretinal hydrodissection to create a controlled, reproducible subtotal retinal detachment, and have abandoned scleral resection during the scleral shortening procedure. They have called their technique limited macular translocation since the operation achieve a smaller degree of postoperative foveal displacement and is less extensive compared to other techniques requiring large retinotomies.

IV. INDICATIONS

The precise indications for limited macular translocation have not been fully ascertained. Currently, limited macular translocation has found its application mainly in the management of recent-onset subfoveal CNV from a variety of etiologies. AMD is the most common indication given the high prevalence of this condition and its poor visual prognosis without treatment. Subfoveal CNV due to other causes such as pathological myopia, ocular histoplasmosis syndrome, angioid streaks, and multifocal choroiditis, as well as idiopathic neovascular membranes, has also been treated with this new procedure (25).

V. PREOPERATIVE CONSIDERATIONS

Proper case selection is crucial to good anatomical and functional outcome following limited macular translocation. A careful and detailed preoperative evaluation is therefore very important, and attention should be paid to the characteristics of the lesion in the macula as well as to concurrent pathology elsewhere in the retina. A recent good-quality fluorescein angiogram, preferably obtained within 1 week of the surgery, is necessary to evaluate the characteristics of the CNV and its precise relationship to the geometrical, center of the foveal avascular zone. Special care should be paid to the retinal periphery during indirect ophthalmoscopy with scleral depression to look for concurrent peripheral retinal pathology that may lead to operative complications.

With increasing experience in limited macular translocation, it appears that several preoperative pathophysiological and anatomical factors are important in determining the postoperative functional and anatomical outcome of patients undergoing the procedure.

A. Pathophysiological Considerations

Several pathophysiological mechanisms responsible for visual loss in eyes with subfoveal CNV may have some bearing on the functional outcome following limited macular translocation. These factors may be broadly divided into "reversible" and "irreversible" components.

1. "Reversible" Components

"Reversible" components of visual loss from subfoveal CNV secondary to AMD include (1) impaired photoreceptor function secondary to abnormal RPE function (retinol metabolism) and impaired nutrient/waste exchange across the RPE and Bruch's membrane, (2) relative retinal ischemia/hypoxia secondary to abnormal RPE–Bruch's membrane–choriocapillaris complex, (3) retinal edema and subretinal fluid, and (4) retinal and subretinal hemorrhages. These problems may be evident early in the course of the disease, resulting in metamorphopsia and central blurring. Their effects are not immediately devastating, and therefore affected eyes do not usually lose foveal fixation. Theoretically, effective macular translocation may, by reestablishing a relatively more normal subretinal space and underlying RPE–Bruch's membrane–choriocapillaris complex, cause one or more of these factors to be reduced or reversed, thereby allowing visual recovery. The best candidates for surgery are therefore those with recent-onset metamorphopsia or disturbance in central vision due to new or recurrent CNV, before massive subretinal fibrosis and degeneration of the photoreceptors permanently destroy the fovea.

2. "Irreversible" Components

Untreated long-standing subfoveal CNV often results in permanent photoreceptor cell loss, an "irreversible" mechanism responsible for visual loss, usually in the late stages of the disease when fibrovascular scarring occurs. Histopathological studies have documented that the size and thickness of the diskiform scar are directly related to the loss of photoreceptors (48). The visual loss associated with photoreceptor cell loss is often severe, but metamorphopsia becomes less prominent. Loss of foveal fixation may result from the severe visual impairment. Such a severely and irreversibly damaged foveal neurosensory retina is unlikely to achieve good functional recovery even after successful relocation to a healthier bed of RPE–Bruch's membrane–choriocapillaris complex, and therefore is a poor candidate for limited macular translocation.

Proper case selection, by identifying patients with good photoreceptor function for surgery and excluding others with irreversible photoreceptor damage from surgery, is of critical importance to achieving good visual outcomes. The foveal function can be assessed preoperatively by a number of means including measurement of visual acuity, scanning laser ophthalmoscope (SLO) microperimetry, and focal electroretinography. An analysis of a large series has shown that preoperative visual acuity is a significant predictor of postoperative visual outcome, with good preoperative visual acuity being associated with better postoperative visual results (49). However, eyes presenting with poorer vision have a greater chance of visual improvement but less likelihood of achieving excellent vision of 20/40 or better.

SLO microperimetry appears to be an excellent way of identifying eyes that have viable foveal photoreceptors (50). It is particularly helpful in identifying patient who have maintained central fixation and may be a better indicator than visual acuity in predicting good visual outcome following macular translocation surgery.

B. Anatomical Considerations

Effective macular translocation may be defined as (1) successful postoperative relocation of the fovea to an area outside the border of the CNV, i.e., a previously subfoveal CNV becomes either juxtafoveal (1–199 microns from the foveal center) or extrafoveal (≥200 microns from the foveal center) following the surgery, or (2) successful postoperative relocation of the fovea to an area outside the border of the RPE defect associated with CNV removal during the surgery. Barring any complication, this anatomical success is dependent on two major factors: (1) the *minimum desired translocation* and (2) the *postoperative foveal displacement* achieved. The minimum desired translocation can be measured prior to surgery and, when taken into consideration with the *median* postoperative foveal displacement normally achieved by the surgeon, can give some idea of the likelihood of achieving effective macular translocation following the surgery.

1. Minimum Desired Translocation

The minimum amount of foveal displacement required to achieve effective macular translocation is the *distance* between the foveal center and a point on either the inferior or superior border of the subfoveal lesion depending on whether the translocation is inferior or superior, all of these points being equidistant from the temporal edge of the optic disk. This distance is the *minimum desired translocation* (Fig. 1). The temporal edge of the optic disk rather than the center of the disk is taken as the pivoting point of the fovea because the papillomacular bundle enters the optic disk from temporally close to this point. This is therefore the point in which the papillomacular bundle would pivot when the fovea is relocated during macular translocation surgery.

Although the size of a subfoveal lesion is intuitively a factor in determining the minimum desired translocation, other factors such as eccentricity and shape of the lesion are important too. For example, in inferior macular translocation, a lesion that is eccentrically centered superiorly relative to the fovea has a smaller minimum desired translocation and is more likely to become juxtafoveal or extrafoveal following surgery compared to another lesion of the same size that is eccentrically centered downward relative to the fovea,

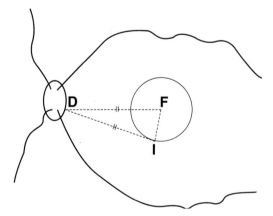

Figure 1 Schematic diagram showing fundus of the left eye. F is the foveal center, D is a point on the temporal edge of the optic disk, and I is a point on the inferior border of the subfoveal lesion (circle) such that DF = DI. The distance FI is the *minimum desired translocation* for an inferior translocation.

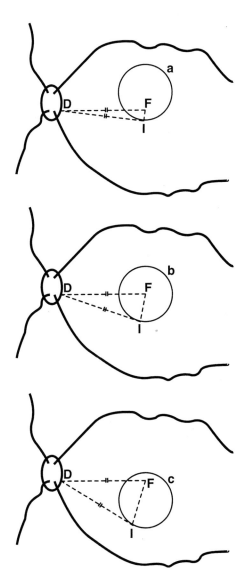

Figure 2 Schematic diagram showing the fundi of three eyes with subfoveal lesions (circles a, b, and c) of equal size but different eccentricity relative to the foveal center (F). Lesion a (top) is centered eccentrically upward relative to the foveal center (F), lesion b (middle) is centered on the foveal center (F), and lesion c (bottom) is centered eccentrically downward relative to the foveal center (F). D is a point on the temporal edge of the optic disk and I is a point on the inferior border of the subfoveal lesions such that DF= DI. The minimum desired translocation (FI) for inferior translocation is smallest for lesion a and greatest for lesion c. Lesion a is therefore more likely to achieve effective macular translocation compared to lesions b and c following inferior macular translocation.

assuming that the net postoperative foveal displacement achieved is identical in both cases (Fig. 2). Lesions of the same size but of different shapes may also have different minimum desired translocations. On the other hand, lesions of different sizes and eccentricities may have the same minimum desired translocation (Fig. 3).

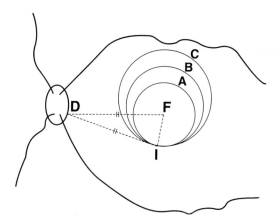

Figure 3   Schematic diagram showing ocular fundus with three possible subfoveal lesions (circles A, B, and C) of different sizes and eccentricities. F is the foveal center, D is a point on the temporal edge of the optic disk, and I is a point on the inferior border of the subfoveal lesions such that DF = DI. The minimum desired translocations (FI) for inferior translocation for lesions A, B, and C are identical. Lesions A, B, and C therefore have the same likelihood of achieving effective macular translocation following inferior macular translocation. Note, however, that the minimum desired translocations for superior translocation for lesions A, B, and C are different.

2. Median Postoperative Foveal Displacement

The *median* postoperative foveal displacement normally achieved by a surgeon can be derived by analyzing data collected either retrospectively or prospectively in a series of consecutive cases operated by the surgeon. To estimate the amount of translocation achieved, we first measure on the preoperative fluorescein angiogram the distance from a predetermined retinal landmark (such as a retinal vascular bifurcation) located superior to the CNV to a specific point along the inferior edge of the CNV. We then use the same points to obtain a similar measurement on the postoperative angiogram. The absolute difference between these two measurements estimates the postoperative foveal displacement achieved (Fig. 4). If the time difference between the preoperative and postoperative angiograms is within 2 weeks, the size and characteristics of the CNV on the postoperative angiogram tend not to change significantly. Although this method of determining the postoperative foveal displacement is not very precise, especially for greater amounts of translocation, it does give useful estimates without the need to resort to sophisticated imaging equipment.

Ideally, a surgeon should have some idea of the *median* postoperative foveal displacement he or she has achieved in previous cases when evaluating potential patients for macular translocation surgery. This information, when considered together with the minimum desired translocation of a particular eye, gives some useful idea of the likelihood of achieving effective macular translocation. If the minimum desired translocation in an eye is *equal* to the median postoperative foveal displacement normally achieved by the surgeon, the eye has an approximately 50:50 chance of achieving effective macular translocation after the surgery, regardless of the other dimensions of the subfoveal lesion. If the minimum desired translocation is less than the median postoperative foveal displacement, the eye has a greater than 50% chance of achieving effective macular translocation. The chance of effective macular translocation is less than 50% if the minimum desired translocation is greater than the median postoperative foveal displacement for the

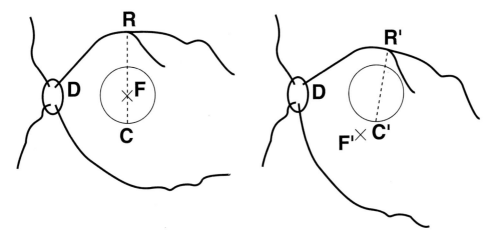

Figure 4 Schematic diagram showing the fundus of an eye before (left) and after (right) inferior macular translocation. R is a point on a retinal vascular bifurcation ("retinal" landmark) situated superior to the subfoveal lesion (circle). C is a point on the inferior border of the subfoveal lesion ("choroidal" landmark) such that the line RC is close to and roughly parallel to the "path" of the foveal displacement. F and F′ are the foveal centers before and after macular translocation, respectively. R′ and C′ are the same "retinal" and "choroidal" landmarks, respectively, following macular translocation. The absolute difference between the distances RC and R'C' estimates the postoperative foveal displacement achieved.

surgeon. If a surgeon has a postoperative foveal displacement greater than the patient's minimum desired translocation in 75% of his previous cases, he could then tell his patient that he has an approximately 75% chance of effective macular translocation following surgery in his hands. If the macular translocation surgery is combined with CNV removal, this rule may not apply if the area of the RPE defect accompanying the CNV removal differs greatly from the area of the original CNV. It is important to remember that the median postoperative foveal displacement for a particular surgeon is not static and may change with modifications or refinements in techniques.

VI. OPERATIVE TECHNIQUE

Since the initial publications of the procedure (24,25,28), a number of modifications have been adopted to improve the amount of translocation, while reducing the incidence of complications (33,42,49). Unlike other techniques of macular translocation surgery that require the creation of large retinotomies to allow foveal displacement (27,36), limited macular translocation relies on scleral imbrication to shorten the outer eyewall (sclera, choroid, and RPE), creating redundancy of the neurosensory retina relative to the eyewall. Instead of large retinotomies, small self-sealing posterior retinotomies are used, reducing the chance of intraoperative and postoperative complications.

Limited macular translocation may be either inferior or superior. Inferior limited macular translocation causes inferior movement of the neurosensory macula relative to the underlying tissues, and vice versa. Our experience with this surgery demonstrates that inferior limited macular translocation achieves a greater median postoperative foveal displacement than superior translocation for the same amount of scleral imbrication used. When the patient's head is upright postoperatively, the buoyancy of the intravitreal air bubble supports the superior retina while the weight of the subretinal fluid stretches the retina inferiorly. These forces probably contribute to the greater downward displacement of the fovea during inferior macular translocation and reduce the upward displacement of the fovea during superior translocation. For this reason, inferior limited macular translocation is currently our preferred technique for the majority of eyes undergoing macular translocation surgery and we restrict superior limited macular translocation to the occasional case in which the CNV is markedly eccentrically centered inferiorly relative to the fovea. The subsequent discussion in this chapter will be limited in scope to the procedure of inferior limited macular translocation.

A. Overview/Equipment

Inferior limited macular translocation by means of scleral imbrication is essentially a five-step procedure (Table 2). The first step *is placement of scleral imbricating sutures*. The second step is a *three-port pars plana vitrectomy* with separation of the posterior hyaloid face from the retina. The third step is *creation of a neurosensory retinal detachment,* with or without subretinal manipulation. The fourth step is *tightening of the scleral imbricating sutures.* The final step in the procedure is a *subtotal fluid-air exchange.*

The equipment necessary to perform this procedure includes a standard three-port pars plana vitrectomy equipment. Additional devices that are unique to this procedure include (1) a 41-gauge retinal hydrodissection cannula (MADLAB retinal hydrodissection cannula, Bausch & Lomb Surgical, St. Louis, MO) for subretinal hydrodissection to create a detachment of the neurosensory retina (Fig. 5), (2) a specially designed retinal manipulator (Bausch & Lomb Surgical, St. Louis, MO) for gently grasping the detached retina, aiding in the separation of the macular neurosensory retina from the RPI, and also

Table 2 Key Surgical Steps in Inferior Limited Macular Translocation

Key surgical steps
Placement of imbricating sutures
Pars plana vitrectomy
Planned neurosensory retinal detachment
Tightening of imbricating sutures
Subtotal fluid-air exchange

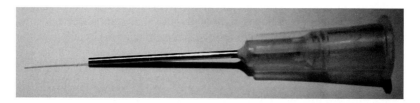

Figure 5 Forty-one-gauge retinal hydrodissection cannula (MADLAB retinal hydrodissection cannula, Bausch & Lomb Surgical, St. Louis, MO).[Courtesy of the Johns Hopkins Microsurgery Advanced Design Laboratory (http://www.madlab.jhu.edu), the Wilmer Ophthalmological Institute, the Johns Hopkins University School of Medicine, Baltimore, MD.]

permitting fluid-air exchange (Fig. 6), and (3) a subretinal pick for subretinal dissection to break firm subretinal adhesions. In addition, we use an air humidifier (MoistAir humidifying chamber, RetinaLabs.com, Atlanta, GA) that minimizes posterior capsular opacification in phakic patients (51) and potentially reduces excessive nerve fiber layer dehydration during the fluid-air exchanges (Fig. 7).

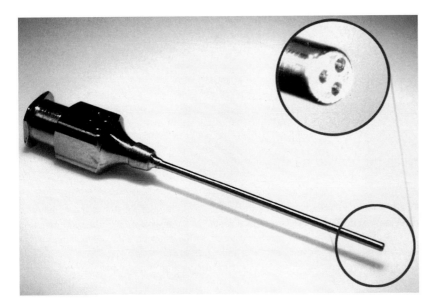

Figure 6   Retinal manipulator (Bausch & Lomb Surgical, St. Louis, MO). The tip of the instrument is enlarged to show the three small openings of the retinal manipulator. [Courtesy of the Johns Hopkins Microsurgery Advanced Design Laboratory (http://www.madlab.jhu.edu), the Wilmer Ophthalmological Institute, the Johns Hopkins University School of Medicine, Baltimore, MD.]

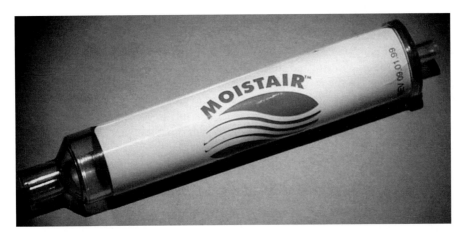

Figure 7   Air humidifier (MoistAir humidifying chamber, RetinaLabs.com, Atlanta, GA). [Courtesy of the Johns Hopkins Microsurgery Advanced Design Laboratory (http://www.madlab.jhu.edu), the Wilmer Ophthalmological Institute, the Johns Hopkins University School of Medicine, Baltimore, MD.]

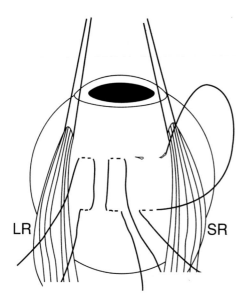

Figure 8 Nonabsorbable imbricating sutures are placed straddling the equator of the globe prior to pars plana vitrectomy. The anterior scleral bites are placed 3 mm posterior to the recti insertion and the posterior scleral bites are placed 6 mm posterior to the anterior bites. Three imbricating sutures are placed between the superior rectus (SR) and lateral rectus (LR). The fourth imbricating suture is placed medial to the superior rectus and the final one is placed inferior to the lateral rectus (not shown).

B. Steps of Inferior Limited Macular Translocation

1. Placement of Imbricating Sutures

For inferior limited macular translocation, we place three imbricating sutures in the superotemporal quadrant between the superior and lateral recti, one suture just nasal to the superior rectus in the superonasal quadrant, and one suture just inferior to the lateral rectus in the inferotemporal quadrant (Fig. 8). The number and actual location of the sutures have been selected in part empirically and are not based on precise data. The purpose of the imbricating sutures is to cause anterior-posterior shortening of the eyewall (sclera, choroid, and RPE) relative to the neurosensory retina. We used to remove a section of the sclera during scleral imbrication (25) but we no longer feel that this is necessary. The sutures are placed in a mattress fashion and we use the same nonabsorbable sutures that we normally use for scleral buckling, i.e., either 4-0 silk or 5-0 dexon. The sutures are placed 6 mm apart from the anterior to posterior extent with the sutures straddling the equator. These sutures are not tightened until later in the procedure. We acknowledge that this technique imbricates the eyewall structures inward into the vitreous cavity and that although this can result in scleral shortening, a more effective scleral shortening would occur if these structures could be evaginated away from the vitreous cavity.

2. Pars Plana Vitrectomy

Following preplacement of the imbricating sutures, vitrectomy is initiated. We prefer to fit the sclerostomies with metal cannulas for limited macular translocation because a "leaky"

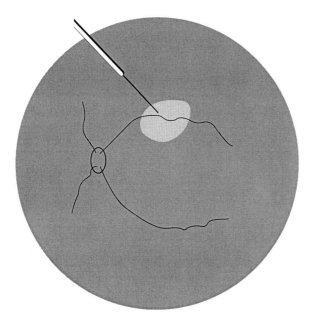

Figure 9   The first retinotomy for subretinal hydrodissection is placed near the superotemporal vascular arcade to detach the superior retina.

system is desirable during the creation of retinal detachment when balanced salt solution is injected into the subretinal space and during tightening of the imbricating sutures when the eye is deliberately kept soft. The metal cannula also facilitates the insertion of the delicate 41-gauge retinal hydrodissection cannula. A subtotal vitrectomy is then performed. It is critical in these cases to be certain that the posterior hyaloid face is separated from the posterior pole, preferably up to the retinal periphery but at least past the intended positions of the posterior retinotomies. It appears that when the posterior hyaloid face has not been separated from the neurosensory retina, it tethers the neurosensory retina and reduces the amount of macular translocation. It is not necessary to trim the vitreous gel down to the vitreous base but the vitreous cavity needs to be debulked sufficiently to achieve a good air or gas fill.

3.   Planned Neurosensory Retinal Detachment

To detach the retina, anywhere from three to eight retinotomies are necessary. The preferred locations of initial retinotomy placement are just superior to the superotemporal vascular arcade and just inferior to the inferotemporal vascular arcade (Fig. 9). A third retinotomy is often necessary and is placed temporal to the macula (Fig. 10). The retinal detachments should be relatively large and need to extend in the superotemporal quadrant past the zone of intended imbrication. The 41-gauge retinal hydrodissection cannula is connected to an infusion pump to actively infuse balanced salt solution under the retina (Fig. 11). Prior to entering the vitreous cavity, the rate of infusion is set so that there is a steady drip of approximately 2 or 3 drops of balanced salt solution per second from the cannula. To initiate the subretinal blister, the 41-gauge retinal hydrodissection cannula is placed

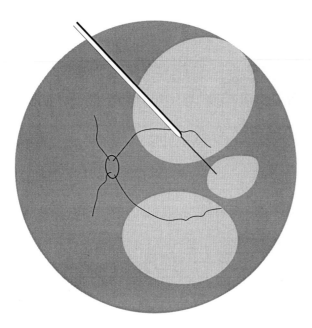

Figure 10 The third retinotomy for subretinal hydrodissection is placed a few disk diameters temporal to the fovea to detach the temporal retina. The inferior retina had earlier been detached with a retinotomy placed near the inferotemporal vascular arcade. Note that the retinal detachment from the first retinotomy extends anteriorly beyond the zone of intended scleral imbrication.

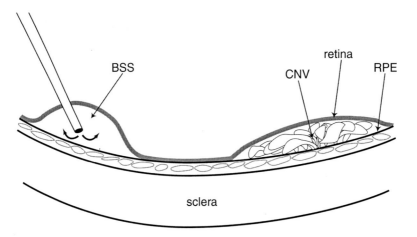

Figure 11 The retina is detached by injecting balanced salt solution (BSS) between the neurosensory retina and the retinal pigment epithelium (RPE) with a 41-gauge retinal hydrodissection cannula through a tiny retinotomy. CNV, choroidal neovascularization.

through the retina with the infusion running. The neurosensory retinal detachment will initially progress rapidly and tends to expand toward the retinal periphery. As the blister becomes larger, the expansion of the blister is slower although the infusion rate remains constant. If the cannula inadvertently becomes dislodged from the retinotomy during the

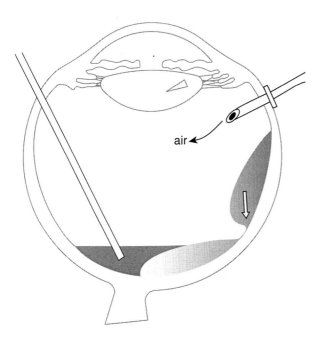

Figure 12   A complete fluid-air exchange allows the subretinal fluid to gravitate posteriorly (white arrow) and dissect the macula off the underlying retinal pigment epithelium.

procedure, one can usually reenter the same retinotomy and continue with the detachment. If this is not possible, a new retinotomy can be made in another site nearby. It is uncommon for the macula to become completely detached during this maneuver since the detachments have a tendency to progress anteriorly, presumably because the macula is relatively more adherent to the RPE than the retinal periphery.

The key to successful macular translocation is to completely detach the macula up to the temporal edge of the optic disk. At the same time, we try to limit detachment of the superonasal aspect of the retina because detachment of this area is associated with a higher risk of macular fold formation. The first step in completely detaching the macula is to perform a complete fluid-air exchange. The subretinal fluid will gravitate posteriorly and will usually dissect the macula off the underlying RPE (Fig. 12). When the macula is detached, the retinal bullae should extend to the optic nerve. However, this does not assure that all subretinal adhesions have been released. At this point, the air is exchanged for fluid and inspection of the posterior retina with the aid of the retinal manipulator will confirm whether or not the macula is completely detached. If adhesions are present, the retinal manipulator can be activated with low suction to grasp a part of the detached retina. Gentle traction is then exerted with the retinal manipulator to release any persistent subretinal adhesion (Fig. 13). Care should be taken when using the retinal manipulator as it may result in iatrogenic retinal breaks, hemorrhage, macular hole, and nerve fiber layer injury. If despite these maneuvers the retina is still not completely detached, a repeat fluid-air exchange can be performed. If repeated attempts fail to free a localized area of subretinal adhesion such as a laser scar, a small retinotomy is created eccentrically in the macula through which a retinal pick can be used to break the adhesions (Fig. 14).

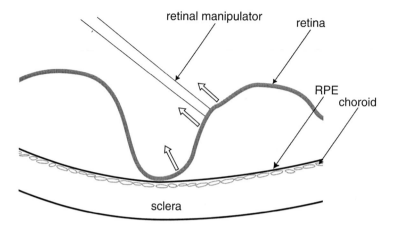

Figure 13   Gentle traction on the retina (white arrows) with a retinal manipulator helps to break abnormal chorioretinal adhesions and fully detach the macula from the retinal pigment epithelium (RPE).

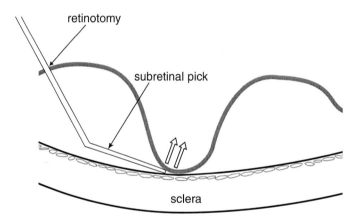

Figure 14   Subretinal blunt dissection (white arrows) with a pick through a small eccentric retinotomy may be necessary to break abnormal chorioretinal adhesions in the macula.

4.   Tightening of the Imbricating Sutures

Following the neurosensory retinal detachment (Fig. 15), when there is still fluid in the vitreous cavity, the imbricating sutures are tightened (Fig. 16). We tighten the sutures while the eye is filled with fluid rather than air to imbricate the eyewall under the bullous retina. Tightening the sutures while the eye is filled with air may cause the retina lying on the eyewall to be "caught" in the crevices of the imbrication and thus reduce the amount of retinal movement relative to the eyewall. To achieve adequate imbrication, the globe should be softened by either clamping the fluid infusion or leaving a sclerotomy open or both. One must consider, however, that this state of hypotony may increase the risk of intraocular hemorrhage such as suprachoroidal hemorrhage. There is also possibly a higher risk of

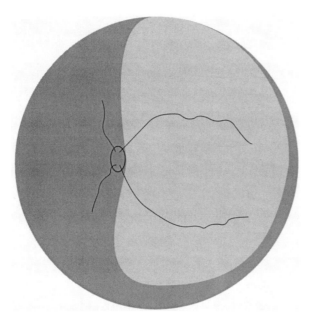

Figure 15 A large retinal detachment temporal to an imaginary vertical line bisecting the optic disk is obtained following coalescence of the multiple smaller localized retinal detachments. It is important to ensure that the macula is completely detached and that the retinal detachment extends anteriorly beyond the zone of intended scleral imbrication.

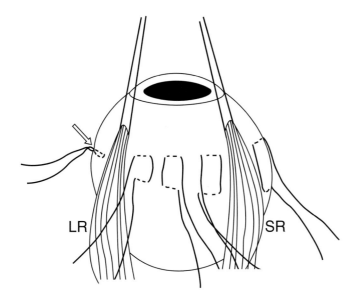

Figure 16 Tightening the imbricating sutures causes the sclera to be imbricated under the Detached retina and creates redundancy of the retina relative to the eyewall (sclera, choroid, and RPE). The imbricating suture inferior to the lateral rectus has been tightened (white arrow), and as a result of the scleral shortening, the spacings between the anterior and posterior scleral bites of other imbricating sutures adjacent to this suture appear decreased. LR, lateral rectus; SR, superior rectus.

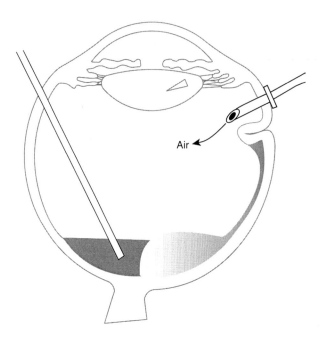

Figure 17   Following scleral imbrication, a final subtotal fluid-air exchange is performed without draining the subretinal fluid.

postoperative endophthalmitis should fluid from outside the eye be aspirated into the eye by negative pressure within the eye.

Although we perform anterior-posterior shortening of the eye wall with scleral imbrication in the majority of our cases of inferior limited macular translocation, it is interesting to note that this is not always necessary, and effective macular translocation may still be achieved without employing scleral imbrication for very small subfoveal lesions (33).

5.   Subtotal Fluid-Air Exchange

The sclerostomy sites and peripheral retina are inspected for inadvertent retinal breaks prior to the final fluid-air exchange. If present, they should be treated with laser retinopexy or cryoretinopexy and a longer-acting gas such as sulfur hexafluoride is then used instead of air for internal tamponade.

The final fluid-air exchange is performed following tightening of the imbricating sutures (Fig. 17). Generally an estimated 75–90% exchange is performed and air is left in the eye unless inadvertent peripheral retinal breaks have been created. We do not reattach the retina by draining the subretinal fluid because this tends to result in a smaller amount of macular translocation. After the sclerostomies and conjunctival incisions have been closed, a combination corticosteroid-antibiotic subconjunctival injection is given. We routinely give our patient intravenous corticosteroids during the procedure to reduce the incidence of PVR.

C.   Patient Positioning

After the eye is patched, the patient is turned on the operative side for about 5 min. This allows the subretinal fluid to gravitate temporally to detach the temporal peripheral retina.

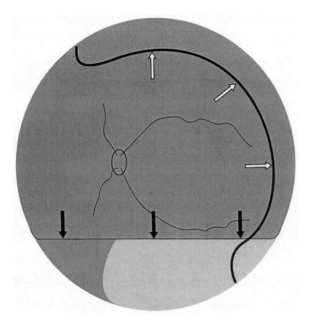

Figure 18 The immediate postoperative head-positioning maneuver (see text) causes all the subretinal fluid to accumulate under the inferior retina. The inferior retina is detached. Note the scleral imbrication (white arrows) and the fluid–air interface in the vitreous cavity (black arrows).

From this position (without turning the patient on his or her back), the patient is sat upright and instructed to keep his or her head upright overnight. Besides allowing the temporal peripheral retina to be completely detached, this maneuver also causes all the subretinal fluid to accumulate in the inferior retina, reducing the incidence of a postoperative macular or foveal fold (Fig. 18). If the superonasal retina has been inadvertently detached during the surgery, sitting the patient upright from the supine position may cause some subretinal fluid to become trapped under the superonasal retina, causing a retinal bulla or retinal fold to overhang from the superonasal retina. This bulla or fold will often cause a retinal fold to stretch from the superior margin of the optic disk into the macula. When such a macular or foveal fold persists postoperatively, undesirable visual consequences occur and remedial surgery is usually necessary to unfold the macula.

The buoyancy of the intravitreal air bubble when the patient's head is upright, coupled with the weight of the subretinal fluid inferiorly, stretches the retina in a downward fashion (Fig. 19). The superior retina is the first to become reattached, and this is quickly followed by the macula and the rest of the retina over the next several days.

D. Combined Removal of CNV and Limited Macular Translocation

Some surgeons have advocated surgically removing the CNV at the time of limited macular translocation (32). We tend not to favor this approach, particularly in patients with AMD, because of the uncertainty in the size of the RPE defect that will occur. Thus even though the preoperative CNV may be of a size and location that effective macular translocation would have a good chance of being achieved, the RPE defect created during

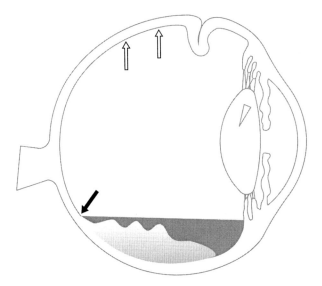

Figure 19   With the head in an upright position following the surgery, the buoyancy of the air bubble supports the superior retina (white arrows) while the weight of the subretinal fluid stretches the retina downward (black arrow), causing the fovea to be displaced downward relative to the underlying eyewall (sclera, choroid, and RPE).

submacular surgical excision may be significantly larger and therefore jeopardize the chances of anatomical success. We feel that laser ablation is a much more precise method of treating the CNV.

VII.   POSTOPERATIVE MANAGEMENT

A.   Postoperative Review, Fluorescein Angiography, and Laser Photocoagulation

On the first postoperative day, the inferior retina is generally still detached but the macula is now attached. Given the presence of the intravitreal air bubble, the view is often too poor to perform fluorescein angiography. Until the retina is completely attached, we prefer that the patient continues to position in such a way as to maintain the attachment of the macula and to lessen the contact between the intravitreal air and the crystalline lens. Complete retinal reattachment generally occurs within 2–3 days. Usually by 3–7 days following the procedure, the air bubble has become small enough that it no longer covers the macula when the patient is upright. At this point, it is appropriate to consider fluorescein angiography so as to identify the postoperative location of the CNV.

Interpretation of the postoperative fluorescein angiograms can be difficult in some cases given the additional retinal pigment epithelial changes induced by the surgical procedure. It is particularly important to obtain good-quality stereoscopic angiograms and to compare the preoperative and postoperative angiograms to determine the actual location and extent of the CNV.

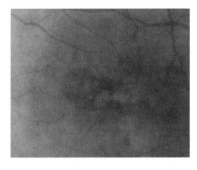 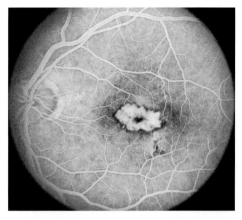

Figure 20 Fundus photograph (left) and fluorescein angiogram (right) at presentation demonstrate a subfoveal choroidal neovascular membrane approximately one MPS disk area in size under the geometrical center of the foveal avascular zone in the left eye. Visual acuity is 20/200-1. See also color insert, Fig. 16.20.

Laser photocoagulation of the entire CNV lesion is considered following effective macular translocation when the CNV no longer lies under the geometrical center of the foveal avascular zone. We follow the guidelines for laser treatment outlined in the Macular Photocoagulation Study (52). Following laser photocoagulation, the patient will be followed up in about 3–4 weeks with repeat fluorescein angiography to detect persistent or recurrent CNV.

1. Clinical Example

A 63-year-old man with 5-month history of decreased vision in his left eye due to neovascular age-related macular degeneration presented for consideration of macular translocation surgery. His best corrected visual acuity at presentation was 20/200-1. Clinical examination and fluorescein angiography confirmed a subfoveal CNV approximately one MPS disk area in size (Fig. 20). After written informed consent was obtained, inferior limited macular translocation was performed without complication. Clinical examination and fluorescein angiography on the third postoperative day disclosed effective inferior translocation of the fovea relative to the CNV (Fig. 21). The postoperative foveal displacement achieved was approximately 700 microns. Laser photocoagulation was applied to the area of the CNV. The best corrected visual acuity improved to 20/60 + 2 and 20/40 at 4 and 8 months, respectively, after the surgery. The patient had no postoperative complication or recurrence of the CNV during the follow-up period (Fig. 22).

B. Management of Persistent Subfoveal CNV

When some of the CNV remains under the center of the fovea owing to insufficient macular translocation, the patient and physician must choose between a number of options including observation, laser ablation of the fovea, surgical resection of CNV, or photodynamic therapy. The potential role of photodynamic therapy in an eye that has undergone translocation has not been determined but remains a reasonable consideration for the postoperative treatment of lesions that remain subfoveal, are possibly subfoveal, or recur

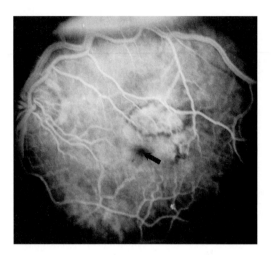

Figure 21 Three days following inferior limited macular translocation, fluorescein angiogram demonstrates effective macular translocation with displacement of the geometrical center of the foveal avascular zone (arrow) to an area inferior to the choroidal neovascular membrane. The postoperative foveal displacement is approximately 700 microns.

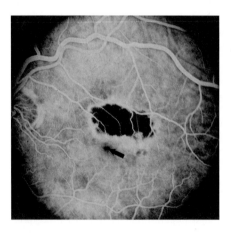 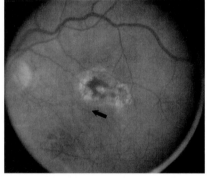

Figure 22 Postoperative fundus photograph (right) and fluorescein angiogram (left) show successful laser ablation of the choroidal neovascular membrane with no evidence of recurrence. The geometrical center of the foveal avascular zone (arrow) is preserved. Visual acuity is 20/40. See also color insert, Fig. 16.22 (right).

subfoveally following laser treatment. We tend not to advocate partial laser treatment of the CNV because it has been shown to be ineffective by the Macular Photocoagulation Study Group (53). We also tend not to make repeat attempts at macular translocation because initial efforts resulted in retinal detachment with significant PVR in some patients. One must consider that even though the CNV lesion has not completely moved out of the foveal center, the partial movement my still benefit the patient as less of the perifoveal retina will need laser ablation.

C. Management of Recurrent CNV

A significant proportion of patients will develop recurrent neovascularization following effective macular translocation and laser photocoagulation. If the recurrence is extrafoveal or juxtafoveal, further laser photocoagulation is indicated. For recurrent lesions that have just extended under the fovea, we sometimes recommend ablating the lesion in an effort to contain the potential damage. Observation, submacular surgery, and photodynamic therapy are other management options. Repeat macular translocation is not recommended.

D. Postoperative Sensory Adaptation

The displacement of the fovea following limited macular translocation causes some patients to experience postoperative diplopia and/or cyclotropia. Our experience and that of Lewis and associates show that because the degree of foveal displacement is small following limited macular translocation, the incidence of postoperative diplopia and/or cyclotropia is low and the symptoms tend to disappear spontaneously within a few months in most of these patients (32). In those with more persistent symptoms, treatment with prisms has been found to be satisfactory. In Lewis and associates' series, only three out of 10 patients experienced either distortion or tilting of image postoperatively and these symptoms persisted at 6 months postoperatively in only one patient (32). This is unlike the considerable disorientation caused by postoperative diplopia and cyclotropia after macular translocation with 360-degree circumferential peripheral retinotomy when the macula may be rotated 30–50 degrees (35). Eckardt and associates have developed torsional muscle surgery for counterrotation of the globe, sometimes with additional muscle surgery on the fellow eye, to reduce this complication (35). We have not found corrective muscle surgery to be necessary for patients following limited macular translocation.

VIII. OUTCOME

The greatest advantage of macular translocation surgery over many other experimental or established treatments is that it offers the potential for improvement in visual acuity. There are very few reports on limited macular translocation for the treatment of subfoveal CNV secondary to AMD in the published literature (25,32,33,42,49). While the results of limited macular translocation have been encouraging in some cases (25,33,49), some surgeons have found the surgery unpredictable (32).

Currently, the largest series on limited macular translocation is by Pieramici and associates, who analyzed the outcomes of 102 consecutive eyes of 101 patients aged 41–89 years (median, 76 years) who underwent inferior translocation by one surgeon for new or recurrent AMD-related subfoveal CNV (49). The median postoperative foveal displacement achieved in the series was 1200 microns (range, 200–2800 microns). Seventy-five percent of the patients experienced at least 900 microns of postoperative foveal displacement and 25% achieved 1500 microns or more of foveal displacement. Sixty-two percent of the patients achieved effective macular translocation. At 3 and 6 months postoperatively, 31% and 49% of the eyes, respectively, achieved a visual acuity better than 20/100 while 37% and 48% of the eyes, respectively, experienced two or more Snellen lines of visual improvement. Sixteen percent of the eyes experienced six more Snellen lines of visual improvement.

Pieramici and associates found that good preoperative visual acuity, achieving the desired amount of postoperative foveal displacement, a greater amount of postoperative foveal displacement, and recurrent CNV at baseline were associated with better visual acuity at 3 and 6 months postoperatively (49). The reason patients with recurrent CNV achieved better outcome was thought to be due to the fact that this select group of patients, having undergone previous laser photocoagulation for a juxtafoveal or extrafoveal lesion, were better educated about the necessity to see their ophthalmologist for any new visual change and were already on close follow-up by the ophthalmologist treating them. The subfoveal disease in this group of patients may therefore be of a shorter duration and less severe than that seen in patients who never had prior laser photocoagulation. Poor preoperative visual acuity and the development of a complication either during or after surgery were associated with worse visual acuity at 3 and 6 months postoperatively.

A smaller series of 10 eyes of 10 patients with subfoveal CNV secondary to AMD treated by one surgeon was reported by Lewis and associates (32). The median postoperative foveal displacement in this series was 1286 microns (range, 114–1919 microns). The best-corrected visual acuity, as measured with the Early Treatment Diabetic Retinopathy Study chart, improved in four eyes (median, 10.5 letters) and decreased in six eyes (median, 14.5 letters). The median change in visual acuity for the entire series was a decrease of five letters. The final visual acuity at 6 months postoperatively was 20/80 in two eyes, 20/126 in one eye, 20/160 in four eyes, 20/200 in one eye, 20/250 in one eye, and 20/640 in one eye.

In our experience, the most important aspects of this procedure are patient selection, achieving the desired amount of macular translocation, and avoiding complications. If this procedure is performed on a patient without viable foveal photoreceptors, there is no chance for visual improvement. If the minimum desired translocation is not achieved, we are left with a persistent subfoveal CNV lesion that will likely result in continued photoreceptor cell damage and visual deterioration. Development of a complication is associated with a poorer prognosis, particularly when retinal detachment occurs (49). To improve on the outcome of this surgery, we must find ways to select the appropriate patients and reduce the incidence of complications. In addition, improvements in the surgical technique that will afford larger and more predictable macular translocation will improve the chances of success and increase the number of patients for whom the procedure is a realistic option.

IX. COMPLICATIONS

The usual risks inherent to pars plana vitrectomy exist for all patients undergoing inferior limited macular translocation surgery since posterior vitrectomy is an integral part of the procedure. In addition, for the majority of patients who also have scleral imbrication, additional risks similar to those associated with scleral buckling surgery are present (Table 3). Table 4 shows the intraoperative and postoperative complications documented in Pieramici and associates' series (49).

A. Intraoperative

Placement of sutures on the sclera for scleral imbrication may cause inadvertent scleral perforation. This may be associated with suprachoroidal hemorrhage, vitreous hemorrhage, and retinal break. Retinal break can also occur during the later stages of the operation. The retina may be inadvertently cut or traumatized during vitrectomy. Vitreous traction near the

Table 3 Complications Associated with Limited Macular Translocation

Timing of complication	Complication
Intraoperative	Scleral perforation
	Unplanned retinal break
	Suprachoroidal hemorrhage
	Subretinal hemorrhage
	Vitreous hemorrhage
	Macular hole
	Unplanned translocation of retinal pigment epithelium
Postoperative	Rhegmatogenous retinal detachment
	Proliferative vitreoretinopathy
	Endophthalmitis
	Cataract
	Vitreous hemorrhage
	Macular or foveal fold
	New choroidal neovascularization at site of retinotomy
	Acute angle-closure glaucoma
	Transient formed visual hallucinations

Table 4 Intra- and Postoperative Complications Associated with Inferior Limited Macular Translocation in Pieramici and Associates' Series ($n = 102$) (49)

Type of complication	Intraoperative (no. of eyes)	Postoperative (no. of eyes)	Total (no. of eyes)
Macular hole	9	0	9
Scleral perforation	2	0	2
Choroidal hemorrhage	1	0	1
Subretinal hemorrhage	1	0	1
Unintended retinal break	6	4	10
Vitreous hemorrhage	2	2	4
Unplanned retinal detachment	0	9	9
Macular fold	0	3	3
New choroidal neovascularization at site of retinotomy	0	2	2

sclerostomies, retinal incarceration at the sclerostomies, and retinal manipulation during planned retinal detachment (32) may also tear the retina. Unintended retinal breaks occurred in 10 of 102 consecutive eyes in Pieramici and associates' series. Unintended non-self-sealing break(s) should receive laser retinopexy or cryoretinopexy during the surgery or in the early postoperative period. Longer-acting gas such as sulfur hexafluoride may also be necessary for internal tamponade. Macular hole formation is another complication that may also require longer-term internal tamponade.

During planned detachment of the retina, subretinal hemorrhage may occur if the retinal hydrodissection cannula used for subretinal hydrodissection or the subretinal pick used for blunt dissection traumatizes the vascular choroid. Unplanned translocation of the RPE can occur when a patch of RPE adherent to the underlying surface of the neurosensory retina detaches with the retina (42).

While the eye is deliberately kept soft momentarily to allow the imbricating sutures to be tightened, the eye is at risk of retinal incarceration at the sclerostomies and severe intraocular hemorrhage including suprachoroidal hemorrhage. It is possible that negative pressure within the eye during this maneuver may aspirate fluids or air from outside the eye into the eye and increase the risk of postoperative endophthalmitis.

B. Postoperative

Rhegmatogenous retinal detachment is the most common serious complication of limited macular translocation. Nine of 102 eyes in Pieramici and associates' series developed persistent postoperative retinal detachment (49). Additional surgery is usually necessary to reattach the retina should this complication occur. Pneumoretinopexy may be effective in treating some cases with retinal breaks in the superior two-thirds of the retinal periphery. The retinal detachment may be associated with PVR, especially if a repeat limited macular translocation has been performed for persistent subfoveal CNV. Postoperative endophthalmitis is another potentially devastating complication of limited macular translocation.

The incidence of cataract formation appears to be similar to that following other vitrectomy procedures. However, long-term follow-up is necessary to determine its exact incidence. Should cataract formation occur soon after limited macular translocation such as following intraoperative lens touch, it can impair visualization of the fundus postoperatively and interfere with clinical examination, fluorescein angiography, and laser photocoagulation. Early cataract surgery is indicated in such cases. Postoperative vitreous hemorrhage can also impair visualization and close follow-up with ultrasonography is warranted to look for associated retinal detachment.

Folds running across the fovea are associated with poor vision, and reoperation to remove the fold may be necessary. A foveal fold formed postoperatively in three of 10 eyes reported by Lewis and associates (32). Rarely, new CNV can occur at the site of the retinotomy used for retinal detachment, presumably as a result of iatrogenic focal defect in Bruch's membrane caused by the retinal hydrodissection cannula. Acute angle-closure glaucoma may follow limited macular translocation, and this may be related to shortening of the axial length from scleral imbrication. We have also seen two patients who developed formed visual hallucinations within 24 h following the procedure. The visual hallucinations ceased completely 3–7 days postoperatively following retinal reattachment.

X. CONCLUSION

Macular translocation surgery has generated excitement and hope for a community frustrated with the lack of a good treatment for subfoveal CNV. Already some surgeons such as Machemer have expressed hope that it may one day also be applied as prophylaxis in diseases such as relentlessly progressive dry AMD or other inherited subfoveal diseases such as Best disease, Stargardt disease, and central areolar chorioretinal dystrophy (30). Although it remains to be seen whether macular translocation surgery will finally find its place as a routine operation for subfoveal diseases, its initial results are encouraging and it remains the only treatment that offers potential for recovery of good visual acuity. Further refinements in surgical techniques with reduction of intraoperative and postoperative complications will make the procedure safer and more predictable. Hopefully, its precise role in ophthalmology will be established with further experience and more controlled evaluation of this procedure.

> *Rationale:* To displace the foveal neurosensory retina in an eye with recent-onset subfoveal CNV to a presumably healthier bed of RPE–Bruch's membrane–choriocapillaris complex devoid of CNV before permanent retinal damage occurs; the foveal displacement allows the destruction of the CNV by laser photocoagulation without damaging the foveal center.
>
> *Indications:* Subfoveal CNV secondary to a variety of etiologies.
>
> *Preoperative Considerations: Favorable factors:* recent-onset CNV, small minimum desired translocation; *Unfavorable factors:* diskiform scarring, photoreceptor loss, large minimum desired translocation.
>
> *Operation: Inferior* limited macular translocation achieves a greater postoperative foveal displacement compared to *superior* limited macular translocation and is the operation of choice in the majority of cases.
>
> *Postoperative Management:* Fluorescein angiography and, if possible, laser photocoagulation of "displaced" CNV.
>
> *Complications: Intraoperative:* scleral perforation, unplanned retinal break, intraocular hemorrhage, macular hole, unplanned translocation of RPE; *postoperative:* rhegmatogenous retinal detachment, proliferative vitreoretinopathy, endophthalmitis, cataract, intraocular hemorrhage, foveal fold, new CNV at site of retinotomy, acute angle-closure glaucoma, transient formed visual hallucinations.

ACKNOWLEDGMENTS

The authors wish to thank Morvarid Behmanesh, M.A., from the Johns Hopkins Microsurgery Advanced Design Laboratory (http://www.madlab.jhu.edu), the Wilmer Ophthalmological Institute, the Johns Hopkins University School of Medicine, Baltimore, Maryland, for the illustrations. K-G Au Eong was supported by a National Medical Research Council-Singapore Totalisator Board Medical Research Fellowship.

REFERENCE

1. Leibowitz HM, Krueger DE, Maunder LR, Milton RC, Kini MM, Kahn HA, Nickerson RJ, Pool J, Colton TL, Ganley JP, Loewenstein JI, Dawber TR. The Framingham Eye Study monograph: an ophthalmological and epidemiological study of cataract, glaucoma, diabetic retinopathy, macular degeneration, and visual acuity in a general population of 2631 adults, 1973–1975. Surv Ophthalmol 1980;24 (Suppl):335–610.
2. Klein R, Klein BEK, Linton KLP. Prevalence of age-related maculopathy: the Beaver Dam Eye Study. Ophthalmology 1992;99:933–943.
3. Macular Photocoagulation Study Group. Laser photocoagulation of subfoveal neovascular lesions in age-related macular degeneration. Results of a randomized clinical trial. Arch Ophthalmol 1991;109:1220–1231.
4. Macular Photocoagulation Study Group. Laser photocoagulation of subfoveal recurrent neovascular lesions in age-related macular degeneration. Results of a randomized clinical trial. Arch Ophthalmol 1991;109:1232–1241.

5. Macular Photocoagulation Study Group. Laser photocoagulation of subfoveal neovascular lesions of age-related macular degeneration. Updated findings from two clinical trials. Arch Ophthalmol 1993;111:1200–1209.

6. Beatty S, Au Eong KG, McLeod D, Bishop PN. Photocoagulation of subfoveal choroidal neovascular membranes in age related macular degeneration: the impact of the macular photocoagulation study in the United Kingdom and Republic of Ireland. Br J Ophthalmol 1999;83:1103–1104.

7. Pharmacological Therapy for Macular Degeneration Study Group. Interferon alfa-2a is ineffective for patients with choroidal neovascularization secondary to age-related macular degeneration: results of a prospective randomized placebo-controlled clinical trial. Arch Ophthalmol 1997;115:865–872.

8. Thomas MA, Ibanez HE. Interferon alfa-2a in the treatment of subfoveal choroidal neovascularization. Am J Ophthalmol 1993;115:563–568.

9. Poliner LS, Tornambe PE, Michelson PE, Heitzmann JG. Interferon alpha-2a for subfoveal neovascularization in age-related macular degeneration. Ophthalmology 1993;100:1417–1424.

10. Chan CK, Kempin SJ, Noble SK, Palmer GA. The treatment of choroidal neovascular membranes by alpha interferon. An efficacy and toxicity study. Ophthalmology 1994;101:289–300.

11. Spaide RF, Guyer DR, McCormick B, Yannuzzi LA, Burke K, Mendelsohn M, Haas A, Slakter JS, Sorenson JA, Fisher YL, Abramson D. External beam radiation therapy for choroidal neovascularization. Ophthalmology 1998;105:24–30.

12. Char DH, Irvine AI, Posner MD, Quivey J, Phillips TL, Kroll S. Randomized trial of radiation for age-related macular degeneration. Am J Ophthalmol 1999;127:574–578.

13. Thomas MA, Ibanez HE. Subretinal endophotocoagulation in the treatment of choroidal neovascularization. Am J Ophthalmol 1993;116:279–285.

14. Lambert HM, Capone A Jr, Aaberg TM, Sternberg P Jr Mandell BA, Lopez PF. Surgical excision of subfoveal neovascular membranes in age-related macular degeneration. Am J Ophthalmol 1992;113:257–262.

15. Thomas MA, Grand MG, Williams DF, Lee CM, Pesin SR, Lowe MA. Surgical management of subfoveal choroidal neovascularization. Ophthalmology 1992;99:952–968.

16. Berger AS, Kaplan HJ. Clinical experience with the surgical removal of subfoveal neovascular membranes: short-term postoperative results. Ophthalmology 1992;99:969–976.

17. Thomas MA, Dickinson JD, Melberg NS, Ibanez HE, Dhaliwal RS. Visual results after surgical removal of subfoveal choroidal neovascular membranes. Ophthalmology 1994;101:1384–1396.

18. de Juan E Jr, Machemer R. Vitreous surgery for hemorrhagic and fibrous complications of age-related macular degeneration. Am J Ophthalmol 1988;105:25–29.

19. Blinder KJ, Peyman GA, Paris CL, Gremillion CM Jr. Submacular scar excision in age-related macular degeneration. Int Ophthalmol 1991;15:215–222.

20. Miller JW, Schmidt-Erfurth U, Sickenberg M, Pournaras CJ, Laqua H, Barbazetto I, Zografos L, Piguet B, Donati G, Lane A.-M, Birngruber R, van den Berg H, Strong A, Manjuris U, Gray T, Fsadni M, Bressler NM, Gragoudas ES. Photodynamic therapy with verteporfin for choroidal neovascularization caused by age-related macular degeneration: results of a single treatment in a phase 1 and 2 study. Arch Ophthalmol 1999;117:1161–1173.

21. Schmidt-Erfurth U, Miller JW, Sickenberg M, Laqua H, Barbazetto I, Gragoudas ES, Zografos L, Piguet B, Pournaras CJ, Donati G, Lane A.-M, Birngruber R, van den Berg H, Strong HA, Manjuris U, Gray T, Fsadni M, Bressler NM. Photodynamic therapy with verteporfin for choroidal neovascularization caused by age-related macular degeneration: results of retreatments in a phase 1 and 2 study. Arch Ophthalmol 1999;177:1177–1187.

22. Treatment of Age-Related macular degeneration with photodynamic therapy (TAP) Study Group. Photodynamic therapy of subfoveal choroidal neovascularization in age-related macular degeneration with verteporfin: one-year results of 2 randomized clinical trials—TAP report. Arch Ophthahlmol 1999;117:1329–1345.

23. Lindsey P, Finkelstein D, D'Anna S. Experimental retinal relocation. ARVO asbtracts. Invest Ophthahlmol Vis Sci 1983;24 (Suppl):242.

24. Imai K, Loewenstein A, de Juan E Jr. Translocation of the retina for management of subfoveal choroidal neovascularization. I. Experimental studies in the rabbit eye. Am J Ophthahlmol 1998;125:627–634.

25. de Juan E Jr. Loewenstein A, Bressler NM, Alexander J. Translocation of the retina for management of subfoveal choroidal neovascularization. II. A preliminary report in humans. Am J Ophthalmol 1998;125:635–646.

26. Machemer R, Steinhorst UH. Retinal separation, retinotomy, and macular relocation. I. Experimental studies in the rabbit eye. Graefes Arch Clin Exp Ophthalmol 1993;231:629–634.

27. Machemer R, Steinhorst UH. Retinal separation, retinotomy, and macular relocation. II. A surgical approach for age-related macular degeneration? Graefes Arch Clin Exp Ophthalmol 1993;231:635–641.

28. Imai K, de Juan E Jr. Experimental surgical macular relocation by scleral shortening. ARVO abstracts. Invest Ophthalmol Vis Sci 1996;37 (suppl):Sl16.

29. Seaber JH, Machemer R. Adaptation to monocular torsion after macular translocation. Graefes Arch Clin Exp Ophthalmol 1997;235:76–81.

30. Machemer R. Macular translocation (editorial). Am J Ophthalmol 1998;125:698–700.

31. Wolf S, Lappas A, Weinberger AWA, Kirchhof B. Macular translocation for surgical management of subfoveal choroidal neovascularizations in patients with AMD: first results. Graefes Arch Clin Exp Ophthalmol 1999;237:51–57.

32. Lewis H, Kaiser PK, Lewis S, Estafanous M. Macular translocation for subfoveal choroidal neovascularization in age-related macular degeneration: a prospective study. Am J Ophthalmol 1999;128:135–146.

33. de Juan E Jr, Vander JF. Effective macular translocation without scleral imbrication. Am J Ophthalmol 1999;128:380–382.

34. Akduman L, Karavellas MP, MacDonald J C OlK RJ, Freeman WR. Macular translocation with retinotomy and retinal rotation for exudative age-related macular degeneration. Retina 1999;19:418–423.

35. Eckardt C, Eckardt U, Conrad H-G. Macular rotation with and without counterrotation of the globe in patients with age-related macular degeneration. Graefes Arch Clin Exp Ophthalmol 1999;237:313–325.

36. Ninomiya Y, Lewis JM, Hasegawa T, Tano Y. Retinotomy and foveal translocation for surgical management of subfoveal choroidal neovascular membranes. Am J Ophthalmol 1996;122:613–621.

37. Fujikado T, Ohji M, Saito Y, Hayashi A, Tano Y. Visual function after foveal translocation with scleral shortening in patients with myopic neovascular maculopathy. Am J Ophthalmol 1998;125:647–656.

38. Fujikado T, Ohji M, Hayashi A, Kusaka S, Tano Y. Anatomic and functional recovery of the fovea after foveal translocation surgery without large retinotomy and simultaneous excision of a neovascular membrane. Am J Ophthalmol 1998;126:839–842.

39. Ohji M, Fujikado T, Saito Y, Hosohata J, Hayashi A, Tano Y. Foveal translocation: a comparison of two techniques. Semin Ophthalmol 1998;13:52–62.

40. Cekic O, Ohji M, Hayashi A, Fujikado T, Tano Y. Foveal translocation surgery in age-related macular degeneration. Lancet 1999;354:340.

41. Toth CA, Machemer R. Macular translocation. In: Berger JW, Fine SL, Maguire MG, eds. Age-Related Macular Degeneration. St Louis: Mosby, 1999;353–362.

42. Harlan JB, de Juan E Jr. Bressler NM. Retinal translocation with unplanned translocation of the retinal pigment epithelium. Wilmer Retina Update 1999;5:3–8.

43. Tso MOM, Friedman E. The retinal pigment epithelium. I. Comparative histology. Arch Ophthalmol 1967;78:641–649.

44. Yoneya S, Tso MOM. Angioarchitecture of the human choroid. Arch Ophthalmol 1987;105:681–687.

45. Toller KK, Hainsworth DP. Traumatic foveal relocation with good visual acuity. Arch Ophthalmol 1998;116:1536–1537.

46. Gass JDM. Biomicroscopic and histopathologic considerations regarding the feasibility of surgical excision of subfoveal neovascular membranes. Am J Ophthalmol 1994;118:285–298.

47. Tiedeman J, de Juan E Jr, Machemer R, Hatchell DL, Hatchell MC. Surgical relocation of the macula. ARVO asbtracts. Invest Ophthalmol Vis Sci 1985;26 (Suppl):59.

48. Green WR, Enger C. Age-related macular degeneration histopathologic studies. The 1992 Lorenz E Zimmerman lecture. Ophthalmology 1993;100:1519–1535.

49. Pieramici DJ, de Juan E Jr., Fujii GY, Reynolds MA, Melia M, Humayun MS, Schachat AP, Hartranft CD. Limited inferior macular translocation for the treatment of subfoveal choroidal neovascularization secondary to age-related macular degeneration. Am J Ophthalmol 2000; 130:419–428.

50. Loewenstein A, Sunness JS, Bressler NM, Marsh MJ, de Juan E. Scanning laser ophthalmoscope fundus perimetry after surgery for choroidal neovascularization. Am J Ophthalmol 1998;125:657–665.

51. Harlan JB Jr, Lee ET, Jensen PS, de Juan E Jr. Effect of humidity on posterior lens opacification during fluid-air exchange. Arch Ophthalmol 1999;117:802–804.

52. Macular Photocoagulation Study Group. Krypton laser photocoagulation for neovascular lesions of age-related macular degeneration. Results of a randomized clinical trial. Arch Ophthalmol 1990;108:816–824.

53. Macular Photocoagulation Study Group. Occult choroidal neovascularization. Influence on visual outcome in patients with age-related macular degeneration. Arch Ophthalmol 1996;114:400–412.

17

Use of Adjuncts in Surgery for Age-Related Macular Degeneration

Lawrence P. Chong

Doheny Retina Institute of the Doheny Eye Institute, University of Southern California Keck School of Medicine, Los Angeles, California

I. INTRODUCTION

Adjuncts that have been used surgery for age-related macular degeneration (AMD) include tissue plasminogen activator, balance salt solution (BSS), and calcium-and-magnesium-free retinal detachment-enhancing solutions. The surgeries in which these solution have been used include submacular surgery to excise choroidal neovascular membranes, large-scale macular translocation surgery, limited macular translocation surgery, evacuation, or displacement of submacular hemorrhages.

II. TISSUE PLASMINOGEN ACTIVATOR

Tissue plasminogen activator (tPA) is a polypeptide of 527 amino acids that cleaves the Arg560–Val561 bond of plasminogen. Because of its high affinity for fibrin, its enhancement of binding of plasminogen to fibrin clot, and potentiation of its activity in the presence of fibrin, fibrinolysis occurs almost exclusively in fibrin clots.

Commercial tPA (Activase, Genentech, Inc.; Actilyse, Boehringer Ingelheim International, GmbH) is a 70,000-MW, single-chain protein produced from a cloned human tPA gene using Chinese hamster ovary cells (1). Endogenous tPA is secreted in its single-chain form to be enzymatically converted by plasmin to its two chain form. Both forms of tPA are equally active. The vehicle consists of L-arginine phosphate, phosphoric acid, and polysorbate 80.

tPA has been used both intracamerally and subretinally. The utility of intracameral tPA was demonstrated in animal models of fibrin (2–4), hyphema (5), vitreous hemorrhage (6–8), and subretinal hemorrhage (9,10). The utility of subretinal injection of tPA was demonstrated in animal models of subretinal hemorrhage (11–13).

In the anterior chamber 0.05 mL containing up to 200 µg and 0.10 mL containing up to 36 µg have been injected without unusual inflammation or toxicity to the cornea or lens.

In the vitreous cavity 0.10 mL containing up to 25 μg has been injected without cornea or retinal toxicity. Repetitive injections (three times, separated by 7-day intervals) of 3 μg tPA also did not show retinal toxicity (8). A single report suggested probable retinal toxicity of 0.1 mL containing 25 μg (14). Dose-dependent retinal toxicity was seen with 0.10-mL injections of 50, 75, and 100 μg into the vitreous cavity (15). Traction retinal detachments were seen following 100-mg (6) and 200-μg (16) tPA injections.

In the subretinal space no retina toxicity was seen after subretinal injection of 25 and 50 μg of tPA in 0.1 mL of volume (11,12).

Lewis and colleagues demonstrated in rabbits that subretinal clots 30 min old cleared faster after a 0.1-mL subretinal injection of 25 μg tPA as compared to an equivalent volume of BSS (11). However, the subretinal tPA could not completely prevent retinal damage. Both BSS and tPA decreased the toxic effect of blood partly on the basis of dilution of the subretinal blood. Johnson and colleagues showed a similar effect for lower doses of tPA (2.5 μg in 0.05 mL) on clots that were 24 h old, but severe progressive retinal degeneration was still seen (12). An ultrasurgical approach using a microinfusion of 0.5–5 μg of tPA facilitated lysis of 1- and 2-day-old clots and their removal through micropipettes under stereotactic control. Good preservation of the retinal architecture was seen compared to untreated controls (13).

The ability of intravitreal injections of tPA to lyse subretinal clots has been explored. Coll and colleagues found that 0.1 mL 50 μg of tPA facilitated the lysis and absorption of 1 day-old subretinal clots compared to equivalent volume injections of saline (9). Unfortunately, retinal damage was not prevented. Boone and colleagues injected 25 μg of tPA into the vitreous space and found only partial clot lysis that was not enough to allow removal by aspiration alone (10). The inability of labeled tPA injected into the vitreous to penetrate the intact neural retina or a subretinal clot in rabbits was demonstrated by Kamei and colleagues (17). Some labeled tPA was able to penetrate into eyes with vitreous hemorrhage presumably from the microdefects through which blood escaped from the subretinal space into the vitreous.

The previous studies spurred simultaneous interest in the clinical use of tPA to assist in the removal of subretinal hemorrhage. These techniques involved the injection of 6.25–12.5 μg of tPA in a volume of 0.05–0.05 mL into the subretinal space and then waiting 10–45 min before aspiration of the liquefied blood. Injections into the subretinal space were accomplished with a glass pipette (18), 33-gauge cannula (19), or bent-tipped 30-gauge needle (20,21). Aspiration was performed with double-barrel subretinal-injector aspirator (19), soft-tipped cannula (18,22), tapered 20-gauge Charles flute needle (21), or 30-gauge subretinal cannula (23). Liquefied subretinal blood was also manipulated with a small perfluorocarbon liquid bubble (20,24,25).

In addition to intravitreal injection of tPA during the pars plana vitrectomy procedure, the injection of 0.1 mL of 25 μg of tPA into the subretinal clot by passing a 30-gauge needle through the pars plana under indirect ophthalmoscopy the day before pars plana vitrectomy has also been described (26).

An intravitreal injection consisting of 6 μg of tPA in 0.1 mL was injected into the midvitreous cavity to liquefy subretinal clots 12–36 h prior to vitrectomy and removal of blood through a retinotomy using perfluorocarbon liquid manipulation (27). Intravitreal injections of 0.1–0.2 mL containing 25–100 μg of tPA into the vitreous cavity have been given either the day before (28) or immediately before (29,30) injection of intravitreal gas to displace submacular hemorrhage. Exudative retinal detachments seen after 100-μg injections were attributed to tPA toxicity (29).

A number of investigators have injected 25–50 µg tPA into the subretinal space following pars plana vitrectomy (31–33). An air fluid exchange was performed and the patient was kept erect to pneumatically displace the liquefied blood from the fovea.

Lewis injected tPA into the subretinal space before excision of the choroidal neovascular membrane but found no improvement compared with injection of BSS into the subretinal space in a randomized

III. CALCIUM- AND MAGNESIUM-FREE RETINAL DETACHMENT–ENHANCING SOLUTIONS

Marmor had discovered that removing calcium and magnesium from a solution that bathed eye wall sections in vitro weakened retinal adhesive force (35). Wiedemann described a "detachment infusion" for macular translocation surgery that was calcium and magnesium free (36). Substituted for conventional vitrectomy infusion fluid, this solution enabled the immediate detachment of the retina from its peripheral, diathermy-induced perforation site to the center of the macula or macular area. He described its use in retinal organ culture and creation of experimental retinal detachment in rabbits and in human surgery.

We hypothesized that BSS Part A might be an ideal retinal detachment-enhancing solution and studied its safety and efficacy in rabbits before using it clinically in humans. BSS was developed as an improvement over normal saline, lactated Ringer's, and Plasma-lyte 148 as a physiologically compatible solution to be used in the eye during surgery (37,38). To further improve the physiological compatibility of BSS, glutathione, glucose, and bicarbonate buffer system were added (39–41) resulting in BSS Plus. BSS Plus consists of two parts, which are reconstituted just prior to use in surgery. These two parts consist of Part B, a sterile 480-mL solution in a 500-mL single-dose bottle to which Part A, a sterile concentrate in a 20-mL single-dose vial, is added. Compared to BSS, BSS Part A lacks magnesium and calcium, and the citrate and acetate buffers of BSS have been replaced with bicarbonate buffer. BSS Part B contains the calcium and magnesium as well as the dextrose and the glutathione, which are unique to BSS Plus. We hypothesized that BSS Part A alone could be used safely in the human eye since it contained almost all the ingredients of BSS except for the calcium and magnesium with a different buffering system and a pH of 7.4. A tremendous advantage to the vitreous surgeons is the commercial availability of BSS. We felt that all these qualities plus the historical use of the solution in the operating room (albeit reconstituted with Part B) could make it an ideal solution to enhance retinal detachment during macular translocation surgery. We showed the safety and efficacy of a calcium- and magnesium-free macular translocation solution by comparing the results of injecting BSS Part A or BSS solution into the subretinal space of rabbit eyes using a 39-gauge cannula (41). No difference was seen in fundus appearance, fluorescein angiography, ERG, or light or electron microscopy in rabbit retinas that had been detached using retinal detachment solution compared to commercially available solution. Using a manual infusion system no more than 100 µg of BSS compared to a much larger volume of retinal detachment solution could be infused into the subretinal space. The diameter of BSS retinal detachments was always less than that of BSS Part A retinal detachments after injection of 100-µg of subretinal fluid.

Aaberg et al. have similarly shown the safety of subretinal BSS Part A in the subretinal space of the rabbit using transscleral infusion (42).

We have used a 39-gauge cannula to atraumatically infuse BSS Part A underneath the retina in macular translocation surgery and to displace submacular hemorrhage.

Clinically, we have found that macular translocation surgery requires only one or two penetrations through the retina with a 39-gauge cannula to detach the posterior retina sufficiently. We have used BSS Part A to displace submacular hemorrhages by performing pars plana vitrectomy, injecting the solution to detach the posterior pole of the retina, performing partial gas-fluid exchange, and then positioning the patient in an erect position for 24 h to displace blood away from the fovea.

IV. SUMMARY

Adjuncts are used primarily in the subretinal space during surgery for AMD. Tissue plasminogen activator can be infused into the subretinal space to liquefy subretinal blood. Tissue plasminogen activator may penetrate human retina after injection into the vitreous cavity through microperforations to liquify subretinal blood. Calcium- and magnesium-free solutions enhance retinal detachment. BSS Plus Part A is a safe and readily available retinal detachment solution. Calcium- and magnesium-free solutions can aid macular translocation surgery and the displacement of submacular hemorrhage.

REFERENCES

1.   Pennica D, Holmes WE, Kohr WJ, Harkins RN, Vehar GA, Ward CA, Bennett WF, Yelverton E, Seeburg PH, Heyneker HL, Goeddel DV, Collen D. Cloning and expression of human tissue type plasminogen activator with DNA in E coli. Nature 1983; 301:214–221.
2.   Johnson RN, Olsen K, Hernandez E. Tissue plasminogen activator treatment of postoperative intraocular fibrin. Ophthalmology 1988; 95:592–596.
3.   Lambrou FH, Snyder RW, Williams GA, Lewandowski M. Treatment of experimental intravitreal fibrin with tissue plasminogen activator. Am J Ophthalmol 1987; 104:619–623.
4.   Snyder RW, Lambrou FH, Williams GA. Intraocular fibrinolysis with recombinant human tissue plasminogen activator. Arch Ophthalmol 1987; 105:1277–1280.
5.   Lambrou FH, Snyder RW, Williams GA. Use of tissue plasminogen activator in experimental hyphema. Arch Ophthalmol 1987; 105:995–997.
6.   Johnson RN, Olsen DR, Hernandez E. Intravitreal tissue plasminogen activator treatment of experimental vitreous hemorrhage. Arch Ophthalmol 1989; 107:891–894.
7.   Min WK, Kim YB, Lee KM. Treatment of experimental vitreous hemorrhage with tissue plasminogen activator. Korean J Ophthalmol 1990; 4:12–15.
8.   Min WK, Kim YB, Ahn BH, Seong GH. Repetitive low-dose tissue plasminogen activator for the clearance of experimental vitreous hemorrhage. Korean J Ophthalmol 1994; 8:45–48.
9.   Coll GE, Sparrow JR, Marinovic A, Chang S. Effect of intravitreal tissue plasminogen activator on experimental subretinal hemorrhage. Retina 1995; 15:319–326.
10. Boone DE, Boldt HC, Ross RD, Folk JC, Kimura AE. The use of intravitreal tissue plasminogen activator in the treatment of experimental subretinal hemorrhage in the pig model. Retina 1996; 16:518–524.
11. Lewis H, Resnick SC, Flannery JG, Straatsma BR. Tissue plasminogen activator treatment of experimental subretinal hemorrhage. Am J Ophthalmol 1991; 111:197–204.
12. Johnson MW, Olsen DR, Hernandez E. Tissue plasminogen activator treatment of experimental subretinal hemorrhage. Retina 1991;11:250–258.
13. Toth CA, Benner JD, Hjelmeland LM, Landers III M.B., Morse LS. Ultramicrosurgical removal of subretinal hemorrhage in cats. Am J Ophthalmol 1992; 113:175–182.

14. Min WK, Kim YB. Resolution of experimental intravitreal fibrin by tissue plasminogen activator. Korean J Ophthalmol 1990; 4:58.

15. Johnson MW, Olsen KR, Hernandez E, Irvine WD, Johnson RJ. Retinal toxicity of recombinant tissue plasminogen activator in the retina. Arch Ophthalmol 1990; 108:259–263.

16. Min WK, Kim YB, Lee KM. Treatment of experimental vitreous hemorrhage with tissue plasminogen activator. Korean J Ophthalmol 1990; 4:12–15.

17. Kamei M, Misono K, Lewis H. Study of the ability of tissue plasminogen activator to diffuse into the subretinal space after intravitreal injection in rabbits. Am J Ophthalmol 1999; 128:739–746.

18. Peyman GA, Nelson NC, Alturki W, FlinderKJ, Paris CL, Desai UR, Harper, III CA. Tissue plasminogen activating factor assisted removal of subretinal hemorrhage. Ophthalm Surg 1991; 22:575–582.

19. Lewis H. Intraoperative fibrinolysis of submacular hemorrhage with tissue plasminogen activator and surgical drainage. Am J Ophthalmol 1994; 118:559–568.

20. Vander JF. Tissue plasminogen activator irrigation to facilitate removal of subretinal hemorrhage during vitrectomy. Ophthalmic Surg 1992; 23:361–363.

21. Moriarty AP, McAllister IL, Constable IJ. Initial clinical experience with tissue plasminogen activator (tPA) assisted removal of submacular haemorrhage. Eye 1995; 9:582–588.

22. Manning LM, Contrad DK. Tissue plasminogen activator in the surgical management of subretinal haemorrhage. Aust NZ J Ophthalmol 1994; 22:59–63

23. Ibanez HE, Williams DF, Thomas MA, Ruby AJ, Meredith TA, Boniuk I, Grand MG. Surgical management of submacular hemorrhage: a series of 47 consecutive cases. Arch Ophthalmol 1995; 113:62–69.

24. Lim JI, Drews-Botsch C, Sternberg, Jr P, Capone, Jr A, Aaberg, Sr TM. Submacular hemorrhage removal. Ophthalmology 1995; 102:1393–1399.

25. Kamei M, Tano Y, Maeno T, Ikuno Y, Mitsuda H, Yuasa T. Surgical removal of submacular hemorrhage using tissue plasminogen activator and perfluorocarbon liquid. Am J Ophthalmol 1996; 121:267–275.

26. Chaudhry NA, Mieler WF, Han DP, Alfaro, III VD, Liggett PE. Preoperative use of tissue plasminogen activator for large submacular hemorrhage. Ophthalmic Surg Lasers 1999; 30:176–180.

27. Kimura AE, Reddy CV, Folk JC, Farmer SG. Removal of subretinal hemorrhage facilitated by preoperative intravitreal tissue plasminogen activator. Retina 1994; 14:83–84.

28. Heriot W. Intravitreal gas and tPA: an outpatient procedure for subretinal hemorrhage. Vail Vitrectomy Meeting, March 10–15, 1996, Vail, Co.

29. Hesse L, Schmidt J, Kroll P. Management of acute submacular hemorrhage using recombinant tissue plasminogen activator and gas. Graefe's Arch Clin Exp Ophthalmol 1999; 202:273–277.

30. Hassan AS, Johnson MW, Schneiderman TE, Regillo CD, Tornambe PE, Poliner LS, Blodi BA, Elner SG. Managment of submacular hemorrhage with intravitreous tissue plasminogen activator injection and pneumatic displacement. Ophthalmology 1999; 106:1900–1907.

31. Connor TB. Surgical displacement of submaclar hemorrhage Vail Vitrectomy Meeting, March 15, 2000, Vail, CO.

32. Federman JL. Variation in surgical management of sub-macular hemorrhage. Vail Vitrectomy Meeting, March 15, 2000,Vail, CO.

33. McCuen BW. A new concept in the treatment of submacular hemorrhage in AMD. Vail Vitrectomy Meeting, March 14, 2000 Vail, CO.

34. Lewis H. VanderBrug Medendorp S. Tissue plasminogen activator-assisted surgical excision of subfoveal choroidal neovascularization in age-related macular degeneration: a randomized, double-masked trial [Clinical Trial. Journal Article. Randomized Controlled Trial]. Ophthalmology 1997; 104(11):1847–1851; discussion 1852.

35. Yao Xiao-Ying, Endo Eric G and Marmor Michael F. Reversibility of retinal adhesion in the rabbit. Invest Ophthalmol Vis Sci 1989; 30:220–224.

36. Faude F, Reichenbach A, Wiedemann P. A detachment infusion for macular translocation surgery. Retina 1999; 19(2):173–174.
37. Edelhauser HF, Van Horn DL, Hyndiuk RA, Schultz RO. Intraocular irrigating solutions: their effect on the corneal endothelium. Arch Ophthalmol 1975; 93:648–657.
38. Waltman SR, Carroll D, Schinimelpfenning W, Okun E. Intraocular irrigating solutions for clinical vitrectomy. Ophthalmic Surg 1975; 6(4):90–94.
39. Benson WE, Diamond JG, Tasman W. Intraocular irrigating solutions for pars plana Vitrectomy: a prospective, randomized, double-blind study. Arch Ophthalmol 1981; 99:1013–1015.
40. Glasser DB, Matsuda M, Ellis JG, Edelhauser HF. Effect of intraocular irrigating solutions on the corneal endothelium after in vivo anterior chamber irrigation. Am J Ophthalmol 1985; 99:321–328.
41. Makoto, Araie MD. Barrier function of corneal endothelium and the intraocular irrigating solutions. Arch Ophthalmol 1986; 104:435–438.
42. Aaberg TM, Sharara NA, Edelhauser HF, and Grossniklaus HE. Hydroseparation of the neurosensory retina with calcium free BSS Plus. September 3, 2000. XXIInd Meeting of the Club Jules Gonin, Taormina, Italy, September 2–6, 2000.

18
Argon Laser to Drusen

Frank J. McCabe
Retina Consultants of Worcester, Worcester, Massachusetts

Allen C. Ho
Wills Eye Hospital, Thomas Jefferson University School of Medicine, Philadelphia, Pennsylvania

I. INTRODUCTION

Age-related macular degeneration (AMD) is the leading cause of visual loss in people older than 65 years in the United States (1). Currently, approximately 200,000 Americans per year lose central vision due to AMD and 50,000 will lose vision in both eyes. Today, there are 38 million American seniors and this number will expand to 88 million by 2030 with a proportional increase in the population at risk from vision loss due to AMD. Ninety percent of the severe visual loss from AMD results from choroidal neovascularization (CNV) (2). Drusen have been shown to be a risk factor for CNV. In 1973, Gass described the disappearance of drusen after laser photocoagulation (3). Subsequently, laser photocoagulation to promote drusen resorption has been examined in numerous studies as prophylaxis against CNV. A preventive treatment of 33% efficacy in the population with bilateral soft drusen would halve the rate of legal blindness from CNV (4).

II. ANATOMY AND PATHOPHYSIOLOGY

To rationalize the potential therapeutic role of prophylactic laser photocoagulation for drusen resorption, it is necessary to define drusen and understand the anatomy and pathophysiology of the outer retina, retinal pigment epithelium (RPE), Bruch's membrane (BM), and choriocapillaris. The RPE, a monolayer of hexagonal-shaped cells external to the neurosensory retina and internal to Bruch's membrane, is intrinsically involved in the outer retina's metabolism. Its functions include phagocytosis of photoreceptor outer segments, maintenance of the blood-retinal barrier, and the transportation of nutrients and waste products (5–7). Bruch's membrane is not a true membrane but a five-layered connective tissue sheet (9). The basal lamina of the RPE is the most internal layer. The inner collagenous layer, elastic lamina, and outer collagenous layer comprise the middle elements. The basal lamina of the choriocapillaris (CC) is the final structure. The choriocapillaris is the innermost layer of the choroid and is composed of an anastomosing sheet of large, fenestrated capillaries. The blood flow in the choroid is one of the highest in the body, largely to meet the high metabolic needs of the outer retina/RPE. Nutrients and waste products pass through the fenestrations of the choriocapillaris. Typically, the BM is not a barrier to these molecules and the RPE transports them to and from the outer retina via active and passive mechanisms (8).

Druse (plural drusen) is a German-derived word meaning nodule. Literally, drusen are crystalline nodules found in stones. In the ophthalmic literature, there have been numerous clinical and histopathological definitions of drusen (9). The lack of standard terminology for drusen makes interpretation of the literature difficult. Recently, a clinical classification and grading for AMD was developed. In this system, drusen are whitish-yellow spots external to the retina or RPE (10). Hard drusen are less than 63 microns, well defined, and yellow-white. Soft drusen are greater than 63 microns. They can have indistinct and distinct borders, may coalesce to form larger, confluent drusen, and typically are white-yellow in color. Pathologically, three types of soft drusen have been described: (1) localized detachments of RPE and basal linear deposit in eyes with diffuse basal linear deposit; (2) localized detachments of the RPE and basal laminar deposit in eyes with diffuse basal laminar deposits; and (3) localized RPE detachments due to focal accumulation of basal linear deposit in eyes without diffuse basal linear deposit (11,12). Ultrastructurally, basal laminar deposits consist of membrane-bound vesicles, wide-spaced collagen, and amorphous, granular material located between the plasma membrane and basal lamina of the RPE. Basal linear deposits are located external to the RPE's basal lamina in the inner collagenous zone. They consist of vesicular and granular electron-dense material and small foci of wide-spaced collagen (11–16). Histochemically, drusen have been shown to consist of lipids, mucopolysaccharides, and glycoconjugates (17–19).

As stated above, the RPE is a metabolically active tissue layer and, most likely, drusen are derived from RPE (20–22). Studies have demonstrated that RPE cells over time accumulate intracellular lipofuscin and other by-products of the catabolism of photoreceptor outer segments (23). It has been shown that the RPE deposits cellular material into the sub-RPE space via evagination of its plasma membrane. This probably is the deposition of the intracellular accumulation of its phagocytic by-products. These plasma-membrane-bound vesicles break down into drusenoid material (22). With normal aging, Bruch's membrane also undergoes ultrastructural and histochemical changes (24–27). BM increases in thickness, accumulates lipids, and develops protein cross-linking. The hydraulic conductivity (flow per unit pressure) of BM in normal eyes decreases with age (26). Similar to drusen, these alterations in BM may also represent the accumulation of waste products from the RPE. The basal linear/laminar deposits and the alterations in BM may impair the flow of fluid to and from the choriocapillaris. The reduced flow of nutrients and oxygen and the impaired removal of waste products may impose a metabolic strain on the outer retina from an enlarged, hydrophobic (lipid-laden) BM and drusen may induce the formation of angiogenic factors and may promote the formation of CNV (28).

III. DRUSEN AS A RISK FACTOR FOR CNV

Laser to drusen has generated investigation because soft drusen are risk factors for CNV and subsequent visual loss. In 1973, Gass noted that nine of 49 (18%) patients with bilateral macular drusen developed visual loss in one eye secondary to "diskiform detachment or degeneration" over an average of 4.5 years (3). Smiddy and Fine followed 71 patients with bilateral macular drusen for an average of 4.3 years. Eight eyes of seven patients (9.9%) developed exudative maculopathy. Severe visual loss (>6 lines) occurred in seven eyes and the 5-year cumulative risk of developing severe visual loss was 12.7% (29). Holz et al. prospectively followed 126 patients with bilateral drusen and "good visual acuity." The 3-year cumulative incidence of developing CNV or pigment epithelial detachment was 13.3% (30). The risk for CNV is higher in patients with drusen in one eye and CNV in the other eye. In Gass' study, 31 of 91 patients lost central vision from CNV in their fellow eye over an average of 4 years (3). The Macular Photocoagulation Study Group followed 127 patients who had an extrafoveal CNV in one eye. In the fellow eye, the risk of developing a CNV was 58% over 5 years if large drusen and RPE hyperpigmentation were present. The risk dropped to 10% if no drusen or hyperpigmentation was present (31). In another study, the Macular Photocoagulation Study Group verified that large drusen are a significant independent risk factor for CNV. In this same study, the risk for CNV jumped to 87% in eyes with five or more drusen, focal hyperpigmentation, one or more large drusen, and systemic hypertension (32). In the study of Sandberg et al., 127 patients with unilateral CNV were followed for an average of 4.5 years; 8.8% per year developed CNV in their fellow eye. Macular appearance, which included large drusen, was significantly associated with CNV (33). One prospective study followed 101 patients with unilateral CNV and drusen in the fellow eye for up to 9 years. The yearly incidence of CNV varied between 5% and 11%. Significant risk factors were the number, size, and confluence of drusen (34).

Numerous pathological studies have shown the correlation of drusen and AMD. Spraul and Grossniklaus examined 51 eyes with AMD and 40 age-matched control eyes. Soft, confluent, and large drusen and basal (linear) deposits correlated with AMD (15). Curcio and Millican demonstrated that basal linear deposits and large drusen are 24 times more likely to be found in eyes with AMD than age-matched control eyes (13).

IV. ARGON LASER PHOTOCOAGULATION

To understand how laser results in drusen resorption, it is necessary to examine the cellular effects of argon laser on the outer retina, RPE, BM, and choriocapillaris. The argon-green laser emits a wavelength of 514 nm. This laser wavelength is largely absorbed by the melanin of the RPE and choroid. Absorption of the laser light elevates the tissue temperature 10–20 °C and causes denaturation of proteins. This thermal effect is called photocoagulation (35,36). The histopathological characteristics of an argon laser burn depend on the power, spot size, and duration of the laser burn. Smiddy et al. examined the light microscopic changes to a human retina 24 h after argon laser application. The juxtafoveal region was treated with laser spots 200 microns in size and 0.5 s in duration. The power ranged between 200 and 400 milliwatts (mW). Histopathologically, there was a choroidal infiltrate of mononuclear and polymorphonuclear cells. The choriocapillaris (CC) was acellular at the center of the burn. The RPE was disrupted and the outer and inner retinal nuclear layers were pyknotic. The ganglion and nerve fiber layers were also affected (37). Thomas et al. conducted a similar study. They examined a human eye 24 h after argon laser. One laser spot of power 310 mW, 100 microns, and 0.5 s was applied in the superonasal quadrant. There was variable RPE necrosis and advanced CC necrosis. A second argon laser burn of 210 mW, 500 microns, and 0.5 s in the peripapillary region demonstrated significant RPE disruption, CC necrosis, and BM disruption (38).

There have been a number of studies with argon laser on cynomologus monkeys, whose fovea is similar to the human fovea. Smiddy et al. placed a 13-spot burn in the juxtafoveal region of a cynomologus monkey with argon green laser and examined the histopathological effects at 1 and 7 days. They used a 200-micron spot size, 0.2-s duration, and power between 100 and 200 mW. The desired reaction was a laser burn that turned the retina light gray. At day 1, the ganglion cell layer was partially preserved but all deeper layers were necrotic with RPE hyperplasia. At day 7, there was disruption of the retina up to the ganglion cell layer (39). In a second study, Smiddy et al. demonstrated that the RPE undergoes cellular proliferation after argon laser (40). Peyman et al. examined the histopathological effects of argon blue-green laser to the parafoveal area of cynomologus monkeys. They used a 100-micron spot size, 0.1-s duration, and a power of 100 mW. At day 1, there was coagulative necrosis of the RPE, outer nuclear layer, and outer plexiform layer. The choroid was minimally affected. At days 12 and 21, glial tissue had replaced the outer retina. There was an inflammatory infiltrate and the RPE was hyperplastic. If the power was increased to 320 mW, the basement membrane was ruptured and choroidal hemorrhages developed (41). Coscas and Soubrane treated the parafoveal region of adult baboons with argon green laser and examined the light and electron microscopic changes at 1 h, 3 weeks, and 6 weeks. As in the above studies, they showed disruption of the outer retina, necrosis of the RPE, and a macrophage response. Depending on the laser settings, there was variable involvement of the choriocapillaris (42). In a review of macular photocoagulation, Swartz states, "The histologic characteristics of a moderate argon-green burn show a typical cone-shaped lesion sparing the inner retina" (43). The laser intensities of these studies exceed those in most human laser-to-drusen trials.

There have been no histopathological studies on human eyes examining the effects of laser on drusen. However, there have been a number of studies involving primates. Duvall and Tso applied argon-green laser directly to drusen in two eyes of a rhesus monkey and noted the light microscopic and ultrastructural characteristics of drusen resorption. At 0–2 days, there was outer-segment retinal disruption, RPE necrosis, and fibrin deposition. The drusen were still present. At 3–8 days, two types of macrophages were present. One type was in the outer retina and subretinal space and their appearance was consistent with blood-borne monocytes. The second type of macrophage contained cell processes that surrounded the drusen material. These cell processes were traced by serial sectioning to the pericytes of the choriocapillaris. At 9 days and beyond, there was resorption of the drusen. Blood-borne monocytes were densely packed in the subretinal space. The cell processes of the choroidal pericytes contained drusenoid material. The authors postulated that the fibrin deposition from the laser photocoagulation initiated a phagocytic response, which resulted in clearance of the drusen by choroidal pericytes. Perry et al. examined the choroidal microvascular response to argon laser in cats. They demonstrated activation of the endothelial cells in the choriocapillaris after laser photocoagulation (44). Della et al. treated a rhesus monkey with soft large drusen. They used an argon laser to apply a grid pattern in the macula. Six weeks after laser, the directly treated drusen had disappeared (45).

V. THEORIES ON DRUSEN REDUCTION AND CNV PREVENTION

Drusen disappearance after laser photocoagulation is clearly documented in the literature. (46–59). However, the mechanism of drusen disappearance is not well understood. Several theories have been proposed: (1) phagocytosis of drusen; (2) decreased deposits by removal of RPE; (3) release of soluble mediators; (4) thinning of Bruch's membrane; and (5) mechanical alteration of the structure of Bruch's membrane. It is clear from the above studies that argon laser induces an inflammatory response and the intensity of the reaction depends on the laser settings. The laser settings in the studies, as well as the laser subjects, are variable, which makes interpretation difficult (6,37–40,42–44,48). Furthermore, in most of the clinical studies of laser to drusen, the calibrated intensity is minimal whitening. This is different from the above studies where stronger intensities where evaluated. However, despite these limitations, we can postulate that laser-induced phagocytosis of drusen occurs. Blood-borne inflammatory cells may ingest the drusen material. Studies certainly indicate their presence after laser. Duvall and Tso noted drusenoid material in cell processes after laser photocoagulation and attributed the origin of these cell processes to choroidal pericytes (48). Dysfunctional RPE, destroyed by laser, is replaced by proliferating RPE, (40). The RPE has phagocytic ability and the proliferating RPE may be involved in drusen resorption (52). Also, the removal of dysfunctional RPE cells may halt further drusen development and allow removal of accumulated material. After laser-induced tissue damage, the RPE and other cells may produce soluble mediators. For instance, Glaser et al. showed that RPE cells release an inhibitor of neovascularization (60). These soluble mediators may enhance the natural processes that result in spontaneous drusen resorption (3,61). They might also account for the observation that drusen distant from laser burns disappear after photocoagulation.

Bruch's membrane in AMD eyes is diffusely thickened and hydrophobic. The structural effect on BM by argon laser is variable. Thomas et al. showed that BM's integrity depended on the energy density of the laser (38). Photocoagulation may thin the abnormally thick BM and, in theory, improve its hydraulic conductivity. The increased metabolic transport could improve drusen clearance and decrease drusen formation. The laser could also exert a mechanical effect on BM, causing contraction of collagen and elastin (similar to laser trabeculoplasty) and improving egress of material through a more permeable BM. Peyman et al. showed that photocoagulation may improve perioxidase diffusion from the vitreous to the choroid (62).

Similar to drusen reduction, it is unclear how laser to drusen might prevent CNV. Some of the same theories on the mechanism of drusen reduction apply to CNV prevention. Improved transport of nutrients across BM might reduce the metabolic strain on the RPE/outer retina and stop the production of angiogenic factors from the RPE. Indeed, laser might even induce the production of vasoinhibitory growth factors from the RPE. Gass postulated that laser "tacks" down the RPE to BM, eliminating a potential cleavage plane for CNV (3). Proliferating RPE, induced by the laser, may envelop early CNV and prevent further growth.

VI. UNCONTROLLED STUDIES AND CASE REPORTS

Since Gass described the disappearance of drusen after laser photocoagulation, a number of case reports and uncontrolled clinical studies have examined the prophylactic treatment of drusen. Cleasby et al. treated 29 eyes in patients with "exudative senile maculopathy (ESM)" in the fellow eye. They treated one eye of 25 patients with "nonexudative senile maculopathy (NSM)" in both eyes. They defined NSM as the presence of drusen, retinal pigment atrophy, and clumping and/or cholesterol deposits in the macula in individuals older than 50. They used the argon laser to directly treat drusen "within a broad ring around the fovea." The desired intensity was a minimally visible reaction in the retina. The laser parameters were a spot size of 50–100 microns, power between 100 and 150 mW, and duration of 0.05–0.1 s. The number of applications was approximately 200–300 shots. In the group of 29 patients with ESM in one eye, three developed ESM in the treated eye over an average follow-up of 28.4 months. This represented a 4.4% yearly rate of ESM formation, which is less than the natural history of AMD. In the NSM group, neither the control eyes nor the treated eyes developed ESM over an average follow-up of 27.3 months. All 25 treated eyes and five control eyes showed a reduction in drusen. There were no reported complications from the laser (47). Despite a small number of patients, no control group for the ESM eyes, and no randomization for NSM eyes, this study suggested prophylactic laser to drusen might be beneficial.

Wetzig treated 42 eyes of 27 patients with prophylactic laser in a retrospective, nonrandomized study. All patients had macular soft drusen and recent visual changes (visual loss or metamorphopsia). The vision ranged from 20/20 to 20/400. Only 25% of eyes had a best-corrected prelaser visual acuity of 20/40 or better. The mean age at treatment was 69 years. Eyes with CNV or hemorrhagic/exudative changes were excluded. Thirty-one eyes were treated with krypton red laser, one eye with a combination of xenon and krypton, eight eyes with argon laser, and two eyes with a combination of argon and krypton laser. Both eyes were treated in some patients and several eyes were retreated. The desired intensity of the laser reaction was a faint, white-gray spot. The spots, approximately 50–75, were applied in a scatter pattern around the fovea. The vision improved, remained stable, or worsened by one line in 22 eyes (52%) over an average follow-up of 3.7 years. Twelve percent developed choroidal neovascularization. The drusen disappeared in these treated eyes, usually beginning at 3 months (58). Wetzig published a follow-up of these patients 6 years after the original publication. The average follow-up time was 120 months. Thirty-three percent of the treated eyes remained stable or lost one line of visual acuity, 21% lost two to three lines, and 46% lost three or more lines. Twenty-one percent of treated eyes developed CNV during the follow-up and several patients developed progressive enlargement of the treatment scars. There was no control group but seven eyes with drusen were untreated. In this untreated group, three eyes retained 20/40 or better visual acuity, two eyes lost two or more lines, and two eyes worsened to 20/400 or less. This study was limited, as it was a retrospective, nonrandomized study with a small number of eyes. Also, it included many patients with poor vision and selected patients with visual symptoms. These patients may have harbored subtle occult CNV. Overall, this study did not show a clear beneficial effect of prophylactic laser (59).

Figueroa et al. treated 20 patients with argon laser. Group 1 consisted of 14 patients with bilateral drusen. One eye was randomly assigned to receive laser treatment. Group 2 consisted of six patients with CNV in one eye and drusen in the fellow eye. The ages ranged from 55 to 80 years and the average follow-up was 18 months. Drusen temporal to the fovea were directly treated with the argon green laser at a power of 100 mW, duration of 0.1 s, and spot size of 100 microns. The desired laser intensity was calibrated to achieve a light gray-white lesion. The mean number of laser spots was 30. Treated drusen disappeared at approximately 2 months while surrounding, untreated drusen disappeared at a mean of 10 months. Visual acuity improved in 30% of eyes by one line or more. This was secondary to the resorption of untreated subfoveal drusen. The visual acuity remained unchanged in 65% of eyes and decreased in 5% (one eye). The one eye that worsened developed a choroidal neovascular membrane away from the laser scars (49). Figueroa et al. updated these results and presented new data in a second publication (50). The laser settings were the same as described above. All treated drusen disappeared at an average of 3.5 months. In all but three patients, the untreated drusen resolved at an average of 8.6 months. The drusen disappearance progressed in a temporal-to-nasal direction. Superonasal drusen persisted the longest time. Two of the 30 control eyes in Group 1 (bilateral drusen) demonstrated spontaneous drusen resolution. After an average of 3 years, one control eye and no treated eyes developed a choroidal neovascular membrane. Three fellow eyes (18%) in Group 2 developed CNV. In one eye, the CNV developed adjacent to the laser scars. Again, it was difficult to draw any conclusions from this study because of the small numbers. But, despite drusen resorption, the laser prophylaxis did not appear to prevent CNV in Group 2.

Sarks et al. treated 18 eyes of 16 patients with bilateral drusen and one eye of 10 patients with exudative changes in the other eye. Patients were 55 years or older and followed for a mean of 16.8 months. Inclusion criteria included visual acuity 20/40 or better and no evidence of atrophy or CNV. A ring of 40–50 nonconfluent laser burns was applied approximately 1500 microns from the foveal center. Drusen were not directly targeted. The argon green laser settings were a spot size of 100 microns, duration from 0.05 to 0.1 s, and a power calibrated to produce "a barely discernible whitening of the RPE." In 14 of the 16 patients with bilateral drusen, only one eye was treated. In these treated eyes, the vision remained stable in 10 eyes and improved in four eyes. The vision decreased in four eyes and remained stable in 10 eyes in the untreated group. Overall, in the two treated groups, visual acuity improved in 12 eyes (40%), remained unchanged in 16 eyes (53%) and worsened in two eyes (7%). Visual improvement was secondary to foveal drusen resorption, which occurred in all treated eyes and not at all in the untreated eyes. Two treated patients developed choroidal neovascular membranes. They developed at 7 and 8 months in retina adjacent to laser burns. Expansion of laser-induced atrophy was minimal in this study (57).

Guymer et al. treated one eye of 12 patients at high risk for visual loss secondary to AMD. All 12 treated eyes demonstrated macula drusen and visual acuity of 20/40 or better. Ten patients had end-stage lesions in one eye and two patients had bilateral soft confluent drusen. Twelve laser spots were placed in a ring 750–1000 microns from the fovea. The argon green laser settings were a spot size of 200 microns, duration of 0.2 s, and power calibrated to achieve faint blanching of the RPE (80–300 mW). The average follow-up was 16 months. Visual acuity remained the same or improved in 11 patients. Nine of the 11 patients had a reduction in drusen size, number, and confluence. One patient lost four lines secondary to CNV membrane development. This membrane did not originate from a laser site. Two patients developed profound atrophy at the laser site and four others developed RPE pigmentary changes at the laser sites. This study showed that a small number of laser applications could promote drusen disappearance. It also showed no correlation between resolution of drusen and improvement or deterioration of dark-adapted retinal thresholds (54).

Sigelman published a case report of a 58-year-old woman with a diskiform scar secondary to AMD in the right eye and confluent soft drusen in the left eye. The patient's vision dropped to 20/40 with metamorphopsia in the left eye. There was no CNV but an increased density and size of foveal drusen. Using a wavelength of 576 nm (yellow), power of 180 mW, duration of 0.3 s, and spot size of 200 microns, he directly treated drusen and also applied a parafoveal grid for a total of 56 spots. Treated and untreated drusen disappeared and the vision returned to 20/20 1 year after treatment (63).

VII. CONTROLLED STUDIES

Information from the above studies confirmed that laser can promote drusen reduction. However, the visual benefit of prophylactic laser was not proven. These reports do not provide enough evidence to support laser treatment in eyes with drusen outside the context of a clinical trial. Frennesson and Little conducted small randomized trials. The Choroidal Neovascularization Prevention Trial (CNVPT) is the largest clinical trial to date. These studies are described below.

Frennesson and Nilsson conducted a randomized, prospective study of prophylactic laser treatment (51). One eye of 13 patients with bilateral soft drusen was treated. In a second group, the fellow eye of six patients with a diskiform lesion in the other eye was treated. The control group consisted of 19 patients who had been randomized to observation. The groups were matched for age and visual acuity but there were more men in the treatment group. The visual acuity in all treated eyes was 20/25 or better. Patients with macular pigment clumping, atrophy, pigment epithelial detachments, or exudative AMD were excluded. A horseshoe-shaped grid pattern with direct drusen treatment as well as scatter treatment was applied with argon green laser. Laser parameters were a spot size of 200 microns, duration of 0.05 s, and power of 100–200 mW. The number of laser spots varied from 51 to 154. The intensity was calibrated to achieve a "grayish reaction." Drusen area on color fundus photographs and fluorescein angiograms was calculated at baseline and follow-up for both groups. Follow-up results were published at 6 months, 12 months, and 3 years (51–53). The mean drusen area significantly decreased in the treated eyes and significantly increased in the control eyes. Over 3 years, five eyes (33%) in the control group developed CNV, while no eyes did in the treatment group. This study demonstrated that laser treatment promotes drusen resorption, which had also been shown in the above studies. Importantly, it suggested that laser prophylaxis might prevent the exudative complications of AMD. However, as with the above studies, the sample size was small and the confidence interval large, which made it difficult to draw valid conclusions (53).

Little et al. randomized one eye of 27 patients with bilateral confluent soft drusen to prophylactic treatment. The mean age of patients was 69.7 years. The minimal visual acuity was 20/60 and the mean follow-up time 3.2 years. Foveal atrophy, pigment epithelial detachments, and exudative changes were exclusionary criteria. Drusen were directly treated. Laser settings for the dye laser (577–620 nm) were a spot size of 100–200 microns, power of 100–200 mW (calibrated to induce a slight lightening of the RPE/outer retina), and duration of 0.05–0.1 s. No laser spots were applied within 300 microns of the foveal center and rarely within 500 microns. Twenty-three to 526 laser spots were applied. Thirty-seven percent of eyes were treated with more than one session. Six treated eyes and no control eyes improved (2) or more lines. Sixteen treated and 17 control eyes remained stable. Five treated and 10 control eyes lost two or more lines. Drusen resorption within 1500 microns of the fovea occurred "more completely" in the treated eyes than control eyes in 22 eyes. In five eyes of both groups, there was equal drusen disappearance. Four control patients and two treated patients developed CNV. Laser scar enlargement occurred in three eyes. It was again difficult to draw conclusions from this study because of a small sample size but visual acuity and drusen resorption were significantly better in the treated eyes (56).

The Choroidal Neovascularization Prevention Trial is the largest pilot study to date to examine the potential treatment benefit of laser to drusen (46,55,64). A total of 156 patients without exudative AMD and with 10 or more large drusen (>63 microns) in each eye were enrolled in the Bilateral Drusen Study and 120 patients with exudative AMD in one eye and with 10 or more large drusen in the other eye were enrolled in the Fellow Eye Study through 16 clinical studies across the United States. Both eyes of patients enrolled in the Bilateral Drusen Study and the eye without exudative AMD of patients enrolled in the Fellow Eye Study were study eyes. The primary criterion for study eyes was 10 or more large (>63 microns) drusen within 3000 microns of the center of the foveal avascular zone. Study eyes also had to have visual acuity of 20/40 or better and no evidence of current or past CNV and progressive ocular disease. Patients had to be 50 years of age or older. In addition, the nonstudy eye of patients enrolled in the Fellow Eye Study had to have evidence of current or past exudative AMD defined as CNV or pigment epithelial detachment. Each patient underwent fluorescein angiography to exclude CNV in the study eye at baseline. The Bilateral Drusen Study included 312 eye of 156 patients and the Fellow Eye Study included 120 eyes of 120 patients. Fifty-nine of the eyes in the Fellow Eye Study were assigned to laser treatment and 61 were assigned to observation (65).

Patients enrolled in the Bilateral Drusen Study had one eye randomized to laser treatment and the other eye served as a control eye. Patients enrolled in the Fellow Eye Study had that eye randomly assigned to either the laser treatment group or the control group. The primary laser protocol, Laser 20, comprised the vast majority of treatments (85%). Laser 20 specified that 20 laser burns, 100 microns in diameter, be placed in a pattern of three rows between 12 o'clock and 6 o'clock beyond the temporal perimeter of the fovea. The burns forming the innermost row were to be placed no closer than 750 microns from the foveola. The duration of each burn was to be 0.1 s with the goal of creating a light gray-white lesion. Direct application of laser burns over drusen was avoided whenever possible without deviating substantially from the desired pattern of burns (Figs. 1–5). At 6 months after the initial treatment, a second laser treatment of 20 burns would be placed on the nasal side of the fovea in a mirror-image pattern to the first treatment if there had been less than a 50% reduction in the amount of drusen present within 3000 microns of the foveola (65) (Fig. 6A and B).

The primary outcome of the study was visual acuity. The incidence of late AMD complications such as CNV, changes in contrast threshold, and change in critical print size for reading were secondary outcomes. The development of CNV after baseline was con-

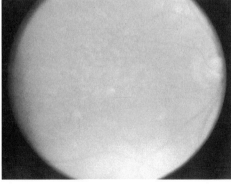
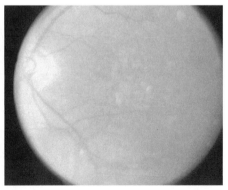

A   B

Figure 1 Baseline color fundus photographs of a patient with (A) age-related macular degeneration and (B) bilateral drusen. Visual acuity is 20/30 OU. Multiple, soft, confluent drusen are noted. See also color insert, Fig. 18.1A, B.

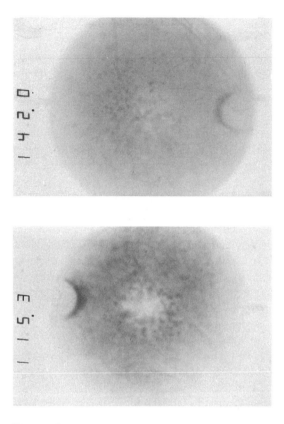

Figure 2   Baseline recirculation phase fluorescein angiography images of the right and left eye show some drusen staining, but no evidence of choroidal neovascularization.

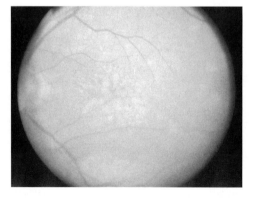

Figure 3   The left eye is randomized to low-intensity laser treatment. Twenty gray-white laser spots are placed in temporal arc in the macula. The laser spots are subtle. See also color insert, Fig. 18.3.

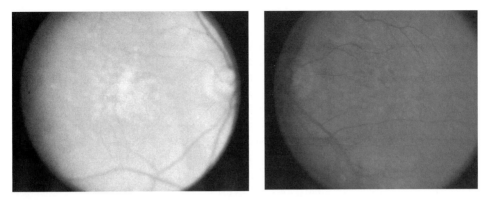

Figure 4 Six-month color fundus photographs show no significant change in drusen in either eye. Visual acuity remains 20/30 OU. See also color insert, Fig. 18.4.

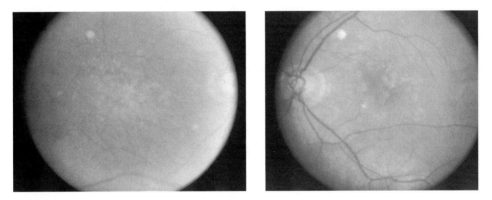

Figure 5 Twelve-month color fundus photographs show marked resolution of drusen in the treated left eye. The right eye remains stable with no significant change in dursen. Visual acuity is 20/30 OD and 20/20 OS. See also color insert, Fig. 18.5.

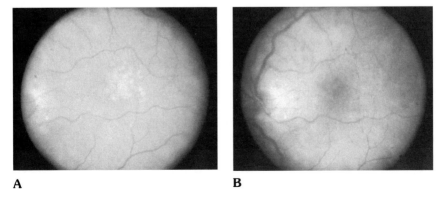

A   B

Figure 6 (A) Baseline fundus photograph demonstrating multiple, large drusen. The eye was treated with 20 laser spots in the temporal macula per the CNVPT protocol. (B) Six months later there is significant drusen reduction and the vision has changed from 20/32 to 20/25. See also color insert, Fig. 18.6A, B.

sidered as having occurred only when there was evidence of dye leakage on fluorescein angiography. Changes in drusen characteristics also were assessed through a comparison of photographs taken at baseline and the particular follow-up visit under consideration. These comparisons were performed to determine whether the total area of drusen was the same as, more, or less than at baseline and whether there were new areas of drusen or areas of drusen that had disappeared. Each eye was also graded for reduction of 50% or more in the area of drusen relative to baseline (65).

The CNVPT protocol specified that eyes assigned to treatment be retreated at 6 months if the area of drusen had not decreased by 50% from baseline. At 6 months, 28% of 78 eyes in the Bilateral Drusen Study and 41% of 37 eyes in the Fellow Eye Study had a 50% reduction in drusen and were exempt from retreatment. By 12 months, 54% of 35 eyes in the Bilateral Drusen Study and 27% of 11 in the Fellow Eye Study had a 50% reduction. One eye in the observed group had a 50% reduction in drusen area. Less than 10% of treated eyes and more than 90% of observed eyes showed no reduction in the area of drusen at 12 months (46).

Recruitment was halted for both the Bilateral Drusen Study and the Fellow Eye Study because of increased rates of CNV formation in the Fellow Eye Study. In the Fellow Eye Study, there were 10 treated eyes and two observed eyes with CNV development ($p = 0.02$). In the Bilateral Drusen Study, there were four treated eyes and two observed eyes that developed CNV ($p = 0.69$) (46). The estimated cumulative proportion of eyes with CNV in each treatment group was calculated. For eyes in the Bilateral Drusen Study, the estimated percentage of eyes with CNV at 1 year was 5% in the treated group and 2% in the observed group ($p = 0.42$). The relative risk estimate was 2.00 (95% confidence interval: 0.37, 10.96). For eyes in the Fellow Eye Study, the estimated percentage of eyes with CNV at 1 year was 24% in the treated group and 2% in the observed group ($p = 0.02$). The relative risk estimate was 4.86 (95% confidence interval: 1.10, 21.57). Thus, although a statistically significant imbalance of CNV between treatment and observed groups was noted for the Fellow Eye Study, this was not the case for the Bilateral Drusen Study (64).

The simultaneous influence of selected baseline covariates and treatment group on the incidence of CNV was examined with the Cox proportional hazards model. The intensity of the laser burns applied at baseline and 6 months had been graded for 74% of the eyes assigned to laser treatment. Eleven of these eyes had developed CNV. Four of the 11 eyes had burns graded as below the intensity standard. The other seven eyes had laser burns graded as meeting the intensity standard. From this information, laser intensity as determined in the CNVPT did not seem to have a significant effect on the development of CNV. Patient age, gender, hypertension status, aspirin use, vitamin and mineral supplement usage, cigarette smoking history, drusen number and size, and presence of focal hyperpigmentation were also examined. None of the factors other than treatment group had a significant effect on the incidence of CNV (65).

Only one (7%) of the 14 eyes assigned to treatment that developed CNV had a lesion with a purely classic pattern of fluorescein leakage on angiography; this eye had a lesion < 1 disk area that appeared to emanate from a treatment burn. The majority of eyes, laser treated or control, that developed CNV revealed at least some occult pattern of leakage (Fig. 7A and B). At the time the CNV was first documented, three (21%) of the 14 eyes assigned to treatment had subfoveal involvement and nine (90%) of the 10 eyes for which location could be determined accurately had CNV within the general area of laser treatment. All but one of the eyes in the group assigned to treatment had been treated under the Laser

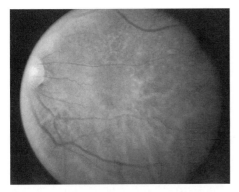

A

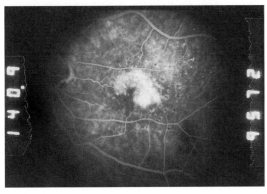

B

Figure 7 (A) Color fundus photograph 6 months after CNVPT laser treatment showing submacular fluid and the visual acuity has dropped from 20/20 to 20/60. (B) Fluorescein angiography shows a fibrovascular pigment epithelial detachment. See also color insert, Fig. 18.7A.

20 protocol. Three of the four eyes that developed CNV in the group assigned to observation had subfoveal involvement (64).

Because follow-up of patients in the CNVPT remains limited beyond 1 year, only preliminary information regarding visual acuity and change in visual acuity are available. In the Bilateral Drusen Study, there was little change in the distribution of visual acuity through 12 months. In the Fellow Eye Study, the proportion of observed eyes with 20/20 or better visual acuity decreased over follow-up time, while the proportion of such eyes in the treated group remained relatively stable.

The distributions of the change in visual acuity at follow-up examinations through 18 months were examined. There were no substantial differences between treated and untreated eyes in the Bilateral Drusen Study at any of the follow-up times. The eyes in the Fellow Eye Study showed a different pattern. There was a higher percentage of eyes with a decrease in visual acuity in the group assigned to observation at 12 and 18 months. The difference achieved nominal statistical significance ($p = 0.02$) at 18 months. The reasons for the loss of two or more lines of visual acuity at 18 months for the six observed eyes were investigated. Two of the eyes had increased pigment, nongeographical atrophy, or drusen; and one each developed CNV, was classified ineligible at baseline because of geographical atrophy within 500 microns of the foveal center, or had a drusenoid pigment epithelial detachment. No reason for the loss in visual acuity could be identified for one eye. Four of the eyes in the Fellow Eye Study assigned to treatment that developed CNV had not yet had additional follow-up after the CNV was noted and only two had 12 months of follow-up.

Interestingly, a comparison of eyes with laser-induced drusen reduction to eyes without drusen reduction showed that eyes with drusen reduction had modest improvements of visual acuity at 1 year (55). These preliminary results do not justify laser treatment of drusen, particularly since eyes that developed CNV were excluded from this analysis, but they certainly are intriguing early observations. Longer follow-up is required.

With the efforts of 16 clinical centers from around the country, the CNVPT Study Group has enrolled 276 patients. The increased incidence of CNV in laser-treated eyes of the Fellow Eye Study prompted the halting of new recruitment in December 1996. Follow-up will continue to determine whether the relative rates of CNV in laser-treated and control eyes will change or remain consistent with the preliminary data described above. Most importantly, these patients will be followed to determine long-term visual results.

The initial increased incidence of CNV in laser-treated eyes in the Fellow Eye Study is intriguing. Although fellow eyes are known to be at a higher risk for development of CNV than eyes with bilateral drusen, the results thus far with laser treatment were unexpected. Interestingly, fellow eyes and bilateral drusen eyes were similar from the standpoint of clinical fundus features as measured in the CNVPT. It may be that some of the fellow eyes harbored undetected CNV, which was then stimulated by laser photocoagulation. We did not perform indocyanine green (ICG) angiography in this study, although recent reports have suggested that eyes with drusen may demonstrate plaque lesions that go on to frank CNV (66). Fellow eyes may represent a group of patients with more advanced AMD who are less amenable to prophylaxis, as suggested by Sarks et al. (20,57). Other groups have specifically targeted macular drusen with laser treatment while the CNVPT treatment strategy resulted in laser treatment between and sometimes directly on drusen. It is possible that differences in laser intensity or laser treatment strategy could account for the increased rate of CNV observed in the CNVPT Fellow Eye Study.

VIII. COMPLICATIONS

The above studies showed that prophylactic laser to drusen can be associated with CNV and atrophy. Furthermore, Hyver et al. reported the development of a granular subfoveal material after laser photocoagulation. The patient had CNV in one eye and large, confluent soft drusen in the fellow eye. Twenty-four burns were placed in the temporal macula. There was no direct drusen treatment. The burn intensity was calibrated to create barely visible whitening. Using a 630-nm wavelength, the setting was a power of 200 mW, duration of 0.05 s and spot size of 200 microns. Ten months after treatment the visual acuity had dropped from 20/25 to 20/60 and there was a granular subfoveal material. There was no CNV on fluorescein angiography (67). The Drusen Laser Study reported seven eyes that developed CNV after laser photocoagulation for drusen. No control eyes in this randomized, controlled trial developed CNV (68). Brancato et al. reported a case of CNV that developed 7 months after prophylactic laser to drusen. The patient had a baseline fluorescein

(FA) and (ICG) angiography. The FA had no CNV but the ICG showed a suspicious one-disk area of hyperfluorescence. The drusen temporal to the fovea were directly treated with krypton red laser. At 7 months, the patient's vision dropped secondary to an occult CNV by fluorescein angiography. The ICG showed a two-disk-area plaque of hyperfluorescence whose border corresponded to the lesion observed on the baseline ICG. The laser was felt to have possibly exacerbated an underlying occult CNV (66). Indeed, laser photocoagulation is used to induce experimental CNV (69). Seven days after krypton photocoagulation to the posterior fundus of rats, Pollack et al. showed full-thickness defects in BM. It was unclear whether laser photocoagulation or cellular processes caused the defects (70). Regardless, full-thickness breaks are associated with CNV development.

IX. FUTURE DEVELOPMENTS

Because the randomized results from the CNVPT Bilateral Drusen Study and the results from the other groups suggest no harm and possibly even visual benefit, the CNVPT Study Group is planning a definitive trial of laser treatment in patients with bilateral drusen. At this time, our inability to manage exudative AMD effectively and the potential public health impact of a prophylactic therapy for AMD are very compelling reasons to continue to investigate this potential therapy. It is estimated that a 33% reduction of the rate of development of CNV in patients with bilateral drusen could halve the rate of bilateral blindness in this population (4).

The Complications of Age-Related Macular Degeneration Prevention Trial (CAPT), a National Eye Institute sponsored clinical trial, will enroll 1000 patients with bilateral drusen and assign one eye of each patient to light laser photocoagulation and the other eye to observation. Approximately 24 clinical centers around the United States will participate to determine the value of this therapy. As in the CNVPT, visual acuity will be the primary outcome of interest.

X. SUMMARY

A prophylactic treatment for AMD is highly desirable and would have significant public health impact. Laser photocoagulation to eyes with large drusen can induce dissolution of drusen. Although the optimal laser delivery characteristics are not known, lower intensity laser is preferred. Laser-induced drusen reduction may effect modest improvements in visual function.

The overall value of laser to drusen still requires study within the context of well-designed clinical trials. We need to evaluate results from definitive clinical trials before we can routinely recommend laser to drusen for our patients.

REFERENCES

1. Kini M. et al. Prevalance of senile cataract, diabetic retinopathy, senile macular degeneration and open-angle glaucome in the Framingham Eye Study. Am J Ophthalmol 1978;85:28–34.
2. Leibowitz H, et al. The Framingham Eye Study monograph. Surv Ophthalmol 1980;24:335–610.

3. Gass JD Drusen and disciform macular detachment and degeneration. Arch Ophthalmol 1973;90(3):206–217.

4. Lanchoney DM, Maguire MG., Fine, SL. A model of the incidence and consequences of choroidal neovascularization secondary to age-related macular degeneration. Comparative effects of current treatment and potential prophylaxis on visual outcomes in high-risk patients. Arch Ophthalmol 1998;116(8):1045–102.

5. Bok D Retinal photoceptor-pigment epithelium interactions. Invest Ophthalmol Vis Sci 1985;26:1659–1694.

6. Marshall J. Interactions between sensory cells, glial cells and the retinal pigment epithelium and their response to photocoagulation. Dev Ophthalmol 1981;2:308–317.

7. Young R. The daily rhythm of shedding the degradation of rod and cone outer segment membranes in the chick retina. Invest Ophthalmol Vis Sci 1978;17:10–116.

8. Foulds W. The choroidal circulation and retinal metabolism: an overview. Eye 1990;4:242–248.

9. Loeffler KU Terminology of sub-RPE deposits: do we all speak the same language? Br J Ophthalmol 1998;82:1104–1105.

10. Group IAES. An international classification and grading system for age-related maculopathy and age-related macular degeneration. Surv Ophthalmol 1995;39:367–374.

11. Bressler NB, et al. Clinicopathologic correlation of drusen and retinal pigment epithelial abnormalities in age-related macular degeneration. Retina 1994;14:130–142.

12. Green W,R, Enger C. Age-related macular degeneration histopathologic studies: the 1992 Lorenz E. Zimmerman Lecture. Ophthalmology 1993;100:1519–1535.

13. Curcio C, Millican C. Basal linear deposit and large drusen are specific for early age-related maculopathy. Arch Ophthalmol 1999;117:329-339.

14. Russell S, et al. Location, substructure and composition of basal laminar drusen compared with drusen assoicated with aging and age-related macular degeneration. Am J Ophthalmol 2000;129:205-214.

15. Spraul C, Grossniklaus H. Characteristics of drusen and Bruch's membrane in postmortem eyes with age-related macular degeneration. Arch Ophthalmol 1997;115:267–283.

16. van der Schaft T, et al. Is basal laminar deposit unique for age-related macular degeneration. Arch Ophthalmol 1991;109:420–425.

17. Farkas T, Syvlester V, Archer D. The ultrastructure of drusen. Am J Ophthalmol 1971;71:1196–1205.

18. Farkas T, et al. The histochemistry of histochemistry of drusen. Am J Ophthalmol 1971;71:1206–1215.

19. Mullins R, Johnson L, Anderson D. Characterization of drusen-associated glycoconjugates. Ophthalmology 1997;104:288–294.

20. Sarks J, Sarks S, Killingsworth M. Evolution of soft drusen in age-related macular degeneration. Eye 1994;8:269–283.

21. Ishibashi T, et al. Pathogenesis of drusen in the primate. Invest Ophthalmol Vis Sci 1986;27:184–193.

22. Ishibashi T, et al. Formation of drusen in the human eye. Am J Ophthalmol 1986;101: 342–353.

23. MJ H. Role of the retinal pigment epithelium in macular disease. Trans Am Acad Ophthalmol Otolarnygol 1972;76:64–80.

24. Feeney-Burns L Ellerisieck M. Age-related changes in the ultrastructure of Bruch's membrane. Am J Ophthalmol 1985;100:686–697.

25. Pauleikhoff D, et al. Correlation between biochemical composition and fluorescein binding of deposits in Burch's membrane. Ophthalmology 1992;99:1548–1553.

26. Moore D, Hussain A, Marshall J. Age-related variation in the hydraulic conductivity of Bruch's membrane. Invest Ophthalmol Vis Sci 1995;36:1290–1297.

27. Pauleikhoff D, et al. Aging changes in Bruch's membrane: histochemical and morphologic study. Ophthalmology 1990;97:171–178.

28. Zarbin M. Age-related macular degeneration: review of pathogenesis. Eur J Ophthalmol 1998;8:199–206.

29. Smiddy W, Fine S. Prognosis of patients with bilateral macular drusen. Ophthalmology 1984;91:271–277.

30. Holz F, et al. Bilateral macular drusen in age-related macular degeneration: prognosis and risk factors. Ophthalmology 1994;101:1522–1528.

31. Bressler SB, et al. Relationship of drusen and abnormalities of the retinal pigment epithelium to the prognosis of neovascular macular degeneration. The Macular Photocoagulation Study Group. Arch Ophthalmol 1990;108:1442–1447.

32. Risk factors for choroidal neovascularization in the second eye of patients with juxtafoveal or subfoveal choroidal neovascularization in the second eye of patients with juxtafoveal or subfoveal choroidal nevasularization secondary to age-related macular degeneration. Macular Photocoagulation Study Group. Arch Ophthalmol 1997;115(6):741–747.

33. Sandberg M, et al. High-risk characteristics of fellow eye of patients with unilateral neovascular age-related macular degeneration. Ophthalmology 1998;105:441–447.

34. Sarraf D, et al. Long-term drusen study. Retina 1999;19:513–519.

35. Mainster M Wavelength selection in macular photocoagulation. Ophthalmology 1986;93:952–958.

36. Peyman G Raichand M, Zeimer R. Ocular effects of various laser wavelenghts. Surv Ophthalmol 1984;28:391–404.

37. Smiddy W, et al. Clinicopathologic correlation of krypton red, argon blue-green, and argon green laser photocoagulation in human fundus. Retina 1984;4:1–21

38. Thomas E, et al. Histopathology and ultrastructure of krypton and argon laser lesions in a human retina-choroid. Retina 1984;4:22–39.

39. Smiddy W, et al. Comparson of krypton and argon laser photocoagulation. Arch Ophthalmol 1984;102:1086–1092.

40. Smiddy W et al. Cell proliferation after laser photocoagulation in primate retina. Arch Ophthalmol 1986;104:1065–1069.

41. Peyman G, et al. Fundus photocoagulation with the argon and krypton lasers: a comparative study. Ophthalm Surg 1981;12:481–490.

42. Coscas G, Soubrane G. The effects of red krypton and green argon laser on the foveal region. Ophthalmology 1983;90:1013–1022.

43. Swartz M Histology of macular photocoagulation. Ophthalmology 1986;93:99–963.

44. Perry D, Reddick R, Risco, J. Choroidal microvascular repair after argon laser photocoagulation. Invest Ophthalmol Vis Sci 1984;25:1019–1026.

45. Della N, et al. Clinical and pathologic effects of grid macular laser in aged primate eyes containing drusen. Invest Ophthalmol Vis Sci 1997;39(Suppl):S18.

46. Laser treatment in eyes with large drusen: short-term effects seen in a pilot randomized clinical trial. Choroidal Neovascularization Prevention Trail Research Group. Ophthalmology 1998;105(1):11–23.

47. Cleasby G, Nankanishi A, Norris J. Prophylactic photocoagulation of the fellow eye in exudative senile maculopathy. Mod Probl Ophthal 1979;20:141–147.

48. Duvall J, Tso, MO. Cellular mechanisms of resolution of drusen after laser coagulation; an experimental study. Arch Ophthalmol 1985;103(5):694–703.

49. Figueroa MS, Regueras A, Bertrand J. Laser photocoagulation to treat macular soft drusen in age-related macular degeneration. Retina 1994;14(5):391–396.

50. Figueroa MS, et al. Laser photocoagulation for macular soft drusen :updated results. Retina 1997;17(5):378–384.

51. Frennesson I, Nilsson S., Effects of argon (green) laser treatment of soft drusen in early age-related maculopathy: a 6 month prospective study. Br J Ophthalmol 1995;79:905–909.

52. Frennesson I,C, Nilsson SE. Laser photocoagulation of soft drusen in early age-related maculopathy (ARM). The one-year results of a prospective, randomised trial. Eur J Ophthalmol 1996;6(3):307–314.

53. Frennesson C Nilsson SE. Prophylactic laser treatment in early age related maculopathy reduced the incidence of exudative complications. Br J Ophthalmol 1998;82(10):1169–1174.

54. Guymer RH, et al. Laser treatment in subjects with high-risk clinical features of age-related macular degeneration: posterior pole appearance and retinal function. Arch Ophthalmol 1997;11(5):595–603.

55. Ho AC, et al. Laser-induced drusen reduction improves visual function at 1 year. Choroidal Neovascularization Prevention Trial Research Group [see comments]. Ophthalmology 1999;106(7):1367–1376; discussion 1374.

56. Little HL, Showman JM, Brown BW. A pilot randomized controlled study on the effect of laser photocoagulation of confluent soft macular drusen [see comments]. Ophthalmology 1997;104(4):623–631.

57. Sarks S, et al. Prophylactic perifoveal laser treatment of soft drusen. Aust Ophthalmol 1996;24:15–26.

58. Wetzig PC. Treatment of drusen-related aging macular degeneration by photocoagulation. Trans Am Ophthalmol Soc 1988;86:276–290.

59. Wetzig PC. Photocoagulation of drusen-related macular degeneration: a long-term outcome. Trans Am Ophthalmol Soc 1994;92:299–303.

60. Glaser B,Campochiaro, P, Davis, S. Retinal pigment epithelial cells release an inhibitor of neovascularization. Arch Ophthalmol 1985;103:1870–1875.

61. Bressler N, et al. Five-year incidence and disappearance of drusen and retinal pigment epithelial abnormalities; Waterman study. Arch Ophthalmol 1995;113:301–308.

62. Peyman G, Spitznas M, Straatsma B. Chorioretinal diffusion of perioxidase before and after photocogulation. Invest Ophthalmol Vis Sci 1971;10:489.

63. Sigelman J. Foveal drusen resorption one year after perifoveal laser photocoagulation. Ophthalmology 1991;98(9):1379–1383.

64. Choroidal neovascularization in the Choroidal Neovascularization Prevention Trial. The Choroidal Neovascularization Prevention Trial Research Group [see comments]. Ophthalmology 1998;105(8):1364–1372.

65. Ho A,C. Laser treatment in eyes with drusen. Curr Opin Ophthalmol 1999;10(3):204–208.

66. Brancato R, et al. Hyperfluorescent plaque lesions in the late phases of indocyanine green angiography: a possible contraindication to the laser treatment of drusen. Am J Ophthalmol 1997;124(4):554–557.

67. Hyver SW, et al. A case of visual acuity loss following laser photocoagulation for macular drusen [letter]. Arch Ophthalmol 1997;115(4):554-555.

68. Owens SL, et al. Fluorescein angiographic abnormalities after prophylactic macular photocoagulation for high-risk age-related maculopathy. Am J Ophthalmol 1999;127(6):681–687.

69. Miller H, et al. Pathogenesis of laser-induced choroidal subretinal neovascularization. Invest Ophthalmol Vis Sci 1990;31:899–908.

70. Pollack A, Heriot W, Henkind, P. Cellular processes causing defects in Burch's membrane following krypton laser photocoagulation. Ophthalmology 1986;93:1113–1119.

19

Treatment of Nonexudative Age-Related Macular Degeneration with Infrared (810 nm) Diode Laser Photocoagulation

Thomas R. Friberg

University of Pittsburgh, Pittsburgh, Pennsylvania

I. INTRODUCTION

When the retina is stimulated by light, the photopigments located within the outer segments of the retinal rod and cone cells release energy. These photopigments are maintained in a high-energy state so that when they are triggered by incident photons, further energy release occurs, which ultimately results in neuronal transmission of the stimulus along the visual pathways. Intense metabolic activity is necessary to keep the outer segments and the visual pigments functioning properly, and the by-products of this metabolism must be recycled. As photoreceptor outer segments contain high concentrations of polyunsaturated fats whose molecules are susceptible to photooxidative injury, the photoreceptors are subject to considerable damage over their lifetime.

With age, the recycling of spent photoreceptor debris becomes imperfect, partly because the enzymes within the retinal pigment epithelium (RPE) become less effective (1). Lipofuscin and other membranous debris then build up within or at the base of the RPE cells or are deposited as basal laminar material along Bruch's membrane (2) (Fig. 1). When these deposits are of sufficient size, they appear clinically as amorphous yellowish deposits beneath the sensory retina, which we call drusen (Fig. 2, left). If these deposits coalesce, their borders may appear fuzzy and indistinct, and they are then termed soft drusen (Fig. 2, right). The presence of macular drusen in an eye of an older adult is pathognomonic for the diagnosis of age-related macular degeneration (AMD). Drusen probably interfere with the nutrient exchange between the sensory retina, RPE, and choriocapillaris, leading to alterations in the photoreceptors and RPE, thereby promoting loss of vision. Clinical and epidemiological studies have clearly established that the presence of drusen in an eye is a significant risk factor for future visual loss from AMD, particularly from choroidal neovascularization (3).

Drusen range in size from a few microns to confluent patches hundreds or even thousands of microns in diameter, and may appear clinically as a localized detachment of the

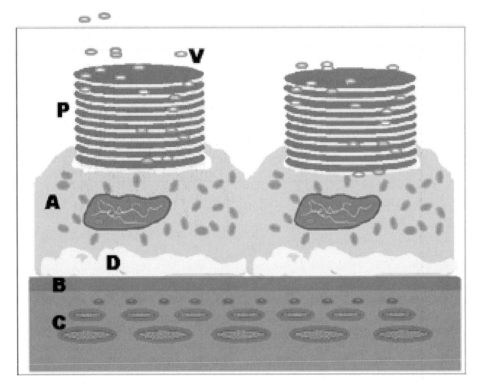

Figure 1   In this anatomical schematic diagram, retinal, pigment epithelial cells (A) must recycle debris produced by the photoreceptor outer segments (P) on which the visual pigments (V) reside. With aging, lipofusion and other membranous debris is deposited along Bruch's membrane (B) and at the base of the RPB cells, forming drusen (D). The choriocapillaris (C) lies below Bruch's membrane.

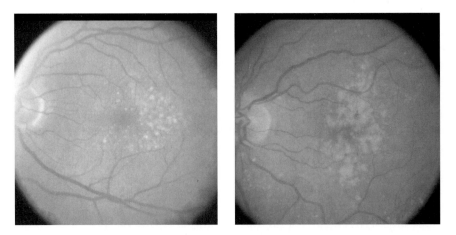

Figure 2   (Left) Fundus of an eye with many macular drusen of a variety of sizes. (Right) Fundus of another eye showing very large confluent drusen. See also color insert, Fig. 19.2.

RPE. Large subfoveal drusen often are associated with decreased visual acuity, diminished contrast sensitivity, impairment of color vision, and metamorphopsia.

Approximately 90% of the severe loss of visual function from macular degeneration occurs secondary to the subsequent development of choroidal neovascularization or exudative lesions. For patients over 65 years of age with drusen present in both eyes, the risk of developing severe visual loss is estimated to be about 18% over 3-years (3–5). Patients who have already had an exudative event in one eye are at an especially high risk of losing vision in the fellow eye; this risk approaches 60% over a 5-year period (6). Because of the risks associated with drusen, investigators have sought to improve the visual prognosis of eyes with dry age-related macular degeneration by using various potentially prophylactic measures. Vitamins, minerals, and other micronutrients may reduce the risks of blindness, but the positive impact of these does not appear striking (7,8). Plasmapheresis (9), or the removal of certain unwanted components from the blood, requires complex, expensive equipment, and has not been shown to be clinically efficacious in any large controlled study despite its promotion by some advocates. Finally, pharmacological approaches that seek to prevent choroidal neovascularization using antiangiogenic drugs are also under study.

Historically, laser photocoagulation has been observed to promote the resorption of drusen even when the laser lesions are placed some distance away from the drusen themselves. However, the precise mechanism of such drusen resolution remains elusive. Duvall and Tso (10) have postulated that laser photocoagulation induces pericytes from the underlying choriocapillaris to form phagocytes, which in turn remove the amorphous drusen debris. Other research suggests that local and circulating antibodies to certain drusen components may also play a role (11).

Until recently, virtually all the clinical studies regarding the prophylactic photocoagulation of eyes with drusen have dealt with small numbers of patients and were of a pilot nature. All used laser light in the visible spectrum, usually the argon and krypton wavelengths. For example, Wetzig (12) used moderate intensity argon or krypton lesions in 42 eyes and noted that drusen resorbed in about half of the eyes over a 3-year period. Cleasby et al. (13) suggested that such prophylactic laser treatment might prevent the development of choroidal neovascularization. A favorable effect on visual acuity was suggested by Frennesson and Nilsson (14), who showed a 50% reduction in drusen area at 12 months. Improved visual acuity after laser photocoagulation was also described by Figueroa et al. (15) and by Little et al. (16). Finally, Guymer et al. (17) demonstrated improved scotopic thresholds after laser photocoagulation of eyes with high-risk clinical features of AMD.

The safety and efficacy of laser treatment placed directly over the drusen themselves versus treatment of the RPE in their vicinity has been debated. Advocates of direct treatment argue that the RPE and underlying Bruch's membrane are thicker at the drusen site so that treatment at the drusen is less likely to induce choroidal neovascularization. Advocates of the 810-nm laser argue that very minimal lesions are clinically effective in inducing drusen absorption, even when lesions are placed in a grid without regard to precise drusen location.

II. PILOT STUDIES

A. Argon Laser Photocoagulation

The Choroidal Neovascularization Prevention Trial (CNVPT) used argon laser photocoagulation (18) to induce drusen disappearance. Patients were divided into two groups; bilaterally eligible patients were defined as those with at least 10 large drusen ($\geq$63 microns in diameter) in the macula of each eye and vision of 20/40 or better. In the unilateral (fellow eye) group, one eye had to have had a previous exudative event prior to entry into the study, so that only the remaining eye with multiple large drusen was eligible for randomization. The eye to be treated was randomly selected for a bilaterally eligible patient, while in the fellow eye group, the eligible eye was randomized to either observation or treatment. Treatment was performed using argon green laser photocoagulation with 100-micron spots placed in one of four separate patterns. The intensity of lesions varied from gray-white to white depending upon the treatment protocol selected. In most cases, a C-pattern located just temporal to the foveola was placed. If there was not an observable reduction of drusen of at least 50% at 6 months' time in the CNVPT, the eye typically was retreated with another C-pattern located nasal to the fovea to, in essence, completely surround the foveola with laser treatment.

After 1 year, the CNVPT study showed paradoxically that treated eyes in the fellow eye group unfortunately had a significantly higher incidence of choroidal neovascularization than observed eyes (16.9% vs 3.2%). Hence, the study was prematurely halted for safety reasons and the protocol and goals were reassessed. Ultimately, the study was relaunched as a larger randomized trial excluding patients who had, at entry, a diskiform process in one of their eyes. Thus, the fellow eye group of patients was excluded from further study.

B. Infrared (810 nm) Diode Laser Photocoagulation

Concurrently, a group of investigators was evaluating the use of 810-nm infrared laser to prophylactically treat eyes with drusen (19). Very importantly, this group also sought to study the effect of altering the intensity of the laser lesion at the time of treatment. Virtually no retinal photocoagulation studies had prospectively randomized laser lesion intensity to evaluate the effect of minimal versus more typical intensities on clinical outcomes.

1. Study Method

In the infrared diode pilot study, 29 eyes of 152 patients aged 50 years or older met the following inclusion criteria and were randomized: at least five large drusen ($\geq$63 microns in size) in the macula, no substantial geographic atrophy, or confounding ocular diseases, and best corrected visual acuity of 20/63 or better as measured on ETDRS acuity charts. Unilateral patients must have had a previous diskiform or exudative event in one of their eyes while the fellow eye met eligibility criteria (Fig. 3, left), whereas in bilateral patients, both eyes met all eligibility criteria (Fig. 3, right).

Randomization for the study was performed as follows: unilaterally eligible patients had their eligible eye randomized to either treatment or observation and bilaterally eligible patients had one of their eyes randomly selected for treatment with the other eye serving as a control. In all cases, laser treatment consisted of placement of 48 125-micron diameter spots in an annular pattern (Fig. 4) grouped to surround but to avoid the foveola. Retreatments were not allowed. Laser lesion intensity was itself randomized to either threshold or subthreshold levels. The threshold laser lesion protocol required the placement of 48 spots that were barely visible directly after placement whereas the subthreshold treatment protocol called for the use of clinically invisible lesions, which remained invisible even hours after placement. This was accomplished by creating a test laser lesion of 0.2 s duration outside of the macula and increasing the laser power from a minimal amount until the retinal

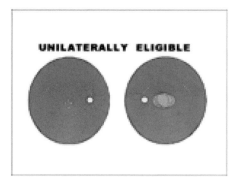 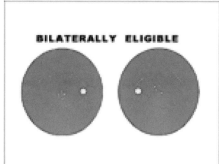

Figure 3 (Left) An eligible patient in the unilateral group has one eye affected by end-stage exudative AMD while the eligible eye has at least 5 drusen 63 microns in size or larger and visual acuity of 20/63 or better. (Right) A bilaterally eligible patient has 5 or more drusen ≥63 microns and 20/63 visual acuity or better in each eye.

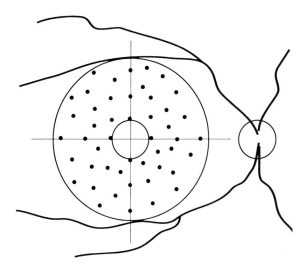

Figure 4 The placement of 48 125-micron laser lesions was done in a grid that surrounded the foveola whereby the lesions were placed in an annulus whose inside radius was one-half an optic disk diameter and whose outside radius was $1^{1}/_{2}$ disk diameters.

lesion could be just barely detected. Keeping the laser power settings constant, the duration of the laser pulse was decreased to 0.1 s, which halved the energy applied to produce the lesion. A subthreshold lesion resulted. These lesions could not be seen directly after treatment. However, they could be placed with reasonable accuracy by dividing the target area into four quadrants and then placing 12 lesions in each section of the treatment annulus. Clinical conformation of lesion placement could be confirmed by fluorescein angiography.

Table 1   PTAMD Pilot Results

	12-month follow-up: CNVM event rates combined	
	Observed	Subthreshold or visible treatment
Unilateral	17%	12%
Bilateral	2.7%	4.0%

	24-month follow-up: CNVM event rates combined	
	Observed	Subthreshold or visible treatment
Unilateral	27%	20%
Bilateral	4.6%	4.0%

	Percentage of diode-treated eyes developing choroidal neovascularization		
	Observation	Visible treatment	Subthreshold treatment
Group at 12 months			
Bilateral	2.7%	8.3%	0%
Unilateral	17%	12%	13%
Group at 24 months			
Bilateral	4.6%	9.7%	0%
Unilateral	27%	16%	27%

2. Results

Choroidal Neovascularization.   At 24 months, the infrared diode pilot study, showed no statistically significant difference in choroidal neovascular event rates in treated versus observed eyes in either the unilaterally eligible or bilaterally eligible patient groups (see Table 1). These results are in contrast to the increased risk of choroidal neovascularization found by the CNVPT study at 12 months in treated eyes of unilaterally eligible patients. The event rates for observed eyes in the unilaterally and bilaterally eligible patients were 27% and 4.6%, respectively, at 24 months. Hence, the risk of choroidal neovascularization was about six times greater in those patients who had already had a previous event in one of their eyes (unilateral group) compared to patients who had both eyes eligible at entry. Prophylactic diode laser treatment did not increase or decrease a patient's chances of developing an exudative event within the follow-up period of 24 months.

Drusen Disappearance.   A total of 43.6% of eyes treated with subthreshold lesions exhibited a 50% reduction in macular drusen area over 24 months compared to 62.3% of eyes treated with more intense (visible) threshold lesions. Overall, at 24 months, diode laser treatment resulted in a 50% reduction in drusen level in 68.3% of eyes compared to virtually no reduction (3.3%) in observed eyes over the same time period. As shown in Figure 5, it was apparent that more intense lesions led to more rapid resolution of drusen, whereas use of more gentle subthreshold spots also resulted in drusen resorption, but at a slower rate.

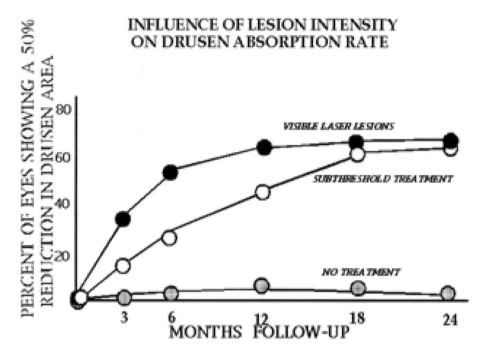

Figure 5 Graph showing the influence of the intensity of the laser lesions used and the time to 50% resolution of drusen area. Subthreshold 811-nm diode laser-treated patients require a longer time, on average, to achieve drusen resorption but at 24 months following treatment, the percentage of eyes showing substantial drusen resorption is similar, regardless of laser treatment intensity.

Visual Improvement.   Although changes in the clinical appearance of drusen can be striking after photocoagulation (Fig. 6), such changes have little relevance to the patient unless they are accompanied by improved visual acuity or reduction of risk of long-term visual loss. A subset of patients in the PTAMD pilot in whom two lines of improvement was possible (20/32–20/63 vision at entry) was analyzed at 24 months. A total of 15.4% of all treated eyes (18.2% of visual treated and 12.5% of subthreshold treated) enjoyed two lines of improvement after 2 years compared to 0% of observation eyes. In the bilateral study arm, 41 patients had initial acuity of 20/32–20/63 and 24.4% of these eyes showed two lines of improvement after treatment compared to 0% of fellow eyes. This visual improvement was statistically significant to the $p < 0.002$ level. These visual results are in harmony with results from several smaller studies that suggest a visual benefit to prophylactic laser treatment to eyes with drusen (15,16,20).

Theoretical Considerations.   The 810-nm-diode wavelength has certain properties that may make it a preferable choice over visible argon or krypton wavelengths for the treatment of drusen. The infrared laser may produce less blood–retinal barrier breakdown because of greater tissue penetration and less thermal disruption, particularly at lower energy levels (21). Pollack et al. (22) concluded that subclinical diode laser photocoagulation of the retina limits damage to the photoreceptors compared to more intense threshold lesions. However, some authors (22) have suggested that the placement of minimal intensity laser lesions is difficult to accomplish in a reproducible manner because of heterogeneity

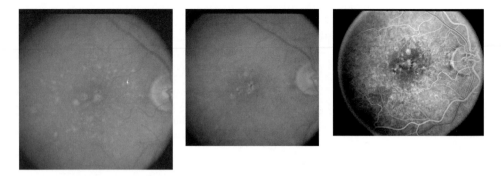

Figure 6 (Left) The right fundus of a patient with multiple, large macular drusen. (Center) Twelve months after treatment with subthreshold laser lesions, drusen resorption has been dramatic. (Right) Fluorescein angiogram of same eye 2 years after treatment. The subthreshold laser scars are virtually undetectable. See also color insert, Fig. 19.6 left and center.

in the RPE cells themselves. Funatsu et al. (23) suggested that diode laser photocoagulation produces a greater increase in preretinal oxygen partial pressure than argon laser photocoagulation, giving the former a theoretical advantage in preventing choroidal neovascularization. Whether or not these potential advantages have clinical relevance remain to be established.

III. PTAMD STUDY

Based on the pilot data, a large multicentered, randomized, controlled trial was initiated using only subthreshold 810-nm-diode laser lesions placed in a single treatment session. To date, approximately 600 patients have enrolled in this study, which is called Prophylactic Treatment of Age-Related Macular Degeneration (PTAMD) Trial. Endpoints being evaluated include choroidal neovascular event rates in both the bilateral and unilateral patient groups, alterations of drusen area and drusen distribution, and changes in best corrected visual acuity.

In designing a prophylactic study, the number of patients required to show potential efficacy is an important figure unlike a therapeutic trial when an intervention or placebo is randomly given to patients identified with a given disease. A prophylactic trial requires a larger patient population. That is, only a minority of patients with AMD would be expected to develop CNVM over a few years' time. Historical estimates can be used, but the data from an available pilot study are partially useful, if the pilot used essentially the same entry criteria and methodology. The choroidal neovascular membrane event rates at 24 months for the PTAMD pilot study are shown in Table 1. If we look only at observed eyes, the unilateral observed eyes had an event rate of 27% over 2 years, or approximately 15% per year; in the bilateral group, the rate was 4.6% over 2 years, or roughly 3% per year. If we then require a 95% confidence interval for detecting significant differences ($\alpha = 0.05$) and a power of 90% (90% confident that if we detect no difference that indeed no difference is present or B = 0.10), we can calculate the estimated number of patients needed in the PTAMD trial. Assume that a patient will be followed for 5 years and that prophylactic treatment reduces the CNVM by a modest 20%. We then would need approximately 200

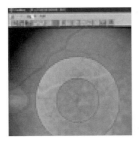
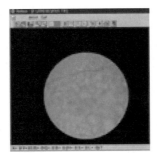
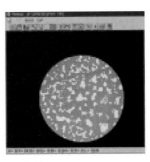

Figure 7 Using a drusen analysis software program, drusen located within the large circle (left) (alzer 1 ring) are selected for analysis and the area of regard is displayed (center). A drusen detection algorithm identifies and displays the drusen it found in false color (right). See also color insert, Fig. 19.7.

patients in the unilaterally eligible group and 2700 patients in the bilaterally eligible group to show such differences. Note that because the CNVM event rate for eyes having already had an exudative event is about six times higher than for an eye of a patient with drusen in both eyes, substantially fewer patients are needed to show treatment efficacy in unilaterally eligible patients. Hence, the continued inclusion of such patients in the PTAMD should facilitate obtaining results over a shorter period of time, in contrast to the CAPT study, which excludes such patients.

IV. FUTURE CONSIDERATIONS

Studies evaluating the effect of laser photocoagulation on drusen disappearance are somewhat hampered by imprecise methods of measuring the drusen themselves. Typically, the total area of drusen in the macula is not a criterion for entry into a study, because methodology to measure drusen area is either rudimentary or depends on the time-consuming placement of templates on images to calculate or measure drusen diameter. Difficulties are compounded by the presence of large geographic patches of confluent drusen. Hence, data relating to drusen disappearance should be considered to be gross estimates rather than objective and precise. Furthermore, the published risk of visual loss in eyes with drusen are projections based on rather gross categorizations of drusen size and extent. Eyes exhibiting even a single large drusen in the macula but far from the fovea have been grouped, in some studies, with eyes that harbor scores of large drusen in the posterior pole. The failure to quantitate drusen size, drusen area, and drusen location is potentially a serious flaw in virtually all clinical studies on the subject, whether the study evaluated the effects of photocoagulation on eyes with drusen or whether it calculated visual loss risk data as a function of the presence of drusen. Automated methods of drusen categorization may make such studies more quantitative and less subjective (Fig. 7).

V. SUMMARY

The presence of drusen in an eye is a significant risk factor for future visual loss from AMD, and in particular from choroidal neovascularization. Prophylactic infrared laser using an 810-nm-diode laser was placed in a grid pattern of 48 spots at a single session to promote drusen disappearance in a prospective randomized pilot study. In the pilot diode laser study, the intensity of laser lesions to be used in a patient's eye was randomized to either threshold (barely visible after placement) or subthreshold (not clinically visible) treatment. At 24 months, there was no significant difference in choroidal neovascular event rates between treated and observed eyes, whether the patient was treated with threshold or subthreshold laser intensity.

In contrast to a similar large pilot study that used argon laser treatment to promote drusen disappearance, diode laser treatment did not lead to significantly higher choroidal neovascular membrane event rates in any patient group. Threshold laser lesions led to a more rapid disappearance of drusen than lighter, subthreshold lesions but both were effective. Overall, diode laser treatment resulted in a 50% reduction of drusen levels in 68% of treated eyes at 24 months.

A total of 15% of patients in the pilot study who had initial visual acuity between 20/32 and 20/63 showed at least two lines of visual acuity improvement after diode laser treatment. A large multicenter randomized study, the Prophylactic Treatment of Age-Related Macular Degeneration (PTAMD), is underway to determine the potential long-term benefits of 810-nm subthreshold laser treatment for patients who have dry AMD and multiple drusen.

REFERENCES

1. Friberg TR. Macular degeneration and its possible relationship to the microcirculation. In: Weinreb RN, Joyner WL, Wheeler LA, eds. Biology of the Ocular Microcirculation. Amsterdam: Excerpta Medica, 1992, pp 173–178.
2. Young RW. Pathophysiology of age-related macular degeneration. Surv Ophthalmol 1987; 31:291–306.
3. Holz FG, Wolfensberger TJ, Piguet B, Gross-Jendroska M, Wells JA, Minassian DC, Chisholm IH, Bird AC. Bilateral macular drusen in age-related macular degeneration prognosis and risk factors. Ophthalmology 1994;101:1522–1528.
4. Bressler SB, Maguire MG, Bressler NB, Fine SL. Relationship of drusen and abnormalities of the retinal pigment epithelium to the prognosis of neovascular macular degeneration. Arch Ophthalmol 1990;108:1442–1447.
5. Smiddy WE, Fine SL. Prognosis of patients with bilateral macular drusen. Ophthalmology 1984;91:271–277.
6. Macular Photocoagulation Study Group. Risk factors for choroidal neovascularization in the second eye of patients with juxtafoveal or subfoveal choroidal neovascularization secondary to age-related macular degeneration. Arch Ophthalmol 1997;115:741–747.
7. Christen WG Jr. Antioxidants and eye disease. Am J Med 1994;97(Suppl 3A):14S–17S.
8. Seddon JM, Ajani UA, Sperduto RD, Hiller R, Blair N, Burton TC, Farber MD, Gragoudas ES, Hiller J, Miller DT, Yannuzzi LA, Willett W. Dietary carotenoids, vitamins A, C, and E, and advanced age-related macular degeneration. JAMA 1994;272:1413–1420.
9. Widder RA, Brunner R, Engels B, Borberg G, Oette K. Changes of hemorheological and biochemical parameters after plasma perfusion using a tryptophan-polyvinyl alcohol adsorber leading to clinical improvement in patients suffering from maculopathy. Blood Purig 1998;16:15–21.
10. Duvall J, Tso MO. Cellular mechanisms of resolution of drusen after laser coagulation: an experimental study. Arch Ophthalmol 1985;103:694–703.
11. Johnson LV, Ozaki S, Staples MK, Erickson PA, Anderson DH. A potential role for immune complex pathogenesis in drusen formation. Exp Eye Res 2000;70:441–449.

12. Wetzig PC. Treatment of drusen-related aging macular degeneration by photocoagulation. Trans Am Ophthalmol Soc 1988;86:276–290.
13. Cleasby GW, Nakanishi AS, Norris JL. Prophylactic photocoagulation of the fellow eye in exudative senile maculopathy: a preliminary report. Mod Probl Ophthalmol 1979;20:141–147.
14. Frennesson IC, Nilsson SE. Effects of argon (green) laser treatment of soft drusen in early age-related maculopathy: a 6-month prospective study. Br J Ophthalmol 1995;79:905–907.
15. Figueroa MS, Regueras A, Bertrand J. Laser photocoagulation to treat macular soft drusen in age-related macular degeneration. Retina 1994;14:391–396.
16. Little HL, Showman JM, Brown BW. A pilot randomized controlled study on the effect of laser photocoagulation of confluent soft macular drusen. Ophthalmology 1997;104:623–631.
17. Guymer RH, Gross-Jendroska M, Owens SL, Bird AC, Fitzke FW. Laser treatment in subjects with high-risk clinical features of age-related macular degeneration: posterior pole appearance and function. Arch Ophthalmol 1997;115:595–603.
18. Choroidal Neovascularization Prevention Trial Research Group. Laser treatment in eyes with large drusen: short-term effects seen in a pilot randomized clinical trial. Ophthalmology 1998;105:11–23.
19. Olk RJ, Friberg TR, Stickney KL, Akduman L, Wong KL, Chen MC, Levy MH, Garcia CA, Morse LS. Therapeutic benefits of infrared (810-nm) diode laser macular grid photocoagulation in prophylactic treatment of nonexudative age-related macular degeneration: two-year results of a randomized pilot study. Ophthalmology 1999;106:2082–2090.
20. Sarks SH, Arnold JJ, Sarks JP, Gilles MC, Walter CJ. Prophylactic perifoveal laser treatment of soft drusen. Aust NZ J Ophthalmol 1996;24:15–26.
21. Sato Y, Berkowitz BA, Wilson CA, de Juan E Jr. Blood-retinal barrier breakdown caused by diode vs argon laser endophotocoagulation. Arch Ophthalmol 1992;110:277–281.
22. Pollack JS, Kim JE, Pulido JS, Burke JM. Tissue effects of subclinical diode laser treatment of the retina. Arch Ophthalmol 1998;116:1633–1639.
23. Funatsu H, Wilson CA, Berkowtiz BA, Sonkin PL. A comparative study of the effects of argon and diode laser photocoagulation on retinal oxygenation. Graefe's Arch Clin Exp Ophthalmol 1997;235:168–175.

20

Risk Factors for Age-Related Macular Degeneration and Choroidal Neovascularization

Kah-Guan Au Eong and Julia A. Haller
*Wilmer Eye Institute, Johns Hopkins University School of Medicine,
Baltimore, Maryland*

I. INTRODUCTION

Age-related macular degeneration (AMD), the most frequent cause of blindness among individuals aged 55 years and older in developed countries, is a major public health problem (1–4). The National Eye Institute estimates that there may be more than 16,000 new cases of legal blindness annually from AMD in the United States. In addition, the prevalence of AMD in the United States is expected to rise as a result of a progressive increase in the life expectancy and the proportion of elderly persons in the population. The increasing impact of AMD, coupled with the limited therapy available for its treatment, has led many investigators to search for factors that could be modified to prevent the onset or alter the natural course and prognosis of AMD. The identification and modification of risk factors has the potential for greater public health impact on the morbidity from AMD than the few treatment modalities at hand.

II. EPIDEMIOLOGICAL STUDIES ON RISK FACTORS FOR AGE-RELATED MACULAR DEGENERATION

Despite the high prevalence and public health importance of AMD, its pathogenesis remains unknown. The types of epidemiological studies that have explored AMD risk factors are *case-control, cross-sectional,* and *prospective cohort studies.* Case-control studies [e.g., the Eye Disease Case-Control Study (5,6)] have compared the frequency of possible risk factors among individuals with AMD to a cohort of control patients without the disease. Cross-sectional studies [e.g., the Framingham Eye Study (2) and the National Health and Nutrition Examination Survey I (NHANES-I) (7) have correlated eye examination data with sociodemographic, medical, and other variables collected as part of larger studies. Prospective cohort studies [e.g., the Physicians' Health Study (8)] collect data in a group of subjects over time. Tables 1, 2, and 3 show some case-control, cross-sectional, and prospective cohort studies that have explored risk factors for AMD.

Table 1 Some Case-Control Studies That Have Investigated the Risk Factors of Age-Related Macular Degeneration

Author(s) (year)	Place/name of study	Design	Study population	Method of diagnosis	Risk factors studied
Maltzman et al. (1979) (60)	Jersey City, NJ	Case-control	30 cases 30 controls	Clinical examination	Various personal and environmental factors
Delaney and Oates (1982) (110)	Syracuse, NY	Case-control	50 cases 50 controls	Clinical examination ± fundus photography	Various personal and environmental factors
Hyman et al. (1983) (48)	Baltimore, MD	Case-control	162 cases 175 controls	Fundus photography	Various personal and environmental factors
Weiter et al. (1985) (61)	Boston, MA and Fort Myers, FL	Case-control	650 cases 363 controls	Fundus photography	Iris color, fundus pigmentation
Blumenkranz et al. (1986) (66)	Miami, FL	Case-control	26 cases 23 controls	Fundus photography	Various personal and environmental factors
Tsang et al. (1992) (69)	Sydney, Australia	Case-control	80 cases 86 controls	Fundus photography	Various personal and environmental factors
Eye Disease Case-Control Study Group (1992 and 1993) (5,6), Seddon et al. (1994) (89)	Baltimore, MD; Boston, MA; Chicago, IL; Milwaukee, WI; and New York, NY/Eye Disease Case-Control Study	Case-control	421 cases 615 controls	Fundus photography	Various personal and environmental factors
Holz et al. (1994) (62)	London, England	Case-control	101 cases 102 controls	Clinical examination and fundus photography for cases. Clinical examination for controls	Iris color

Mares-Perlman et al. (168) (1995)	Beaver Dam, WI Beaver Dam Eye Study	Nested case control within a population-based cohort	167 cases 167 controls	Fundus photography	Antioxidants
Vingerling et al. (126) (1995)	Rotterdam, The Netherlands/Rotterdam Study	Nested case control within a population-based cohort	59 female cases 295 female controls	Fundus photography	Reproductive and related factors
Darzins et al. (152) (1997)	Newcastle, Australia	Case control	409 cases 286 controls	Fundus photography	Sunlight exposure
Tamakoshi et al. (136) (1997)	Kanto district, Japan	Case control	52 male cases 82 male controls	Fundus photography for cases; clinical examination for controls	Cigarette smoking
Chaine et al. (64) (1998)	France/FRANCE-DMLA Study	Case control	1844 cases 1844 controls	Fundus photography	Various personal and environmental factors
Belda et al. (150) (1998)	Valencia, Spain	Case control	25 cases 15 controls	Clinical examination	Serum vitamin E and zinc, sunlight exposure
Hyman et al. (19) (2000)	New York, NY/Age-related Macular Degeneration Risk Factors Study	Case control	182 neovascular AMD cases 227 non-neovascular AMD cases 235 controls	Fundus photography	Systemic hypertension, cardiovascular disease, cholesterol intake

Table 2 Some Cross-Sectional Studies That Have Investigated the Risk Factors of Age-Related Macular Degeneration

Author(s) (year)	Place/name of study	Design	Study population[a]	Method of diagnosis	Risk factors studied
Kahn et al. (1997) (12,26), Leibowitz et al. (1980) (2), Sperduto et al. (1980, 1981 and 1986)(99,100,114)	Framingham, MA/Framingham Eye Study	Population-based cross-sectional	2631 survivors of the Framingham Heart Study cohort, mean age = 65.3 years	Clinical examination	Various personal and environmental factors
Martinez et al. (1982) (27)	Gisborne, New Zealand	Population-based cross-sectional	481 participants aged ≥ 65 years	Clinical examination	Age, sex
Klein and Klein (1982) (10), Goldberg et al. (1988) (7), Liu et al. (1989)(102)	United States/National Health and Nutritional Examination Survey I (NHANES-I)	Population-based cross-sectional	3,082 participants aged ≥ 45 years	Clinical examination	Various personal and environmental factors
Gibson et al. (1986) (33)	Melton Mowbray, England/Melton Mowbray Eye Study	Population-based cross-sectional	529 participants aged ≥ 75 years	Fundus photography	Various personal and environmental factors
West et al. (1989) (67), Bressler et al. (1989) (13), Taylor et al. (1990 and 1992) (96, 97)	Somerset County, MD and lower Dorchester County, MD/Chesapeake Bay Watermen Study	Occupational cross-sectional	782 male watermen aged ≥ 30 years	Fundus photography	Age, sunlight exposure
Vinding (1989, 1990 and 1992) (28,68,130)	Copenhagen, Denmark	Population-based cross-sectional	924 survivors from the Copenhagen City Heart Study aged 60–79 years	Fundus photography	Various personal and environmental factors

West et al. (1994) (161)	Baltimore, MD and Washington, DC/Baltimore Longitudinal Study of Aging	Cross-sectional	916 participants of the Baltimore Longitudinal Study of Aging, aged ≥ 40 years	Fundus photography	Antioxidants
Klein et al. (1992, 1993, and 1994) (14,59,101, 113,124,131), Cruickshanks et al. (1993) (151), Heiba et al. (1994) (42), Mares-Perlman et al. (1995) (118)	Beaver Dam, WI/Beaver Dam Eye Study	Population-based cross-sectional	4926 participants, aged 43–84 years	Fundus photography	Various personal and environmental factors
Schachat et al. (1995) (15)	Barbados, West Indies/Barbados Eye Study	Population-based cross-sectional	3444 participants aged 40–84 years	Fundus photography	Various personal and environmental factors
Vingerling et al. (1995) (29,112)	Rotterdam, The Netherlands/Rotterdam Study	Population-based cross-sectional	6251 participants aged 55–98 years	Fundus photography	Various personal and environmental factors
Mitchell et al. (1995, 1996, 1998 and 1999) (16,63,125,134), Attebo et al. (1996) (3), Smith et al. (1997, 1998, 1999, and 2000) (18,51,119, 165,166), Wang et al. (1998 and 1999) (31,108)	Blue Mountains region, Sydney, Australia/Blue Mountains Eye Study	Population-based cross-sectional	3654 participants aged ≥ 49 years	Fundus photography	Various personal and environmental factors

(continued)

Table 2 *(continued)*

Author(s) (year)	Place/name of study	Design	Study population[a]	Method of diagnosis	Risk factors studied
Hirvela et al. (1996) (30)	Oulu County, Northern Finland	Population-based cross-sectional	500 participants aged ≥ 70 years	Fundus photography	Various personal and environmental factors
Delcourt et al. (1998 and 1999) (17, 128, 137)	Sete, France/POLA (Pathologies Oculaires Liees a l'Age) Study	Population-based cross-sectional	2196 participants aged ≥ 60 years	Fundus photography	Various personal and environmental factors
Friedman et al. (1999) (38)	East Baltimore, MD/Baltimore Eye Study	Population-based cross-sectional	5308 participants aged ≥ 40 years	Fundus photography	Age, race
Klein et al. (1999) (40)	Forsyth County, NC; Jackson, MS; Minneapolis, MN and Washington County, MD/Atherosclerosis Risk in Communities Study	Population-based cross-sectional	11,532 participants aged 48–72 years	Fundus photography	Various personal and environmental factors
Klein et al. (1995 and 1999) (25,39)	United States/National Health and Nutritional Examination Survey III (NHANES-III)	Complex, multistage area probability sample design (certain groups, e.g., Americans ≥ 60 years, Mexican-American, and non-Hispanic blacks, were sampled at a higher probability than other persons	8270 participants aged ≥ 40 years	Fundus photography	Various sociodemographic, ocular, medical, and environmental factors

[a]The sample size may vary slightly among the different reports.

Table 3 Some Prospective Cohort Studies That Have Investigated the Risk Factors of Age-Related Macular Degeneration

Author(s) (year)	Place/name of study	Design	Study population[a]	Method of diagnosis	Risk factors studied
Moss et al. (1996) (190), Klein et al. (1997 and 1998) (23,70,116)	Beaver Dam, WI/Beaver Dam Eye Study	Population-based prospective cohort	3684 participants aged 43–86 years	Fundus photography	Alcohol consumption, cardiovascular disease risk factors
Seddon et al. (1996) (135)	11 states in the United States/Nurses' Health Study	Prospective cohort	31, 843 female registered nurses aged ≥ 50 years	Diagnosis by treating ophthalmologists or optometrists	Cigarette smoking
Christen et al. (1996) (8,133), Ajani et al. (1999) (193)	United States/Physicians' Health Study	Prospective cohort	21,157 male physicians aged 40–84 years at baseline	Diagnosis by treating ophthalmologists or optometrists	Cigarette smoking, antioxidant vitamin supplements, alcohol consumption
Cho et al. (2000) (192)	United States/Nurses' Health Study and Health Professionals Follow-up Study	Prospective cohort	32,764 female registered nurses and 29,488 male health professionals aged ≥ 50 years	Diagnosis by treating ophthalmologists	Alcohol consumption

[a]The sample size may vary slightly among the different reports.

III. PROBLEMS AND LIMITATIONS OF EPIDEMIOLOGICAL STUDIES ON RISK FACTORS FOR AGE-RELATED MACULAR DEGENERATION

There may be different causative factors that damage the macula and result in common clinical manifestations that we recognize as AMD. The analysis of risk factors for AMD is inherently difficult because many of them are closely interrelated, e.g., race, ocular pigmentation, and sunlight exposure, or socioeconomic status, smoking, and nutrition. Studying risk factors such as sunlight exposure includes challenges in measurement of acute and chronic lifetime exposure and the effect of potential confounding factors such as sun sensitivity and sun-avoidance behavior. In addition, the difficulties in establishing a causal link between a chronic disease and a potential risk factor are magnified for a condition such as AMD because it manifests itself late in life. Additional problems in this circumstance include a long lead time, a possible recall bias, and survivor cohort effects.

Despite the extensive past and ongoing research on AMD worldwide, there is currently no universally accepted definition of AMD. Different definitions of early and late signs of AMD have been used in various studies, making direct comparison of the results difficult or impossible (Table 4) (9). The problem is further compounded by differences in methodology used in the various studies. A wide range of different diagnostic tools has been used in different clinical and epidemiological studies (9). For example, NHANES-I, a population-based study of a sample of the noninstitutionalized U.S. population, relied

Table 4   Definitions of and Age Limits in Age-Related Macular Degeneration (Age-Related Maculopathy) Used in Population-Based Studies

1. Framingham Eye Study (2): An eye was diagnosed as having senile macular degeneration if its visual acuity was 20/30 or worse and the ophthalmologist designated the etiology of changes in the macula or posterior pole as senile.
   Age limits: 52–85 years.
2. National Health and Nutrition Eye Study I (7): Age-related diskiform macular degeneration: loss of macular reflex, pigment dispersion and clumping, and drusen associated with visual acuity of 20/25 or worse believed to be due to this disease. Age-related diskiform macular degeneration: choroidal hemorrhage and connective-tissue proliferation beneath retina (this condition should be differentiated from diskiform degenerations of other causes, e.g., histoplasmosis, toxoplasmosis, angioid streaks, and high myopia). Age-related circinate macular degenation: perimacular accumulation of lipoid material within the retina. Age limits: 1–74 years.
3. Gisborne Study (27): Senile macular degeneration: when the visual acuity in the affected eye was 6/9 (20/30) or worse and senile macular degeneration was identified as the probable cause of this visual loss. Age limits: ≥65 years.
4. Copenhagen Study (28): Age-related macular degeneration (AMD): best corrected visual (Snellen) acuity (including pinhole improvement) of 6/9 or less, explained by age-related morphological changes of the macula. Atrophic (dry) changes: disarrangement of the pigment epithelium (atrophy/clustering) and/or a small cluster of small drusen and/or medium drusen and/or large drusen and/or pronounced senile macular choroidal atrophy/sclerosis without general fundus involvement. Exudative (wet) changes: elevation of the neurosensory retina and/or the pigment epithelium and/or hemorrhages, and/or hard exudates and/or fibrovascular tissue. Age-related macular changes without visual impairment (AMCW) is defined as similar morphological lesions but without visual deterioration. Age limits: 60–80 years.

5. Chesapeake Bay Study (13): No specific overall definition. Geographic atrophy: an area of well-demarcated atrophy of the RPE in which the overlying retina appeared thin. Exudative changes: choroidal neovascularization, detachments of the RPE, and diskiform scarring. Grading of AMD in 4 grades:

    Grade 4: geographic atrophy of the RPE or exudative changes.

    Grade 3: eyes with large or confluent drusen or eyes with focal hyperpigmentation of the RPE

    Grade 2: eyes with many small drusen ($\geq$20) within 1500 microns of the foveal center.

    Grade 1: eyes with at least five small drusen within 1500 microns of the foveal center or at least 10 small drusen between 1500 and 3000 microns from the foveal center. No visual acuity included. Age limits: $\geq$30 years.

6. Beaver Dam Eye Study (14): Early age-related maculopathy was defined as the absence of signs of the late age-related maculopathy as defined in table 5 and as the presence of soft indistinct or reticular drusen or by the presence of any drusen type except hard indistinct, with RPE degeneration or increased retinal pigment in the macular area. Late age-related maculopathy was defined as the presence of signs of exudative age-related macular degeneration or geographic atrophy. The grade assigned for the participant was that of the more severely involved eye. No visual acuity included. Age limits: 43–86 years.

7. Rotterdam Study (29): All ARM changes had to be within a radius of 3000 microns of the foveola. No definition of early ARM, but separate prevalence figures for drusen and retinal pigment epithelial hyperpigmentations or hypopigmentations attributable to age-related causes. Late ARM (similar to AMD): the presence of atrophic AMD (well-demarcated area of RPE atrophy with visible choroidal vessels) and/or neovascular AMD (serous and/or hemorrhagic RPE detachment, and/or subretinal neovascular membrane and/or hemorrhage, and/or periretinal fibrous scar) attributable to age-related causes. In a participant the most severely involved eye was taken for the analysis. No visual acuity included. Age limits: $\geq$55 years.

Source: Reprinted from The International ARM Epidemiological Study Group. An international classification and grading system for age-related maculopathy and age-related macular degeneration. Surv Ophthalmol 1995;39(5); 367–374. Copyright 1995, with permission from Elsevier Science.

solely on clinical examinations by multiple independent examiners with varying levels of experience, and standardization of the diagnosis of AMD was uncertain (7,10). Fundus photographs of a subset of the study population were reviewed and discrepancies in the macular gradings were disclosed (11). The Framingham Eye Study, which has provided the most frequently cited prevalence data on AMD to date, was based mainly on clinical examination and fundus photography was performed only on a small subset of the study population (12). More recent studies have used fundus photography to detect and grade AMD but the details were not always standardized among the studies (13–17).

In an effort to standardize disease definition and study methodology, the International Age-Related Maculopathy Epidemiological Study Group published in 1995 an international classification and grading system for AMD in the hope of producing a common detection and classification system for epidemiological studies (9). It defined *age-related maculopathy* (ARM) to include two alternate late lesions *(neovascular maculopathy* and *geographic atrophy),* termed *age-related macular degeneration* (AMD), or *late ARM,* and early lesions (soft or large drusen and retinal pigmentary abnormalities), termed *early ARM* (Table 5). In this definition, visual acuity is not a criterion for the presence or absence of ARM. This new terminology, however, has not been universally accepted. In this chapter,

Table 5   Definitions of Age-Related Maculopathy

Age-related maculopathy (ARM) is a disorder of the macular area of the retina, most often
    clinically apparent after 50 years of age, characterized by any of the following primary items,
    without indication that they are secondary to another disorder (e.g., ocular trauma, retinal
    detachment, high myopia, chorioretinal infective or inflammatory process, choroidal dystrophy,
    etc.):
Drusen, which are discrete whitish-yellow spots external to the neuroretina or the retinal pigment
    epithelium. They may be soft and confluent, often with indistinct borders.
    Soft distinct drusen have uniform density with sharp edges.
    Soft indistinct drusen have decreasing density from center outward with fuzzy edges.
    Hard drusen, usually present in eyes with as well as those without ARM, do not of themselves
    characterize the disorder.
Areas of increased pigment or hyperpigmentation (in the outer retina or choroid) associated with
    drusen.
Areas of depigmentation or hypopigmentation of the retinal pigment epithelium (RPE), most often
    more sharply demarcated than drusen, without any visibility of choroidal vessels associated with
    drusen.
Late stages of ARM, also called age-related macular degeneration.
Age-related macular degeneration (AMD) is a later stage of ARM and includes both "dry" and
    "wet" AMD.
Dry AMD is also called geographic atrophy and is characterized by:
Any sharply delineated roughly round or oval area of hypopigmentation or depigmentation or
    apparent absence of the RPE in which choroidal vessels are more visible than in surrounding
    areas that must be at least 175 microns in diameter on the color slide (using a 30° or 35°
    camera).
Wet AMD is also called "neovascular" AMD, "diskiform" AMD, or "exudative" AMD and is
    characterized by any of the following:
RPE detachment(s), which may be associated with neurosensory retinal detachment, associated
    with other forms of ARM.
Neovascular membrane(s), which may be subretinal or sub-RPE.
Scar/glial tissue or fibrin-like deposits, which may be epiretinal (with exclusion of idiopathic
    macular puckers), intraretinal, subretinal, or subpigment epithelial.
Subretinal hemorrhages, which may be nearly black, bright red, or whitish-yellow and are not
    related to other retinal vascular disease. Hemorrhages in the retina (retinal hemorrhages) or
    breaking through it into the vitreous (vitreous hemorrhages) may also be present.
Hard exudates (lipids) within the macular area related to any of the above, and not to other retinal
    vascular disease.

Source: The International ARM Epidemiological Study Group. An International Classification and
Grading System for Age-Related Maculopathy and Age-Related Macular Degeneration. Surv
Ophthalmol 1995; 39(5): 367–374. Copyright 1995, with permission from Elsevier Science.

we will use the more conventional definition of AMD to include the entire spectrum of the
disease (i.e., equivalent to ARM in the new terminology). Neovascular AMD and geographic atrophy will be collectively termed *late AMD* (equivalent to late ARM) and the
early lesions of AMD will be termed *early AMD* (equivalent to early ARM).

It is possible that the factors associated with early AMD may be different from
those associated with progression to geographic atrophy or neovascular AMD. In
addition, although geographic atrophy and neovascular AMD are termed collectively
as late AMD (or late ARM), they may have different causes (9). For these reasons, it

Table 6   Risk Factors for Age-Related Macular Degeneration

Established risk factors
   Age
   Race/ethnicity
   Heredity
   Smoking
Possible risk factors
   Gender
   Socioeconomic status
   Iris color
   Macular pigment density
   Cataract and its surgery
   Refractive error
   Cup/disk ratio
   Cardiovascular disease
   Hypertension and blood pressure
   Serum lipid levels and dietary fat intake
   Body mass index
   Hematological factors
   Reproductive and related factors
   Dermal elastotic degeneration
   Antioxidant enzymes
   Sunlight exposure
   Micronutrients
   Dietary fish intake
   Alcohol consumption
Factors probably not associated with AMD
   Diabetes and hyperglycemia

may be important to pay attention to the different stages of AMD and to separate the two manifestations of late AMD in epidemiological studies, as has been done in several recent studies (18,19).

Some studies have evaluated huge numbers of variables for possible associations with ocular findings. For example, the Framingham Eye Study correlated its ophthalmic diagnoses with almost all of 667 variables from the Framingham Heart Study (12). Because of the very large number of variables evaluated, it is possible that some of the associations found may be due to chance alone (20). Similarly, while it is plausible that risk factors may be different for the various manifestations of AMD [e.g., drusen, increased retinal pigment, retinal pigment epithelial (RPE) depigmentation, geographic atrophy, and neovascular AMD], simultaneously conducting multiple comparisons within individual studies increases the likelihood of chance findings (21). In fact, one in 20 variables should have a positive association (for $p = 0.05$) by chance alone (22), and this probably contributes partly to the inconsistent results between studies. To provide compelling evidence of a real association between AMD and potential risk factors, repeated findings of the same risk factors in well-designed studies conducted in different populations are necessary.

While results from epidemiological studies may identify risk factors for AMD, proof that modifying a particular established risk factor can influence the course of the disease can emerge only from randomized prospective clinical trials.

IV. RISK FACTORS FOR AGE-RELATED MACULAR DEGENERATION

A number of risk factors for AMD have been incriminated from various epidemiological studies, suggesting that the condition is multifactorial in etiology (Table 6). These risk factors may be broadly classified into personal or environmental factors, and the personal factors may be further subdivided into sociodemographic, ocular, and systemic factors.

V. SOCIODEMOGRAPHIC FACTORS

A. Age

Age is the strongest risk factor associated with AMD. The prevalence, incidence, and progression of all forms of AMD rise steeply with advancing age (14,23). There is a consistent finding across multiple population-based studies of an increase in prevalence of late AMD with age, from near absence at age 50 years to about 2% prevalence at age 70, and about 6% at age 80 (14,24,25). In the Framingham Eye Study, the prevalence of any AMD (defined as degenerative changes of the macula with visual acuity of 20/30 or worse) was 1.6% for persons aged 52–64 years, 11.0% for persons aged 65–74 years, and 27.9% for persons aged 75–85 years (26). Although closely linked to the aging process, AMD is not universal and is not inevitable with increasing age.

B. Gender

Gender has not been consistently found to be a risk factor for AMD. Gender was not associated with AMD in a study in Gisborne, New Zealand (27), the NHANES-I (7), the Copenhagen Study (28), the Rotterdam Study (29), and a Finnish population-based study (30). Frequency estimates for drusen and the high-risk features of AMD among the black participants in the Barbados Eye Study were similar for men and women (15).

In the Blue Mountains Eye Study, there were consistent, although not statistically significant, gender differences in prevalence for most lesions of AMD, with women having higher rates for late AMD and soft indistinct drusen than men, but not retinal pigmentary abnormalities, which were slightly more frequent in men (16). In addition, a significantly higher rate of bilateral involvement in women than men was found for neovascular AMD [odds ratio (OR), 7.7; 95% confidence interval (CI), 1.3–46.7] in the Blue Mountains Eye Study (31). For all other lesions of AMD, nonsignificant increased odds ratios were found for bilateral involvement in women (OR, 2.4; 95% CI, 0.6–10.0 for geographic atrophy and OR, 1.6; 95% CI, 0.7–3.5 for early AMD). In the Beaver Dam Eye Study, exudative AMD was more frequent in women $\geq$ 75 years compared with men in the same age group (6.7% vs. 2.6%, $p = 0.02$) (14). In addition, in an incidence study, after adjusting for age, the incidence of early AMD was 2.2 times (95% CI, 1.6–3.2) as likely in women $\geq$ 75 years of age compared to men this age (23).

Smith and associates pooled data from the Rotterdam Study (29), the Beaver Dam Eye Study (14), and the Blue Mountains Eye Study (16) to determine whether women have a higher age-specific AMD prevalence than men (32). These three recent large-scale, population-based studies used almost identical diagnostic techniques and criteria for AMD, and the published data are presented in identical form for age groups 55–85 years. The overall pooled data show a significant but modest increase in AMD prevalence among women compared to men, with odds ratio of 1.15 (95% CI, 1.10–1.21) adjusting for 10-year age categories. Age stratum-specific pooled odds ratios (95% CI) show an increase in risk, rising from 0.62 (0.35–1.10) for ages 55–64 years to 1.04 (0.87–1.26) for ages 65–74 years and 1.29 (1.20–1.38) for ages 75–84 years.

The Melton Mowbray Eye Study (33) and the Framingham Eye Study (2,34) also found a higher prevalence of AMD among women. In NHANES-III, after controlling for age, white women (OR, 1.32; 95% CI, 1.10–1.61) and black women (OR, 1.39; 95% CI, 1.00–1.92) had statistically significant higher odds of having soft drusen (defined as drusen > 63 microns) than did men of the same race/ethnicity group, respectively (25). White women (OR, 1.24; 95% CI, 1.02–1.51) and black women (OR, 1.47; 95% CI, 1.06–2.03) 2.03) were also more likely to have early AMD present than white and black men, respectively (25).

Further research is necessary to confirm whether true gender differences exist in AMD.

C. Race/Ethnicity

Differences in genetic susceptibility probably explain part of the disparities in the prevalence of AMD in different races. The low numbers of black participants in the Macular Photocoagulation Study (MPS) trials for AMD suggested that the condition is less prevalent in black than in white populations (35). As of July 1, 1991, only one (0.08%) of 1319 patients enrolled in the MPS trials for AMD was black, while 1314 were white and four were listed as "other" (35).

Several studies have suggested that AMD is more prevalent among whites than blacks (15,36–38). Gregor and Joffe, comparing 377 white patients from London, England, with 864 age- and sex-matched black South Africans, found that drusen and pigment epithelial changes were twice as common in whites as in black Africans (18.3% vs. 9.3%, $p < 0.001$ and 11.4% vs. 4.6%, $p < 0.001$, respectively) (36). They also observed that diskiform degeneration was present in 3.5% of white patients compared to 0.1% of South African patients ($p < 0.001$).

In the Baltimore Eye Survey, a cross-sectional, population-based study of black and white residents of East Baltimore, all AMD-related blindness was found in whites (37,38). Drusen > 63 microns were identified in about 20% of individuals in both blacks and whites, but large drusen (>125 microns) were more common among older whites (15% for whites vs. 9% for blacks over 70 years old) (38). Retinal pigmentary abnormalities were also more common among older whites (7.9% for whites vs. 0.4% for blacks over 70 years old) (38). The prevalence ratio (white:black) was 10.7 for geographic atrophy, 8.8 for neovascular AMD, and 10.1 for all late AMD (geographic atrophy plus neovascular AMD) (38).

In the Barbados Eye Study, (15), a population-based study in a large population of persons primarily of African descent, age-related macular changes occurred at a lower frequency than in the predominantly white populations of the Maryland Watermen Study (13) and the Beaver Dam Eye Study (14). At least one small (<63 microns) drusen was present in 66.2% of the Barbados Eye Study participants, which is lower than that of 86% of Maryland Watermen Study participants and 94% of the Beaver Dam Eye Study participants. The frequency of at least one large drusen of 1.1% in the Barbados Eye Study was also lower compared with these other studies, which had rates of 9% and 20% for the Maryland Watermen Study and Beaver Dam Eye Study, respectively. Neovascular AMD was found in

0.6% in the Barbados Eye Study. This was similar to the Maryland Watermen Study but lower than the 1.2% found in the Beaver Dam Eye Study. One caveat in the interpretation of the Barbados Eye Study, which is based on 30° stereoscopic fundus photographic grading, is that because the gradability of the fundus photographs decreased significantly with increasing age, predominantly as a result of an increasing incidence and severity of media opacities, and the participants excluded from the data analyses tended to be older, the frequencies presented in the Barbados Eye Study may underestimate the true frequency of AMD in this population (15).

In NHANES-III, after adjusting for age, the frequency of early AMD was similar in non-Hispanic whites compared with that of non-Hispanic blacks and Mexican-Americans (25). Although the frequencies of soft drusen appear similar among the racial/ethnic groups, retinal pigmentary abnormalities and signs of late AMD are more frequent in non-Hispanic whites than in non-Hispanic blacks and Mexican-Americans. For increased retinal pigment and RPE depigmentation, the odds ratios (95% CI) comparing non-Hispanic blacks to non-Hispanic whites were 0.47 (0.31–0.72) and 0.59 (0.33–1.04), respectively, and for comparing Mexican-Americans to non-Hispanic whites, they were 0.41 (0.21–0.81) and 0.72 (0.44–1.19), respectively. For late AMD, the odds ratio (95% CI) for non-Hispanic blacks compared to non-Hispanic whites was 0.34 (0.10–1.18) and for Mexican-Americans compared to non-Hispanic whites, it was 0.25 (0.07–0.90). Interestingly, before 60 years of age, Mexican-Americans (OR, 1.53; 95% CI, 1.00–2.35) and non-Hispanic blacks (OR, 1.59; 95% CI, 0.86–2.95) had a greater chance of having any AMD than non-Hispanic whites; thereafter, Mexican-Americans (OR, 0.63; 95% CI, 0.44–0.90) and non-Hispanic blacks (OR, 0.50; 95% CI, 0.37–0.68) had a lesser chance than non-Hispanic whites (39). Other Hispanics, Asians, and native Americans were included in NHANES-III but were not reported owing to inadequate sample sizes.

Klein and associates studied the prevalence of a large cohort of black and white participants in the Atherosclerosis Risk in Communities Study and found that the overall prevalence of any AMD was lower in blacks (3.7%) than whites (5.6%) (40). After controlling for age and sex, the odds ratio for any AMD in blacks compared with whites was 0.73 (95% CI, 0.58–0.91). The prevalence of most of the component lesions that define early AMD was also lower in blacks than whites ≥ 60 years of age.

Klein and Klein, using data from NHANES-I, found no difference between whites and blacks in the percentage of patients with AMD (10). Another analysis of the same data came to the same conclusion (7).

It is unclear whether the degree of fundus pigmentation affects the ability to detect lesions such as hyper- and hypopigmentation of the RPE, and soft drusen that characterize AMD. It is plausible that variations in normal fundus pigmentation may lead to errors in detecting subtle early AMD lesions, resulting in apparent differences among the ethnic groups.

Overall, current evidence suggests that early AMD is common among blacks and Hispanics, but less common than among non-Hispanic whites. However, late AMD is less frequent in these groups compared to non-Hispanic whites. Racial differences in AMD support a potential genetic component to this condition.

D. Heredity

Analysis of heredity in the disease process of AMD is limited by the fact that the disorder is associated with aging, frequently causing its most significant phenotypic manifestations in the later years of life. As a result, usually only one generation in the appropriate age range is available for study. The parents of the proband are often deceased, and the children are often too young to manifest the disease. Because information from several generations of families of multiple affected individuals is often lacking, genetic analysis is limited.

Clinical experience indicates that AMD demonstrates familial clustering, suggesting that heredity may be an important factor in the etiology of this condition although the exact role and relative contribution of genetics in the pathogenesis are unknown (41–44). It is believed that this genetic predisposition, in the presence of appropriate environmental influences, causes the aging macula to manifest AMD.

Although Hutchinson and Tay observed a familial occurrence of AMD as early as 1875 (45), the association between heredity and AMD has not been well studied until recently. Bradley in 1966 commented on his patients with AMD that "nearly every patient I have seen has had other members of the family similarly afflicted" (46). In 1973, Gass reported a positive family history of loss of central vision in 10–20% of his patients with AMD (47).

Hyman and associates reported a statistically significant association between AMD and a family history of the disease in either the parents or siblings (OR, 2.9; 95% CI, 1.5–5.5) (48). A significantly higher correlation of number of drusen between siblings than between spouses was found by Piguet and associates (41). The lack of concordance between spouses who have shared a common environment for at least 20 years suggests that environmental factors may not play a key role in the etiology of AMD (41). Seddon and associates found the overall prevalence of AMD was higher among first-degree relatives of cases than among relatives of controls (OR, 2.4; 95% CI, 1.2–4.7) (49). They also found that familial aggregation of AMD was associated with the type of AMD in the proband, i.e., dry AMD (large or extensive macular drusen, RPE abnormalities, and geographic atrophy) versus exudative AMD [RPE detachment or choroidal neovascularization (CNV)]. Relatives of probands with exudative disease were significantly more likely to have AMD than were relatives of control probands after adjusting for age and sex (OR = 3.1, 95% CI = 1.5–6.7). On the other hand, relatives of probands with dry AMD were slightly more likely to have AMD than were relatives of control probands (OR = 1.5, 95% CI = 0.6–3.7), but this difference was not statistically significant. In another study, the odds ratio of siblings for AMD of patients compared to siblings of controls was 25.2 (95% CI = 3.4–519.0) (50).

In the Blue Mountains Eye Study, subjects with signs of AMD (4.5%) were more likely to report a first-degree family history of AMD than subjects without AMD (2.3%) (51). The highest rate was reported by subjects with late AMD (6.9%), particularly those with neovascular AMD (8.2%). After adjusting for age, sex, and current smoking, a clear increase in risk associated with family history, from no AMD [OR, 1.0 (index)] to early AMD (OR, 2.17; 95% CI, 1.04–4.55), late AMD (geographic atrophy or neovascular AMD) (OR, 3.92; 95% CI, 1.344–11.46), and neovascular AMD (OR, 4.30; 95% CI, 1.37–13.45) was observed (51).

Klaver and associates examined the siblings and children of probands derived from the population-based Rotterdam Study (52). First-degree relatives of 87 patients with late AMD (geographic atrophy or neovascular AMD) were compared with those of 135 controls without AMD. For siblings, the prevalence of early AMD was 9.5% for siblings of patients versus 2.9% for siblings of controls ($p = 0.04$, age- and sex-adjusted), and the prevalence of late AMD was 13.4% versus 2.2% ($p = 0.001$, age- and sex-adjusted). For offspring, the prevalence of early AMD was 6.3% for offspring of patients versus 1.9% for offspring of controls ($p = 0.05$, age- and sex-adjusted), and late AMD was present in only

1.4% of offspring of patients ($p = 0.20$, age- and sex-adjusted). The prevalence of early (OR, 4.8; 95% CI, 1.8–12.2) and late (OR, 19.8; 95% CI, 3.1–126.0) AMD was significantly higher in first-degree relatives of patients with late AMD than in relatives of controls. The lifetime absolute risk estimate of developing early AMD was 48% (95% CI, 31–65%) for relatives of patients versus 23% (95% CI, 10–37%) for relatives of controls ($p = 0.001$), yielding a risk ratio of 2.1 (95% CI, 1.4–3.1). The lifetime risk estimate of late AMD was 50% (95% CI, 26–73%) for relatives of patients versus 12% (95% CI, 2–16%) for relatives of controls ($p < 0.001$), yielding a risk ratio of 4.2 (95% CI, 2.6–6.8). The authors calculated that the population-attributable risk related to genetic factors was 23% (52).

No association, however, was found between family history and AMD in the small population-based Melton Mowbray Eye Study (33). It should be pointed out that in studies in which the family history data were ascertained by interview alone, the data should be interpreted with caution since reported histories of ocular disease are unreliable (53).

Three reports of single pairs of monozygotic twins (54–56) and two larger series, with nine (44) and 50 pairs of identical twins (57), described a high concordance of early and late AMD in the twins. Gottfredsdottir and associates examined the concordance of AMD in 100 monozygotic twins (50 pairs) and 47 spouses (57). The average duration of marriage for the twin/spouse pair was 30 years (range, 26–50 years). The concordance of AMD was 90% in monozygotic twin pairs, which significantly exceeded that of 70% for twin/spouse pairs ($p = 0.0279$). In the nine twin pairs that were concordant, fundus appearance and visual impairment were similar. Although the environmental influences are probably more similar for identical twins than for dizygotic twins, other siblings, or unrelated individuals, the strikingly similar incidence of age-related macular changes in these identical twins suggests that a substantial genetic component may exist in some patients with AMD.

Although AMD runs in families, the phenotypic appearance of the macula within families with the disorder tends to be quite variable and representative of the wide range of findings typically associated with AMD; i.e., both neovascular AMD and geographic atrophy and early signs of AMD may be present in different individuals within the families (58). Indeed, neovascular and nonneovascular AMD was observed among different individuals in four of eight families in the study, suggesting that geographic atrophy may be part of the same disease process as neovascular AMD. On the other hand, the distinctly different phenotypes of the two forms of late AMD may also indicate different origins. It is currently unknown why geographic atrophy develops in some instances and neovascular AMD in others, even within the same family.

E. Socioeconomic Status

In NHANES-I, a significant negative trend ($p < 0.03$) of decreased prevalence of AMD was found with increasing levels of education (7). Compared with the least educated group, persons who attended high school have a reduced prevalence of AMD (OR, 0.64; 95% CI, 0.44–0.92) as do persons who have some education beyond high school (OR, 0.71; 95% CI, 0.44–1.15). The Eye Disease Case-Control Study found that persons with higher levels of education had a slightly reduced risk of neovascular AMD, but the association did not remain statistically significant after multiple regression modeling (6).

The Beaver Dam Eye Study found no relation of income, educational level, or marital status to AMD (59). No association between social class and AMD was found in the

Melton Mowbray Eye Study (33). Two case-control studies found no association between AMD and occupation (48,60).

VI. OCULAR FACTORS

A. Iris Color

Iris color is a hereditary factor that may be associated with AMD (61). However, this association has not been consistently found in studies. A number of studies have reported an increased risk of AMD in people with blue or light iris color compared with those with darker iris pigmentation (48,61–64) and one study documented worse AMD in subjects with light iris color (65). Others, however, have found no association between iris color and AMD (6,33,66–70). The Beaver Dam Eye Study did not find any relationship between iris color and the incidence and progression of AMD (70). One histological study found no significant correlation between iris color and macular aging (71). Data from NHANES-III showed that blue iris color was negatively associated with soft drusen in non-Hispanic whites (OR, 0.69; 95% CI, 0.55–0.88) but not in Mexican-Americans (OR, 0.35; 95% CI, 0.05–2.72) (25). The reasons for these disparities are not clear.

Case-control studies by Hyman and associates (48) and Weiter and associates (61) demonstrated a positive association between light iris color and AMD. In Hyman and associates' series, only 9.2% of 162 cases had brown irides compared to 26.4% of 174 controls ($p = 0.0002$) (48). Blue or lightly pigmented irides were associated with a higher risk of AMD, the degree of association being greater for men (OR, 8.3; 95% CI, 2.3–29.7) than for women (OR, 2.4; 95% CI, 1.1–5.0) (48). Weiter and associates found that 76% of 650 patients had light irides compared with 40% of 363 controls ($p = 0.0001$) (61). In addition, patients with AMD and light iris color were found to be significantly younger (mean age, 73.6 ± 7.3 years) than those with dark iris color (mean age, 78.3 ± 5.8 years) ($p = 0.0008$) (61). The FRANCE-DMLA Study Group, comparing 1844 cases of AMD with a similar number of age- and sex-matched controls, found that persons with light iris color (blue, green, and gray) had increased risk of AMD compared to those with dark iris color (OR, 1.22; 95% CI, 1.05–1.42) (64). This concurs with the Blue Mountains Eye Study, which found that blue iris color was significantly associated with an increased risk for both early AMD (OR, 1.5; 95% CI, 1.1–1.9) and late AMD (OR, 1.7; 95% CI, 1.0–2.9) (63).

Holz and associates found that lighter present iris color, but not initial iris color during youth, was associated with an increased risk of AMD (62). They calculated that a history of decreasing iris color was associated with a 5.55-fold (95% CI, 2.03–15.91) increase in risk of AMD ($p = 0.0001$). Some studies have shown that declines in the melanin content of the iris and RPE occur with age (72,73). The Beaver Dam Eye Study showed higher prevalences of blue or gray iris color with increased age, but no relationship was found between iris color and the incidence or progression of AMD in the study (70).

The mechanism by which iris pigmentation might influence AMD is uncertain, but a plausible explanation is that the lower risk for AMD among subjects with darker iris color may be due to the fact that these individuals have more tissue melanin, including the choroid. Indeed, fundus pigmentation was found to correspond closely to iris pigmentation both clinically and by objective histological microdensitometric techniques (61). This increased pigmentation may provide some protection to the retina from exposure to sunlight, reducing direct photooxidative damage and thus reducing the risk of AMD (see below).

This is consistent with the observation in some studies that AMD is more prevalent among whites than among the more pigmented races (15,37,38).

B. Macular Pigment Density

Recently, there is heightened interest in the potential role of macular pigment in protecting against AMD (74). The yellow macular pigment, which characterizes the retinas of primates including man, was shown in 1985 to be composed of two chromatographically separable components, namely lutein and zeaxanthin (75). Although the exact role of the macular pigment remains uncertain, several functions have been hypothesized. These include limiting the effects of light scatter and chromatic aberration on visual performance (76,77), reducing the damaging photooxidative effects of blue light through its absorption (78,79), and protecting against the effects of photochemical reactions by its antioxidant properties (80). There is evidence that oxidative damage plays a role in the pathogenesis of AMD (81–84). Consequently, some have suggested that the absorption characteristics and antioxidant properties of macular pigment may confer protection against AMD (80,85).

The density of macular pigment has been found to be significantly different between men and women. In one study, macular pigment density for men was 38% higher than for women (86). Given the putative protective role of macular pigments (80), this finding may explain the higher prevalence of AMD in women found in some studies (see above). Likewise, a strong inverse relationship between smoking and macular pigment density has been shown by Hammond and associates, and this may explain how smoking increases the risk of AMD (see below) (87).

The density of the macular pigment can be altered by diet. Hammond and associates reported that an average increase of approximately 20% in human macular pigment density was obtained after 4 weeks of a diet enriched in corn and spinach (88). The Eye Disease Case-Control Study reported that a high dietary intake of macular pigments from leafy green vegetables was associated with a reduced risk of neovascular AMD (see below) (89). Sommerburg and associates reported that fruits and vegetables of different colors could be consumed to increase the dietary intake of lutein and zeaxanthin (90). Because human macular pigment can be augmented with dietary modification, the protective effect of macular pigment, if proven, has potential therapeutic implications.

C. Cataract and Its Surgery

Since cataract and AMD are the most frequent causes of visual impairment in older individuals and their prevalence is strongly age-related (91), a possible association between the two conditions has long been debated. There may be potential risk factors that are common to both conditions, such as antioxidant intake (92), cigarette smoking (93), and sunlight exposure (94–98).

The association between cataract and AMD has not been consistently found. In the small population-based study in Melton Mowbray (33) and a case-control study by Tsang and associates (69), no statistically significant association was found between cataract and AMD. Sperduto and Siegel found no association between cataract and AMD when the various age-related lens changes were pooled in the Framingham Eye Study and they concluded that cataract and AMD are unrelated and develop entirely independently (99). However, when they reexamined the same data to study specific types of cataracts, they found a positive association between AMD and cortical changes and a negative association between AMD and nuclear sclerosis (100). In contrast, Klein and associates found a positive association between early or any AMD and nuclear sclerosis but no relationship of cortical cataract or of posterior subcapsular cataract to early or late AMD in the Beaver Dam Eye Study (101). In addition, there was no relationship of nuclear or cortical cataract to the incidence and progression of AMD (70).

An analysis of the data from NHANES-I by Liu and associates found that the odds ratios of having AMD in eyes with lens opacity without visual impairment and cataract when compared to eyes with no lens opacity were 1.80 (95% CI, 1.400–2.30) and 1.14 (95% CI, 0.84-1.55), respectively (102). The authors postulated that the weak association between cataract and AMD may reflect the difficulty of visualizing the ocular fundus in eyes with dense cataract. Other possible theories include retardation of transmission of light to the retina by cataracts, thus decreasing the extent of light damage, and different kinds of cataracts may have differing pathogenesis and for some types, no common factors may be shared with AMD (102). In the FRANCE-DMLA Study Group's case-control study, persons with lens opacities had increased risk of AMD (OR, 1.69; 95% CI, 1.45–1.97) (64).

Several authors have noted deterioration of AMD following cataract surgery (103–107). In one study, Pollack and associates evaluated 47 patients with bilateral, symmetrical, early AMD who underwent extracapsular cataract extraction with intraocular lens implantation in one eye (105). They found that progression to neovascular AMD occurred more often in the operated eyes (19.1%) compared with the fellow eyes (4.3%). This concurs with a histological study that suggested a higher prevalence of diskiform macular degeneration in pseudophakic eyes than in age-matched phakic eyes (71). Interestingly, Pollack and associates found that progression to neovascular AMD occurred significantly more often in men than in women ($p < 0.05$) (105).

In the Beaver Dam Eye Study, eyes that had undergone cataract surgery before baseline, compared with eyes that were phakic at baseline, were more likely to have progression of AMD (OR, 2.71; 95% CI, 1.69–4.35) and to develop signs of late AMD (OR, 2.80; 95% CI, 1.03–7.63) after controlling for age (70). These relationships remained after controlling for other risk factors in multivariate analyses. The FRANCE-DMLA Study Group found an increased risk of AMD in persons with a history of previous cataract surgery compared to those with no lens opacities or cataract surgery (OR, 1.68; 95% CI, 1.45–1.95) (64). Similarly, Liu and associates found that data from NHANES-I suggest the odds ratio of having AMD in eyes with aphakia compared with eyes with no lens opacity was 2.00 (CI, 1.44–2.78) (102). They suggested that an increase in light transmittance following cataract surgery may reinitiate and dramatically accelerate progression to frank AMD. It is also possible that the association is a result of easier visualization and detection of AMD lesions after cataract surgery (70). It has also been hypothesized that inflammatory changes that may occur in eyes following cataract surgery may be related to the development of late AMD (71).

In the Blue Mountains Eye Study, a higher prevalence of late AMD in eyes with past cataract surgery (6.3%) than in phakic eyes (1.3%) was observed. However, the association was primarily an effect of age because the odds ratio for late AMD reduced to 1.3 (CI, 0.6–2.6) and became nonsignificant after adjusting for age and sex, and to 1.2 (CI, 0.5–2.9), after multivariate adjustment (108). Similarly, a higher prevalence of early AMD was found in eyes with a history of cataract surgery (7.1%) than in phakic eyes (4.4%), with a multivariate-adjusted odds ratio of 0.7 (CI, 0.4–0.9), which suggests a protective effect for cataract surgery (108). The Rotterdam Study also did not find any association between cataract surgery and AMD prevalence (109).

It is unclear why the results vary among the studies. It is possible that these variations in findings may have resulted from differences in the study population and/or from differences in methodology and case definitions.

D. Refractive Error

Several case-control studies have found an association between AMD and refractive error, with hyperopic eyes at greater risk of AMD (48,60,64,100). Hyman and associates found that statistically significant differences in mean refractive error were present between female cases and controls ($p = 0.009$), but not between male cases and controls ($p = 0.16$) (48). Female cases had a more positive refractive error (mean = 1.8 diopters) than female controls (mean = 1.1 diopters). The FRANCE-DMLA Study Group found the odds ratios for AMD in hyperopes and myopes, compared to emmetropes, were 1.33 (95% CI, 1.11–1.59) and 0.99 (95% CI, 0.78–1.25) (64). The Eye Disease Case-Control Study found that persons with hyperopia had a slightly higher risk of neovascular AMD, but the association did not remain statistically significant after multivariate modeling (6). One caveat in the interpretation of findings in these case-control studies is that because the controls were recruited from ophthalmological clinics, the control groups may be enriched in the proportion of myopes compared with the general population. In fact, in the case-control study by the FRANCE-DMLA Study Group, the authors stated that "the majority of the control group was seen for refractive problems" (64).

Data from NHANES-I showed that the odd ratios (95% CI) of AMD in hyperopes and myopes, compared to emmetropes, were 1.61 (1.15–2.25) and 1.33 (0.69–2.57), respectively (7). This differs from the Beaver Dam Eye Study, which showed a protective effect of borderline significance of hyperopia at baseline on the incidence of early AMD, but no relationship to the incidence of late AMD or to the progression of AMD (70).

E. Cup/Disk Ratio

The Eye Disease Case-Control Study found that eyes with large horizontal and vertical cup/disk ratios were at reduced risk for neovascular AMD (6). The horizontal cup/disk ratio persisted as statistically significant after multivariate modeling, adjusting for known and potential confounding factors. This finding is consistent with the association between AMD and hyperopia.

VII. SYSTEMIC FACTORS

A. Cardiovascular Disease and Its Risk Factors

A number of documented risk factors for cardiovascular disease, such as age, hypertension, hypercholesterolemia, diabetes, smoking, and dietary intake of fats, alcohol, and antioxidants, have been associated with AMD in some studies (111). This raises the possibility that the causal pathways for cardiovascular disease and AMD may share similar risk factors. Results from studies, however, have not been consistent.

1. Cardiovascular Disease

A number of studies have suggested an association between AMD and various clinical manifestations of cardiovascular disease in a case-control study, Hyman and associates found AMD to be positively associated with a history of three cardiovascular conditions (48). These conditions are arteriosclerosis, circulatory problems, and stroke and/or transient ischemic attacks, with odds ratios (95% CI) of 2.3 (1.9–2.7), 2.0 (1.1–3.5), and 2.9 (1.3–6.9), respectively (48). The FRANCE-DMLA Study Group found an increased risk of AMD in persons with a history of coronary artery disease (OR, 1.31; 95% CI, 1.02–1.68) (64). In NHANES-I, a positive association between AMD and cerebrovascular disease was found, but positive associations with other vascular diseases did not reach statistical significance (7).

The Rotterdam Study found that atherosclerotic plaques in the carotid bifurcation, as assessed ultrasonographically, were associated with a 4.5 times increased prevalence odds (95% CI, 1.9–10.7) of either geographic atrophy or neovascular AMD (112). Those with plaques in the common carotid artery or with lower extremity arterial disease (as measured by the ratio of the systolic blood pressure level of the ankle to systolic blood pressure of the arm) had the same increased prevalence odds of 2.5 (95% CI, 1.4–4.5). From these observations, the authors suggested that atherosclerosis may be involved in the etiology of AMD. However, other cardiovascular disease risk factors, such as hypertension, systolic blood pressure, total cholesterol, and HDL cholesterol, were not associated with AMD in the same study (112). Diastolic blood pressure was marginally higher in AMD cases than in those without AMD, but this did not reach statistical significance (112). In subjects participating in the Atherosclerosis Risk In Communities Study, presence of carotid artery plaque was significantly associated with RPE depigmentation (OR, 1.77; 95% CI, 1.18–2.65) (40). Focal retinal arteriolar narrowing was also associated with RPE depigmentation (OR, 1.79; 95% CI, 1.07–2.98) in the same study. In a Finnish population-based study, a significant correlation between the severity of retinal arteriolar sclerosis and AMD ($p = 0.0034$) was found (30).

Several case-control studies, including the Eye Disease Case-Control Study, found that persons who report a history of cardiovascular disease did not have a significantly increased risk of AMD (6,60,69). The Beaver Dam Study (113), the Atherosclerosis Risk in Communities Study (40), and the Blue Mountains Eye Study also found no statistically significant relationship between a history of stroke or cardiovascular disease and early or late AMD.

2. Hypertension and Blood Pressure

Two large population-based studies showed a small and consistent significant association between AMD and systemic hypertension (7,12,114). Kahn and associates, using the Framingham Heart and Eye Studies data, found a positive association between the presence of AMD and higher levels of diastolic blood pressure measured many years before the eye examination (12). Diastolic blood pressure was also associated with AMD in a small Israeli study (115). Also using data from the Framingham Heart and Eye Studies, Sperduto and Hiller found the age- and sex-adjusted relative risk for any AMD was 1.18 (95% CI, 1.01–1.37) for persons diagnosed with hypertension 25 years before the eye examination and 1.04 (95% CI, 0.96–1.23) for persons with hypertension at the time of the eye examination, when compared to those without hypertension (114). In addition, an increase in the odds ratio of AMD with longer duration of systemic hypertension was documented. The NHANES-I showed that systolic blood pressure and hypertension were associated with AMD (7). Persons with a history of hypertension were 1.36 times (95% CI, 1.00–1.85) more likely to have AMD compared to persons without such a history. In addition, the prevalence of AMD increased with increasing levels of systolic blood pressure although the test for trend was only marginally significant ($p < 0.08$). However, elevated diastolic blood pressure was not associated with AMD.

The Beaver Dam Eye Study found elevated systolic blood pressure to be significantly related to the presence of RPE depigmentation in women (OR, 1.07; 95% CI, 1.00–1.14), but not in men (113). Pulse pressure was also related to the presence of RPE depigmentation (OR, 1.10; 95% CI, 1.01–1.19), increased retinal pigment (OR, 1.07; 95% CI, 1.00–1.15), and pigmentary abnormalities (OR, 1.08; 95% CI, 1.01– 1.15) in women, but not in men (113). However, hypertension or diastolic blood pressure was not related to any sign of early or late AMD in either sex. In an incidence study, after controlling for age and sex, both higher systolic blood pressure (OR per 10 mmHg, 1.16; 95% CI, 1.05—1.27) and uncontrolled "treated" hypertension (OR, 1.98; 95% CI, 1.00–3.94) were related to the incidence of RPE depigmentation, but not development of neovascular AMD (116). Higher pulse pressure was significantly associated with increased incidence of RPE depigmentation (OR per 10 mmHg, 1.27; 95% CI, 1.14–1.42) and neovascular AMD (OR per 10 mmHg, 1.29; 95% CI, 1.02– 1.65) after controlling for age and sex.

Systemic hypertension was found to be a significant risk factor for AMD by the FRANCE-DMLA Study Group (64). Another recent case-control study by the Age-Related Macular Degeneration Risk Factors Study Group analyzed risk factors separately for neovascular and nonneovascular AMD to address the possibility that the two forms of AMD have different risk factors (19). The group showed that neovascular AMD, but not non-neovascular AMD, is associated with moderate to severe hypertension (19). Neovascular AMD was found to be positively associated with diastolic blood pressure greater than 95 mmHg (OR, 4.4; 95% CI, 1.4–14.2), self-reported use of antihypertensive medications more potent than diuretics (OR, 2.1; 95% CI, 1.2–3.0), physician-reported history of hypertension (OR, 1.8; 95% CI, 1.2–3.0), and physician-reported use of any antihypertensive medications (OR, 2.5; 95% CI, 1.5–4.2). The findings in this study suggest that neovascular AMD and hypertension may have a similar systemic process. In addition, they support the hypothesis that neovascular and nonneovascular AMD may arise through different pathogenetic mechanisms.

No association between hypertension and AMD was found in several population-based cross-sectional studies such as the Rotterdam Study (112), the Blue Mountains Eye Study (18), and the Atherosclerosis Risk in Communities Study (40), or in several case-control studies (6;48;60;69). In the Eye Disease Case-Control Study, no significant association was found with hypertension and AMD, but a trend for an increased risk associated with higher systolic blood pressure was seen (6).

3. Serum Lipid Levels and Dietary Fat Intake

Some evidence suggests that dietary fat intake, particularly intake of saturated fat and cholesterol, is associated with an increased risk for atherosclerosis (117). It is biologically plausible that higher dietary saturated fat intake increases the risk of AMD by promoting atherosclerosis.

The Eye Disease Case-Control Study found that persons with midrange (4.889–6.748 mmol/L) and high (≥6.749 mmol/L) total cholesterol levels compared with those with low levels (≤4.888 mmol/L) had odd ratios for neovascular AMD of 2.2 (95% CI = 1.3–3.4) and 4.1 (95% CI = 2.3–7.3), respectively, after controlling for other factors (6). A slight but not statistically significant increased risk of neovascular AMD was seen with increasing levels of serum triglycerides in the same study (6).

In the Beaver Dam Eye Study, after controlling for age, total serum cholesterol was inversely related to early AMD in women (OR, 0.89; 95% CI, 0.80–0.98), whereas the total cholesterol/HDL cholesterol ratio was inversely related (OR, 0.89; 95% CI, 0.84–0.96) and HDL cholesterol was positively related to early AMD in men (113). The reasons for these associations are not clear although a possible explanation is selective survival. Because persons with higher cholesterol levels or lower HDL cholesterol levels are at higher risk of cardiovascular death than persons with normal levels of cholesterol, a positive relationship may have been obscured. Serum cholesterol or HDL cholesterol was not related to neovascular AMD or geographic atrophy in the same study (113).

The Age-Related Macular Degeneration Risk Factors Study Group found neovascular AMD, but not nonneovascular AMD, to be positively associated with high-density lipoprotein level (OR, 2.3; 95% CI, 1.1–4.7), and dietary cholesterol level (OR, 2.2; 95% CI, 1.0–4.8) (19).

In the Beaver Dam Eye Study, persons with intake of saturated fat and cholesterol in the highest compared with the lowest quintile had odds ratio of 1.8 (95% CI, 1.2–2.7) and 1.6 (95% CI, 1.1–2.4) for early AMD, respectively, after adjusting for age and beer intake (118). However, no significant association between these intakes was found with late AMD (118). The findings in this study concur with the Blue Mountains Eye Study, which found that total and saturated fat intake were associated with a borderline significant increase in risk for early AMD [ORs (95% CI) for highest compared to lowest quintiles of intake, 1.60 (0.94–2.73) and 1.50 (0.91–2.48), respectively], but not for late AMD (119). A significant association (p for trend = 0.05) for increasing prevalence of early AMD with increasing monounsaturated fat intake was observed. Cholesterol intake was associated with a borderline significant increase in risk for late AMD [OR (95% CI) for highest compared to lowest quintiles of intake, 2.71 (0.93–7.96); p for trend = 0.04].

The Rotterdam Study (112), the Blue Mountains Eye Study (18), and the Atherosclerosis Risk in Communities Study (40) did not find any association between serum cholesterol or HDL cholesterol with AMD. No significant association between AMD and serum cholesterol was also found in the Framingham Eye Study (12), NHANES-I (7), and several small studies (69, 120, 421). No difference in the levels of plasma cholesterol and fatty acids was found between 65 cases of neovascular AMD and control pairs in a study by Sanders and associates (122).

4. Diabetes and Hyperglycemia

The majority of studies that have investigated the relationship between diabetes and/or hyperglycemia and AMD have found no significant association (6,12,30,40,48,60,69,123).

One small study by Vidaurri and associates observed an association between drusen and serum glucose in women but not in men (115). In the Beaver Dam Eye Study, diabetes was not associated with early AMD (124). In persons ≥ 75 years, those with diabetes had a higher frequency of neovascular AMD (9.4%) than those without (4.7%) but both groups had similar frequencies of geographic atrophy. The relative risk of neovascular AMD in diabetic men compared to nondiabetic men ≥ 75 years was 10.2 (95% CI, 2.4–43.7); for women it was 1.1 (95% CI, 0.4–3.0). The authors suggested that the relationship of neovascular AMD in older men, but not women, might be the result of chance, in the same study, no relationship was found between glycosylated hemoglobin and any signs of AMD in nondiabetic persons (124). The Blue Mountains Eye Study found geographic atrophy to be significantly associated with diabetes (OR, 4.0; 95 CI, 1.6–10.3), but no association was found with either neovascular AMD (OR, 1.2; 95% CI, 0.4–3.5) or early AMD (OR, 1.0;

95% CI, 0.5–1.8 (125). There was also no association found between impaired fasting glucose and AMD (125). The Atherosclerosis Risk in Communities Study (40) did not find any association between AMD and diabetes.

Overall, there is scant evidence in the literature to suggest a real relationship between diabetes and/or hyperglycemia and AMD.

5. Body Mass Index

In the Blue Mountains Eye Study, having a body mass index (BMI) [defined as body weight in kilograms divided by height in meters squared (kg/m^2)] either lower or higher than the accepted normal range (20–25) was associated with a significantly increased risk of early AMD (18). Low BMI (OR, 1.92; 95% CI, 1.16–3.18) conferred an increased risk for early AMD almost equal to that of obesity (OR, 1.78; 95% CI, 1.19–2.68). This association is thus difficult to explain in terms of cardiovascular risk. Although the odds ratios were similar for association with late AMD, they did not reach statistical significance. A Finnish population-based study found that a high BMI was associated with an increased risk of AMD in men but not in women (30). On the other hand, the Beaver Dam Eye Study found that BMI was associated with increased frequency of RPE degeneration, increased retinal pigment, and increased presence of pigmentary abnormalities in women but not in men (113). No association between BMI and AMD was found in the Atherosclerosis Risk in Communities Study (40).

6. Hematological Factors

The Beaver Dam Eye Study found that, after controlling for age, sex, diabetes, and smoking history, neovascular AMD was associated with higher hematocrit values (OR, 1.09; 95% CI, 1.00–1.19) and higher leukocyte count (OR, 1.10; 95% CI, 1.00–1.19) in people 65 years of age or older (113). Blumenkranz and associates also found a higher leukocyte count in patients with neovascular AMD compared to controls (66). No association between hematocrit and AMD was found in NHANES-1 (7).

The Blue Mountains Eye Study found that plasma fibrinogen level was associated with late but not early AMD (18). The Eye Disease Case-Control Study found a nonsignificant increased risk of neovascular AMD with increasing plasma fibrinogen levels (6).

7. Cigarette Smoking

This will be discussed under environmental factors (see below).

B. Reproductive and Related Factors

The relationship of cardiovascular disease to AMD has generated some interest in the effect of estrogen-related variables on the risk of AMD in women. The Eye Disease Case-Control Study found that use of postmenopausal exogenous estrogen was negatively associated with neovascular AMD (6). Current and former users of estrogen had odd ratios of 0.3 (95% CI, 0.1–0.8) and 0.6 (95% CI, 0.3–0.98) for neovascular AMD, respectively, when compared to women who never used estrogen. This is compatible with findings from a nested case-control study within the Rotterdam Study, which suggest that early artificial menopause increases the risk of late AMD (atrophic or neovascular AMD) (126). Women with early menopause after unilateral or bilateral oophorectomies had an increased risk of late AMD compared with women who had their menopause at 45 years or later. No significant excess risk was found for early spontaneous menopause and early hysterectomy. In the Blue Mountains Eye Study, a significant protective association for early AMD was found with increased years from menarche to menopause (OR, 0.97; 95% CI, 0.95–0.99) (32). Other female-specific factors including late menarche, history of hormone replacement therapy, and early menopause were not significantly associated with early or late AMD (32).

No significant relationship, however, was found in the Beaver Dam Eye Study between years of estrogen therapy and neovascular AMD, geographic atrophy, or early AMD (127). It should be noted that because the number of cases of late AMD in the Beaver Dam Eye Study was small, the power to detect a real association is limited.

Women who have ever been pregnant (parity $\geq$ 1) had increased odds of 2.2 (95% CI = 1.3–3.9) compared to women who have never been pregnant (parity = 0) in the Eye Disease Case-Control Study (6). On the other hand, the Beaver Dam Eye Study documented that the number of past pregnancies was significantly inversely related to soft drusen, with odds ratio of 0.94 per pregnancy (95% CI, 0.90–0.98) (127). The relationship with the number of pregnancies to any AMD was of borderline significance, the odds ratio being 0.96 per pregnancy (95% CI, 0.92–1.01). The number of pregnancies was not significantly related to neovascular AMD or geographic atrophy. Past use of birth control pills, age of menarche, or the number of years of menstruation had no significant effect on AMD in the Beaver Dam Eye Study (127).

C. Dermal Elastotic Degeneration

In a small case-control study, Blumenkranz and associates found a correlation between the degree of dermal elastic degeneration in sun-protected skin with the development of neovascular AMD (66). However, there was no significant difference in outdoor sun exposure as estimated by patients. In fact, cases admitted to fewer average hours outdoors weekly than controls. The authors suggested that patients with neovascular AMD may have a generalized systemic disorder characterized by abnormal susceptibility of elastic fibers to photic or other as-yet unrecognized degenerative stimuli.

D. Antioxidant Enzymes

Recently, the POLA (Pathologies Oculaires Liees a l'Age) Study, a large-scale, population-based, cross-sectional study in southern France, found that higher levels of plasma glutathione peroxidase were significantly associated with a ninefold increase in late AMD prevalence, but not with prevalence of early AMD (128). Plasma glutathione peroxidase therefore appears to be one of the strongest indicators of late AMD ever found, but the biological meaning of this finding remains to be elucidated. The authors suggest that oxidative stress may lead to the induction of antioxidant enzymes, and therefore high concentrations of antioxidant enzymes may be indicators of oxidative stress. In the same study, levels of erythrocyte superoxide dismutase activity were not associated with either early or late AMD.

VIII. ENVIRONMENTAL FACTORS

A. Smoking

Of the environmental influences, smoking has most consistently been associated with increased risks of AMD in recent studies (6,48,129–137). However, a number of studies

(30,60,64,66,69), including the Framingham Eye Study (12) and NHANES-III (25), did not find an association between smoking and AMD. In fact, one study by West and associates even showed smoking to be protective (67). However, when this decreased risk of AMD associated with smoking was further investigated, no clear dose-response relationship was demonstrated. In the large case-control study by the FRANCE-DMLA Study Group, a past history of smoking, but not current smoking status, was associated with an increased risk of AMD after univariate analysis (64). After multivariate adjustment, both factors were not significantly associated with AMD.

Paetkau and associates noted in their case series of 114 patients with at least one eye blind from AMD that the mean age at the onset of blindness in the first eye was 64 years in current smokers compared with 71 years in the group that had never smoked (129). However, because there was no control group, confounding factors such as increased mortality in the smoking group cannot be excluded. In a Japanese case-control study, compared to male nonsmokers, the age-adjusted odds ratio of developing neovascular AMD was 2.97 (95% CI, 1.00–8.84) for male current smokers and 2.09 (95% CI, 0.71–6.13) for male former smokers (136). In addition, smoking-habit-related variables, such as use of extra filter, smoke inhalation level, age at starting smoking, duration of smoking, and the Brinkman index, defined as the numbers of cigarette smoked per day times smoking years, were found to be significantly related to an increased risk of neovascular AMD (136).

The Beaver Dam Eye Study found that the relative odds for neovascular AMD in men and women who were current smokers compared with those who were former smokers or who never smoked were 3.29 (95% CI, 1.03–10.50) and 2.50 (95% CI, 1.01–6.20), respectively (131). However, there was no significant relation between smoking status and geographic atrophy. In addition, smoking status, pack-years smoked, and current exposure to passive smoking were not associated with signs of early AMD, except for a higher frequency of increased retinal pigment in men who were former smokers compared with those who had never smoked (131).

The Blue Mountains Eye Study found current cigarette smoking to be significantly associated with both early and late AMD, after adjusting for the effects of age and sex (134). The odds ratio of early and late AMD when comparing current smokers to those who never smoked was 1.89 (95% CI, 1.25–2.84) and 4.46 (95% CI, 2.20–9.03), respectively. A history of having ever smoked was significant for late AMD (OR, 1.83; 95% CI, 1.07–3.13) but not early AMD (134). In addition, passive smoking among subjects who never themselves smoked, but lived with a smoking spouse, incurred a moderate but not statistically significant increase in the risk of late AMD (OR, 1.42; 95% CI, 0.62–3.26).

In the POLA Study, after adjustment for age and sex, current (OR, 3.6; 95% CI, 1.1–12.4) and former smokers (OR, 3.2; 95% CI, 1.3–7.7) had an increased prevalence of late AMD when compared to nonsmokers (137). The risk of late AMD increased with increasing number of pack-years, with up to a 5.2-fold increase in risk among participants (current and former smokers combined) who smoked 40 pack-years or more (OR, 1.9; 95% CI, 0.6–6.4 for 1–19 pack-years, OR, 3.0; 95% CI, 0.9–9.5 for 20–39 pack-years, and OR, 5.2; 95% CI, 2.0–13.6 for 40 pack-years and more). In addition, the risk of late AMD remained increased until 20 years after cessation of smoking. However, the study found no significant associations of smoking with early AMD (soft distinct and indistinct drusen and pigmentary abnormalities) (137).

Two large prospective cohort studies evaluated the relationship between smoking and AMD (133,135). In the Nurses' Health Study with 12 years of follow-up, women who currently smoked ≥ 25 cigarettes per day had a relative risk of AMD of 2.4 (95% CI,

1.4–4.0) compared with women who never smoked (135). Risk of AMD also increased with an increasing number of pack-years smoked (p for trend < 0.001). Past smokers of this amount also had a relative risk of 2.0 (95% CI, 1.2–3.4) compared to women who never smoked. Compared with current smokers, little reduction in risk was found even after quitting smoking for 15 or more years. In the Physicians' Health Study, men who were current smokers of ≥ 20 cigarettes per day had a relative risk of AMD of 2.5 (95% CI, 1.6–3.8) compared with men who never smoked (133). Men who were past smokers had a modest elevation in relative risk of AMD of 1.3 (95% CI, 1.0–1.7).

Some have suggested that the effect of cigarette smoking on the development of AMD may be related to its effect on antioxidants in the body (136). Studies have shown that smokers have much lower plasma levels of β-carotene than do nonsmokers (122,138). Stryker and associates found that men and women who smoked one pack per day had 72% (95% CI, 58–89) and 79% (95% CI, 64–99) of the plasma β-carotene levels of nonsmokers, respectively, after accounting for dietary carotene and other variables (138). Another study also disclosed that smokers had lower plasma concentrations of total carotenoids, α-carotene, and β-carotene than nonsmokers (122). In addition, a recent study found that smokers have significantly lower macular pigment density compared to nonsmoking matched controls (87).

In summary, data from several large population-based studies (131,132,134,137), case-control studies (6,48,36), and two large prospective cohort studies (133,135) provide convincing evidence that cigarette smoking is a risk factor for AMD. The strongest risk is for current smokers, suggesting that there may be potential benefits of targeting antismoking patient education, especially for those who are current smokers and have signs of early AMD (134).

B. Sunlight Exposure

Exposure to sunlight has long been suggested as a risk factor for AMD. Short-term exposures to longer-wavelength ultraviolet and blue light can cause retinal damage in animals (139). There are some similarities between long-term changes seen in laboratory animals exposed to shorter-wavelength visible light and changes seen in patients with AMD (81,140–145). It is theorized that light may lead to the generation of reactive oxygen species in the outer retina and/or choroid (81), perhaps by photoactivation of protoporhyrin (146). The activated forms of oxygen may, in turn, cause lipid peroxidation of the photoreceptor outer segment membranes, leading to the development of AMD.

Tso and Woodford have shown that short exposure of intense visible light can produce atrophy at the photoreceptor level in nonhuman primates (147), but these animals did not develop histopathological changes of drusen, diffuse thickening of Bruch's membrane, or choroidal neovascularization seen in clinicopathological studies of AMD (148). In addition, the short, intense light exposure used in animal studies is different from the typical chronic exposure to light that occurs in people in their lifetime. The only animal model for light-induced deposits in Bruch's membrane is that of Gottsch and co-workers, who have proposed that photosensitization of choriocapillary endothelium with blood-borne photosensitizers such as protoporphyrin IX is a mechanism for the histopathological features seen in AMD (146,149).

The epidemiological evidence of an association between light exposure and AMD is lacking, with only a few clinical studies showing a positive association between sun exposure and late AMD. A small Spanish case-control study found a higher sun exposure index in AMD cases compared to controls (150). In the Chesapeake Bay Watermen Study, an association between late AMD (geographic atrophy or diskiform scarring) and ocular exposure in the previous 20 years to blue or visible light (OR, 1.36; 95% CI, 1.00–1.85) was found in phakic men (96). However, no positive association was seen for early AMD (large drusen or RPE abnormalities) (96). In addition, there was no association between ultraviolet-A or ultraviolet-B exposure and any degree of AMD in the same population (67,96).

The Beaver Dam Eye Study found that leisure time outdoors in summer was significantly associated with the presence of neovascular AMD when both men and women were analyzed together (OR = 2.26, 95% CI = 1.06–4.81) (151). Time spent outdoors in summer was significantly associated with the prevalence of increased retinal pigment in men (OR = 1.44, 95% CI = 1.01–2.04) but not in women (OR = 0.93, 95% CI = 0.63–1.38). Use of sunglasses and hats with brims was inversely associated with the prevalence of soft indistinct drusen in men (OR = 0.61, 95% CI = 0.38–0.98) but not in women (OR = 0.99, 95% CI = 0.69–1.45). The association between light exposure and AMD is not consistent across the study since an association was found in men only, and involved only a specific subset of light exposure (time spent outdoors in summer but not in winter) and a specific subset of early AMD (151).

A number of case-control studies, including the Eye Disease Case-Control Study (6), failed to show an association between sunlight exposure and AMD (48,152). An Australian case-control study in fact showed that control subjects had greater median annual ocular sun exposure (865 h) than cases (723 h) ($p > 0.0001$) (152). Despite analysis stratified by sun sensitivity, sun exposure was greater in control subjects than in cases with AMD (152).

In summary, there is currently no convincing research data to support strategies to reduce light exposure to the eye for the prevention of AMD. However, since there is little, if any, risk to a person wearing sunglasses, and ultraviolet-light exposure has been associated with the presence of cataract (95), it is reasonable to suggest that individuals wear sunglasses for comfort and to reduce exposure of ultraviolet light to ocular structures. It must be emphasized, however, that there is no published data to indicate whether the wearing of sunglasses is of any benefit in preventing any eye disease, including AMD.

C. Nutritional Factors

1. Micronutrients

The potential role of nutritional supplements to reduce the incidence or severity of AMD has received a great deal of attention (80,92). The lack of an effective treatment for the majority of cases of AMD, coupled with the public's perception that over-the-counter nutritional supplements are relatively harmless, creates the potential for widespread use of these supplements in the absence of demonstrated effectiveness (153). Because of possible, but as yet unproven, benefits of antioxidant vitamins in cancer, cardiovascular, and other chronic diseases, vitamin supplement usage in the United States has increased steadily in recent years. It is estimated that more than half of the adult population in the United States uses dietary supplements, including supplements of antioxidant vitamins, at a cost of approximately $12 billion annually (21).

Although epidemiological studies provide support for a protective role of nutritional antioxidants in the prevention of AMD, results of prospective randomized clinical trials are necessary before firm conclusions can be drawn about the balance of benefits and risks of nutritional supplements for the prevention of AMD. In fact, use of nutritional supplement has been shown to have deleterious effects in some nonophthalmic medical trials. The Alpha-Tocopherol, Beta-Carotene (ATBC) Cancer Prevention Study found a higher incidence of lung cancer among men who received β-carotene than among those who did not (change in incidence, 18%; 95% CI, 3–36%) (154). There were also more deaths due to lung cancer, ischemic heart disease, and ischemic and hemorrhagic stroke among recipients of β-carotene, with an increased overall mortality of 8% (95% CI, 1–16%). Those randomized to vitamin E supplementation had higher rates of hemorrhagic stroke, but there was no overall difference in mortality rates or cancer incidence (154). In the Carotene and Retinol Efficacy Trial (CARET), participants who were given β-carotene and vitamin A supplements had a 28% (95% CI, 4–57%) increased incidence of lung cancer and a 17% (95% CI, 3–33%) higher mortality compared to those who were not (155).

a. Antioxidants. Some have suggested that antioxidants and a variety of trace minerals necessary for the proper functioning of some key enzyme systems may reduce the risk of AMD (81, 156, 157). Photochemical damage from light can induce the production of activated forms of oxygen, which in turn can cause lipid peroxidation of the photoreceptor outer segment membranes. Antioxidants, such as vitamin C, vitamin E, β-carotene, and glutathione, and antioxidant enzymes, such as selenium-dependent glutathione peroxidase, in theory could act as singlet oxygen and free-radical scavengers and thereby prevent cellular damage (158). There is considerable interest in determining whether free radicals contribute to the pathogenesis of AMD and whether high levels of these antioxidants may protect against AMD. This hypothesis is supported by findings of disruption of retinal photoreceptors in nonhuman primates with deficiencies of vitamins A and E (159) and a protective effect of vitamin C in reducing the loss of rhodopsin and photoreceptor cell nuclei in rats exposed to photic injury (160).

Many studies have used serum levels of micronutrients to investigate the relationship of these micronutrients and AMD. Unfortunately, high and low levels are defined differently for most studies. Most have defined the high and low categories on the basis of percentile categories, i.e., those individuals with serum concentrations above a given percentile were categorized as high and those below a given percentile were categorized as low.

Blumenkranz and associates reported in their small case-control study that the serum levels of vitamins A, C, and E were not different in cases of neovascular AMD and in controls (66). In another case-control study, serum levels of vitamin E in cases and controls were similar but serum selenium was significantly lower in cases compared to controls ($p = 0.02$) (69). The Eye Disease Case-Control Study found that persons with carotenoid scores in the medium and high percentile groups, compared with those in the low group, had markedly reduced levels of risk of neovascular AMD, with levels of risk reduced to one-half (OR, 0.5; 95% CI, 0.4–0.8) and one-third (OR, 0.3; 95% CI, 0.2–0.6), respectively (5). Similarly, except for lycopene, higher levels of individual carotenoids (lutein/zeaxanthin, β-carotene, α-carotene, or cryptoxanthin) were associated with statistically significant reductions in risk of neovascular AMD. In addition, there was a progressive decrease in risk of neovascular AMD with increasing levels of carotenoids and increasing levels of the antioxidant index. However, no statistically significant overall association was seen with neovascular AMD and serum levels of vitamin C, vitamin E, and selenium in the study (5).

West and associates examined the relationship between plasma levels of retinol, ascorbic acid, α-tocopherol, and β-carotene in 630 participants of the Baltimore Longitudinal Study on Aging (161). They found a favorable association between plasma antioxidants and AMD. Their data suggest that only α-tocopherol was significantly associated with a protective effect (OR for middle vs. lowest quartiles, 0.50; 95% CI, 0.32-0.79; OR for highest vs. lowest quartile, 0.43; 95% CI, 0.25-0.73). This is consistent with findings from a small Spanish case-control study (150). There was a suggestion of a protective effect with ascorbic acid and β-carotene in the Baltimore Longitudinal Study on Aging, but their effects were not statistically significant (161). No protective effect was noted for retinol. For late AMD (neovascular AMD or geographic atrophy), no significant protective effect was observed for any plasma micronutrient. An antioxidant index constructed of ascorbic acid, α-tocopherol, and β-carotene, controlled for age and sex, suggested that high values were protective for AMD compared with low values.

It is now generally recognized that plasma α-tocopherol level should be expressed in terms of its concentration within lipids or lipoproteins (162–164). For this reason, the POLA Study correlated ocular findings with both plasma α-tocopherol and lipid-standardized α-tocopherol levels (17). The study found a weak negative association between late AMD and plasma α-tocopherol level, which was not statistically significant ($p = 0.07$), but this relationship was strengthened when α-tocopherol-lipid ratio instead of plasma level was used ($p = 0.003$). After adjusting for confounding factors, the odds ratios (95% CI) for late AMD in persons with α-tocopherol-lipid ratio in the highest and middle quintiles, compared with those with ratio in the lowest quintile, were 0.18 (0.05–0.67) and 0.46 (0.22–0.95), respectively. The odds ratios (95% CI) for any sign of early AMD in persons with α-tocopherol-lipid ratio in the highest and middle quintiles, compared with those with ratio in the lowest quintile, were 0.72 (0.53–0.98) and 0.78 (0.61–1.00), respectively. No association was found with plasma retinol and ascorbic acid levels or with red blood cell glutathione values (17).

Data from NHANES-I, collected between 1971 and 1972, suggest that the frequency of consumption of fruits and vegetables characterized as rich in vitamin A is inversely related to the prevalence of AMD, after adjustment for medical and demographic factors (7). The Eye Disease Case-Control Study evaluated the relationship of dietary intake of carotenoids, and vitamins A, C, and E, with neovascular AMD (89). Those in the highest quintile of carotenoid intake, after adjusting for other risk factors of AMD, had an odds ratio of 0.57 (95% CI = 0.35–0.92) for neovascular AMD compared with those in the lowest quintile. Among the specific carotenoids, the strongest association with a reduced risk for neovascular AMD was found with lutein and zeaxanthin, which are primarily obtained from dark-green, leafy vegetables. Intake of vitamin C was associated with a small but nonsignificant reduction in risk of neovascular AMD. No reduction in risk was found with intake of vitamin A or E.

The Blue Mountains Eye Study, using a validated 145-item semiquantitative food frequency questionnaire, found no significant associations between early or late AMD and dietary intakes of carotene, vitamin A, or vitamin C, from combined diet and supplement, after adjusting for age, sex, current smoking, and AMD family history (165). There were no statistically significant trends for decreasing AMD prevalence with increasing intake of any antioxidant. Consumption of supplements was also not significantly associated with either early (OR, 1.0; 95% CI, 0.7–1.4) or late (OR, 1.2; 95% CI, 0.6–2.3) AMD. In addition, a nested case-control study within the Blue Mountains Eye Study did not find any association between AMD or serum α-tocopherol or β-carotene (166). Similarly, no significant associations between the intake of vitamin C or E or carotenoids from the diet or supplements and the prevalence of early or late AMD were observed in the Beaver Dam Eye Study (167). However, in a nested case-control study within the Beaver Dam Eye Study population-based cohort, low levels of serum lycopene, but not other carotenoids (α-carotene, β-carotene, β-cryptoxanthin, or lutein and zeaxanthin), was related to an increased likelihood of AMD (OR, 2.2; 95% CI, 1.1–4.5) (168).

The association between self-selection for antioxidant vitamin supplement use and incidence of AMD was examined among 21,120 participants in the Physicians' Health Study I who did not have a diagnosis of AMD at baseline (8). A total of 279 incident cases of AMD with vision loss to 20/30 or worse were confirmed during an average follow-up of 12.5 years. Compared to nonusers of vitamin supplements, persons who reported taking vitamin E supplements at baseline had a nonsignificant 13% reduced risk of AMD (RR, 0.87; 95% CI, 0.53–1.43), after adjusting for other risk factors. Users of multivitamins had a nonsignificant 10% reduced risk of AMD (RR, 0.90; 95% CI, 0.68–1.19). No reduced risk of AMD was observed for users of vitamin C supplements (RR, 1.03; 95% CI, 0.71–1.50).

   b. Zinc.   Zinc has received attention because of its high concentration in ocular tissues, particularly the sensory retina, RPE, and choroid (169), and its role as a cofactor for numerous metalloenzymes, including retinol dehydrogenase and catalase (170). In addition, there are some reports of zinc deficiency in the elderly, the population subgroup at greatest risk of AMD (171). Data from NHANES-III suggest that persons aged ≥71 years, together with young children aged 1–3 years and adolescent females aged 12—19 years, were at the greatest risk of inadequate zinc intakes (172). It has been hypothesized that zinc deficiency in elderly persons may cause the loss of zinc-dependent coenzymes in the RPE, resulting in the development or worsening of AMD (173).

   Newsome and associates conducted a prospective, randomized, double-blind, placebo-controlled trial that investigated the effects of oral zinc administration on the visual acuity outcome in 151 subjects with early to late AMD (174). They showed that eyes in zinc-treated group had significantly less visual loss than the placebo group after a follow-up of 12–24 months. In addition, there was less accumulation of drusen in the zinc-treated group compared with the placebo group. However, in another double-masked, randomized, placebo-controlled trial, oral zinc supplementation did not have any short-term effect on the course of AMD in patients who have neovascular AMD in one eye (175).

   The Beaver Dam Eye Study found that people in the highest quintile, compared to those in the lowest quintile, for intake of zinc from foods had lower risk of early AMD (OR = 0.6, 95% CI = 0.4–1.0) (167). A lower serum level of zinc was found in AMD cases compared to controls in a small Spanish case-control study (150). However, zinc intake was unrelated to late AMD in the same study. The Eye Disease Case-Control Study did not find any significant relationships between serum zinc levels or zinc supplementation and risk of neovascular AMD (6). This concurs with findings from the Blue Mountains Eye Study (165).

   c. Randomized Trials of Antioxidant Vitamins and Age-Related Macular Degeneration.   The most reliable, and only direct, method of testing the potential protective effects of nutritional supplements is to conduct randomized clinical trials. A small prospective randomized clinical trial showed that a specific 14-component antioxidant-mineral capsule (Ocuguard, Twin Lab, Inc., Ronkonkoma, NY) taken twice daily stabilized but did not improve dry AMD over one and a half years (176,177). Several large-scale randomized clinical trials including the Age-Related Eye Disease Study (AREDS) (153,173), the Physicians' Health Study II (PHS II) (178), the Vitamin E, Cataract, and Age-related macular degeneration Trial (VECAT) (179), the Women's Health Study (WHS) (180), and the Women's Antioxidant Cardiovascular Study (WACS) (181), have been designed to address the issue of antioxidant vitamins and AMD (Table 7). Results of these major trials should provide the strongest evidence to support or to refute an association of antioxidant intake with AMD. Of these trials, AREDS, sponsored by the National Eye Institute (National Institutes of Health, Bethesda, MD), is the first to be completed (173).

Table 7 Some Ongoing Large-Scale Randomized Trials Addressing the Balance of Risks and Benefits of Antioxidant Vitamins for Age-Related Macular Degeneration

Name of randomized trial	Details of trial	Remarks
Age-Related Eye Disease Study (AREDS) (153,173)	A multicenter prospective, double-blind, randomized clinical trial evaluating the role of antioxidant micronutrients (β-carotene, vitamins E and C, and/or zinc) in AMD and cataract. Patients with early AMD to advanced unilateral AMD were randomized to receive either antioxidants, minerals, combination therapy, or placebo. 4,757 individuals aged 55–80 years at baseline were enrolled. Morbidity and mortality associated with the supplements were monitored. Endpoints include doubling of visual angle and morphological progression of AMD.	Sponsored by the National Eye Institute of the National Institutes of Health. Trial was completed in 2001 with follow-up of participants currently planned until at least 2006.
Physicians' Health Study II (PHS II) (178)	A randomized, double-blind, placebo-controlled trial enrolling 15,000 willing and eligible physicians 55 years and older. It will test alternate-day β-carotene, alternate-day vitamin E, daily vitamin C, and a daily multivitamin in the prevention of AMD as well as cataract, total and prostate cancer, and cardiovascular disease.	PHS II is sponsored by BASF AG. Approximately half of the PHS II cohort is comprised of participants of the PHS I cohort, which was sponsored by the National Institutes of Health.
Vitamin E, Cataract, and Age-Related Macular Degeneration Trial (VECAT) (179)	A 4-year randomized, placebo-controlled, double-masked trial of vitamin E on the rate of progression of cataract and AMD in 1204 elderly Australian volunteers.	Sponsored by the National Health and Medical Research Council of Australia and other sources.
Women's Health Study (WHS) (21,180)	A randomized, double-blind, placebo-controlled trial of vitamin E and low-dose aspirin in the prevention of cancer and cardiovascular disease among 39,876 apparently healthy, postmenopausal U.S. female health professionals.	Has been funded by the National Eye Institute to extend its investigation to include AMD and cataract.
Women's Antioxidant Cardiovascular Study (WACS (21,181)	A randomized, double-blind, placebo-controlled, secondary prevention trial to test antioxidant vitamins (β-carotene, vitamin C, vitamin E) and a combination of folate, vitamin B$_6$, and vitamin B$_{12}$ among 8171 female health professionals, aged 40 or older, who are at high risk for cardiovascular disease.	Has been funded by the National Eye Institute to extend its investigation to include AMD and cataract.

The AREDS is an 11-center double-masked clinical trial that randomly assigned participants to receive oral total daily supplementation of: (1) antioxidants (vitamin C, 500 mg; vitamin E, 400 IU; and β-carotene, 15 mg); (2) zinc (zinc, 80 mg as zinc oxide, and copper, 2 mg as cupric oxide to prevent potential anemia); (3) antioxidants plus zinc; or (4) placebo (173). Participants from aged 55–80 years were enrolled from November 13, 1992 through January 15, 1998, and followed up until April 16, 2001. Enrolled participants in the AREDS AMD trial had extensive [drusen area $\geq$ 125 μm diameter circle (about 1/150 disk area)] small ($<$63 μm) drusen, intermediate (63-124 μm) drusen, large ($\geq$125 μm) drusen, noncentral geographic atrophy, or pigment abnormalities in one or both eyes, or advanced AMD or vision loss due to AMD in one eye. At least one eye had a best-corrected visual acuity of 20/32 or better (the study eye[s]).

The average follow-up of the 3640 enrolled study participants in the AREDS AMD trial was 6.3 years, with 2.4% lost to follow up. Compared with patients receiving placebo, patients randomized to supplementation with antioxidants plus zinc had a statistically significant odds reduction for the development of advanced AMD (OR, 0.72; 99% CI, 0.52–0.98). Advanced AMD was defined as photocoagulation or other treatment for CNV, or photographic documentation of any of the following: geographic atrophy involving the center of the macula, nondrusenoid RPE detachment, serous or hemorrhagic retinal detachment, hemorrhage under the retina or RPE, and/or subretinal fibrosis. The ORs for zinc alone and antioxidants alone are 0.75 (99% CI, 0.55–1.03) and 0.80 (99% CI, 0.59–1.09), respectively. The study found that participants with extensive small drusen, nonextensive intermediate size drusen, or pigment abnormalities had only a 1.3% 5-year probability of progression to advanced AMD. There was no evidence of any treatment benefit in delaying the progression of these patients to more severe drusen pathology. When these 1063 participants were excluded and analysis performed for the rest of the participants who had more severe age-related macular features (extensive [drusen area $\geq$360 μm diameter circle {about 1/16 disk area} if soft indistinct drusen are present or drusen area $\geq$656 μm diameter circle {about 1/5 disk area} if soft indistinct drusen are absent] intermediate drusen, large drusen, or noncentral geographic atrophy in one or both eyes, or advanced AMD or vision loss [best-corrected visual acuity $<$20/32] due to AMD in one eye) and who are at the highest risk for progression to advanced AMD, the odds reduction estimates increased (antioxidants plus zinc: OR, 0.66; 99% CI, 0.47–0.91; zinc: OR, 0.71; 99% CI, 0.52–0.99; antioxidants: OR, 0.76; 99% CI, 0.55–1.05). Estimates of relative risks derived from the ORs suggested risk reductions for those taking antioxidants plus zinc, zinc alone, and antioxidants alone of 25%, 21%, and 17%, respectively. Both antioxidants plus zinc and zinc significantly reduced the odds of developing advanced AMD in this higher risk group. However, the only statistically significant reduction in rates of at least moderate vision loss (defined as decrease in best-corrected visual acuity score from baseline of 15 or more letters in a study eye [equivalent to a doubling or more of the initial visual angle, e.g., 20/20 to 20/40 or worse, or 20/50 to 20/100 or worse]) occurred in persons randomized to receive antioxidants plus zinc (OR, 0.73; 99% CI, 0.54–0.99) in this same group. The estimated 27% odds reduction of at least moderate vision loss for the combination arm (antioxidants plus zinc) may be the combined benefit of the zinc component (odds reduction of 17%) and the antioxidant component (odds reduction of 15%). There was no statistically significant serious adverse effect associated with any of the formulations.

The study recommended that persons older than 55 years should have dilated eye examinations to determine their risk of developing advanced AMD. Those with extensive intermediate size drusen, at least one large druse, noncentral geographic atrophy in one or

both eyes, or advanced AMD or vision loss due to AMD in one eye, and without contraindications such as smoking, should consider taking a supplement of antioxidants plus
zinc to reduce their risk of progression to advanced AMD and vision loss. Because results
from two other randomized clinical trials suggested increased risk of mortality among
smokers supplementing with β-carotene (154,155), persons who smoke cigarettes should
probably avoid taking β-carotene, and they might choose to supplement with only some of
the study ingredients.

2. Dietary Fish Intake

A high proportion of polyunsaturated ω-3 fatty acids, particularly docosahexaenoic acid, is
present in the human retina and macula (156,182). Docosahexaenoic acid appears to play an
important role in the normal functioning of the retina, and is found predominantly in oily fish
and offal (122). Increased consumption of fish and fish oils containing ω-3 fatty acids has
been associated with a protective effect against atherosclerosis in several studies (183–185).

The Blue Mountains Eye Study found that more frequent consumption of fish appeared to protect against late AMD but not early AMD, after adjusting for age, sex, and
smoking (119). The protective effect of fish intake for late AMD commenced at a relatively
low frequency of consumption (OR for intake 1–3 times/month vs. intake <1 time/month,
0.23 [95% CI, 0.08–0.63]) and overall had an OR of 0.5. A borderline protective effect for
consumption of polyunsaturated fat was also observed (OR for intake in highest vs. lowest
quintile, 0.40 [95% CI, 0.14–1.18]). This concurs with the finding in the Beaver Dam Eye
Study that increased consumption of margarine, which contains higher ratios of polyunsaturated to saturated fatty acids, was associated with a reduction in risk for early AMD (OR
for intakes in highest vs. lowest quintile, 0.5 [95% CI, 0.4–0.8]) (118). However, intake of
seafood, a marker of intake of ω-3 fatty acids, was unrelated to early or late AMD (118).
Sanders and associates also found no association between AMD and the proportion of
polyunsaturated fatty acids in the plasma and erythrocyte phospholipids in a case-control
study (122).

The relation of other dietary fat intake and AMD has been dealt with under cardiovascular disease risk factors (see above).

D. Alcohol Consumption

A recent report by Obisesan and associates, using data from NHANES-I, investigated the
relationship of alcohol consumption and AMD (186). Although the data are not statistically
significant, persons who consumed 12 or fewer drinks of alcohol per year appear to be less
likely to develop AMD when compared to nondrinkers (4% vs. 7%, respectively). Beer
consumption alone did not have a significant effect on the development of AMD (OR, 0.72;
95% CI, 0.45–1.12). After adjusting for the effect of age, gender, income, history of congestive heart failure, and hypertension, wine consumption showed a statistically significant
negative association with AMD (OR, 0.81; 95% CI, 0.67–0.99). In a preliminary report of
the Eye Disease Case-Control Study, higher alcohol intake was also related to a reduced
risk of neovascular AMD (187). Considering that AMD may share similar pathological
processes with cardiovascular diseases (30), the finding that moderate wine consumption
is associated with decreased odds of developing AMD is consistent with reports of a protective effect of moderate alcohol intake for coronary artery disease and stroke (188).

In the Beaver Dam Eye Study, beer consumption was found to be associated with increased prevalence of retinal pigment and neovascular AMD (189). In an incidence study,
beer consumption was found to be positively associated with the incidence of soft indistinct
drusen, increased drusen area, and confluence of soft drusen (190). The Blue Mountains

Eye Study found no association between alcohol consumption and the prevalence of early or late AMD or large drusen, although there was a significant positive association between consumption of distilled spirits and early AMD (191).

Prospective data from 111,238 women and men in the Nurses' Health Study and the Health Professionals Follow-up Study do not support a protective effect of moderate alcohol consumption on the risk of AMD (192). No substantial association between total alcohol intake and incidence of AMD was found from the 697,498 person-years of follow-up in women and 229,180 person-years of follow-up in men. After controlling for age, smoking, and other risk factors, the pooled relative risks (RR) (95% CI) for AMD compared with non-drinkers were 1.0 (0.7–1.2) for drinkers who consumed 0.1–4.9 g/day of alcohol; 0.9 (0.6–1.4) for 5–14.9 g/day; 1.1 (0.7–1.7) for 15–29.9 g/day; and 1.3 (0.9–1.8) for 30 g/day or more. However, there was a modest increased risk of early AMD and geographic atrophy in women who consumed 30 g/day or more of alcohol (RR, 2.04; 95% CI, 1.22–3.42). There was no association between alcohol intake and neovascular AMD in either sex, but it should be pointed out that the number of cases of neovascular AMD was small in the study.

Prospective data of 21,041 male physicians with an average follow-up of 12.5 years in the Physicians' Health Study also indicate that alcohol intake is not appreciably associated with the risk of AMD (193). The overall relative risk of any AMD among men who reported baseline alcohol consumption of ≥ 1 drink/week compared to those drinking <1 drink/week was 0.97 (95% CI, 0.78–1.21) after multivariate adjustment. Similarly, the relative risk of AMD with visual loss and neovascular AMD was 0.99 (95% CI, 0.75–1.31) and 0.87 (95% CI, 0.51–1.51), respectively, after multivariate adjustment. For AMD with vision loss, the relative risks (95% CI) for those reporting <1 drink/week, 1 drink/week, 2–4 drinks/week, 5–6 drinks/week, and ≥1 drink/day at baseline were 1.0 (referent), 0.75 (0.47–1.21), 1.0 (0.69–1.45), 1.20 (0.81–1.78), and 1.19 (0.87–1.61), respectively. Several other smaller studies also found no association between the history of alcohol consumption and AMD (60,69,130).

IX. DEVELOPMENT OF CHOROIDAL NEOVASCULARIZATION IN AGE-RELATED MACULAR DEGENERATION

AMD is a bilateral condition that tends to be fairly symmetrical in its presentation and clinical course (194,195). A study of the symmetry of diskiform scars found a significant correlation between eyes in terms of the final scar size, and large macular scars were more frequent in the second eye if the first eye had a large scar (194). In the Blue Mountains Eye Study, 40% of the neovascular AMD cases were bilateral (31). Once one eye is affected, there is a significant risk for involvement in the fellow eye. Although peripheral vision is almost always retained in late AMD, bilateral central scotomata result in decreased mobility and impaired reading ability, and dramatically impact on occupational and recreational activities.

It has been demonstrated that choroidal neovascular lesions of AMD account for the vast majority of severe visual loss from this condition (196). Seventy-nine percent and 90% of eyes legally blind due to AMD in the Framingham Eye Study (2) and a large case-control study (48), respectively, had choroidal neovascularization (CNV). Thus, patients at risk of bilateral CNV are at the greatest risk of severe visual loss. Because select cases of CNV may be potentially treatable, it is important to identify high-risk patients and educate them about the importance of daily self-monitoring of the central visual field for each eye.

A. Risk of Choroidal Neovascularization in Age-Related Macular Degeneration

A number of studies have reported the natural course of patients with bilateral drusen with good visual acuity (47,197–199) (Table 8) while others have assessed the risk of developing CNV in the fellow eye in patients with age-related CNV in one eye (Table 9) (47,200–209). Variation in the reported risk among the studies is probably due partly to variation in the clinical features of the macula (e.g., drusen size and confluence, presence of focal hyperpigmentation, and/or RPE depigmentation) (210).

Lanchoney and associates (211), using the follow-up studies of Smiddy and Fine (197) and Holz and associates (198), predicted that the proportion of patients with bilateral soft drusen developing CNV in either one or both eyes would be 12.4% within 10 years, but this risk varied from 8.6 to 15.9%, depending on sex and age of the patient. In their model, the rate of development of CNV in the first eye was reduced after 5 years to 75% of the initial rate observed in follow-up studies and to 50% of the initial rate after 10 years (211).

Gass reported that of 91 patients who were seen initially with loss of vision due to diskiform macular detachment or degeneration in one eye, neovascular lesions developed in the second eye in 31 patients (34%) over an average follow-up of 4 years (47). Chandra and associates reported that among 36 patients with unilateral diskiform lesions, bilateral involvement occurred in 13 (36%) after an average follow-up of 22 months (201). Gregor and associates followed 104 patients aged 60–69 years who initially had a diskiform macular degeneration in one eye for between 1 and 5 years (203). From their data, they estimated the annual incidence of developing a diskiform lesion in the fellow eye to be 12% per year in the first 5 years. Strahlman and associates reported that among 84 patients with unilateral exudative AMD, nine (11%) developed bilateral involvement after a mean follow-up of 27 months (204). Baun and associates studied 45 patients with unilateral neovascular AMD for 4 years and documented CNV in the fellow eye in 14 (31%) patients (205). Sandberg and associates found an average of 8.8% of patients with unilateral neovascular AMD develop CNV in the fellow eye each year in their prospective series of 127 patients with 4.5 years of follow-up (206).

The Macular Photocoagulation Study (MPS) Group examined the data of fellow eyes of study participants in the MPS randomized trial for argon laser photocoagulation for extrafoveal CNV secondary to AMD (208) and the randomized trials of laser photocoagulation for new juxtafoveal CNV, new subfoveal CNV, or recurrent subfoveal CNV secondary to AMD (209). In the extrafoveal CNV trial, 128 participants had a fellow eye that was initially free of CNV at baseline (208). During 5 years of follow-up, CNV lesions associated with AMD were observed in 33 (26%) of the 128 fellow eyes. In the other three MPS trials, among 670 patients with no classic or occult CNV in the fellow eye at the time of enrollment, CNV developed in 236 (35%) within 5 years (209). The cumulative incidence rates of CNV in the fellow eye for this group of patients were estimated to be 10%, 28%, and 42% at 1, 3, and 5 years, respectively (Fig. 1).

B. Risk Factors for Progression to Choroidal Neovascularization

The MPS Group evaluated selected risk factors for development of CNV in the fellow eye of patients in the randomized trials of laser photocoagulation for new juxtafoveal CNV, new subfoveal CNV, or recurrent subfoveal CNV secondary to AMD (209). A trend for in-

Table 8 Risk of Developing Choroidal Neovascularization in Age-Related Macular Degeneration Patients with Bilateral Drusen and Good Bilateral Visual Acuity

Study	Number of eyes/patients	Mean age (y)(range)	Initial visual acuity	Mean follow-up (y) (range)	Results
Gass (1973) (47)	98/49	61 (29–81)	20/20 OU in 21 patients (43%) 20/25 to 20/40 OU in 18 patients (37%)	4.9	9 (18%) of 49 patients developed central visual loss in one eye because of CNV
Smiddy and Fine (1984) (197)	142/71	58 (16–78)	20/50 or better in 132 (93%) of eyes studied	4.3 (0.5-8.6)	8 eyes (9.9%) of 7 patients developed CNV over 4.3 y (14.3% cumulative risk) 7 eyes (8.5%) of 6 patients developed severe visual loss (12.7% 5-yr cumulative risk)
Holz et al. (1994) (198)	126 patients	68	"Good"	3	17 (13.5%) of 126 patients developed new lesions[†] Cumulative incidence of new lesions among patients ≥ 63 y old was: 8.55% @ 1 y 16.37% @ 2 y 23.52% @ 3 y
Bressler et al. (1995) (199)	483 patients	NA	NA	5	1 (0.2%) of 483 patients developed CNV 1 (0.2%) of 488 patients developed peripapillary CNV None developed geographic atrophy

* NA = information not available; OU = both eyes.
† Classic or occult CNVs, RPE detachment ± CNVs, or geographic atrophy extending to the fovea.
Reprinted from Abdelsalam A, Del Priore L, Zarbin MA. Drusen in age-related macular degeneration: pathogenesis, natural course, and laser photocoagulation-induced regression. Surv Ophthalmol 1994;44(1):1–29. Copyright 1999, with permission from Elsevier Science.

Table 9 Risk of Developing Choroidal Neovascularization in the Fellow Eye of Age-Related Macular Degeneration Patients with Choroidal Neovascularization in One Eye

Study	Number of eyes/patients	Mean age (y) (range)	Initial visual acuity	Mean follow-up (range)	Results
Gass (1973) (47)	91 patients	67 (49-82)	20/20 in 30 patients (33%) 20/40 or better in all but 7 patients (92%)	4 y	31 eyes (34%) lost central vision because of CNV[a] during follow-up
Teeters and Bird (1973) (200)	42 patients	NA	NA	21 eyes (50%) followed up for 21 mos (range, 7-19 mos)	No change
				16 eyes (38%) followed up for 10 mos (range, 4-19 mos)	Increased drusen and pigmentation
				3 eyes (7%) followed up for 9, 16, and 21 mos	All 3 eyes developed avascular diskiform appearance[b]
				2 eyes (5%) followed up for 19 and 24 mos	Both eyes developed neovascular diskiform appearance
					Overall, 5 (12%) of 42 eyes developed "avascular" and neovascular complications
Gragoudas et al. (1976) (202)	36 patients	NA	"Good"	22 mos (12–48 mos)	13 (36%) of 36 patients developed diskiform macular lesions
Gregor et al. (1977) (203)	104 patients	NA	NA	Up to 5 y	13-15%/ year developed CNV; results were: 9/104 (9.8%) @ 1 y 18/74 (19%) @ 2 y 17/53 (30%) @ 3 y 11/23 (48%) @ 4 y 5/11 (45%) @ 5 y

(continued)

Table 9 (*Continued*)

Study	Number of eyes/patients	Mean age (y) (range)	Initial visual acuity	Mean follow-up (range)	Results
Strahlman et al. (1983) (204)	84 patients	68 (47–91)	NA	27 mos (6-95 mos)	Using Kaplan-Meier technique, the risk of developing exudative maculopathy in fellow eye was estimated to be 3-7% yearly 6/84 (7%) developed CNV[a] 2/84 (2%) developed PED 1/84 (1%) developed geographic atrophy over 18 mos (range, 5-36 mos)
Bressler et al. (1990) (212)	127 patients with extrafoveal CNV[a] in one eye	NA	NA	5 yrs	10% of eyes with no large drusen of RPE hyperpigmentation compared with 58% of eyes with both large-drusen and hyperpigmentation developed CNV in the fellow eye within 5 y
Macular Photocoagulation Study Group (1997) (209)	870 patients with juxtafoveal or subfoveal CNV[a] in one eye	NA	20/400 or better	NA	Estimated 5 y incidence rates ranged from 7% for the subgroup with one risk factor to 87% for the subgroup with all four risk factors[b] The presence of occult CNV[a] in the first eye affected had no influence on the type of CNV[a] in the fellow eye

* NA = Information not available.

[a] Serous RPE detachment of RPE and retina without evidence of CNV.

[b] Five or more drusen, large (> 63 μm in diameter) focal hyperpigmentation systemic hypertension.

Reprinted from Abdelsalam A, Del Priore L, Zarbin MA. Drusen in age-related macular degeneration: pathogenesis, natural course, and laser photocoagulation-induced regression. Surv Ophthalmol 1994;44(1):1–29. Copyright 1999, with permission from Elsevier Science.

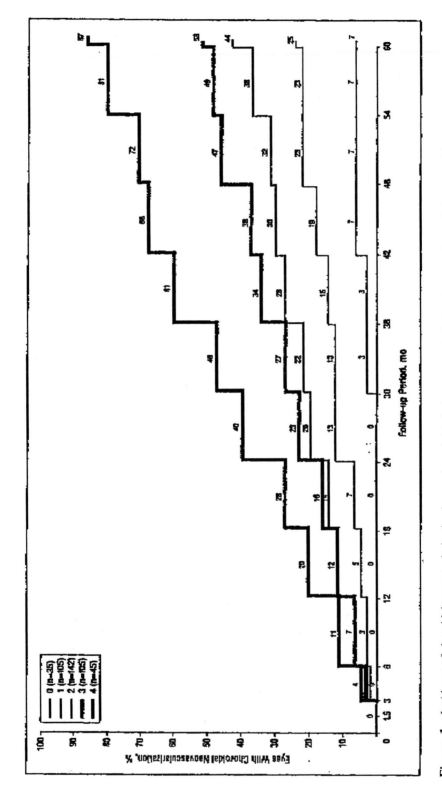

Figure 1 Incidence of choroidal neovascularization by number of risk factors present including hypertension, ≥5 drusen, ≥1 large drusen (greatest linear dimension >63 microns), and focal hyperpigmentation. (Reprinted from Arch Ophthalmol; 1997;115:741–747. Copyright 1997, American Medical Association.)

creased incidence with age ($p = 0.06$) was observed. No strong association was found between female sex, higher frequency of aspirin usage, cigarette smoking, or hyperopia with an increased risk of CNV.

Certain drusen and RPE abnormalities within 1500 microns of the foveal center present in the fellow eye and patient characteristics at baseline were identified as risk factors for the development of CNV in these eyes (209,212). Specific risk factors include the presence of five or more drusen (RR, 2.1; 95% CI, 1.3–3.5), focal hyperpigmentation (RR, 2.0; 95% CI, 1.4–2.9), definite systemic hypertension (systolic pressure ≥ 140 mmHg, diastolic pressure ≥ 90 mmHg, or use of antihypertensive medications) (RR, 1.7; 95% CI, 1.2–2.4), and one or more large drusen (> 63 μm in greatest linear dimension) (RR, 1.5, 95% CI, 1.0–2.2). The risk of CNV developing within 5 years after presenting with CNV in the first eye ranged from 7% if none of these risk factors was present to 87% if all four risk factors were present (Fig. 1).

X. SUMMARY

In summary, several risk factors for AMD have been identified from case-control, cross-sectional, and prospective cohort studies. Risk factors such as increasing age and a family history of the disease cannot be modified. One modifiable well-established risk of AMD to date is cigarette smoking (135). Dietary habits are also modifiable, and findings from AREDS suggest that persons with extensive intermediate size drusen, at least one large druse, noncentral geographic atrophy in one or both eyes, or advanced AMD or vision loss due to AMD in one eye, and without contraindications such as cigarette smoking, should consider taking a supplement of antioxidants plus zinc to reduce their risk of progression to advanced AMD and vision loss. Since sunglasses may protect against cataract formation, are inexpensive, and are not associated with any major side effects, it may be reasonable to wear sunglasses to reduce ultraviolet and other light exposure to ocular structures. The challenge for researchers is to more firmly establish modifiable risk factors and to conduct large-scale prospective intervention trials on these factors so that preventive measures and better treatments can be developed.

The identification and modification of risk factors for AMD has potential for greater public health impact on the morbidity from the disease than the few treatment modalities currently available. Case-control, cross-sectional, and prospective cohort studies can identify risk factors for AMD. Repeated findings of the same risk factors in well-designed studies conducted in different populations are necessary to provide compelling evidence of a real association between AMD and potential risk factors. However, only randomized prospective clinical trials can prove that modifying a particular established risk factor can influence the course of AMD.

Risk factors for AMD may be broadly classified into *personal* or *environmental* factors (e.g., smoking, sunlight exposure, and nutritional factors including micronutrients, dietary fish intake, and alcohol consumption). Personal factors may be further subdivided into *sociodemographic* (e.g., age, sex, race/ethnicity, heredity, and socioeconomic status), *ocular* (e.g., iris color, macular pigment density, cataract and its surgery, refractive error, and cup/disk ratio), and *systemic* factors (e.g., cardiovascular disease and its risk factors, reproductive and related factors, dermal elastotic degeneration, and antioxidant enzymes).

Established risk factors for AMD are age, race/ethnicity, heredity, and smoking. Possible risk factors are sex, socioeconomic status, iris color, macular pigment density, cataract and its surgery, refractive error, cup/disk ratio, cardiovascular disease, hypertension and blood pressure, serum lipid levels and dietary fat intake, body mass index, hematological factors, reproductive and related factors, dermal elastotic degeneration, antioxidant enzymes, sunlight exposure, micronutrients, dietary fish intake, and alcohol consumption. Factors probably not associated with AMD are diabetes and hyperglycemia. Risk factors for progression to choroidal neovascularization include presence of 5 or more drusen, focal hyperpigmentation, systemic hypertension; 1 or more large drusen (763 μm in greatest linear dimension).

A number of well-established factors such as increasing age and a family history of the disease unfortunately cannot be modified. One modifiable well-established risk factor is cigarette smoking. There may be potential benefits of antismoking patient education for primary and secondary prevention of AMD. The Age-Related Eye Disease Study (AREDS) suggested that persons older than 55 years with extensive intermediate size drusen, at least one large druse, noncentral geographic atrophy in one or both eyes, or advanced AMD or vision loss due to AMD in one eye, and without contraindications such as cigarette smoking, should consider taking a supplement of antioxidants plus zinc to reduce their of progression to advanced AMD and vision loss. Although sunlight exposure has not been established as a risk factor for AMD, it may be reasonable to wear sunglasses to reduce ultraviolet and other light exposure to ocular structures since sunglasses may protect against cataract formation, are inexpensive and not associated with any major side effects.

ACKNOWLEDGMENT

K. G. Au Eong was supported by a National Medical Research Council-Singapore Totalisator Board Medical Research Fellowship, Singapore.

REFERENCES

1. Krumpaszky HG, Ludtke R, Mickler A, Klauss V, Selbmann HK. Blindness incidence in Germany. A population-based study from Wurttemberg-Hohenzollern. Ophthalmologica 1999;213:176-182.
2. Leibowitz HM, Krueger DE, Maunder LR, Milton RC, Kini MM, Kahn HA, Nickerson RJ, Pool J, Cotton TL, Ganley JP, Loewenstein JI, Dawber TR. The Framingham Eye Study monograph. An ophthalmological and epidemiological study of cataract, glaucoma, diabetic retinopathy, macular degeneration, and visual acuity in a general population of 2631 adults, 1973–1975. Surv Ophthalmol 1980;24(Suppl):335–610.
3. Attebo K, Mitchell P, Smith W. Visual acuity and the causes of visual loss in Australia. The Blue Mountains Eye Study. Ophthalmology 1996;103:357–364.
4. Hawkins BS, Bird AC, Klein R, West SK. Epidemiology of age-related macular degeneration. Mol Vis 1999;5:26.
5. Antioxidant status and neovascular age-related macular degeneration. Eye Disease Case-Control Study Group. Arch Ophthalmol 1993;111:104–109.
6. Risk factors for neovascular age-related macular degeneration. The Eye Disease Case-Control Study Group. Arch Ophthalmol 1992;110:1701–1708.
7. Goldberg J, Flowerdew G, Smith E, Brody JA, Tso MO. Factors associated with age-related macular degeneration. An analysis of data from the first National Health and Nutritional Examination Survey. Am J Epidemiol 1988;128:700–710.
8. Christen WG, Ajani UA, Glynn RJ, Manson JE, Schaumberg DA, Chew EC, Buring JE, Hen-

nekens CH. Prospective cohort study of antioxidant vitamin supplement use and the risk of age-related maculopathy. Am J Epidemiol 1999;149:476–484.

9   An international classification and grading system for age-related maculopathy and age-related macular degeneration. The International ARM Epidemiological Study Group. Surv Ophthalmol 1995; 39:367–374.

10.   Klein BE, Klein R. Cataracts and macular degeneration in older Americans. Arch Ophthalmol 1982;100:571–573.

11.   Boldt HC, Bressler SB, Fine SL, Bressler NM. Age-related macular degeneration. Curr Opin Ophthalmol 1990;1:247–257.

12.   Kahn HA, Leibowitz HM, Ganley JP, Kini MM, Colton T, Nickerson RS, et al. The Framingham Eye Study. II. Association of ophthalmic pathology with single variables previously measured in the Framingham Heart Study. Am J Epidemiol 1977;106:33–41.

13.   Bressler NM, Bressler SB, West SK, Fine SL, Taylor HR. The grading and prevalence of macular degeneration in Chesapeake Bay watermen. Arch Ophthalmol 1989;107:847–852.

14.   Klein R, Klein BEK, Linton LKP. Prevalence of age-related maculopathy. The Beaver Dam Eye Study. Ophthalmology 1992;99:933–943.

15.   Schachat AP, Hyman L, Leske C, Connell AMS, Wu SY. Features of age-related macular degeneration in a black population. Barbados Eye Study Group. Arch Ophthalmol 1995;113:728–735.

16.   Mitchell P, Smith W, Attebo K, Wang JJ. Prevalence of age-related maculopathy in Australia. The Blue Mountains Eye Study. Ophthalmology 1995;102:1450–1460.

17.   Delkourt C, Cristol JP, Tessier F, Leger CL, Descomps B, Papoz L. Age-related macular degeneration and antioxidant status in the POLA Study Group. Pathologies Oculaires Liees a Age. Arch Ophthalmol 1999;117:1384–1390.

18.   Smith W, Mitchell P, Leeder SR, Wang JJ. Plasma fibrinogen levels, other cardiovascular risk factors, and age-related maculopathy: the Blue Mountains Eye Study. Arch Ophthalmol 1998;116:583–587.

19.   Hyman L, Schachat AP, He Q, Leske C. Hypertension, cardiovascular disease, and age-related macular degeneration. Age-Related Macular Degeneration Risk Factors Study Group. Arch Ophthalmol 2000;118(3):351–358.

20.   Ferris FL. Senile macular degeneration: review of epidemiologic features. Am J Epidemiol 1983;118:132–151.

21.   Christen WG. Randomized trials of antioxidant vitamins and eye disease. Comp Ophthalmol Update 2000;1:55–61.

22.   Bressler NM, Bressler SB, Fine SL. Age-related macular degeneration. Surv Ophthalmol 1988;32:375–413.

23.   Klein R, Klein BE, Jensen SC, Meuer SM. The five-year incidence and progression of age-related maculopathy: the Beaver Dam Eye Study. Ophthalmology 1997;104:7–21.

24.   Vingerling JR, Klaver CCW, Hofman A, de Jong PT. Epidemiology of age-related maculopathy. Epidemiol Rev 1995;17:347–360.

25.   Klein R, Klein BE, Jensen SC, Mares-Perlman JA, Cruickshanks KJ, Palta M. Age-related maculopathy in a multiracial United States population: the National Health and Nutrition Examination Survey III. Ophthalmology 1999;106:1056–1065.

26.   Kahn HA, Leibowitz HM, Ganley JP, Kini MM, Colton T, Nickerson RS, Dawber TR. The Framingham Eye Study. I. Outline and major prevalence findings. Am J Epidemiol 1977;106:17–32.

27.   Martinez GS, Campbell AJ, Reinken J, Allan BC. Prevalence of ocular disease in a population study of subjects 65 years old and older. Am J Ophthalmol 1982; 94:181–189.

28.   Vinding T. Age-related macular degeneration. Macular changes, prevalence and sex ratio. An epidemiological study of 1000 aged individuals. Acta Ophthalmol (Copenh) 1989;67:609–616.

29.   Vingerling JR, Dielemans I, Hofman A, Grobbee DE, Hijmering M, Kramer CF Le Jong PT. The prevalence of age-related maculopathy in the Rotterdam Study. Ophthalmology 1995;102:205–210.

30. Hirvela H, Luukinen H, Laara E, Laatikainen L. Risk factors of age-related maculopathy in a population 70 years of age or older. Ophthalmology 1996;103:871–877.
31. Wang JJ, Mitchell P, Smith W, Cumming RG. Bilateral involvement by age related maculopathy lesions in a population. Br J Ophthalmol 1998;82:743–747.
32. Smith W, Mitchell P, Wang JJ. Gender, oestrogen, hormone replacement and age-related macular degeneration: results from the Blue Mountains Eye Study. Aust NZ J Ophthalmol 1997;25(Suppl 1):S13–S15.
33. Gibson JM, Shaw DE, Rosenthal AR. Senile cataract and senile macular degeneration: an investigation into possible risk factors. Trans Ophthalmol Soc UK 1986;105:463–468.
34. Kini MM, Leibowitz HM, Colton T, Nickerson RJ, Ganley J, Dawber TR. Prevalence of senile cataract, diabetic retinopathy, senile macular degeneration, and open-angle glaucoma in the Framingham eye study. Am J Ophthalmol 1978; 85:28–34.
35. Jampol LM, Tielsch J. Race, macular degeneration, and the Macular Photocoagulation Study. Arch Ophthalmol 1992;110:1699–1700.
36. Gregor Z, Joffe L. Senile macular changes in the black African. Br J Ophthalmol 1978;62:547–550.
37. Sommer A, Tielsch JM, Katz J, Quigley HA, Gottsch JD, Javitt JC, Mortone JF, Royall RM, Witt KA, Ezrine S. Racial differences in the cause-specific prevalence of blindness in East Baltimore. N Engl J Med 1991;325:1412–1417.
38. Friedman DS, Katz J, Bressler NM, Rahmani B, Tielsch JM. Racial differences in the prevalence of age-related macular degeneration: the Baltimore Eye Survey Ophthalmology 1999; 106:1049–1055.
39. Klein R, Rowland ML, Harris MI. Racial/ethnic differences in age-related maculopathy. Third National Health and Nutrition Examination Survey. Ophthalmology 1995;102:371–381.
40. Klein R, Clegg L, Cooper LS, Hubbard LD, Klein BE, King WN, Folsom AR. Prevalence of age-related maculopathy in the Atherosclerosis Risk in Communities Study. Arch Ophthalmol 1999;117:1203–1210.
41. Piguet B, Wells JA, Palmvang IB, Wormald R, Chisholm IH, Bird AC. Age-related Bruch's membrane change: a clinical study of the relative role of heredity and environment. Br J Ophthalmol 1993;77:400–403.
42. Heiba IM, Elston RC, Klein BE, Klein R. Sibling correlations and segregation analysis of age-related maculopathy: the Beaver Dam Eye Study. Genet Epidemiol 1994;11:51–67.
43. Gass JD. Pathogenesis of disciform detachment of the neuroepithelium. Am J Ophthalmol 1967;63(Suppl):1–139.
44. Klein ML, Mauldin WM, Stoumbos VD. Heredity and age-related macular degeneration: observations in monzygotic twins. Arch Ophthalmol 1994;112:932–937.
45. Hutchinson J, Tay W. Symmetrical central chorio-retinal disease in senile persons. R Lond Ophthalmol Hosp Rep 1875;8:231–244.
46. Bradley AE. Dystrophy of the macula. Am J Ophthalmol 1966;61:1–24.
47. Gass JD. Drusen and disciform macular detachment and degeneration. Arch Ophthalmol 1973;90:206–217.
48. Hyman LG, Lilienfeld AM, Ferris FL, Fine SL. Senile macular degeneration: a case-control study. Am J Epidemiol 1983;118: 213–227.
49. Seddon JM, Ajani UA, Mitchell BD. Familial aggregation of age-related maculopathy. Am J Ophthalmol 1997;123:199–206.
50. Silvestri G, Johnston PB, Hughes AE. Is genetic predisposition an important risk factor in age-related macular degeneration? Eye 1994;8:564–568.
51. Smith W, Mitchell P. Family history and age-related maculopathy: the Blue Mountains Eye Study. Aust NZ J Ophthalmol 1998;26:203–206.
52. Klaver CC, Wolfs RC, Assink JJ, Duijn CM, Hofman A, de Jong PT. Genetic risk of age-related maculopathy. Population-based familial aggregation study. Arch Ophthalmol 1998;116:1646–1651.

53. Linton KL, Klein BE, Klein R. The validity of self-reported and surrogate-reported cataract and age-related macular degeneration in the Beaver Dam Eye Study. Am J Epidemiol 1991;134:1438–1446.

54. Melrose MA, Magargal LE, Lucier AC. Identical twins with subretinal neovascularization complicating senile macular degeneration. Ophthalm Surg 1985;16:648–651.

55. Meyers SM, Zachary AA. Monozygotic twins with age-related macular degeneration. Arch Ophthalmol 1988;106:651–653.

56. Dosso AA, Bovet J. Monozygotic twin brothers with age-related macular degeneration. Ophthalmologica 1992;205:24–28.

57. Gottfredsdottir MS, Sverrisson T, Musch DC, Stefansson E. Age related macular degeneration in monozygotic twins and their spouses in Iceland. Acta Ophthalmol Scand 1999;77(4):422–425.

58. De La Paz MA, Pericak-Vance MA, Haines JL, Seddon JM. Phenotypic heterogeneity in families with age-related macular degeneration. Am J Ophthalmol 1997;124(3):331–343.

59. Klein R, Klein BEK, Jensen SC, Moss SE, Cruickshanks KJ. The relation of socioeconomic factors to cataract, maculopathy, and impaired vision: the Beaver Dam Eye Study. Ophthalmology 1994;101(12):1969–1979.

60. Maltzman BA, Mulvihill MN, Greenbaum A. Senile macular degeneration and risk factors: a case-control study. Ann Ophthalmol 1979;11(8):1197–1201.

61. Weiter JJ, Delori FC, Wing GL, Fitch KA. Relationship of senile macular degeneration to ocular pigmentation. Am J Ophthalmol 1985;99(2):185–187.

62. Holz FG, Piguet B, Minassian DC, Bird AC, Weale RA. Decreasing stromal iris pigmentation as a risk factor for age-related macular degeneration. Am J Ophthalmol 1994;117(1):19–23.

63. Mitchell P, Smith W, Wang JJ. Iris color, skin sun sensitivity, and age-related maculopathy: the Blue Mountains Eye Study. Ophthalmology 1998;105(8):1359–1363.

64. Chaine G, Hullo A, Sahel J, Soubrane G, Espinasse-Berrod M-A, Schutz D et al. Case-control study of the risk factors for age-related macular degeneration. Br J Ophthalmol 1998;82(9):996–1002.

65. Sandberg MA, Gaudio AR, Miller S, Weiner A. Iris pigmentation and extent of disease in patients with neovascular age-related macular degeneration. Invest Ophthalmol Vis Sci 1994;35(6):2734–2740.

66. Blumenkranz MS, Russell SR, Roeby MG, Kott-Blumenkranz R, Penneys N. Risk factors in age-related maculopathy complicated by choroidal neovascularization. Ophthalmology 1986;96(5):552–558.

67. West SK, Rosenthal FS, Bressler NM, Bressler SB, Munoz B, Fine SL et al. Exposure to sunlight and other risk factors for age-related macular degeneration. Arch Ophthalmol 1989;107(6):675–879.

68. Vinding T. Pigmentation of the eye and hair in relation to age-related macular degeneration: an epidemiological study of 1000 aged individuals. Acta Ophthalmol (Copenh) 1990;68(1):53–58.

69. Tsang NCK, Penfold PL, Snitch PJ, Billson F. Serum levels of antioxidants and age-related macular degeneration. Doc Ophthalmol 1992;81(4):387–400.

70. Klein R, Klein BEK, Jensen SC, Cruickshanks KJ. The relationship of ocular factors to the incidence and progression of age-related maculopathy. Arch Ophthalmol 1998;116(4):506–513.

71. van der Schaft TL, Mooy CM, de Bruijn WC, Mulder PGH, Pameyer JH, de Jong PTVM. Increased prevalence of disciform macular degeneration after cataract extraction with implantation of an intraocular lens. Br J Ophthalmol 1994; 78(6):441–445.

72. Feeney-Burns L, Hilderbrand ES, Eldridge S. Aging human RPE: morphometric analysis of macular, equatorial, and peripheral cells. Invest Ophthalmol Vis Sci 1984;25(2):195–200.

73. Bito LZ, Matheny A, Cruickshanks KJ, Nondahl DM, Carino OB. Eye color changes past early childhood: the Louisville Twin Study. Arch Ophthalmol 1997; 115(5):659–663.

74. Beatty S, Boulton M, Henson D, Koh H-H, Murray IJ. Macular pigment and age-related macular degeneration. Br J Ophthalmol 1999;83(7):867–877.

75. Bone RA, Landrum JT, Tarsis SL. Preliminary identification of the human macular pigment. Vision Res 1985;25(11):1531–1535.

76. Nussbaum JJ, Pruett RC, Delori FC. Historic perspectives: macular yellow pigment: the first 200 years. Retina 1981;1(4):296–310.

77. Reading VM, Weale RA. Macular pigment and chromatic aberration. J Optom Soc Am 1974;64(2):231–234.

78. Kirschfeld K. Carotenoid pigments: their possible role in protecting against photooxidation in eyes and photoreceptor cells. Proc R Soc Lond B Biol Sci 1982; 216(1202):71–85.

79. Bone RA, Landrum JT. Macular pigment in Henle fiber membranes: a model for Haidinger's brushes. Vision Res 1984;24(2):103–108.

80. Snodderly DM. Evidence for protection against age-related macular degeneration by carotenoids and antioxidant vitamins. Am J Clin Nutr 1995;62(Suppl):1448S– 1461S.

81. Young RW. Solar radiation and age-related macular degeneration. Surv Ophthalmol 1988;32(4):252–269.

82. De La Paz MA, Anderson RE. Regional and age-dependent variation in susceptibility of the human retina to lipid peroxidation. Invest Ophthalmol Vis Sci 1992;33(13):3497–3499.

83. Winkler BS, Boulton ME, Gottsch JD, Sternberg P. Oxidative damage and age-related macular degeneration. Mol Vis 1999; 5:32.

84. Cai J, Nelson KC, Wu M, Sternberg P, Jones DP. Oxidative damage and protection of the RPE. Prog Retin Eye Res 2000;19(2):205–221.

• 85. Landrum JT, Bone RA, Kilburn MD. The macular pigment: a possible role in protection from age-related macular degeneration. Adv Pharmacol 1997;38:537– 556.

86. Hammond BR, Curran-Celentano J, Judd S, Fuld K, Krinsky NI, Wooten BR et al. Sex differences in macular pigment optical density: relation to plasma carotenoid concentrations and dietary patterns. Vision Res 1996;36(13):2001– 2012.

87. Hammond BR, Wooten BR, Snodderly DM. Cigarette smoking and retinal carotenoids: implications for age-related macular degeneration. Vision Res 1996; 36(18):3003–3009.

88. Hammond BR, Johnson EJ, Russell RM, Krinsky NI, Yeum KJ, Edwards RB et al. Dietary modification of human macular pigment density. Invest Ophthalmol Vis Sci 1997;38(9):1795–1801.

89. Seddon JM, Ajani UA, Sperduto RD, Hiller R, Blair N, Burton TC et al. Dietary carotenoids, vitamins A, C, and E, and advanced age-related macular degeneration. JAMA 1994;272(18):1413–1420.

90. Sommerburg O, Keunen JEE, Bird AC, van Kuijk FJ. Fruits and vegetables that are sources for lutein and zeaxanthin: the macular pigment in human eyes. Br J Ophthalmol 1998;82(8):907–910.

91. Klaver CCW, Wolfs RCW, Vingerling JR, Hofman A, de Jong PTVM. Age-specific prevalence and causes of blindness and visual impairment in an older population: the Rotterdam Study. Arch Ophthalmol 1998;116(5):653–658.

92. Jacques PF. The potential preventive effects of vitamins for cataract and age-related macular degeneration. Int J Vitam Nutr Res 1999;69(3):198–205.

93. Christen WG, Manson JE, Seddon JM, Glynn RJ, Buring JE, Rosner B et al. A prospective study of cigarette smoking and risk of cataract in men. JAMA 1992;268(8):989–993.

94. Hiller R, Sperduto RD, Ederer F. Epidemiologic associations with nuclear, cortical, and posterior subcapsular cataracts. Am J Epidemiol 1986;124(6):916–925.

95. Taylor HR, West SK, Rosenthal FS, Munoz B, Newland HS, Abbey H et al. Effect of ultraviolet radiation on cataract formation. N Eng J Med 1988; 319(22):1429–1433.

96. Taylor HR, West SK, Munoz B, Rosenthal FS, Bressler SB, Bressler NM. The long-term effects of visible light on the eye. Arch Ophthalmol 1992;110(1):99–104.

97. Taylor HR, Munoz B, West S, Bressler NM, Bressler SB, Rosenthal FS. Visible light and risk of age-related macular degeneration. Trans Am Ophthalmol Soc 1990;88:163–173.

98. Delcourt C, Carriere I, Ponton-Sanchez A, Lacroux A, Covacho MJ, Papoz L et al. Light ex-

posure and the risk of cortical, nuclear, and posterior subcapsular cataracts. Arch Ophthalmol 2000;118(3):385–392.

99. Sperduto RD, Seigel D. Senile lens and senile macular changes in a population-based sample. Am J Ophthalmol 1980;90(1):86–91.

100. Sperduto RD, Hiller R, Seigel D. Lens opacities and senile maculopathy. Arch Ophthalmol 1981;99(6):1004–1008.

101. Klein R, Klein BEK, Wang Q, Moss SE. Is age-related maculopathy associated with cataracts? Arch Ophthalmol 1994;112(2):191–196.

102. Liu IY, White L, LaCroix AZ. The association of age-related macular degeneration and lens opacities in the aged. Am J Public Health 1989;79(6):765–769.

103. Oliver M. Posterior pole changes after cataract extraction in elderly subjects. Am J Ophthalmol 1966;62(6):1145–1148.

104. Blair CJ, Ferguson J. Exacerbation of senile macular degeneration following cataract extraction. Am J Ophthalmol 1979;87(1):77–83.

105. Pollack A, Marcovich A, Bukelman A, Oliver M. Age-related macular degeneration after extracapsular cataract extraction with intraocular lens implantation. Ophthalmology 1996;103(10):1546–1554.

106. Pollack A, Marcovich A, Bukelman A, Zalish M, Oliver M. Development of exudative age-related macular degeneration after cataract surgey. Eye 1997;11(Pt 4):523–530.

107. Pollack A, Bukelman A, Zalish M, Leiba H, Oliver M. The course of age-related macular degeneration following bilateral cataract surgery. Ophthalmic Surg Lasers 1998;29(4):286–294.

108. Wang JJ, Mitchell P, Cumming RG, Lim R. Cataract and age-related maculopathy: the Blue Mountains Eye Study. Ophthalmic Epidemiol 1999; 6(4):317–326.

109. Vingerling JR, Klaver CCW, Hoffman A, de Jong PTVM. Cataract extraction and age-related macular degeneration: the Rotterdam Study [abstract]. Invest Ophthalmol Vis Sci 1997;38(Suppl):S472.

110. Delaney WV, Oates RP. Senile macular degeneration: a preliminary study. Ann Ophthalmol 1982;14(1):21–24.

111. Snow KK, Seddon JM. Do age-related macular degeneration and cardiovascular disease share common antecedents? Ophthalmic Epidemiol 1999;6(2):125–143.

112. Vingerling JR, Dielemans I, Bots ML, Hofman A, Grobbee DE, de Jong PTVM. Age-related macular degeneration is associated with atherosclerosis: the Rotterdam Study. Am J Epidemiol 1995;142(4):404–409.

113. Klein R, Klein BE, Franke T. The relationship of cardiovascular disease and its risk factors to age-related maculopathy. The Beaver Dam Eye Study. Ophthalmology 1993;100:406–414.

114. Sperduto RD, Killer R. Systemic hypertension and age-related maculopathy in the Framingham Study. Arch Ophthalmol 1986;104:216–219.

115. Vidaurri JS, Pe'er J, Halfon ST, Halperin G, Zauberman H. Association between drusen and some of the risk factors for coronary artery disease. Ophthalmologica 1984;188:243–247.

116. Klein R, Klein BE, Jensen SC. The relation of cardiovascular disease and its risk factors to the 5-year incidence of age-related maculopathy: the Beaver Dam Eye Study. Ophthalmology 1997;104:1804–1812.

117. Willett WC. Diet and health: what should we eat? Science 1994;264:532–537.

118. Mares-Perlman JA, Brady WE, Klein R, VandenLangenberg GM, Klein BEK, Palta M. Dietary fat and age-related maculopathy. Arch Ophthalmol 1995;113:743–748.

119. Smith W, Mitchell P, Leeder SR. Dietary fat and fish intake and age-related maculopathy. 2000;118:401–404.

120. Landolfo V, Albini L, DeSimone S. Senile macular degeneration and alteration of the metabolism of the lipids. Ophthalmologica 1978;177:248–253.

121. Albrink MJ, Fasanella RM. Serum lipids in patients with senile macular degeneration. Am J Ophthalmol 1963;55:709–713.

122. Sanders TAB, Haines AP, Wormald R, Wright LA, Obeid O. Essential fatty acids, plasma cholesterol, and fat-soluble vitamins in subjects with age-related maculopathy and matched control subjects. Am J Clin Nutr 1993;57:428–433.

123. Pauleikhoff D, Wormald RP, Wright L, Wessing A, Bird AC. Macular disease in an elderly population. Ger J Ophthalmol 1992;1:12–15.

124. Klein R, Klein BE, Moss SE. Diabetes, hyperglycemia, and age-related maculopathy. The Beaver Dam Eye Study. Ophthalmology 1992;99:1527–1534.

125. Mitchell P, Wang JJ. Diabetes, fasting blood glucose and age-related maculopathy. The Blue Mountains Eye Study. Aust NZ J Ophthalmol 1999;27:197–199.

126. Vingerling JR, Dielemans I, Witteman JCM, Hofman A, Grobbee DE, de Jong PTVM. Macular degeneration and early menopause: a case-control study. Br Med J 1995;310:1570–1571.

127. Klein BEK, Klein R, Jensen SC, Ritter LL. Are sex hormones associated with age-related maculopathy in women? The Beaver Dam Eye Study. Trans Am Ophthalmol Soc 1994;92:289–295.

128. Delcourt C, Cristol J-P, Leger CL, Descomps B, Papoz L. Associations of antioxidant enzymes with cataract and age-related macular degeneration. The POLA Study. Pathologies Oculaires Liees a I'Age. Ophthalmology 1999;106:215–222.

129. Paetkau ME, Boyd TA, Grace M, Bach-Mills J, Winship B. Senile disciform macular degeneration and smoking. Can J Ophthalmol 1978;13:67–71.

130. Vinding T, Appleyard M, Nyboe J, Jensen G. Risk factor analysis for atrophic and exudative age-related macular degeneration. An epidemiological sutdy of 1000 aged individuals. Acta Ophthalmol (Copenh) 1992;700:66–72.

131. Klein R, Klein BE, Linton KL, DeMets DL. The Beaver Dam Eye Study: the relation of age-related maculopathy to smoking. Am J Epidemiol 1993; 137:190–200.

132. Vingerling JR, Hofman A, Grobbee DE, de Jong PT. Age-related macular degeneration and smoking. The Rotterdam Study. Arch Ophthalmol 1996;114:1193–1196.

133. Christen WG, Glynn RJ, Manson JE, Ajani UA, Buring JE. A prospective study of cigarette smoking and risk of age-related macular degeneration in men. JAMA 1996;276:1147–1151.

134. Smith W, Mitchell P, Leeder SR. Smoking and age-related maculopathy. The Blue Mountains Eye Study. Arch Ophthalmol 1996;114:1518–1523.

135. Seddon JM, Willett WC, Speizer FE, Hackinson SE. A prospective study of cigarette smoking and age-related macular disease in women. JAMA 1996; 276:1141–1146.

136. Tamakoshi A, Yuzawa M, Matsui M, Uyama M, Fujiwara NK, Ohno Y et al. Smoking and neovascular form of age related macular degeneration in late middle aged males: findings from a case-control study in Japan. Research Committee on Chorioretinal Degenerations. Br J Ophthalmol 1997;81:901–904.

137. Delcourt C, Diaz JL, Ponton-Sanchez A, Papoz L. Smoking and age-related macular degeneration. The POLA study. Pathologies Oculaires Liees l'Age. Arch Ophthalmol 1998; 116(8):1031–1035.

138. Stryker WS, Kaplan LA, Stein EA, Stampfer MJ, Sober A, Willett WC. The relation of diet, cigarette smoking, and alcohol consumption to plasma beta-carotene and alpha-tocopherol levels. Am J Epidemiol 1988;127:283–296.

139. Ham WT, Mueller HA, Ruffolo JJ, Guerry D, Guerry RK. Action spectrum for retinal injury from near-ultraviolet radiation in aphakic monkey. Am J Ophthalmol 1982;93:299–306.

140. Tso MO. Pathogenetic factors of aging macular degeneration. Ophthalmology 1985;92:628–635.

141. Noell WK. Possible mechanisms of photoreceptor damage by light in mammalian eyes. Vis Res 1980;20:1163–1171.

142. Lawwill T. Three major pathologic processes caused by light in the primate retina: a search for mechanisms. Trans Am Ophthalmol Soc 1982;80:517–579.

143. Borges J, Li ZY, Tso MO. Effects of repeated photic exposures on the monkey macula. Arch Ophthalmol 1990;12:17–33.

144. Tso MO. Photic maculopathy in rhesus monkey. A light and electron microscopic study. Invest Ophthalmol 1973;12:17–34.

145. Ewald RA, Ritchey CL. Sun gazing as the cause of foveomacular retinitis. Am J Ophthalmol 1970;70:491–497.
146. Gottsch JD, Bynoe LA, Harlan JB, Rencs EV, Green WR. Light-induced deposits in Bruch's membrane of protoporphyric mice. Arch Ophthalmol 1993; 111:126–129.
147. Tso MO, Woodford BJ. Effect of photic injury on the retinal tissues. Ophthalmology 1983;90:952–963.
148. Green WR, Enger C. Age-related macular degeneration histopathologic studies. The 1992 Lorenz E. Zimmerman lecture. Ophthalmology 1993;100:1519–1535.
149. Gottsch JD, Pou S, Bynoe LA, Rosen GM. Hematogenous photosensitization. A mechanism for the development of age-related macular degeneration. Invest Ophthalmol Vis Sci 1990;31:1674–1682.
150. Belda JI, Roma J, Vilela C, Puertas FJ, Diaz-Llopis M, Bosch-Morell F, Romero FJ. Serum vitamin E levels negatively correlate with severity of age-related macular degeneration. Mech Ageing Dev 1999;107:159–164.
151. Cruickshanks KJ, Klein R, Klein BE. Sunlight and age-related macular degeneration. The Beaver Dam Eye Study. Arch Ophthalmol 1993;111:514–518.
152. Darzins P, Mitchell P, Heller RF. Sun exposure and age-related macular degeneration. An Australian case-control study. Ophthalmology 1997;104:770–776.
153. Sperduto RD, Ferris FLI, Kurinij N. Do we have a nutritional treatment for age-related cataract or macular degeneration? Arch Ophthalmol 1990;108:1403–1405.
154. The effect of vitamin E and beta carotene on the incidence of lung cancer and other cancers in male smokers. The Alpha-Tocopherol, Beta Carotene Cancer Preventation Study Group. N Engl J Med 1994;330:1029–1035.
155. Omenn GS, Goodman GE, Thornquist MD, Balmes J, Cullen MR, Glass A, Keogh JP, Meyskens FL, Valanis B, Williams JH, Barnhart S, Hammer S. Effects of a combination of beta carotene and vitamin A on lung cancer and cardiovascular disease. N Engl J Med 1996;334:1150–1155.
156. Robison WG, Kuwabara T, Bieri JG. The roles of vitamin E and unsaturated fatty acids in the visual process. Retina 1982;2:263–281.
157. Christen WG. Antioxidants and eye disease. Am J Med 1994; 97(Suppl 3A):14S–17S.
158. Frei B. Reactive oxygen species and antioxidant vitamins: mechanisms of action. Am J Med 1994;97(Suppl 3A):5S–13S.
159. Hayes KC. Retinal degeneration in monkeys induced by deficiencies of vitamin E or A. Invest Ophthalmol 1974;13:499–510.
160. Organisciak DT, Wang HM, Li ZY, Tso MO. The protective effect of ascorbate in retinal light damage of rats. Invest Ophthalmol 1985;26:1580–1588.
161. West S, Vitale S, Hallfrisch J, Munoz B, Muller D, Bressler S, Bressler NM. Are antioxidants or supplements protective for age-related macular degeneration? Arch Ophthalmol 1994;112:222–227.
162. Horwitt MK, Harvey CC, Dahm CH, Scarey MT. Relationship between tocopherol and serum lipid levels for determination of nutritional adequacy. Ann NY Acad Sci 1972;203:223–236.
163. Thurnham DI, Davies JA, Crump BJ, Situnayake RD, Davis M. The use of different lipids to express serum tocopherol: lipid ratios for the measurement of vitamin E status. Ann Clin Biochem 1986;23:514–520.
164. Jordan P, Brubacher D, Moser U, Stahelin HB, Gey KF. Vitamin E and vitamin A concentrations in plasma adjusted for cholesterol and triglycerides by multiple regression. Clin Chem 1995;41:924–927.
165. Smith W, Mitchell P, Webb K, Leeder SR. Dietary antioxidants and age-related maculopathy: the Blue Mountains Eye Study. Ophthalmology 1999;106:761–767.
166. Smith W, Mitchell P, Rochester C. Serum beta carotene, alpha tocopherol, and age-related maculopathy: the Blue Mountains Eye Study. Am J Ophthalmol 1997; 124:838–840.

167. Mares-Perlman JA, Klein R, Klein BEK, Greger JL, Brady WE, Palta M, et al. Association of zinc and antioxidant nutrients with age-related maculopathy. Arch Ophthalmol 1996;114:991–997.
168. Mares-Perlman JA, Brady WE, Klein R, Klein BE, Bowen P, Stacewicz-Sapuntzakis M, Palta M. Serum antioxidants and age-related macular degeneration in a population-based case-control study. Arch Ophthalmol 1995;113:1518–1523.
169. Galin MA, Nano HD, Hall T. Ocular zinc concentration. Invest Ophthalmol Vis Sci 1962;1:142–148.
170. Sigel H. Zinc and Its Role in Biology and Nutrition. New York: Marcel Dekker, 1983.
171. Silverstone BZ, Landau L, Berson D, Sternbuch J. Zinc and copper metabolism in patients with senile macular degeneration. Ann Ophthalmol 1985;17:419–422.
172. Briefel RR, Bialostosky K, Kennedy-Stephenson J, McDowell MA, Ervin RB, Wright JD. Zinc intake of the U.S. population: findings from the Third National Health and Nutrition Examination Survey, 1988–1994. J Nutr 2000;130(5S Suppl):1367S–1373S.
173. Age-Related Eye Disease Study Research Group. A randomized, placebo-controlled, clinical trial of high-dose supplementation with vitamins C and E, beta carotene, and zinc for age-related macular degeneration and vision loss: AREDS report no. 8. Arch Ophthalmol 2001;119(10):1417–1437.
174. Newsome DA, Swartz M, Leone NC, Elston RC, Miller E. Oral zinc in macular degeneration. Arch Ophthalmol 1988;106(2):192–198.
175. Stur M, Tittl M, Reitner A, Meisinger V. Oral zinc and the second eye in age-related macular degeneration. Invest Ophthalmol Vis Sci 1996;37(7):1225–1235.
176. Richer S. Multicenter ophthalmic and nutritional age-related macular degeneration study - part 1: design, subjects and procedures. J Am Optom Assoc 1997;67(1):12–29.
177. Richer S. Multicenter ophthalmic and nutritional age-related macular degeneration study - part 2: antioxidant intervention and conclusions. J Am Optom Assoc 1996;67(1):30–49.
178. Christen WG, Gaziano JM, Hennekens CH. Design of Physicians' Health Study II —a randomized trial of beta-carotene, vitamins E and C, and multivitamins, in prevention of cancer, cardiovascular disease, and eye disease, and review of results of completed trials. Ann Epidemiol 2000;10:125–134.
179. Garrett SK, McNeil JJ, Silagy C, Sinclair M, Thomas AP, Robman LD, McCarty CA, Tikellis G, Taylor HR. Methodology of the VECAT study: vitamin E intervention in cataract and age-related maculopathy. Ophthalm Epidemiol 1999;60:195–208.
180. Buring JE, Hennekens CH. The Women's Health Study: summary of the study design. J Myocard Ischem 1992;4(3):27–29.
181. Manson JE, Gaziano JM, Spelsberg A, Ridker PM, Cook NR, Buring JE, Willett WC, Hennekens CH. A secondary prevention trial of antioxidant vitamins and cardiovascular disease in women. Rationale, design, and methods. Ann Epidemiol 1995;5:261–269.
182. van Kuijk FJ, Buck P. Fatty acid composition of the human macula and peripheral retina. Invest Ophthalmol Vis Sci 1992;33:3493–3496.
183. Kromhout D, Bosschieter EB, de Lezenne Coulander C. The inverse relation between fish consumption and 20-year mortality from coronary heart disease. N Engl J Med 1985;312:1205–1209.
184. Sanders TA, Sullivan DR, Reeve J, Thompson GR. Triglyceride-lowering effect of marine polyunsaturates in patients with hypertriglyceridemia. Arteriosclerosis 1985;5:459–465.
185. Katan MB. Fish and heart disease. N Engl J Med 1995;332:1024–1025.
186. Obisesan TO, Hirsch R, Kosoko O, Carlson L, Parrott M. Moderate wine consumption is associated with decreased odds of developing age-related macular degeneration in NHANES-1. J Am Geriatr Soc 1998;46:1–7.
187. Ajani U, Willett W, Miller D, Haller J, Yannuzzi L, Blair N, Burton T, Seddon J. Alcohol consumption and neovascular age-related macular degeneration (abstr). Am J Epidemiol 1993;138:646.

188. Gaziano JM, Buring JE, Breslow JL, Goldhaber SZ, Rosner B, VanDenburgh M, Willett W, Hennekens CH. Moderate alcohol intake, increased levels of high-density lipoprotein and its subfractions, and decreased risk of myocardial infarction. N Engl J Med 1993;329:1829–1834.

189. Ritter LL, Klein R, Klein BE, Mares-Perlman JA, Jensen SC. Alcohol use and age-related maculopathy in the Beaver Dam Eye Study. Am J Ophthalmol 1995;120:190–196.

190. Moss SE, Klein R, Klein BE, Jensen SC, Meuer SM. Alcohol consumption and the 5-year incidence of age-related maculopathy: the Beaver Dam eye study. Ophthalmology 1998;105:789–794.

191. Smith W, Mitchell P. Alcohol intake and age-related maculopathy. Am J Ophthalmol 1996;122:743–745.

192. Cho E, Hankinson SE, Willett WC, Stampfer MJ, Spiegelman D, Speizer FE, Rimm EB, Seddon JM. Prospective study of alcohol consumption and the risk of age-related macular degeneration. Arch Ophthalmol 2000;118:681–688.

193. Ajani UA, Christen WG, Manson JE, Glynn RJ, Schaumberg D, Buring JE, Hennekens CH. A prospective study of alcohol consumption and the risk of age-related macular degeneration. Ann Epidemiol 1999;9:172–177.

194. Lavin MJ, Eldem B, Gregor ZJ. Symmetry of disciform scars in bilateral age-related macular degeneration. Br J Ophthalmol 1991;75:133–136.

195. Chang B, Yannuzzi LA, Ladas ID, Guyer DR, Slakter JS, Sorenson JA. Choroidal neovascularization in second eyes of patients with unilateral exudative age-related macular degeneration. Ophthalmology 1995;102:1380–1386.

196. Ferris FL, Fine SL, Hyman L. Age-related macular degeneration and blindness due to neovascular maculopathy. Arch Ophthalmol 1984;102:1640–1642.

197. Smiddy WE, Fine SL. Prognosis of patients with bilateral macular drusen. Ophthalmology 1984;91:271–277.

198. Holz FG, Wolfensberger TJ, Piguet B, Gross-Jendroska M, Wells JA, Minassian DC, Chisholm IH, Bird AC. Bilateral macular drusen in age-related macular degeneration. Prognosis and risk factors. Ophthalmology 1994;101:1522–1528.

199. Bressler NM, Munoz B, Maguire MG, Vitale SE, Schein OD, Taylor HR, West SK. Five-year incidence and disappearance of drusen and retinal pigment epithelial abnormalities. Waterman study. Arch Ophthalmol 1995;113:301–308.

200. Teeters VW, Bird AC. The development of neovascularization of senile disciform macular degeneration. Am J Ophthalmol 1973;76:1–18.

201. Chandra SR, Gragoudas ES, Friedman E, Van Buskirk EM, Klein ML. Natural history of disciform degeneration of the macula. Am J Ophthalmol 1974;78:579–582.

202. Gragoudas ES, Chandra SR, Friedman E, Klein ML, Van Buskirk EM. Disciform degeneration of the macula. II. Pathogenesis. Arch Ophthalmol 1976;94:755–757.

203. Gregor Z, Bird AC, Chisholm IH. Senile disciform macular degeneration in the second eye. Br J Ophthalmol 1977;1977:141–147.

204. Strahlman ER, Fine SL, Hillis A. The second eye of patients with senile macular degeneration. Arch Ophthalmol 1983;101:1191–1193.

205. Baun O, Vinding T, Krogh E. Natural course in fellow eyes of patients with unilateral age-related exudative maculopathy. A fluorescein angiographic 4-year follow-up of 45 patients. Acta Ophthalmol 1993;71:398–401.

206. Sandberg MA, Weiner A, Miller S, Gaudio AR. High-risk characteristics of fellow eyes of patients with unilateral neovascular age-related macular degeneration. Ophthalmology 1998;105:441–447.

207. Roy M, Kaiser-Kupfer M. Second eye involvement in age-related macular degeneration: a four-year prospective study. Eye 1990;4:813–818.

208. Macular Photocoagulation Study Group. Five-year follow-up of fellow eyes of patients with age-related macular degeneration and unilateral extrafoveal choroidal neovascularization. Arch Ophthalmol 1993;111:1189–1199.

209. Macular Photocoagulation Study Group. Risk factors for choroidal neovascularization in the second eye of patients with juxtafoveal or subfoveal choroidal neovascularization secondary to age-related macular degeneration. Arch Ophthalmol 1997;115:741–747.

210. Abdelsalam A, Del Priore L, Zarbin MA. Drusen in age-related macular degeneration: pathogenesis, natural course, and laser photocoagulation-induced regression. Surv Ophthalmol 1999;44:1–29.

211. Lanchoney DM, Maguire MG, Fine SL. A model of the incidence and consequences of choroidal neovascularization secondary to age-related macular degeneration. Comparative effects of current treatment and potential prophylaxis on visual outcomes in high-risk patients. Arch Ophthalmol 1998;116:1045–1052.

212. Bressler SB, Maguire MG, Bressler NM, Fine SL. Relationship of drusen and abnormalities of the retinal pigment epithelium to the prognosis of neovascular macular degeneration. The Macular Photocoagulation Study Group. Arch Ophthalmol 1990;108:1442–1447.

21

The Psychosocial Consequences of Vision Loss

Gretchen B. Van Boemel
Doheny Retina Institute of the Doheny Eye Institute, University of Southern California Keck School of Medicine, Los Angeles, California

I. INTRODUCTION

As routine as the words "there is nothing more that can be done to correct your vision" seem to us, these words can have devastating consequences on those on the receiving end. These words can cause feelings of hopelessness, helplessness, despair, shock, and a host of other feelings (1). Individuals who were vulnerable to such things as illness, family violence, feelings of depression, or social isolation may be at greater risk after learning of the permanence of the vision problem, as chronic vision loss seems to exacerbate other situations that may put an individual at risk (2). It therefore becomes part of our responsibility as eye care professionals to initiate the discussion of the consequences of vision loss, as well as low vision rehabilitation services with our patients within the clinical setting. An open and sensitive discussion of these issues, where we listen as much as we speak, can be very therapeutic for our patients with low vision (3,4). This chapter will be dedicated to exploring the psychosocial consequences that vision loss has on our patients with age-related macular degeneration (AMD) so as to help facilitate the physician/patient interaction. This chapter will outline situations concerning an older low-vision patient group. It is designed as an introductory text to this subject. It will be presented in sections dealing with specific topics of concern and will include both anecdotal and scientific information from a wide variety of fields. It will include a review of the eye care professional's role in interacting with those with vision loss. It will also include a review of some of the more pressing psychological issues affecting the individual with vision loss, a review of interpersonal relationships and family support issues, and will conclude with community interventions for those with low vision.

II. THE PRIMARY EYE CARE PROFESSIONAL'S ROLE IN PATIENT ADJUSTMENT

A. Breaking the News

The most important discussion an eye care professional may ever have with a patient is breaking the news that the patient's vision loss is permanent and uncorrectable. A frank and honest discussion of the subject is very important. Initiating the discussion regarding vision loss and low vision rehabilitation with a question about reading ability, driving, or other daily living activities should both decrease the anxiety and increase the comfort of both the patient and the physician. The eye care professional may want to conduct this conversation early in the disease process when vision is only moderately affected, such as vision loss of 20/60 in the better eye after correction. Waiting until the person is legally blind or profoundly visually impaired may result in poorer rehabilitation outcomes. A referral to the low-vision specialist when vision is only moderately affected should result in tremendous satisfaction on the part of the patient, as these individuals have the easiest vision to improve. The initial referral to the low-vision ophthalmologist or optometrist when successful fitting is possible will contribute to a good patient/practitioner relationship between the two of them. The individual with low vision can start to get used to adaptive devices such as high plus readers in the +6– +10 diopter range. When lower-powered readers and magnifiers no longer work successfully and the individual needs strengths in the +12–+20 diopter range, the focal distance needed will not be as foreign to the individual and adjustment to and utilization of such devices will be much greater. Adjustment to vision loss may be more successful if the individual has been able to make both psychological and daily living skill adjustments on an incremental basis (5). Moreover, an early referral may reduce the patient's sense of anger toward us. Waiting until the patient is legally blind in both eyes results in many years of missed opportunities and much frustration on the part of the patient.

In addition to discussing problems of daily living, the initial discussion should include a full description of AMD, its visual prognosis and any treatment options that may be available, a definition of low vision and legal blindness, and an opportunity for the patient and his/her family to ask questions. This should help the patient better understand his/her disease, reduce any unrealistic hopes for a cure the patient or the family may still harbor, and start the patient on the road to recovery. It will legitimize the concerns the person with AMD may have about vision loss, while at the same time dispelling some of the myths and misconceptions the person or his/her family has about vision loss. It may also reduce the fear the patient may have about becoming totally blind from AMD. Referrals to other professionals if necessary (such as psychologists when coping strategies are limited or orientation and mobility specialists when vision loss is profound and safety is an issue) should complete the conversation. This will introduce the concept of low-vision rehabilitation to the patient and his/her family and should reduce frustration within the individual and the family unit if done appropriately and in a timely manner. Low-vision rehabilitation has been shown to be effective in both promoting adjustment to vision loss and enhancing daily living abilities in those with vision loss (6–9), providing a further reason to approach this subject with our patients.

Certainly we cannot address every issue surrounding vision loss in the initial conversation but we can start the dialog. Much of the discussion surrounding vision loss includes the more psychologically based aspects of vision loss. This is an area that many of us are uncomfortable with or feel is outside our scope of practice (10). Our understanding of the psychosocial issues associated with vision loss and our knowledge of the resources available to those with vision loss will assist us in these difficult conversations. By providing this in-depth conversation to our patients with AMD, we will reduce much of the patient's anxiety and will eliminate their "having to find things out on their own." This should reduce their need to "doctor shop" as full disclosure will result in their believing that they have been fully cared for by us. If we do not address these issues within the clinical setting, we are implying that there is, in fact, nothing more that can be done and the individual must do everything on his or her own to cope with vision loss. The elderly person with insufficient information about low-vision rehabilitation may fall prey to those within the eye care community who are not fully reputable or ethical. (I have seen very unrealistic advertisements suggesting that 80-year-olds who are legally blind should still be able to drive with the right adaptive devices. These devices cost about $3000.) Reassurance from the eye care professional that he or she will always be available for consultation reduces the patient's fear of physician abandonment. Even a little encouragement and information from a health care professional will have tremendous benefits for our patients (11). Moreover, many older adults prefer to have their health care decisions made for them by a physician (12). This decision-making preference makes the initial discussion of low-vision rehabilitation even more important for the older person with low vision, as that individual may not seek rehabilitative services without the input of the primary eye care professional.

Unfortunately, we may underestimate the effects vision loss has on our patients (13). We must be careful not to tell our patients that their vision problems or situation as a result of their vision problems could be worse. These types of statements usually result in the patient feeling resentful of us. They may feel misunderstood or minimalized. It also reduces the person's willingness to ask questions, as the patient may now feel as if his/her "insignificant" vision problem should not warrant a lengthy discussion from the eye care professional. Assuring our patients that they will not go totally blind from macular degeneration and then giving them the opportunity to ask questions is more beneficial than telling them not to worry about their vision problems.

Moreover, as practitioners we do not want to encourage self-blame. For example, the "if only I had quit smoking I would not have developed macular degeneration" scenario does not improve the possibility of rehabilitation. To reduce self-blame, I tell my patients that almost everyone will develop macular degeneration if he lives long enough. This suggestion helps the individual realize that macular degeneration is a "natural" part of the aging process, and since they would not blame themselves for developing wrinkles, they should not blame themselves for macular degeneration.

We need to be mindful that many patients will not be "ready" for either a discussion about low vision or a referral to a low-vision specialist. This is a perfectly normal reaction to devastating news. If this is the case, a follow-up appointment about 2 months after the initial conversation may be necessary. Two months usually is enough time to result in a change of heart and a willingness to accept a referral. Subsequent yearly or half-yearly follow-up visits help maintain a relationship between the patient and the low-vision specialist.

B. Understanding Vision Loss

Probably the most difficult challenge facing those of us within the field of ophthalmology is ensuring that our patients and their families understand the meaning of vision loss. Most individuals think of vision as being dichotomous—either perfect 20/20 vision or "no light perception" vision. Very few individuals are aware that visual acuity is actually on a continuum, ranging from 20/20 to no light perception. Helping the patient and the family understand the concept of vision as being on a continuum will help us work more effectively with them. Many family members do not fully understand the meaning of low vision and as a result the family members may not know what to expect from their loved ones with low vision (12). Family members may feel that the person with low vision is "faking" symptoms to get out of doing unpleasant chores around the home. Explaining, fully, to both the patient and his/her family that vision may fluctuate, that under certain conditions the person's vision will appear better, and that high-contrast objects will be easier for the individual with poor vision to see will help eliminate friction within the family unit. The ophthalmologist's explanation of this to the family legitimizes the experiences of those with low vision, thus making it easier for the individual with low vision to interact with his/her family.

C. The "Blindness" Word

Along the same vein, the word "blindness" may produce excessive anxiety that could be eliminated if the words "low vision" were used. Most individuals do not understand the meaning of the term "legal blindness" and hear only the word "blindness," since most individuals are familiar with that term. If we do not provide information on the concept of legal blindness, then much of the time spent during the first visit with the low-vision specialist may consist of them explaining the term legal blindness to our patients. Legal blindness is an important classification as it means that the individual with vision loss is eligible for special services such as state and federal paid vision rehabilitation, income tax deductions, and no-cost "411" service, to name a few. However, if a patient hears only the word "blindness," we have increased his or her anxiety significantly, as the individual may think that he/she will be going totally blind in the very near future. By using the term low vision, we will reduce our patients' anxiety about total vision loss as the ultimate outcome of macular degeneration. When a person does become legally blind, we should discuss this information openly with our patients. We need to make sure that each patient obtains all of the benefits to which he or she is entitled. We must make sure that we have sufficient time to spend with our patients when this discussion becomes necessary. Rescheduling the discussion to a later date when necessary ensures that we have enough time to fully discuss the issue with our patients and their families.

III. PSYCHOLOGICAL REACTIONS TO VISION LOSS

Aging and vision loss can result in feelings of change and loss. These feelings of loss can range from loss of a spouse to loss of a career. The person may feel that he/she is living longer but not better or may feel fearful of having to relocate to an assisted-living facility (5). This section will review several areas of concern to those who are both aged and visually impaired.

A. Losing Independence, Privacy, and Self-Worth

The loss of independence and privacy can be very debilitating to those who are elderly. These losses can result in the individual becoming depressed and less likely to seek rehabilitative care, thus further increasing isolation and dependence on others (14). For those who cannot see adequately and who have not undergone daily living skills training, the level of independence that can be successfully exhibited is minimal. The individual cannot drive, cook, or read mail, and often cannot perform hygienic activities or maintain a household on his/her own. This results in the individual having to seek assistance from family members, friends, or paid attendants. Those with macular degeneration and low vision may not seek assistance from others, as this may signal impending decline and death. Certainly, the mere presence of these helping individuals implies that the person with low vision can no longer live or function independently. Moreover, the individual has now lost all of his/her privacy. This comes in the form of having others read personal mail and assist in keeping financial records. In some instances, it may include assistance with hygiene as well. Unfortunately, the absence of these helpful individuals can mean the person with low vision is living in squalid or unsafe conditions.

Individuals who have low vision and who can no longer live independently may choose to live in assisted-living facilities if financial resources are available. This further suggests a loss of independence, as the person is no longer able to inhabit the home he/she has lived in for many years. The loss of a home and a move to a retirement home or assisted-living facility may imply eminent death to the individual with low vision (5). Vision loss is frequently cited as the reason for moving from the family home to an assisted-living facility (5). The move to a retirement community can have deleterious effects on an individual's health (5). The person may feel that he is now at the "end of the line" and that death is imminent. Therefore, it is the goal of many low-vision specialists to keep those with low vision in their own homes for as long as possible.

Vision loss may also lead to feelings of limited self-worth (1). Individuals currently affected by AMD report feeling useful primarily while working (5). These individuals may volunteer their time after retirement and may be as busy as they were prior to retirement. However, if the person is plagued with vision loss, he/she may not be able to continue to pursue retirement activities. If the person is not adaptable and does not know how to modify his/her life to make accommodations for the vision loss, the likelihood of continuing with the old regime is unlikely. The inability to work or pursue retirement activities may lead to feelings of limited self-worth. The person's role within the family may change, further affecting the sense of self-worth. Feelings of self-worth are highly desirable and lead to increased well-being and improved psychological functioning. Those with reduced feelings of self-worth are at risk for such things as despair and depression (5).

B. Depression, Isolation, and Loneliness

Depression, isolation, and loneliness are a very unfortunate, but real, part of aging. These conditions may be as a result of losing family and friends to death, or may be due to disabling features of aging, such as vision loss or other chronic or disabling conditions that keep the individual home-bound. Vision loss, in and of itself, can cause psychopathological symptoms such as anxiety, adjustment disorder, major depression, suicidal ideation and attempt, and phobia (15–21). Psychological symptoms may range from mild problems of maladjustment to significant problems of a psychopathological nature. Those with minor adjustment problems usually regain psychological normalcy after adjustment to vision loss occurs (16). Symptoms may include feelings of dependence on others or frustration at having to ask for assistance to help with things that were done with ease previously. The individual who is adjusting poorly may also have a sense of diminished well-being. This may be further exacerbated if the individual lives in a relatively low-vision-unfriendly apartment (one with poor lighting and numerous stairs for example) (19,20). Treatment should include daily living skill enhancement that will likely be sufficient to help the individual adjust better to the vision loss.

For those at risk for more severe psychological problems, the presence of permanent vision loss may result in chronic mental health problems. Individuals who are at risk should be referred to appropriate professionals as soon as symptoms start to appear (18). In those who are depressed, symptoms of feeling blue, feelings of lethargy, and poor sleep patterns are frequently observed. Suicidal ideation and rarely suicide may occur as a result of permanent vision loss (16). For at-risk individuals, a referral to a mental health practitioner who is familiar with the effects of chronic illness on individuals, as well as being sensitive to the needs of a geriatric patient population, is essential.

If a patient needs psychotropic medication to relieve symptoms, a referral to a psychiatrist should be considered. If the patient needs to talk with someone about feelings of frustration about his/her inability to perform daily living tasks, a referral to a psychologist is more appropriate. If the patient is having specific problems with a family member, a referral to a marriage and family counselor may be the most appropriate. Referrals to mental health care practitioners who are not familiar with both the effects of vision loss and the needs of geriatric patients will likely be less than beneficial. Having a good understanding of what types of referrals our colleagues want and the types of services that our colleagues have to offer our patients should enhance our referral patterns to mental health professionals.

Vision loss is frequently accompanied by a sense of isolation from others and from society (1). The person who is visually impaired is frequently unable to drive (or drive a great distance), resulting in an isolation from the community. Individuals with vision problems may feel embarrassed about their visual disabilities and this may further remove them from society. Those who are visually impaired may be isolated from their natural support groups of family and friends. Moreover, the person with vision loss may be unable to read a newspaper or book, further adding to the sense of isolation from society (14). The sense of social isolation can exacerbate the psychological problems faced by our patients with vision loss. Those who are isolated may have reduced feelings of well-being and may have increased problems with adjustment over time (19,20). Assisting low-vision patients with community involvement can result in improved psychological well-being and functioning (22).

For many individuals, isolation is accompanied by a sense of loneliness. Individuals who are homebound have little means by which to access the company of others. The individual who is homebound must rely on others to come to visit him/her and is forced to rely on others for transportation to doctor appointments (23).

C. Denial

Denial is a strong and natural human response to a risky or unpleasant situation. It may, in fact, be a self-protective behavior (24). Psychologists have suggested that if we believed that we were at great risk of being in a car accident every time we got into a car, we probably would not drive. Unfortunately denial can also be deleterious to our health and well-being. This is exemplified in the following case history. Several years ago, I was coordinating an outreach program to assist eligible individuals receive blind disability benefits. I interviewed a patient who had end-stage glaucoma and vision of hand motions in both eyes. I suggested that she might be eligible for these benefits and she replied to me that she was not blind. She had not sought any type of rehabilitation services for those with vision loss, such as orientation and mobility training (white cane training) as she believed that her ophthalmologist would cure her of her vision problems. Not only was she unwilling to pursue obtaining blind disability benefits, she could not conceive of the possibility that her ophthalmologist could not cure her eye problems. She was in very serious denial. She was relying on others for assistance in daily living tasks, as well as putting herself at risk for attempting to do things that were beyond her visual ability. Many individuals who are totally blind are able to do everything that can be done by those with normal sight, with a few exceptions. But this requires rehabilitation techniques and training. Denial of the permanence of her vision loss allowed this patient to be unsafe in many situations and overly dependent on people in other situations.

This type of scenario can be repeated over and over again when describing the newly (or not so newly) visually impaired. Individuals may continue to drive even though they cannot see well. Men are far more likely than women to insist upon driving even when their vision is in the 20/200 range (23). On the other hand, women may continue to cook elaborate meals even when they cannot see well. People may be so fearful of going totally blind that they do not seek care, or they will downplay the severity of their vision loss to their family members and friends. People do not want to disappoint others, lose their independence, or change their lifestyles. They may believe that the next surgery will finally cure their vision problems, thus maintaining unrealistic expectations of what ophthalmologists are able to do. They may seek opinion after opinion until they hear the news that they want—that a cure is available for their particular problem. They may undergo unnecessary, expensive, or ill-advised treatments, and may not take "no" as an answer when requesting another opinion.

We cannot make people move beyond denial, but we can encourage them to seek appropriate care from rehabilitation specialists or psychologists. Involving family members in this process may also be helpful, Family members should be counseled on the extent of vision loss and the limitations of the individual with vision loss. Unfortunately, family members may actually impede the process of moving past denial, as they may be in denial themselves and may inadvertently influence those with vision problems to remain in denial as well.

D. Why Me? Making Meaning Out of Misfortune

One of the first questions asked by someone who has experienced a tragedy is "why me?" As health care professionals we have heard our patients ask this question on many occasions. Elizabeth Kubler-Ross revolutionized our ideas about the "why me?" question with her studies on death and dying with the terminally ill in the mid-1960s. She suggested that individuals go through a specific process to answer this question and to ultimately accept their own mortality and death. Much of her work was anecdotal and more recent work has suggested that the process is much more individualized than she proposed (25). However, one aspect of the grieving process is virtually universal; that is the process of making meaning out of misfortune. Although little research has been conducted to look at the specific reactions of those with low vision, one should be able to assume that vision loss is considered a personal tragedy, and as such, the need by patients to make meaning out of its presence should be expected. Helping a patient come to terms with vision loss and make meaning of it may be an important part of the rehabilitation process.

Most individuals will try to explain to themselves why something bad has happened to them. Those who are religious may show improvement in psychological well-being and improvement in health when faced with disabling or chronic illness (26,27), and as a result, more and more physicians are discussing religious beliefs and ideas with their patients (28). Those who are not as religious may look for some "good" to come from their experience with vision loss. The ability to find something good in a bad situation is frequently associated with positive affectivity. Those with a positive affect will be very optimistic about life, whereas those with a negative affect will be very pessimistic about life. The presence of a positive affect has been associated with improved health and well-being (29). Some will spend months feeling depressed, with little time spent on the "why me?" question, while others will immediately focus on the process of making meaning out of misfortune. Those who are unaware that their vision loss is permanent may not try to make meaning out of it and may feel that it is just an extremely annoying part of the aging process that will eventually resolve. They may feel disillusioned with their ophthalmologist and depressed about their situation, especially when they feel that no one is talking with them. Feelings of depression can overwhelm the individual, thus making it even more difficult for him/her to adapt to vision loss. Since the elderly are prone to depression with the onset of chronic illness and disability, the lack of a conversation with the ophthalmologist about one's visual prognosis may result in serious health and mental health problems.

E. Adaptability in the Elderly

The saying "you can't teach an old dog new tricks" is very applicable in the realm of low-vision rehabilitation for those with AMD. Many individuals with AMD have vision loss of 20/200 or greater in the better eye after correction. To assist the person with reading tasks, the dioptric strength needed is along the lines of +10 or stronger. This results in a focal distance of 10 cm or less. The question facing the low-vision practitioner is "how can I get my patient to hold that book next to her nose?" In many instances, the older individual with low vision will not tolerate the short focal distance. Others will not have the capacity to hold their reading material steadily (such as those with Parkinson's disease) and the focal range is very narrow and success is therefore limited. The individual may only be able to read word by word or, worse, letter by letter, with a high-plus add thus making functional reading ability very limited. For individuals with very few health-related comorbid symptoms, reading in this manner is difficult.

For the individual with memory loss, this type of reading is impossible as the individual will forget the words first read before finishing the sentence.

Many patients with AMD just want regular glasses and do not want "those strange-looking glasses." The person may be annoyed at the focal range, may dislike the weight of the low-vision device, may be embarrassed at its appearance, or may be unwilling to spend the money on the device. Most just want their vision "back the way it was." Choosing a successful low-vision rehabilitation candidate from among our patients with AMD may be quite difficult. I used to believe that those individuals who had a positive affect were more successful candidates for optical low-vision aids and other types of low-vision rehabilitative strategies. I have found very positive people doing poorly with their aids and more negative people doing quite well. What I have since learned is that acceptance of low-vision aids has little to do with affectivity and much more to do with motivation and adaptability.

Adaptability is very beneficial for seniors, as it may result in the older person learning new skills such as how to use a computer. More and more seniors are finding computer technologies fun and easy to learn. However, elderly individuals with low vision may not readily accept newer computerized technologies. Many may not have sufficient computer skills to use the Internet or World Wide Web, so learning how to use a computer after vision loss to function better at home is unlikely. Access to computers by normally sighted senior citizens should eventually help individuals who develop vision loss to better utilize newer computerized technologies. Since many of the newer low-vision technologies are utilizing computer technology, knowledge of computers will be essential for full access to low-vision devices by the elderly.

Younger individuals with low vision adapt to aids and technologies relatively easily. However, those who are elderly may have difficulty changing the way that they do things to accommodate the low-vision aid. This is especially true if the individual is trying to use a high plus spectacle correction for reading. Let's say that a patient can read newsprint with a +20.00 D lens. The focal distance is about 5 cm. How likely will the person "accept" this aid? Not likely. That is because the way that he holds the paper to read (almost against his nose) is not the way he has done it for the last 75 years. Either a gradual increase in near correction or concentrated reading rehabilitation and training is necessary for acceptance (30). Prescribing a +20.00 D the first time a low-vision aid is prescribed is a formula for disaster if the correct training does not accompany the prescription. The knowledge that reading is possible (although uncomfortable) is invaluable, however. The individual may never use the device, but has now become aware that reading is possible. The person is simply choosing not to read. This information provides a feeling of self-efficacy in the person's life and is rehabilitative in and of itself.

Determining which patients are adaptable and which ones are not is not an easy task. Asking about positive thinking will not help. Asking the person whether he/she feels that using any technique to regain reading ability is acceptable may be a place to start, but this does not guarantee success either. Many of my patients have reported that they want to read more than anything, that they have waited all their lives to spend their retirement reading. This level of desire to read does not necessarily guarantee success. The patient may still be unwilling to accept the short focal distance or may be unwilling to spend the money necessary to purchase a closed-circuit television that magnifies text. Even though a patient has been successful using a device does not mean that the individual will actually purchase and use the device. The person may not want to spend the family's inheritance, the person may not have cash readily available, or the person may not feel as if he/she deserves the money to be spent on him/her. All of these barriers reduce the success of low-vision rehabilitation. If the person is also unwilling to try new techniques to cope with vision loss, he will not be a successful low-vision rehabilitation candidate (31–33).

Although adaptability and willingness to try are essential for good low-vision rehabilitation to occur, we should refer all of our patients to low-vision specialists regardless of their apparent adaptability. The low-vision practitioner may be able to convince the individual of the benefits of low-vision aids and may be able to "teach our patients new tricks." If we screen our patients too closely, we will likely not refer an individual who has the potential of being assisted.

IV. INTERPERSONAL RELATIONSHIPS AFTER VISION LOSS

A. The Role of Family and Friends in Vision Rehabilitation

Adaptation to chronic illness rarely occurs in a vacuum. This can certainly be said for vision loss. In fact, family and friends are often a very necessary part of coping with vision loss (34). Individuals with supportive families and friends frequently cope better with vision loss than do those without supportive networks. Those who are married may cope better with vision loss, but this is more likely to occur if the individual with vision loss is male (23). In fact, many men who are visually impaired do not feel "handicapped" by their vision loss because their wives are there assisting them with daily living tasks as usual. On the other hand, women who are visually impaired with normally sighted husbands may have tremendous difficulties coping, as they must continue to perform activities of daily living without spousal support (2). If the woman has an adult daughter living nearby, the daughter may be the one to assist her visually impaired mother cope with vision loss. Familial patterns of behavior can be amplified if a visually impaired individual lives within the household (35). If the family is loving and supportive, that support will likely translate into the new living arrangements with husbands taking over certain domestic responsibilities. If the family unit is dysfunctional, the familial problems can be exacerbated. I had a patient who had been abused by her husband for years. She reported that the abuse had worsened after she lost her vision. He would not allow anyone to assist his wife nor would he allow her to undergo low-vision rehabilitation training. She therefore reported living in a very unsafe environment. As this constituted spousal and elder abuse, the authorities were notified. However, many visually impaired seniors do not receive any intervention and live precarious lives.

Many cultures believe that elderly family members should not have to work or care for the family. This is generally done out of respect for the elderly individual. However, those with vision loss may not be allowed to do anything, as they may be viewed as unsafe to do so. Unfortunately, they also are not allowed to obtain low-vision rehabilitation training, thus making them more dependent on their younger family members than their age alone would warrant.

V. COMMUNITY RESOURCES FOR THOSE WITH VISION LOSS

A. Resources for People with Vision Loss

Numerous resources are available for those with vision loss. They include local resources, county resources, state and federal resources, as well as national not-for-profit organizations and medical organizations such as the American Academy of Ophthalmology. To best assist our patients with low vision, we should attempt to create a personalized reference guide that includes all of these resources. In this way, we will actually be able to screen the type of information that we provide to our patients and their families. We may not want them to access certain types of organizations, whereas we may want them to utilize the resources of other organizations.

A search on the World Wide Web (Internet) may be a great starting point. Searching under the term "low vision" or "blindness" should lead to numerous organizations serving the visually impaired. A review of these sites should help us determine whether or not we wish our patients to access the information. By utilizing the Internet, we will reduce the time we spend searching for these organizations, and we should be able to find the most up-to-date information about each organization. In addition, a call to local senior citizen groups may lead us to social support groups serving the visually impaired. Social support groups may be extremely effective since social support has been shown to increase coping skills and psychological well-being in those who are visually impaired (34,36). A call to the local department of Rehabilitation should finish our search for local services for the blind and visually impaired. The Department of Rehabilitation provides low-vision devices, orientation and mobility training, and other services to the visually impaired. Generally, those with more severe visual impairment are given preferential treatment, as are those who plan to go back to work. However, if state moneys are available, any individual who is legally blind should be eligible for the services provided by the Department of Rehabilitation.

B. Finding a Good Low-Vision Practitioner

The biggest question facing my colleagues who see patients with low vision is "how do I find a good low-vision practitioner?" This is a very important question, as our reputations are associated with the individuals to whom we refer our patients. Because of this, we must carefully develop a referral list of practitioners we trust. Individuals should only appear on the list ideally after we have had a chance to interview them. During the interview we should ask about such things as training, length of time serving those with low vision, participation in national meetings or activities, membership in professional organizations, and the like. Does this person meet our standards as a specialist in the field? If the answer is "no," then it may be best to find someone else to provide the services. If we cannot find a specialist we trust who fits low-vision aids, then we might want to consider providing the aids ourselves. In this way we can have control over what our patients receive. If that does not seem feasible, we should make sure that the person doing the fitting has a money-back guarantee on all products sold. This reduces the likelihood that our patients will purchase devices that are of little use.

VI. SUMMARY

Patients need sufficient information regarding AMD to understand their prognosis and to be able to seek appropriate low-vision care. This information is best delivered by the patient's own ophthalmologist. Patients frequently misunderstand the concept of low vision and legal blindness. Many focus on the word "blindness" and believe that if they become legally blind they will eventually go totally blind. A thorough explanation of what constitutes low vision should eliminate this confusion.

Profound vision loss can result in the individual needing assistance from others for such simple things as writing a check, reading a bank statement, or picking out a good piece of meat at the market. Dependence on others can make the person with low vision feel worthless. Individuals with low vision, who can no longer drive or take the bus easily, must depend on others for transportation and socializing. Those with limited support networks may become very depressed as a result of social isolation.

Those with macular degeneration may deny the seriousness of their vision loss to maintain their independence and driver's license. Denial can have very deleterious consequences on the individual and his/her family. Individuals who have experienced a serious loss will search for meaning in their misfortune and will frequently need to answer the "why me?" question.

Those who are elderly frequently have difficulty accepting low-vision aids. This is often due to the fact that the individual must read in a fashion that is very unfamiliar. Many refuse to use low-vision aids because they cannot read in the way "normal people" can. Family and friends who are supportive of the person with AMD are necessary for quick acceptance and recovery on the part of the patient. A good low-vision practitioner should be willing to offer patients a money-back guarantee on all low-vision items sold.

REFERENCES

1. Alien M, Birse E. Stigma and blindness. J Ophthalm Nurs Technol 1991;10(4):147–152.
2. VanBoemel GB, Lee PP, Tansman MS. When Family Support Isn't: Dynamics in Households of Low Vision Diabetics. Fort Lauderdale, FL: Association for Research in Vision and Ophthalmology, 1998.
3. Faye EE. Living with low vision. What you can do to help patients cope. Postgrad Med 1998;103(5):167–70,175–178.
4. Fletcher DC. Low vision: the physician's role in rehabilitation and referral. Geriatrics 1994;49(5):50–53.
5. Orr AL. The psychosocial aspects of aging and vision loss. In: Webber N, ed. Vision and Aging: Issues in Social Work Practice. New York: Haworth Press, 1991, pp 1–4.
6. Bachar E, Shanan J. Long lasting blindness, availability of resources, and early aging. Percept Mot Skills 1997;84(2):675–688.
7. Brody BL, Williams RA, Thomas RG, Kaplan RM, Chu RM, Brown SI. Age-related macular degeneration: a randomized clinical trial of a self-management intervention Ann Behav Med 1999;21(4):322–329.
8. Kleinschmidt JJ. An orientation to vision loss program: meeting the needs of newly visually impaired older adults. Gerontologist 1996;36(4):534–538.
9. Miller HL Jr. Legally blind veterans—the link between appropriate referral and the ability to cope. J Miss State Med Assoc 1999;40(2):48–50.
10. VanBoemel GB, Fowler LM. Education and Outreach: Extending SSI benefits to the blind, newly blind aged, and visually disabled. (Contract number 14-S-10041-9-1). Social Security Administration, Department of Health and Human Services, Baltimore, MD, 1994.
11. Roe B. Effective and ineffective management of incontinence: issues around illness trajectory and health care. Qual Health Res 2000;10(5):677–690.
12. Arora NK, McHorney CA. Patient preferences for medical decision making: who really wants to participate? Med Care 2000;38(3):335–341.
13. Brown GC, Brown MM, Sharma S. Difference between ophthalmologists' and patients' perceptions of quality of life associated with age-related macular degeneration. Can J Ophthalmol 2000;35:127–133.
14. Hershberger PJ. Information loss: the primary psychological trauma of the loss of vision. Percept Mot Skills 1992;74(2):509–510.
15. Cox DJ, Kiernan BD, Schroeder DB, Cowley M. Psychosocial sequelae of visual loss in diabetes. Diabetes Educ 1998;24(4):481–484.
16. DeLeo D, Hickey PA, Meneghel G, Cantor CH. Blindness, fear of sight loss, and suicide. Psychosomatics 1999;40(4):339–344.
17. Fagerstrom R. Correlation between psychic and somatic symptoms and vision in aged patients before and after a cataract operation. Psychol Rep 1991;69(3 Pt 1):707–721.
18. Leinhaas MA, Hedstrom NJ. Low vision: how to assess and treat its emotional impact. Geriatrics 1994;49(5):53–56.
19. Wahl HW, Heyl V, Oswald F, Winkler U. Deteriorating vision in the elderly: double stress? Ophthalmology 1998;95(6):389–399.
20. Wahl HW, Schilling O, Oswald F, Heyl V. Psychosocial consequences of age-related visual impairment: comparison with mobility-impaired older adults and long-term outcome. J Gerontol

B Psychol Sci Soc Sci 1999;54(5):304–316.

21. Yoshida T, Ichikawa T, Ishikawa T, Hori M. Mental health of visually and hearing impaired students from the viewpoint of the University Personality Inventory. Psychiatry Clin Neurosci 1998;52(4):413–418.

22. Van Boemel GB, Rozee PD. Treatment for psychosomatic blindness among Cambodian refugee women. Women Ther 1992;13(3):239–266.

23. Van Boemel GB, Iwai LS, Yoshinaga P, Vartanian J, Walonker F. Does adherence to traditional sex roles influence low vision rehabilitation? Vision '99, sponsored by Lighthouse International, New York, July 1999.

24. Weinstein N. Unrealistic optimism about susceptibility to health problems. J Behav Med 1982;2:11–20.

25. Wortman CB, Silver RC. The myths of coping with loss. J Consult Clin Psychol 1989;57(3):349–357.

26. Silver RL, Boon C, Stones MH. Searching for meaning in misfortune: making sense of incest. Social Issues 39(2):81–102.

27. Mackenzie ER, Rajagopal DE, Meibohm M, Lavizzo-Mourey R. Spiritual support and psychological well-being; older adults' perceptions of the religion and health connection. Altern Ther Health Med 2000;6(6):37–45.

28. Post SG, Puchalski CM, Larson DB. Physicians and patient spirituality: professional boundaries, competency, and ethics. Ann Intern Med 2000;132(7):578–883.

29. Erdal KJ, Zautra AJ. Psychological impact of illness downturns: a comparison of new and chronic conditions. Psychol Aging 1995;10(4):570–577.

30. Nilsson UL, Nilsson SEG. Rehabilitation of the visually handicapped with advanced macular degeneration. Docum Ophthalmol 1986;62:345–367.

31. Burckhardt CS. Coping with chronic illness. Nurs Clin North Am 1987;22(3):543–550.

32. Gignac MA, Cott C, Badley EM. Adaptation to chronic illness and disability and its relationship to perceptions of independence and dependence. J Gerontol B Psychol Sci Soc Sci 2000;55(6):362–372.

33. Epker J, Gatchel RJ. Dysfunctional coping strategies are associated with chronic psychosocial difficulties. Psychosom Med 2000;62(1):69–75.

34. Reinhardt JP. The importance of friendship and family support in adaptation to chronic vision impairment. J Gerontol B Psychol Sci Soc Sci 1996;51(5):268–278.

35. Bernbaum M, Albert SG, Duckro PN, Merkel W. Personal and family stress in individuals with diabetes and vision loss. J Clin Psychol 1993;49(5):670–677.

36. Raleigh ED: Sources of hope in chronic illness. Oncol Nurs Forum 1992;19(3):443.

22

Clinical Considerations for Visual Rehabilitation

Susan A. Primo

Emory University School of Medicine, Atlanta, Georgia

I. INTRODUCTION

While the trauma of macular degeneration is difficult enough for some patients to cope with, the visual impairment left afterward is even tougher. Patients must not only learn to accept the fate of retinal disease, but must also summon the strength to accept the fact that they will surrender a certain degree of independence as visual acuity declines. The visual rehabilitative process helps the visually impaired patient to regain a satisfactory level of independence and can be achieved by assisting the patient in learning to cope with the psychological, emotional, and economic aspects of vision loss, as well as through the use of optical, nonoptical, and electronic devices. Typically, this type of integrated rehabilitative process is necessary for patients with severe and profound visual impairment, i.e., legal blindness.

The term "legal blindness" as defined is a visual acuity of 20/200 or worse in the best corrected better eye or a visual field of 20 degrees or less in the widest diameter of vision. A patient cannot have poor vision in one eye only and be considered legally blind. This classification becomes a part of the patient's permanent record and has implications for eligibility for state financial assistance, tax benefits, reduced public transportation fares, and other circumstances. In addition, in many states that have "commissions" for the blind, reporting of legal blindness may cause a driver's license to be revoked. For many people, maintaining a driver's license, whether they are actually driving or not, has significant meaning and serves as a form of identification. The practitioner should be aware of these issues when designating this classification.

II. REHABILITATIVE EVALUATION

The low-vision examiner begins the evaluation with a complete understanding of the patient's ocular history. Detailed documentation of surgical history and stage of pathology are important components. Typically, a low-vision evaluation, should not commence until a patient has undergone all surgical and nonsurgical attempts at restoring visual function. The reasons for this are twofold. First, the low-vision examiner is concerned with performing an extensive evaluation often using state-of-the-art devices, which can be quite expensive. If the patient's final visual acuity is in question, these devices may not be suitable once the visual acuity has reached its final level and has stabilized. Second, the patient needs to have gone through the "mourning process" of losing sight with the understanding that the next step must be taken to begin the visual rehabilitative process. This is not to say that if miracle breakthroughs become available, a patient should not have access to any possibility of restoring sight. However, success with low-vision devices is completely dependent upon: (1) a patient's full acceptance of his or her visual impairment and (2) the ability and desire to move on.

A. History

During the history, the patient is asked about aspects of vision loss. These aspects include duration, symmetry, fluctuations, stability, loss of ability to discriminate color, effects of various illuminations or lighting conditions, and mobility concerns. These questions assist patients in learning to talk about the effects of the visual impairment on their lifestyle, an important step in beginning the rehabilitative process. While ascertaining this information, the low-vision examiner also documents any current devices, including glasses, that may already be in the patient's possession. Frequently a well-meaning spouse or relative has already offered the patient a magnifier of some sort. It is important to categorize all such devices for type, style, and power. It is also important to determine the usefulness of these devices. For example, can the patient read large print or headlines of a newspaper with glasses and/or a magnifier? Often, patients will say that all devices are useless, but in reality, they may be able to see large print and not regular print. While this may be considered useless to them, it is important to the examiner.

Perhaps the last and most important part of the history is an expression by the patient of his or her goals and expectations. During this portion, the examiner determines whether the patient has realistic goals and expectations or whether the desire is to "just see again." A detailed list of desired activities is recorded in order of importance to the patient. Sometimes it takes a little prodding, but virtually all patients' primary desire is to be able to read again. It is important to determine whether a patient simply wants to read mail or bills to be able to handle his or her own finances and/or the patient wants to continue leisurely reading of printed materials such as newspaper, novels, etc. Second to a desire to read is usually improvement of distance vision. Again, specific distant activities (watching television, bird watching, or driving) need to be discussed. The driving issue is an extremely sensitive area and the examiner must use compassion and sensitivity in discussing this topic. A more detailed discussion of driving will follow later in this chapter. Using a checklist approach is a quick and easy method for determining the patient's current level of vision and subsequently any special material the patient wishes to read or certain activities the patient wishes to engage in, i.e., playing cards, sewing, drawing or painting, golf, etc. (Fig. 1). Finally, maximizing an education environment is critical for a young child or adult, as is attention to a patient's workplace if he or she is employed or seeking gainful employment.

B. Visual Acuity Testing

Although there is a standard format to the low-vision evaluation, the examiner always bears in mind a goal-oriented approach. For example, if a patient expresses the desire to read

Checklist for current level of vision/goals

	YES	NO	DESIRES
Headlines	___	___	___
Magazines	___	___	___
Regular Newsprint	___	___	___
Labels, price tags	___	___	___
Money	___	___	___
Recognize faces	___	___	___
Watch TV	___	___	___
Cooking	___	___	___
Sew, knit, etc.	___	___	___
Housekeeping	___	___	___
Hygiene	___	___	___
Handiwork	___	___	___
Garden/yard work	___	___	___
Sports (golf, etc.)	___	___	___
Play cards	___	___	___
Driving	___	___	___
Other			
	___	___	___
Glare	___	___	

Figure 1   Checklist for current level of vision.

only, the focus will be on achieving this goal. The examiner might explain possibilities for improvement in distance vision, but if a patient is still uninterested, the telescopic evaluation is probably unnecessary. Likewise, if a patient's only desire is to drive, a short near evaluation may be performed to demonstrate possibilities, but clearly the emphasis in this case would be on the telescopic evaluation. As the examiner notices head and body movements as the patient initially walks into the examination room, these seemingly minor observations provide information not only about visual status, but also about a patient's level of adaptation to the vision loss. In addition, before visual acuity testing begins, any auxiliary testing is performed, which may include contrast sensitivity, Amsler grid, visual fields, etc. These tests can shed light on the size and extent of the central scotoma as well as other subjective aspects to the acuity loss.

As clear-cut as it may seem, visual acuity testing is an extremely important (and often long) part of the rehabilitative examination. Evaluating a patient with reduced visual acuity requires that basic examination techniques be modified. It is generally recommended that vision testing be done at 10 ft with a self-illuminated, portable eye chart. The Early Treatment Diabetic Retinopathy Study (ETDRS) chart is the most widely used. A projector chart is the least favorable means of measuring acuity in a patient with reduced vision. Not only is contrast not constant with a projector chart depending on the level of room illumination, but a patient would also have to be moved closer to the chart if vision was worse than 20/400. Moving a visually impaired patient only reinforces awareness of the vision loss and causes stress and negative feelings during the examination.

The ETDRS chart has several advantages. It is self-illuminated with high contrast and is on wheels so that it could be moved closer than 10 ft if necessary. Also, the chart has a wide spectrum of visual acuity values, ranging from a "Snellen 200-ft" equivalent to a 10-

ft equivalent. Since the testing distance is always recorded as the numerator of the Snellen fraction, this chart gives an acuity range (at 10 ft) from 10/200 (20/400) to 10/10 (20/20). If the chart is moved closer, the test distance is again recorded as the numerator. It is best not to convert the acuity to the 20-ft equivalent when recording vision so that the examiner may always know the test distance for subsequent evaluations. "Counting fingers" vision for measurement is generally not used during a low-vision evaluation. The fingers subtend approximately the same visual angle as a 200-ft Snellen figure. Therefore, a patient should be able to read the top line of the ETDRS chart at a closer distance. Recording visual acuity as "3/200" instead of counting fingers at 3 ft is much more accurate, which is important in determining which optical devices may be appropriate.

Determination of eccentric view, if suspected, is done during acuity testing. The easiest method is called the clock-face method. The patient is asked to keep his or her head still and to face straight ahead. The examiner then asks the patient to imagine that the eye chart is at the center of a clock. The patient is asked to move his/her eye in various positions of the clock until the top line becomes the clearest and most complete. Typically, but not always, a patient with acquired macular disease will attempt to place the image on the temporal retina where the most room is; i.e., the right eye will eccentrically view toward the right (3 o'clock) and the left eye will view toward the left (9 o'clock). This position should be demonstrated to the patient several times and recorded next to visual acuity. The knowledge of the exact location of the eccentric view will become useful for the remainder of the evaluation with devices.

Manifest refraction in a trial frame is generally the rule. In this case, the examiner can observe the patient's eyes particularly to reinforce the eccentric view. A phoropter does not allow a patient's eyes to be observed and the use of an eccentric view by the patient becomes quite difficult. In addition, the lens increments may be too small for a patient to determine any subjective difference; i.e., a patient with 20/200 vision will not appreciate a difference of ±.25D. The examiner cannot easily make large increments of change in the phoropter for patients with poorer vision. Generally, a patient whose vision is less than 20/100 will appreciate .50D lens changes. For vision between 20/100 and 20/200, the examiner should use .75–1.50D changes. If a patient's vision is 20/200–20/400, 1.50–2.00D lens increments should be used. This technique is called lens bracketing and is the most time efficient and effective. Likewise, when measuring astigmatic corrections, a higher-powered Jackson Cross Cylinder (.75–2.00D) is employed to ensure the patient appreciates the lens changes for power and axis refinements. To ensure that large refractive errors are not missed, keratometry, retinoscopy, and/or autorefraction offer a starting point. A scrupulous refraction is crucial before low-vision devices are demonstrated. Spectacles should always be prescribed using polycarbonate lenses even if there seems to be a minimal increase in visual acuity; they serve as an important source of protection particularly when the patient is engaged in activities where there may be hanging branches, flying objects, chemicals, etc., or simply unfamiliar terrain.

Depending on the patient's expression of initial goals, either a brief or extensive telescopic evaluation is performed next. Improvement of distance vision may have not initially been an expressed goal since a patient may be mostly tuned in to reading concerns. In any event, a brief introduction of a 3 or 4× powered telescope in the trial frame will demonstrate not only the device to the patient, but also the possibility of enhancing distance vision. Vision should generally improve proportionately to the power of the scope. For example, if a patient has best-corrected vision of 20/200, vision should improve to 20/50 with a 4× telescope. Exceptions to this rule may be a large or irregular central scotoma or the coexistence of other media opacities. Generally speaking, most distance activities usually require visual acuity of 20/30–20/50. It is rare that an individual would need to be corrected to 20/20 or better with a telescope. The aim should be to prescribe the lowest-powered telescope to achieve the required vision. The reasons for this are that as a telescope power becomes greater, the smaller the field of view and the more difficult it becomes to use effectively. If visual acuity is near equal between the two eyes, the examiner may choose to prescribe a binocular system, which will give a much larger field of view for activities such as watching television, going to shows, etc. As vision approaches 20/400 and worse, standard telescopic devices may not be useful; more advanced technological devices may be indicated.

C. Driving

The driving issue remains controversial and requires special mention. Driving is an important component of everyday life for most patients. The inability to drive has psychological implications in terms of limited independence. The subject must be treated with extreme carefulness and sensitivity. Visual acuity requirements vary from state to state, typically from 20/40 to 20/70. Currently 37 states allow bioptic telescopes for driving if visual acuity falls below the state's legal limit. The term "bioptic" simply implies two (bi-)optical centers. This form of a telescope is mounted several millimeters above the distance optical center. Therefore, a patient looks through his/her natural prescription through the carrier lens housing the telescope. When sharper acuity is needed for viewing street signs, etc., the patient lowers the chin and spots through the scope. This manner of use is similar to the fashion in which a driver would use the rearview mirror; the telescope is used only approximately 10–15% of the time while driving. This point is an extremely important one and often confused because it is thought that since there is a reduced field through the telescope, one could not possibly drive safely. Again, the driver is primarily looking through the carrier lens, not the telescopic device.

Although visual acuity is a fundamental part of safe driving, several studies have demonstrated that peripheral field (or vision) appears to play a more critical role in driving than visual acuity (1–3). All states allowing bioptic telescopes have a minimum visual field requirement without the telescope (usually between 120 and 140 degrees). Other requirements include maximum acuity without the telescope (usually 20/200) and minimum visual acuity with the telescope (20/40–20/60). Certainly, there are issues that go beyond visual acuity and peripheral field in determining whether any given driver will drive safely, particularly one with a visual impairment. Factors such as age, experience, visual attention and processing, reaction times, and cognitive deficits all inarguably affect an individual's ability to drive safely. Recent research has led to the development of mechanism called the Useful Field of View test (Visual Resources, Inc., Chicago, IL). This test requires higher-order processing skills and not only determines a conventional visual field, but also allows for the assessment of the visual field area over which rapid stimuli are flashed, i.e., a car or other object moved into a cluttered background (4). Simulating the "real" driving experience with this test, an association has been shown between elderly drivers who have reductions in their useful field of view and crash involvement (5). This test is invariably more important in determining driving safety than traditional assessments of visual acuity and peripheral field. Although the test is not commercially available yet, its software is being piloted.

Most drivers with visual impairment do limit driving exposure and tend to avoid challenging driving situations, i.e., driving at night, on interstate highways, during inclement weather, etc. No association has been found between drivers with macular degeneration and increased accident rates/fatalities; however, driving exposure is taken into account (6). One study has demonstrated that, although patients with macular degeneration performed more poorly on driver simulator and on-the-road tests compared to a control group, this did not translate into an increased risk of real-world accidents (7). Hence it still remains unclear whether reduced exposure decreases a driver's risk or whether any association exists between increased injurious accidents and visual impairment secondary to macular degeneration. The decision to prescribe a telescopic device for a patient to legally maintain a driver's license is a joint decision best left to doctors, patient, and family; the decision should be made on an individual basis.

D. Near Evaluation

Following refraction and distance evaluation is the near evaluation. Near visual acuity is most appropriately measured and evaluated with continuous-text reading cards. These cards test a patient's functional ability to read versus the ability to read a line of numbers or letters. Both Designs for Vision and Sloan make continuous-text near cards. "M" notation is generally used for recording near acuity. This notation uses the metric system, is standardized, and does not require a fixed testing distance. To begin the near evaluation, a reading lens addition should always be in place when testing patients greater than 50 years of age and test distance must be appropriate for the power of the add. For example, the test distance for a +2.50D add should be 40 cm or 16 in. (100/2.50 = 40 cm; 40/2.50 = 16 in.); test distance for a +4.00D add should be 25 cm or 10 in. (100/4.00 = 25; 40/4.00 = 10 in.). Distance and near visual acuities (with standard +2.50D add) should be approximately the same so that if a patient's best corrected vision is 20/200 in the distance, the near vision with standard add should also be 20/200. Pupil size, asymmetry, significant media opacities, and large central scotomas may create disparities; however, large differences between distance and near acuities should alert the examiner to an inaccurate manifest refraction.

   Once initial near acuity has been determined, the examiner increases the power of the add until the appropriate acuity is obtained. The approximate add it will take for any given patient to read newspaper size print (1M or 20/50) can be predicted by calculating the reciprocal of the distance or near acuity. For example, if a patient's vision is 20/200, it would take at least a +10.00D add (200/20 = 10) for this patient to read newspaper-size print. This value may be modified depending upon the patient's initial expression of goals for reading. If a patient wishes to read the stock pages, more plus may be needed; if a patient only wishes to read large-print text, less plus is needed.

E. Binocular Adds

Binocular adds are typically prescribed when the acuity is equal or near equal between the two eyes. Base-in prism is always required in binocular adds greater than +6.00D because fusional vergence is exhausted and the eyes drift toward an exophoric posture. The amount of prescribed prism is 2 prism diopters more than the amount of plus. For example, if the examiner wishes to prescribe a +8.00D-add OU, the prescribed prism should be 10 prism diopters base-in total split equally between the two eyes. Glasses should be prescribed in a half-eye frame size owing to the thickness and heaviness of the lenses. Because the nasal edge of the lens becomes quite thick with increased prism, adds greater than +12.00D should be prescribed monocularly with the eye not being used either occluded or the lens frosted to avoid diplopia. If a patient has one eye that is considerably better, the high add is prescribed monocularly. However, there may still be a "ghost" image or halo around letters or words coming from the poorer eye. In this instance, the lens of the poorer eye can be frosted (or occluded).

For higher adds, most patients continually need reinforcement regarding the appropriate and close working distance. Most people are able to conceptualize inches rather than centimeters. Conversion of reading distance into inches requires the power of the add to be divided into 40. For example, if a $+7.50D$-add has been prescribed, the patient must hold all reading material at $5^1/_3$ in. $(40/7.5 = 5.33)$. The patient should begin with larger text initially to become adjusted to the closer-than-usual reading distance and probably increased fatigue. If a patient has not yet accepted his/her visual loss, success with high adds and close reading distances is virtually impossible.

For those patients rejecting the close reading distance of high adds, other alternatives exist. Telemicroscopes (surgical loupes/telephoto lens) can be made with a specified reading distance. The patient, however, must weigh the benefit of the increased distance versus the reduction in field of view experienced. Although every attempt is made to prescribe a spectacle-borne reading device, electronic devices such as the closed-circuit television (CCTV) are good alternatives to spectacles. A patient can sit back at a comfortable distance and is able to magnify print large enough to read easily. Clearly, a CCTV is not a portable device and can cost several thousands of dollars, but can have a tremendous impact in allowing a patient to read (or work) again. Handheld or stand magnifiers are prescribed in conjunction with spectacles. These devices are most useful for spot reading rather than extended reading. However, for those patients rejecting spectacles, these devices are quite effective.

F. Contrast Enhancement, Glare Reduction, and Nonoptical Devices

Contrast enhancement and glare reduction provide the final steps to the low-vision evaluation. Patients with macular degeneration often experience a loss of contrast. Contrast enhancement lenses shield the eyes from too much shorter wavelengths of light. These shorter wavelengths consist of high-energy visible blue light and can cause loss of contrast as well as glare, which reduces the eye's overall function. The Corning GlareControl family of lenses consists of nine filters that selectively block specific wavelengths of blue light while transmitting light at other wavelengths. There are eight graduated filter levels, each numbered to block below the corresponding wavelength (CPF 450, 450X, 511, 511X, 527, 527X, 550, and 550XD). The filters range in color from yellow (450) to deep red (550). The ninth filter is called the GlareCutter lens and is for patients with beginning to moderate light sensitivity. The lens color is more cosmetically appealing because it has more of a brownish hue rather than orange/red. All of the filters are photochromatic easing the transition between different light levels. These lenses are very helpful to patients with macular degeneration. In addition to providing benefits for protection from ultraviolet light, they provide contrast enhancement as well as glare reduction. Although the full range of filters are suitable for many ocular pathologies, usually the CPF 511 and 527 lenses work best in patients with moderate to advanced macular degeneration. Since the lenses are glass (and not high-impact polycarbonate plastic), they are best prescribed in the clip-on variety.

Other nonoptical devices that might be considered are large-print books, check register, clock, watch, playing cards, etc., to name a few. There are talking books, watches, and clocks as well as specialized appliances for diabetics. Catalogs of such devices can be

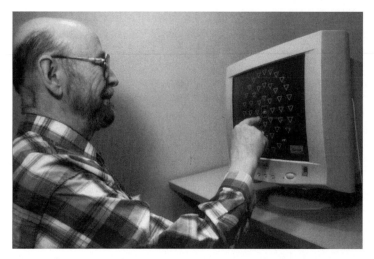

Figure 2   Useful Field of View Visual Attention Analyzer. (Courtesy of Visual Awareness, Inc.)

given to the patient and family. Occupational rehabilitation to assist in training of optical devices as well as activities of daily life is often quite useful for most patients with varying levels of visual impairment.

III.   FUTURE IMPLICATIONS AND IMPROVEMENTS

A.   New Applications

The Useful Field of View test (Fig. 2), as mentioned, is an extremely important tool in determining driving safety of older patients particularly those with visual impairment. Many times, the patient has expressed an interest to continue driving, but the examiner feels the patient may not be a good candidate even with a bioptic telescope. This test gives objective results informing both patient and family whether the patient will be at risk for injurious accidents.

Scanning laser ophthalmoscope (SLO) macular perimetry (Fig. 3) allows for the characterization of central field defects, i.e., macular scotomata. The presence or absence of macular scotomata and their characteristics are extremely important indicators of reading success and speed with low-vision devices as well as performance with activities of daily living (8). The confocal SLO has graphic capabilities that allow a retinal map of the scotomata to be drawn by determining the retinal location of visual stimuli directly on the retina. The instrument obtains retinal images continuously using near-infrared (780 nm) laser while scanning graphics onto the retina with a modulated vision HeNe (633 nm) laser at the same time (9). Thus the patient can see the stimuli and the investigator can view the stimuli on the retina. From these capabilities, a preferred retinal locus (PRL) can be identified and both relative and dense scotomata can be mapped.

Patients with macular scotomata do not often perceive black spots. Rather they say that letters or words are missing in their central vision while reading or they simply have difficulties functioning. The presence of these scotomata can decrease many areas of visual

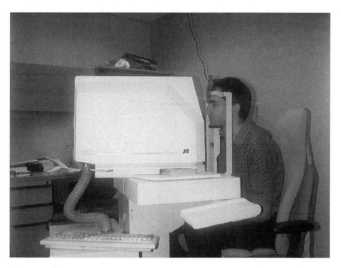

Figure 3   Scanning laser ophthalmoscope.

performance although the specific relationships between macular scotoma characteristics and visual performance have not been identified (10). Therefore, it becomes useful to be able to map out the scotomata and to know the exact location of preferred retinal loci before beginning the rehabilitative process. Traditional approaches attempt to establish a direction of the eccentric view and then to basically repeat this direction to the patient during training, etc. Many times this technique is effective, but often patients do not respond as well as predicted to the devices, training, visual performance task, and/or during activities of daily living. The SLO can essentially determine the characteristics of the scotomata and their relationship to the PRL. Once the PRL is identified, the rehabilitative team can instruct and train the patient on better use of the PRL.

Studies with the SLO have shown that there are different shapes and patterns of scotomata from round centered on a nonfunctioning fovea to ring scotoma surrounding a functioning fovea to highly complex amoeboid shapes (8). While the majority of patients do have dense scotomata, it was found that if the scotomata are complex and surround the PRL by more than two of its borders, these patients have the most difficulties in performing visual tasks as compared to those with less-encumbered PRLs (8). This knowledge will aid in prediction of patient success.

B.   New Technologies

Enhanced Vision (Huntington Beach, CA) has perhaps made some of the greatest breakthroughs for enhancing the quality of life of visually impaired patients. They have developed three important devices utilizing the latest advances in optical technology.

1.   The JORDY II is an amazing "virtual reality" system that immerses the patient in a video image. A tiny, color television camera is mounted in a head-borne device weighing less than 10 oz, (Fig. 4). Designed for patients whose vision is worse than 20/200, this device ranges in power from as little as 1× to as much as 24× for distance and up to 50 times for reading. It is considered the all-in-

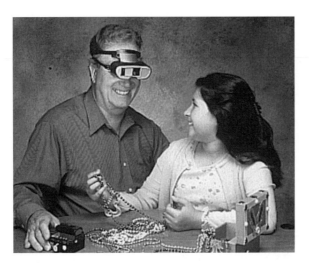

Figure 4 The JORDY II.

one system because it enhances distance, can attach to a television set or computer, and has closed-circuit television capabilities for reading or writing. For distance viewing, there is a wide (44 in.) field of view. The autofocus magnification has preset settings as well as zoom switches that are operated from an easy-to-use handheld control unit.   Both contrast and brightness controls make the color image quite clear. For near viewing, the closed-circuit television feature allows the device to be placed in a portable docking stand. The image is magnified depending on the size of the television screen or computer monitor. The light requirements are low, with the system requiring no additional light thereby resulting in minimum glare. The device is not designed to be used while walking, driving, or during any mobility.

2. The MaxPort is a device that allows the visually impaired patient to read with the ease of a closed-circuit television set, but is portable. The system consists of two components: a digital magnifier that captures the information and a pair of lightweight (4 oz) glasses that display the magnified image (Fig. 5). The patient would simply place the magnifier on any surface, either curved or straight, and view the magnified image on the glasses. The image can be magnified up to 28 times and is available in black and white or color and is most suitable for patients whose vision is 20/100 or worse. It is a great solution for professional, students, and seniors. Concise brightness control makes the image clear and crisp. There is also a special tracking guide (MaxTrak) that makes the magnifier move straight across the page. The device is very easy to use as no connections or assembly is required. It operates on a rechargeable battery and comes in a sleek carrying case.

3. The Max is another innovative, but lower-priced, magnifying system. It is a portable, handheld magnifier that easily connects to any television set or computer monitor to magnify words, pictures, and more (Fig. 6). Using a 20-in. television set, the device will magnify in both black and white and color from 16 to 28 times. It is quite easy to use with either the right or left hand and the image is virtually distortion free; it can also be used on any surface, curved or

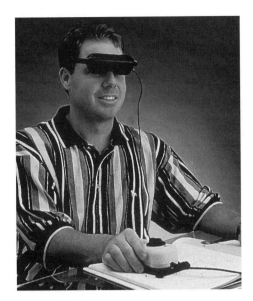

Figure 5 The Maxport.

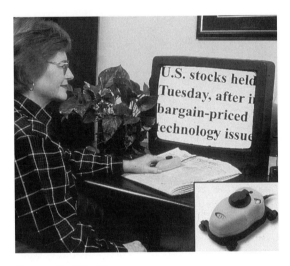

Figure 6 The Max.

straight. The three viewing options (low contrast/photo, high contrast/positive, high contrast/negative) make it suitable for most patients whose vision is 20/100 or worse.

Ocutech, Inc. (Chapel Hill, NC) has recently made advances with several new telescopic devices.

1. The VES-AF (Vision Enhancing System-Auto Focus) is the first autofocus telescope available. It has extremely high optical quality and consists of 4×

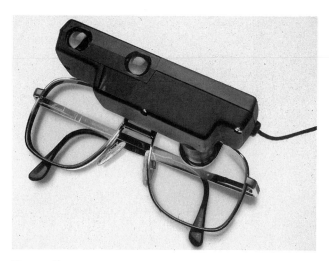

Figure 7 VES-Autofocus. (Courtesy of Ocutech, Inc.)

telescope focusing from as close as 12 in. to optical infinity (Fig. 7). The autofocus component works through computer-controlled infrared electrooptics, which measure the focusing distance, and another computer, which moves the focusing lens to the proper position. The 4× telescope has an amazing 12.5 degrees of field and is lightweight (2.5 oz). The device is worn on the top of a frame and is connected to a rechargeable battery pack, which can be worn around the waist or in a pocket or purse. This device is useful for distance, intermediate, and limited near vision including activities such as driving, card/music playing, birdwatching, golf, etc., and works best for patients who have vision between 20/80 and 20/200.

2. Currently under development is a binocular autofocus telescope. This device has the same quick automatic focusing at distance and near, but has the added capability of binocular viewing for an enhanced field of view through the telescopes. Still under development, the device would be most beneficial for patients who have equal or near-equal acuity in both eyes and wish to use the device for both distance and reading.

3. The VES-II is a bioptic telescope that was designed to address some of the major drawbacks of conventional bioptic telescope systems, namely, poor acceptance by patients and fitting problems by the prescriber (Fig. 8). It offers significant improvements in field of view, image brightness, and contrast as compared to conventional bioptics of similar powers. Probably the nicest feature is the fully adjustable mounting design, which gives the prescriber full control over the positioning of the telescope. Available in 4× and 6×, this innovative telescope is best prescribed for patients with visual acuity between 20/80 and 20/400. Although needing to be manually focused, it offers a less expensive alternative to the autofocus telescope.

4. The VES-MINI, also an innovative design, is a miniature 3× expanded field telescope (Fig. 9). It has wide 15-degree field of view combined with a very compact physical design. The telescope is equivalent in size to small focusing galilean telescopes, but is half the size of most expanded field telescopes. The

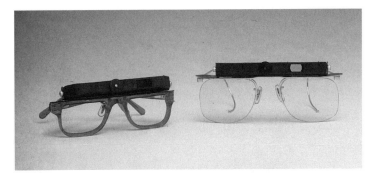

Figure 8 VES-II. (Courtesy of Ocutech, Inc.)

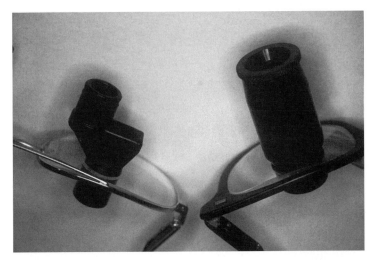

Figure 9 VES-MINI (left) as compared to a standard (right) expanded-field telescope. (Courtesy of Ocutech, Inc.)

optics are quite crisp and bright and can be prescribed for monocular or binocular use. Other special features are its unique design that minimized the ring scotoma that can be characteristic of many telescopic systems. Also, its field of view has been expanded horizontally to provide extra added vision in the most important lateral fields. The manual focus is quite fast with capabilities of focusing from optical infinity down to 12 in. covered in less than one complete turn. In addition to being extremely lightweight, it has internal refractive corrections from $+12D$ to $-12D$; eyepiece corrections are available for other refractive errors. This telescope is a good option for patients whose vision is better than 20/200.

Optelec, a leader in closed-circuit television, has developed a new line of these most popular electronic devices. Their new ClearView line has an ergonomic design and is user friendly. The best features are the fingertip controls that give instant focus, one-touch zoom, push-button brightness level, normal text and reverse-contrast modes, and a position locator.

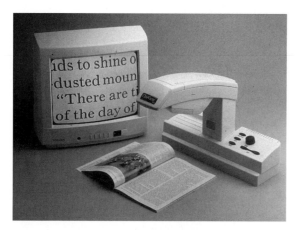

Figure 10   Clearview 100 series with attachment to standard television.

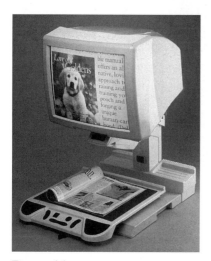

Figure 11   Clearview 517 with integrated tiltable monitor.

1. The simplest and least expensive 100 series is a lightweight and portable unit that connects easily to any television video input jack (Fig. 10). Although black and white only, it will enlarge text depending on the size of the television screen. This very affordable system has the push-button instant focus and fingertip zoom control features; the image is very sharp.
2. The ClearView 300 series also connects easily to a television set, but has an ergonomically designed table that allows for ease of use while reading or writing. The ClearView 317 features an integrated 17-in. black-and-white monitor that tilts to provide a comfortable viewing angle.
3. Probably the best of the line, the ClearView 517 has all the bells and whistles with the ergonomically designed table, instant focus, one-touch zoom, push-button brightness level, positive and negative contrast, and the position locator (Fig. 11). The device delivers a full-color performance on an integrated 17-in.

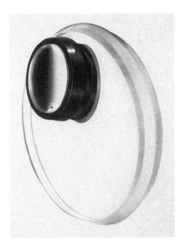

Figure 12   Designs for Vision standard 2.2× BIO II bioptic telescope.

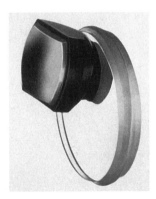

Figure 13   Designs for Vision 3× bioptic telescope.

tiltable monitor. Additionally, this system has an affordable price compared to other comparable systems on the market.

Designs for Vision, Inc. (Ronkonkoma, NY) has always been at the forefront for producing high-optical-quality devices for visually impaired patients. In addition to their traditional line of bioptics (Fig. 12 and 13), they have also become quite innovative with reading devices. The ClearImage II telephoto microscope and high-power microscopes (Fig. 14) are higher-powered reading microscopes available in powers 8× (+32D) to 20× (+80D). These lenses allow low-vision patients to read at a greater distance from the eye than any other comparable systems. The fields of view are quite large and lenses are virtually distortion free from edge to edge, which is what makes them innovative. Because of the higher powers, they are most suitable for patients whose vision is worse than 20/400.

Corning Medical Optics (Corning, NY) has added four new filters to its line of GlareControl lenses. The X (extra) filters (450X, 511X, 527X) are slightly darker than their corresponding filters. These filters work extremely well for increased contrast enhancement and add additional glare reduction in patients with beginning to advanced macular de-

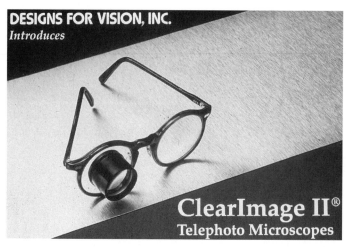

Figure 14   Designs for Vision ClearImage II telephoto microscope.

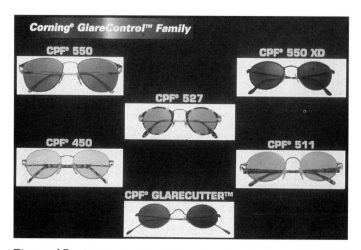

Figure 15   Corning family of filters. See also color insert, Fig. 22.15.

generation. The fourth newest filter is called the CPF GlareCutter lens. This lens is excellent for patients with early macular degeneration who do not need quite as much contrast enhancement, but who definitely need glare reduction. The lens also has less color distortion and a more attractive color for patients who reject the cosmetic appearance of the CPF 511 and 527 series. Blocking 99% UVA and 100% UVB rays, the lens transmits 18% of light in its lightened state and 6% in its darkened state (Figs. 15 and 16).

Zeiss Optical has launched a new line of handheld magnifiers and telescopes. Although the new devices are traditional, Zeiss has utilized its expertise in high-quality lens design and incorporated it into some sleek new devices. Of particular interest is its line of handheld magnifiers with an added patented antireflection coating (Fig. 17). These magnifiers have high optical quality giving edge-to-edge, crisp, clean, and bright images. Also in Zeiss's line is an inconspicuously designed, lightweight 5X penlight telescope that can be easily carried in the pocket and used for spotting both indoors and outdoors (Fig. 18).

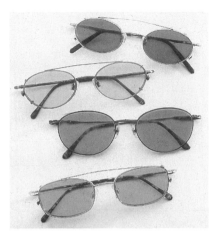

Figure 16 Corning's X series, which are slightly darker than their corresponding filters. See also color insert, Fig. 22.16.

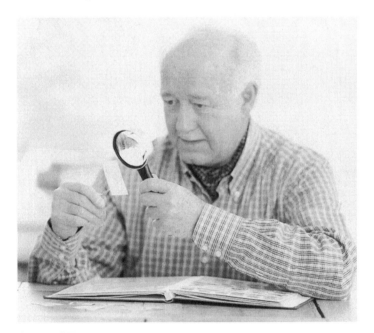

Figure 17 Zeiss handheld magnifier.

IV. SUMMARY

Patient success with low-vision devices is dependent upon a number of factors including age, physical and mental status, level and stability of visual acuity, patient's dependency on others, and the interval since visual loss. Resistance to low-vision devices and thus limited success tend to be seen in those patients who have not yet accepted or mourned their visual loss. Generally speaking, the more profound the visual loss, the more difficult it becomes to find means of enhancing vision. Nonoptical devices may be the only mechanism acceptable to the patient to regain a small degree of independence.

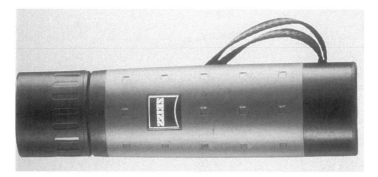

Figure 18   Zeiss 5× Mini quick penlight telescope.

The role of vocational rehabilitation and occupational therapy for orientation/mobility training, activities of daily living, etc., should always be considered for patients with advanced macular degeneration. Support groups may also provide comfort and new friendships in helping to cope with the visual impairment. Sometimes it is best to wait for a low-vision consultation until the patient seeks this care voluntarily after it has been suggested. Success with visual rehabilitation is always based on identification and satisfaction of the visual requirements and goals of the patient.

There are exciting new applications and devices in the field of low vision/visual rehabilitation. Much of the novelty utilizes the latest technology and will no doubt be of great benefit to many visually impaired patients suffering from macular degeneration.

Websites of companies for further information:

Enhanced Vision Systems—www.enhancedvision.com
Optelec—www.optelec.com
Ocutech, Inc.—www.ocutech.com
Designs for Vision—www.designsforvision.com
Corning Medical Optics—www.corning.com
Carl Zeiss, Inc.—www.zeiss.com

REFERENCES

1. Kelleher DK. Driving with low vision. J Vis Impair Blind 1968;11:345–350.
2. Lovsund P, Hedin A. Effect on driving performance of visual field defect. In: Gale A, Freeman MH, Haslegrave CM, et al., eds. Vision in Vehicles. Amsterdam: Elsevier, 1989.
3. Wood JM, Dique T, Troutbeck R. The effect of artificial visual impairment on functional visual fields and driving performance. Clin Vis Sci 1993;8:563–575.
4. Ball K, Beard B, Roenker D. Age and visual search: expanding the useful field of view. J Opt Soc Am 1988;5:2210–2219.
5. Owsley C., Ball K, Sloane ME, et al. Visual/cognitive correlates of vehicle accidents in older drivers. Psychol Aging 1991;6:403–415.
6. McCloskey LW, Koepsell TD, Wolf ME, Buchner DM. Motor vehicle collision injuries and sensory impairments of older drivers. Age Aging 1994;23:267–272.
7. Szkyk JP, Pizzimenti CE, Fishman GA, et al. A comparison of driving in older subjects with and without age-related macular degeneration. Arch Ophthalmol 1995;113:1033–1040.

8. Fletcher DC, Schuchard RA, Livingston CL, et al. Scanning laser ophthalmoscope macular perimetry and applications for low vision rehabilitation clinicians. Ophthalmol Clin North Am 1994;7(2):257–265.
9. Schuchard RA, Fletcher DC, Maino J. A scanning laser ophthalmoscope (SLO) low-vision rehabilitation system. Clin Eye Vis Care 1994;6(3):101–107.
10. Fletcher DC, Schuchard RA. Preferred retinal loci relationship to macular scotomas in a low-vision population. Ophthalmology 1997;104:632–638.

23
Retinal Prosthesis

Kah-Guan Au Eong and Eyal Margalit
Wilmer Eye Institute, Johns Hopkins University School of Medicine, Baltimore, Maryland

James D. Weiland, Eugene de Juan, Jr., and Mark S. Humayun
Doheny Retina Institute of the Doheny Eye Institute, University of Southern California Keck School of Medicine, Los Angeles, California

I. INTRODUCTION

There is currently no treatment for blindness due to neural diseases affecting the different parts of the visual system. These include a variety of conditions such as outer retinal damage secondary to age-related macular degeneration (AMD) and retinitis pigmentosa, inner retinal damage from severe diabetic retinopathy, and optic nerve disorders including glaucomatous optic neuropathy. Efforts to transplant photoreceptors and retinal pigment epithelial cells and gene therapy have not been successful to date (1–7). Recent advances in microtechnology, computer science, optoelectronics, and neurosurgical and vitreoretinal surgery have encouraged some researchers to investigate the feasibility of building a visual prosthesis to treat some of these disorders (8–27).

It has been well demonstrated both experimentally and clinically that nerve cells respond to externally applied electric current on a long-term basis. The cochlear implant is an accepted therapy for treatment of profound deafness. Other applications of neural stimulation include pain management, vagus nerve stimulation for sleep apnea, and treatment of Parkinsonian tremor. The visual prosthesis aims to bypass damaged portions of the visual system by directly stimulating the more proximal functional portions of the system.

The visual prosthesis will have to interface with the neural system at some location along the visual pathway. There are at least several potential sites for neurostimulation: the retina, the optic nerve, the lateral geniculate body, and the visual cortex (Fig. 1). In theory, the more proximal the interface is to the visual cortex, the more diseases the visual prosthesis can potentially treat. For example, a cortical visual prosthesis can potentially treat conditions due to damage anywhere along the afferent visual pathway provided the visual cortex is intact (9–11). However, there are many challenges the cortical visual prosthesis will have to overcome. First, the convoluted surface of the visual cortex, a large part of which is buried in the sulci on the medial surface of the occipital lobe, is not readily accessible, and the need for a craniotomy to gain access to an otherwise normal brain is at least a major psychological barrier. Second, the mobility of the brain and the subsurface input

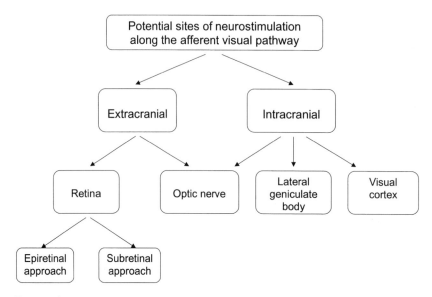

Figure 1 Approaches to building a visual prosthesis.

layer to the visual cortex makes the maintenance of a stable interface difficult. Third, complications such as infection of the brain and its meninges can cause significant morbidity and are potentially life-threatening. Other intracranial portions of the visual pathways such as the lateral geniculate body and the optic nerve are even less accessible than the visual cortex. Although cortical responses to electrical stimulation of the optic nerve have been measured by Shandurina and Lyskov (28), the densely packed axons of the optic nerve make selective stimulation of the axons difficult. One group recently reported chronic implantation of a self-sizing spiral cuff electrode with four contacts around the optic nerve of a 59-year-old volunteer blind from retinitis pigmentosa (29). Electrical stimuli applied to the optic nerve produced visual sensations that were broadly distributed throughout the visual field and could be varied by changing the stimulating conditions.

Compared to the intracranial locations, the retina is relatively more accessible with current vitreoretinal techniques and its topographic mapping of the visual space is fairly well defined. A number of groups including ours are currently evaluating the possibility of restoring sight by using a retinal prosthesis that would electrically stimulate the remaining retinal neural element (16–19, 23, 27, 30–36). An electronic device placed either in a subretinal or epiretinal location to replace the photoreceptors may be able to provide useful vision to patients blind from photoreceptor loss. However, any intraocular retinal prosthesis interfacing with the visual system at this distal location will not be able to treat disorders proximal to the interface such as patients blind from inner retinal or optic nerve damage.

This chapter reviews past efforts and the current state of the art, and considers the obstacles that must be overcome to bring the retinal prosthesis to fruition.

II. RATIONALE

The success of the cochlear implant by bypassing distal damaged or absent receptors and electrically stimulating more proximal neurons has prompted investigators to embark on the idea of the retinal prosthesis. In the normal retina, light stimulus causes the photoreceptors to initiate a neural response that is conducted to the inner retinal layers and via the nerve fiber layer to the optic nerve. Degenerative diseases of the outer retina such as retinitis pigmentosa and AMD share similarities in that the photoreceptors are almost completely absent in the retina in eyes with end-stage retinitis pigmentosa (37,38) and in the macula in some patients with advanced age-related diskiform scarring (39). Green and Enger have observed greater photoreceptor loss in diskiform scars secondary to AMD that are large and thick (39). The retinal prosthesis aims to replace lost or damaged photoreceptors by directly stimulating the inner retinal layer.

III. HISTORICAL BACKGROUND

The concept of a visual prosthesis for the blind or partially sighted is not new (40–42). Surgeons have been aware that electrical stimulation of the brain can produce physical or psychophysical effects as early as 1874 (43). Experiments by Foerster and Breslau in 1929 (44) as well as more recent work by others (45–50) have shown that phosphenes can be produced through electrical stimulation of the occipital cortex.

Button and Putnam reported implanting surface electrodes over the visual cortex of three blind patients in 1962 (51). With a manually operated photocell that sent signals directly to the brain through a wire traversing the scalp and skull, two of the three patients were able to locate grossly a light source by scanning the visual field with the photocell. However, the implants were of limited practical use because the resolution power was negligible.

The development of the first meaningful visual prosthesis was made by Brindley and associates in the late 1960s (48, 52–54). They implanted their first cortical visual prosthesis in a human in 1967. The subject was a 52-year-old nurse blind from bilateral severe glaucoma and retinal detachment in the left eye. Following an occipital craniotomy, a silicone plate carrying 80 platinum surface electrodes was placed in direct contact with the medial occipital cortical surface and the occipital cerebral pole. Wires through a burr hole in the bone flap connected each electrode to a radio receiver screwed to the outer bony surface. To activate a given receiver and to stimulate the cortex, an oscillator coil was placed above the receiver over the scalp and radio signals were sent inward. With this system, the patient was able to see light points in 40 positions of the visual field, demonstrating that half of the implanted electrodes were functional. A second cortical visual prosthesis was implanted in 1972 in a 64-year-old man blind from retinitis pigmentosa for over 30 years (33).

Following several early reports on attempts to develop a cortical visual prosthesis in the 1970s (8–10, 55), Dobelle reported recently a visual prosthesis providing useful artificial vision to a volunteer blind in both eyes by connecting a digital video camera, computer, and associated electronics to his visual cortex (11). The volunteer is a 66-year-old man who lost his vision in one eye from trauma at the age of 22 and in the opposite eye from a second injury at the age of 36. In 1978, at the age of 41 years, he had an intracranial electrode array implanted under local anesthesia on the medial side of his right occipital cortex. The implanted pedestal and electrode array has been used to experimentally stimulate the visual cortex over a period of more than 20 years. The external electronics package and software used in the recent report, however, were entirely new (11). Each electrode produces 1–4 closely spaced phosphenes when stimulated. The phosphene map occupies an area roughly 8 in. in height and 3 in. wide, at arm's length. The map and the parameters for stimulation have been stable over the last two decades. With scanning, the patient can recognize a

6-in.-square "tumbling E" at 5 ft, corresponding to a visual acuity of approximately 20/1200, and count fingers. He is also able to travel alone in the New York metropolitan area, and to other cities, using public transport (11,56). For more details of the early development of the cortical visual prosthesis, the reader is referred to an excellent comprehensive review by Karny (40) and an editorial by Kolff (42).

Experimental work toward a functional retinal prosthesis is a more recent development. Several groups of investigators have been making steady progress toward this end in the last decade. Some of these more important studies are discussed below. Work in this area has shifted from feasibility studies to implanting a retinal prosthesis on a long-term basis. In fact, at the time of this writing, this major milestone has been reached. On June 28, 2000, Jose S. Pulido, Gholam A. Peyman, and Alan Y. Chow implanted silicon chips into the subretinal space of two patients with retinitis pigmentosa. A third patient also received the retinal prosthesis on June 29, 2000. The retinal prosthesis, measuring 2 mm in diameter and one-thousandth of an inch thick, contains 3500 solar cells that generate power from light received by the eye (57).

IV. INDICATIONS

The proposed retinal prosthesis aims to replace lost photoreceptors and will stimulate the ganglion cells and/or the nerve fiber layer of the inner retina. It requires that the visual pathway proximal to the inner retina be largely intact. For this reason, it is likely to be useful only for diseases of the outer retina such as retinitis pigmentosa and AMD. Diseases more distal to this prosthesis–neural interface such as glaucomatous optic neuropathy and intracranial lesions will not benefit from the retinal prosthesis.

V. PRINCIPLES OF THE RETINAL PROSTHESIS

The human visual system is one of the most highly developed sensory systems found in nature. Human vision is a multimodal sensation and includes quality such as spatial resolution, color, contrast, movement, and depth perception. Spatial information is the most fundamental of these, and allows a person to perceive the basic shape of visual images. Current approaches are based on the hypothesis that electrical stimulation of selected points on the retina with a two-dimensional array of microelectrodes will create a spatial image not unlike the formation of a letter from single dots on a dot-matrix printer, or an image on a stadium scoreboard. The engineering of the system is considered feasible with available technology, much of which is currently used in the cochlear implant for the hearing impaired.

The retinal prosthesis proposed by Humayun, also known as the multiple-unit artificial retinal chipset (MARC) (Fig. 2) (58), consists of several components:

1. A video camera external to the eye and body captures the visual environment and electronic image-processing circuitry reduces the resolution and complexity of the image. Both components are mounted on an eyeglass frame worn by the patient.
2. The image data are digitally encoded and fed via a telemetry link (laser or radio frequency modulated signal) to a decoder chip implanted in the eye. Besides

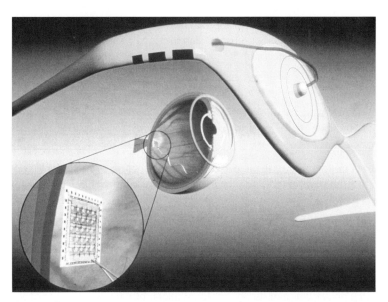

Figure 2 Diagram of the proposed retinal prosthesis by Humayun and associates. The external components (camera, video processor, power, and data transmitter) are mounted on an eyeglass frame. The implanted components (receiver coil and intraocular electronics) positioned over the retina decode the received signal and produce the appropriate pattern of electrical stimulus at the electrode array.

transmitting image data, the transmission beam will be used to supply power to the implanted circuitry,

3. The decoder chip inside the eye converts the transmitted image data and produces the necessary pattern of small electrical currents to be applied to the retina through a two-dimensional array of electrodes positioned at the inner retinal surface. Each individual electrode directly stimulates the underlying retinal neurons that then relay this information to the visual cortex, resulting in perception of a dot of light at a point in the visual field corresponding to the retinal location. Simultaneous activation of multiple electrodes in the array will create a pattern of individual dots of light.

At first glance, it may appear preferable to engineer a single implantable retinal prosthesis with all system components for light detection, image processing, current generation, and electrode stimulation. However, a prototype device with discrete subsystems with a majority of the electronics outside the eye will reduce the size and heat dissipation of the intraocular components, and allow the external components to be repaired, modified, or upgraded without additional surgery.

VI. CHALLENGES IN THE DEVELOPMENT OF A USEFUL RETINAL PROSTHESIS

An implanted retinal prosthesis must be both safe and effective. The integration of electronic devices with neural tissue requires special design considerations to ensure that the device that is communicating with the tissue does not damage the tissue. This damage could result from mechanical or electrical interactions between the device and the tissue. Several prerequisites are paramount to the success of the proposed retinal prosthesis. Each will be dealt with briefly.

Prerequisite 1: There must be a sufficient number of intact retinal neural cells in eyes with photoreceptor loss.

The survival of neurons in the inner retina is paramount to the success of the retinal prosthesis. After the death of photoreceptors (primary neurons), secondary visual neurons undergo transneuronal degeneration due to the withdrawal of synaptic input or trophic factors (37). Morphometric studies on the macula of eyes with retinitis pigmentosa have confirmed loss of neurons in the inner nuclear layer and ganglion cell layer (37, 38). However, this transneuronal degeneration is incomplete, and at least 30–75% of nuclei in the ganglion cell layer and as much as 78–88% of the nuclei in the inner nuclear layer were preserved in the macula (Fig. 3). Morphometric analysis of extramacular regions of eyes with retinitis pigmentosa disclosed some preservation of the inner retinal nuclei but the preservation of the inner nuclear layer and ganglion cell layer was less than that found in the macula (59). In AMD, the inner retina is relatively preserved over diskiform scars in spite of photoreceptor loss (39). Since these neural elements proximal to the photoreceptors remain viable in large numbers, it may be possible for the surface electrodes of a retinal prosthesis to electrically evoke a response from the remaining retinal neurons and relay visual information to the visual cortex.

Prerequisite 2: The device implanted into the eye must be biocompatible.

The first safety concern that must be addressed is material biocompatibility. The current prototype retinal prosthesis array will have a platinum and silicone electrode array and a silicone-coated electronic device. Both of these materials have been demonstrated as compatible for use in the eye. Further, platinum has a proven record as a stimulating electrode material from the cochlear implant and other implantable stimulating devices. Titanium nitride is a material proposed for use as a stimulating material, but it has been shown to have an adverse reaction in cell culture (27).

An important consideration for a stimulating electrode is the material that forms the interface to the tissue. Since the electrode must conduct a large amount of electricity, metals are best suited for this purpose. A basic property the material must have is that it will not corrode under physiological conditions. Second, the metal must not be neurotoxic. The noble metals (gold, platinum, iridium) satisfy these first two constraints. The metal must withstand large amounts of current applied without inducing undesirable corrosion reactions. Gold has been shown to dissolve when stimulating currents are applied. However, platinum and iridium can withstand high-intensity stimulating current.

Another biocompatibility question involves electrical biocompatibility. The ideal electrical stimulus pulse would be a single negative-current pulse. It would require the least amount of power and result in depolarization of the cell membrane under the electrode. However, current pulses are typically applied in trains so that a stimulus appears continuous to the cell and hence is perceived as continuous. If a stimulus waveform consists of a

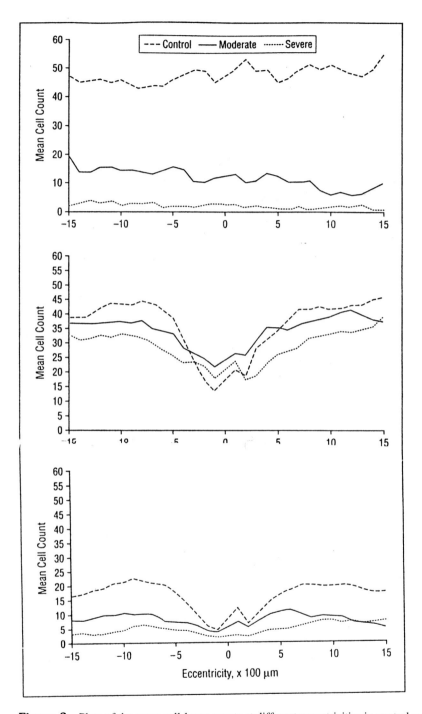

Figure 3 Plots of the mean cell-layer counts at different eccentricities in control eyes, eyes with moderate retinitis pigmentosa, and eyes with severe retinitis pigmentosa. Top: Outer nuclear layer. Middle: Inner nuclear layer. Bottom: Ganglion-cell layer. (From Santos A, Humayun MS, de Juan E, Jr, et al. Preservation of the inner retina in retinitis pigmentosa: a morphometric analysis. Arch Ophthalmol 1997;115:511–515, with permission.

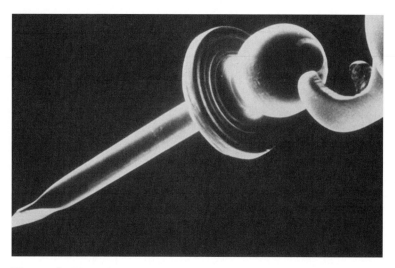

Figure 4 The retinal tack is the only proven method for attaching a retinal prosthesis in an epiretinal location to date.

repeated, cathodic pulse, residual electrical charge will remain on the electrode. Net charge on the electrode displaces the electrode potential from equilibrium. Continued charge accumulation will increase the electrode potential eventually resulting in the evolution of gaseous hydrogen or oxygen (gassing or bubbling) (60). To reduce net charge accumulation, a stimulus pulse must be charge balanced. This can be accomplished by either capacitively coupling the electrode or using a charge-balanced stimulus pulse. At the end of the current pulse, the capacitor discharges so that no net current is applied to the electrode. A more common method is actively reversing the charge by applying a positive current pulse after the negative pulse, again resulting in no net charge.

Prerequisite 3: The device must be stable in its position after implantation.

The retina is a delicate tissue that can be easily torn or detached. Positioning a stimulating array on the retinal surface will require a balancing act that seeks to find the closest proximity for the electrodes without being too close to exert deleterious pressure on the retina. Furthermore, some mechanical means must be used to secure the stimulating array to the retina since saccadic eye movement and head movement may dislodge the device if it is not firmly held. To date, the only proven method for attaching a prosthesis to the retina is a retinal tack. (26,61) (Fig. 4). These tacks were initially developed for use inside the eye as an aid in repair of retinal detachments. There are no material biocompatibility concerns. The stimulating array is secured to the retina with a tack in much the same way a piece of paper is secured to a bulletin board with a thumb tack. This results in destruction of the retina underneath or in close proximity to the tack. However, if the stimulating electrodes are a sufficient distance from the tack, the retina targeted for neurostimulation is spared.

Walter and associates have reported successful long-term implantation of electrically inactive epiretinal microelectrode arrays in rabbit eyes using retinal tacks (26). Their experiments involved two operations. During the first operation, a lens-sparing three-port core vitrectomy was performed and the prospective fixation area inferior to the optic nerve was coagulated with an infrared diode endolaser. Three weeks later, a second vitrectomy was performed to remove residual cortical vitreous and the microelectrode array was implanted and a retinal tack made of titanium (Geuder, Heidelberg, Germany) was used to fixate the implant by penetrating the area of the laser scar. Tack fixation of the microelectrode array was successful in nine out of 10 eyes. In one case, a total retinal detachment with dense cataract formation occurred after implantation. Throughout 6 months of follow-up, the implant remained at its original fixation area in the nine eyes with no dislocation. The retina remained attached in the nine eyes but in two cases, epiretinal membranes were seen around the tack.

Majji and associates also tested the feasibility of using retinal tacks to fix a 5 × 5 microelectrode array (25 platinum disk-shaped electrodes in a silicone matrix) onto the retinal surface of normal dogs (61). The retinal tacks and the microelectrode arrays remained firmly affixed to the retina up to 1 year of follow-up. No side effect of the tack or microelectrode array was observed clinically. Histological examination disclosed near-total preservation of the retina underlying the microelectrode array, demonstrating that epiretinal fixation of the array is surgically feasible with insignificant damage to the underlying retina. In addition, the study also shows that the retinal tacks as well as the platinum and silicone microelectrode arrays are biocompatible.

Another method of fixation under development is the use of biocompatible adhesives (25, 62). In one study, nine commercially available compounds were examined for their suitability as intraocular adhesives in rabbits (62). The materials studied included commercial fibrin sealant (Heamacure Co.), autologous fibrin, Cell-Tak (Becton Dickinson), three different photocurable glues (Star Technology Inc., Lightwave Energy Systems Co.-LESCO, and Loctite Co.), and three different polyethylene glycol hydrogels (Shearwater Polymers, Cohesion Technologies Inc.). Hydrogels were shown to have 2–39 times more adhesive force than the other glues tested. One type of hydrogel (SS-PEG, Shearwater Polymers, Cohesion Technologies Inc.) proved to be nontoxic to the rabbit retina.

Prerequisite 4: Stimulation of viable retinal layers must result in visual perception.

The question of whether or not a retinal prosthesis will produce a usable image in a blind individual has been addressed in part by Humayun and associates. While the final answer will not be known for some time until more retinal prostheses are implanted in humans, animal studies and short-term human experiments to date have produced encouraging results.

Electrical stimulation of the retina using a bipolar contact-lens electrode in rabbits with monoiodoacetic acid– or sodium iodate–induced experimental outer retinal degenerations, absent or markedly reduced electroretinogram, and severely damaged photoreceptor layer has been shown to produce evoked potentials from the visual cortex (63). In a series of human experiments, Humayun and associates have shown that controlled electrical signals applied with a microelectrode positioned near the retina in individuals blind from end-stage retinitis pigmentosa and AMD results in the perception of a spot of light that correlates both spatially and temporally to the applied stimulus (12,13,20,24). They were able to obtain resolution compatible with a Snellen visual acuity of 4/200 (crude ambulatory vision) using a two-point discrimination test (20). In addition, they showed that subjects were able to perceive simple forms in response to pattern electrical stimulation of the retina using wire electrodes or electrode arrays consisting of nine (3 × 3 array) or 25 (5 × 5 array) individual stimulating electrodes (Fig. 5) (14).

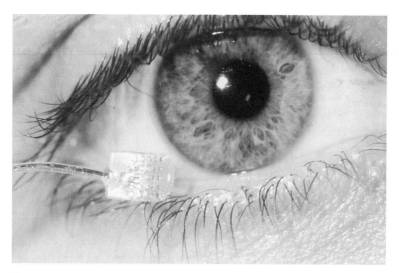

Figure 5   A 5 × 5 array of platinum electrodes in a silicone matrix held near an eye. The square formed by the array is approximately 3 mm on a side. A cable extends from the end opposite to the electrode sites to allow connection to the electronics.

Recent work in human volunteers by Weiland and associates has shown that visual percepts caused by electrical stimulation change depending on the neural element(s) stimulated (22). In this study, normal retina as well as two areas of laser-induced retinal damage (argon green and krypton red) in one eye of two subjects who were scheduled for exenteration due to recurrent cancer near the eye were stimulated. Significantly different visual percepts resulted from electrical stimulation of the normal retina and the laser-damaged retina. A dark perception in normal retina and a white perception in an area where the outer segments of the photoreceptors were damaged were reported by both volunteers.

These experiments demonstrate the ability to create the perception of a spot of light by electrically stimulating a retinal area that contains no photoreceptors (14,22). The perception of a spot of light corresponds with the stimulus time and location (14), suggesting that the brain, with no training, is capable of responding to a presumably unfamiliar signal from a retina with no photoreceptors. However, it remains to be determined whether the human brain can piece together hundreds of input channels from a two-dimensional electrode array into a useful visual image when the brain normally receive signals from 100 million photoreceptors. In this regard, the experience from the cochlear implant is encouraging. The cochlear implant bypasses damaged cochlear hair cells and directly electrically stimulates the auditory nerve to produce the sensation of sound. Using only six electrical inputs to the auditory nerve, which contains approximately 30,000 nerve fibers, with several months of training and adaptation, patients can learn to understand this reduced input with sufficient clarity to enable them to converse on an ordinary telephone (64).

Thompson and associates evaluated reading speed and facial recognition in four normally sighted subjects using simulated pixelized prosthetic vision (65). Parameters such as dot size, gray levels, dropout of pixels, and contrast were studied. Their study suggests that with pixelized vision parameters such as 25 × 25 grid in a 10° field, high contrast imaging, and four or more gray levels, a fair level of visual function can be achieved for facial recognition and reading large print text. Similarly, work by Cha and associates on normally sighted human subjects has shown that reduction of visual input to a 25 × 25 array of pixels distributed within the foveal visual area could provide useful visually guided mobility in environments not requiring a high degree of pattern recognition (66,67). The ability to perceive light may in itself be useful for some totally blind subjects (68).

VII. EPIRETINAL VERSUS SUBRETINAL APPROACH IN THE RETINAL PROSTHESIS

The stimulating electrodes could be placed in the subretinal (34,35) or epiretinal location (21,30–33,36,69) (Table 1). One potential advantage of placing the prosthesis in the subretinal space over an epiretinal location is that the electrodes will stimulate neural elements more peripheral in the afferent visual pathway. This may have the theoretical advantage of capturing some of the early neural processing that occurs in the middle layer of the retina. With current vitreoretinal techniques, it is easier to place a prosthesis in the subretinal space than to fix it onto the epiretinal surface. However, a subretinal prosthesis is a highly unnatural bed for the overlying neural elements. Exchange of nutrients and waste material between the retina and its underlying retinal pigment epithelium and choroidal circulation may be disrupted or impaired by the subretinal prosthesis. How well the retina will survive the separation from its underlying retinal pigment epithelium and choriocapillaris by an interposed prosthesis is also relatively unknown. In fact, experiments in rats by Zrenner and associates disclosed photoreceptor degeneration most likely related to reduced transport of nutrients from the choroid to the outer retina caused by the nonperforated subretinal prosthesis (27). Zrenner and associates believe that "thinner, flexible, and better designed retinal prosthesis with openings to allow diffusion should alleviate these problems." In addition, because the lateral extensions of horizontal cells are extremely long, it is not known how stimulation of these cells will impact the transfer of spatially detailed visual information.

The epiretinal approach places the stimulating electrodes in contact with the internal limiting membrane and an array of nerve fibers or ganglion cell bodies to transmit information to the visual cortex. Although free of some of the potential problems associated with the subretinal prosthesis, it has its own challenges. The prosthesis must remain in its position to ensure a stable electrode–neural elements relationship. There is currently no good technique to fix the retinal prosthesis at a predetermined distance from the retina. The inertial force from the mass of the retinal prosthesis and the fluid drag from intraocular fluid are two forces arising from angular acceleration during saccadic movements that would tend to shear the prosthesis from the retinal surface. It is possible that stimulation of Muller and other cells could lead to the formation of epiretinal membranes and fibrous cocoons surrounding the retinal prosthesis, not unlike the situation seen in chronic intraocular foreign bodies. These membranes could interfere with the function of the prosthesis by becoming a barrier of high electrical resistance between the prosthesis and the inner retina. No fibrous encapsulation of the microelectrode array, however, was observed in Majji and associates' experiments in dogs (61).

VIII. CONCLUSION

The results of feasibility studies to develop the retinal prosthesis have been encouraging, and have culminated in a phase I clinical trial in three patients (57). The knowledge gained from these early and more recent studies, when combined with technological advances in

Table 1   Advantages and Disadvantages of Subretinal Versus Epiretinal Approach for the Retinal Prosthesis

Subretinal approach	Epiretinal approach
Advantages	Advantages
Prosthesis is located at the physiological position of photoreceptors	Prosthesis is not interposed between retina and underlying retinal pigment epithelium and choroid, and therefore is less likely to interfere with retinal metabolism
Remaining retinal neuronal network that is responsible for processing information from photoreceptors can be utilized	
Retinal implant does not cover any possibly intact photoreceptors	
Subretinal space provides technically easier fixation	
Proliferative vitreoretinal reaction is possibly less common and less severe in the subretinal location than the epiretinal location	
Disadvantages	Disadvantages
Visual prosthesis, being interposed between retina and underlying retinal pigment epithelium and choroid, may disrupt the metabolism of the retina.	Prosthesis is not situated at the physiological location of photoreceptors
	Remaining retinal neural network that is responsible for processing information from photoreceptors not utilized
	Prosthesis may cover any possibly intact photoreceptors
	Epiretinal fixation is technically challenging and will require a balancing act that seeks to find the closest proximity to the retina without exerting deleterious pressure on the retina
	Proliferative vitreoretinal reaction is possibly more common and more severe in the epiretinal location than in the subretinal location

electronics, prosthetic manufacturing, and surgical techniques, is likely to bring a useful retinal prosthesis to fruition in the near future. However, much work remains to be done and it is prudent for both clinicians and the public to maintain realistic expectations for the degree of benefit to the initial patients using any prototype retinal prosthesis. Some have suggested that a hierarchical approach whereby we endeavor to provide restoration of light perception first, followed thereafter by higher visual functions (41), is a reasonable approach to treat those blind from outer retinal disease.

IX. SUMMARY

The retinal prosthesis is intended to replace lost or damaged photoreceptors by directly stimulating the inner retinal layer. It is indicated for outer retinal diseases such as age-related macular degeneration and retinitis pigmentosa.

A video camera external to the eye captures the visual environment and electronic image-processing circuitry reduces the resolution and complexity of the image. The image data are fed via a telemetry link to a decoder chip implanted in the eye. The decoder chip converts the image data and produces the necessary pattern of small electrical currents to be applied to the retina through a two-dimensional array of electrodes positioned at the inner retinal surface. Each individual electrode directly stimulates the underlying retinal neurons, resulting in perception of a dot of light at a point in the visual field corresponding to the retinal location. Simultaneous activation of multiple electrodes in the array creates a pattern of individual dots of light.

Encouraging results of feasibility studies have culminated in a phase I clinical trial in three patients.

ACKNOWLEDGMENT

K-G. Au Eong was supported by a National Medical Research Council-Singapore Totalisator Board Medical Research Fellowship, Singapore.

REFERENCES

1. del Cerro M, Gash DM, Rao GN, Notter MF, Wiegand S J, Gupta M. Intraocular retinal transplants. Invest Ophthalmol Vis Sci 1985;26:1182–1185.
2. Gouras P, Du J, Kjeldbye H, Kwun R, Lopez R, Zack DJ. Transplanted photoreceptors identified in dystrophic mouse retina by transgenic receptor gene. Invest Ophthalmol Vis Sci 1991;32:3167–3174.
3. Blair JR, Gaur VP, Laedtke TW, Lil, Yamaguchi K, Yamaguchi K. In oculo transplantation studies involving the neural retina and its pigment epithelium. Prog Retin Res 1991;10:69–88.
4. Silverman MS, Hughes SE, Valentine TL, Liu Y. Photoreceptor transplantation: anatomic, electrophysiologic, and behavioral evidence for the functional reconstruction of retinas lacking photoreceptors. Exp Neurol 1992;115:87–94.
5. Bok D. Retinal transplantation and gene therapy. Present realities and future possibilities. Invest Ophthalmol Vis Sci 1993;34:473–476.
6. Weisz JM, Humayun MS, de Juan E Jr, Del Cerro M, Sunness JS, Dagnelie G, Soylu M, Rizzo L, Nussenblatt RB. Allogenic fetal retinal pigment epithelial cell transplant in a patient with geographic atrophy. Retina 1999;19:540–545.
7. Humayun MS, de Juan E Jr, del Cerro M, Dagnelie G, Radner W, Sadda SR, del Cerro C. Human neural retinal transplantation. Invest Ophthalmol Vis Sci 2000;41:3100–3106.
8. Dobelle WH, Mladejovsky MG, Evans JR, Roberts TS, Girvin JP. "Braille" reading by a blind volunteer by visual cortex stimulation. Nature 1976;259:111–112.
9. Dobelle WH, Mladejovsky MG, Girvin JP. Artificial vision for the blind: electrical stimulation of visual cortex offers hope for a functional prosthesis. Science 1974; 183:440–444.
10. Dobelle WH, Quest DO, Antunes JL, Roberts TS, Girvin JP. Artificial vision for the blind by electrical stimulation of the visual cortex. Neurosurgery 1979;5:521–527.
11. Dobelle WH. Artificial vision for the blind by connecting a television camera to the visual cortex. ASAIO J 2000;46(Jr.):3–9.
12. Humayun MS, de Juan E Jr. Artificial vision. Eye 1998;12:605–607.
13. Humayun M, de Juan E Jr, Greenberg R, Dagnelie G, Rader RS, Katona S. Electrical stimulation of the retina in patients with photoreceptor loss. Invest Ophthalmol Vis Sci 1997;38(Suppl):S39.

14. Humayun MS, de Juan E Jr, Weiland JD, Dagnelie G, Katona S, Greenberg R, Suzuki S. Pattern electrical stimulation of the human retina. Vis Res 1999;39:2569–2576.
15. Normann RA, Maynard EM, Rousche PJ, Warren DJ. A neural interface for a cortical vision prosthesis. Vis Res 1999;39:2577–2587.
16. Rizzo JF, Loewenstein J, Wyatt J. Development of an epiretinal electronic visual prosthesis: the Harvard Medical School–Massachusetts Institute of Technology Research Program. In: Hollyfield JG, Anderson RE, LaVail MM, eds. Retinal Degenerative Diseases and Experimental Therapy. New York: Kluwer Academic/Plenum Publishers, 1999, pp 463–469.
17. Peachey NS, Chow AY, Pardue MT, Perlman JI, Chow VY. Response characteristics of subretinal microphotodiode-based implant-mediated cortical potentials. In: Hollyfield JG, Anderson RE, LaVail MM, eds. Retinal Degenerative Diseases and Experimental Therapy. New York: Kluwer Academic/Plenum Publishers, 1999, pp 471–477.
18. Eckmiller R. Goals, concepts, and current state of the retina implant project: EPI-RET. In: Hollyfield JG, Anderson RE, LaVail MM, eds. Retinal Degenerative Diseases and Experimental Therapy. New York: Kluwer Academic/Plenum Publishers, 1999, pp 487–496.
19. Zrenner E, Stett A, Brunner B, Gabel VP, Graf M, Graf HG et al. Are subretinal microphotodiodes suitable as a replacement for degenerated photoreceptors? In: Hollyfield JG, Anderson RE, LaVail MM, eds. Retinal Degenerative Diseases and Experimental Therapy. New York: Kluwer Academic/Plenum Publishers, 1999, pp 497–505.
20. Humayun MS, de Juan E Jr, Dagnelie G, Greenberg RJ, Propst RH, Phillips DH. Visual perception elicited by electrical stimulation of retina in blind humans. Arch Ophthalmol 1996;114:40–46.
21. Humayun MS, de Juan E Jr, Weiland JD, Suzuki S, Dagnelie G, Katona J, Greenberg RJ. Visual perceptions elicited in blind patients by retinal electrical stimulation: understanding artificial vision (ARVO abstracts). Invest Ophthalmol Vis Sci 1998; 39(Suppl):S902.
22. Weiland JD, Humayun MS, Dagnelie G, de Juan E Jr, Greenberg RJ, Iliff NT. Understanding the origin of visual percepts elicited by electrical stimulation of the human retina. Graefe's Arch Clin Exp Ophthalmol 1999;237:1007–1013.
23. Humayun MS, Santos A, Weiland JD, de Juan E. Retinal-based visual prosthesis. In: Quiroz-Mercado H, Alfaro DVI, Liggett PE, Tano Y, de Juan E, eds. Macular Surgery. Philadelphia: Lippincott, Williams & Wilkins, 2000:387–391.
24. Humayan MS, Weiland JD, de Juan E Jr. Electrical stimulation of the human retina. In: Hollyfield JG, Anderson RE, La Vail MM, eds. Retinal Degenerative Diseases and Experimental Therapy. New York: Kluwer Academic/Plenum Publishers, 1999:479–485.
25. Walter P, Szurman P, Krott R, Baum U, Bartz-Schmidt K-U, Heimann K. Experimental implantation of devices for electrical retinal stimulation in rabbits: preliminary results. In: Green K, Edelhauser HF, Hackett RB, Hull DS, Potter DE, Tripathi RC, eds. Advances in Ocular Toxicology. New York: Plenum Press, 1997:113–120.
26. Walter P, Szurman P, Vobig M, Berk H, Ludtke-Handjery H-C, Richter H, Mittermayer C, Heimann K, Sellhaus B. Successful long-term implantation of electrically inactive epiretinal microelectrode arrays in rabbits. Retina 1999;19:546–552.
27. Zrenner E, Stett A, Weiss S, Aramant RB, Guenther E, Kohler K, Miliezek KD, Seiler MJ, Haemmerle H. Can subretinal microphotodiodes successfully replace degenerated photoreceptors? Vis Res 1999;39:2555–2567.
28. Shandurina AN, Lyskov EB. Evoked potentials to contact electrical stimulation of the optic nerves. Hum Physiol 1986;12:9–16.
29. Veraart C, Raftopoulos C, Mortimer JT, Delbeke J, Pins D, Michaux G, Vanlierde A, Parrini S, Wanet-Defalgue MC. Visual sensations produced by optic nerve stimulation using an implanted self-sizing spiral cuff electrode. Brain Res 1998;813:181–186.
30. Wyatt J, Rizzo J. Ocular implants for the blind. IEEE Spectrum 1996;33:47–53.
31. Mann J, Edell D, Rizzo JF, Raffel J, Wyatt JL. Development of a silicon retinal implant: microelectronic system for wireless transmission of signal and power (ARVO abstracts). Invest Ophthalmol Vis Sci 1994;35(Suppl):1380.

32. Wyatt JL, Rizzo JF, Grumet A, Edell D, Jensen RJ. Development of a silicon retinal implant: epiretinal stimulation of retinal ganglion cells in the rabbit (ARVO abstracts). Invest Ophthalmol Vis Sci 1994;35(Suppl):1380.

33. Narayanan MV, Rizzo JF, Edell D, Wyatt JL. Development of a silicon retinal implant: cortical evoked potentials following focal stimulation of the rabbit retina with light and electricity (ARVO abstracts). Invest Ophthalmol Vis Sci 1994; 35(Suppl):1380.

34. Chow A, Chow V. Subretinal electrical stimulation of the rabbit retina. Neurosci Lett 1997;225:13–16.

35. Zrenner E, Miliczek KD, Gabel VP, Graf HG, Guenther E, Haemmerle H, Hoefflinger B, Kohler K, Nisch W, Schubert M, Stett A, Weiss S. The development of subretinal microphotodiodes for replacement of degenerated photoreceptors. Ophthalm Res 1997;29:269–280.

36. Eckmiller R. Learning retina implants with epiretinal contacts. Ophthalm Res 1997;29:281–289.

37. Stone JL, Barlow WE, Humayun MS, de Juan E, Milam AH. Morphometric analysis of macular photoreceptors and ganglion cells in retinas with retinitis pigmentosa. Arch Ophthalmol 1992;110:1634–1639.

38. Santos A, Humayun MS, de Juan E, Greenburg RJ, Marsh MJ, Klock IB, Milam AH. Preservation of the inner retina in retinitis pigmentosa. A morphometric analysis. Arch Ophthalmol 1997;115:511–515.

39. Green WR, Enger C. Age-related macular degeneration histopathologic studies. The 1992 Lorenz E Zimmerman lecture. Ophthalmology 1993;100:1519–1535.

40. Karny H. Clinical and physiological aspects of the cortical visual prosthesis. Surv Ophthalmol 1975;20:47–58.

41. Suaning GJ, Lovell NH, Schindhelm K, Coroneo MT. The bionic eye (electronic visual prosthesis): a review. Aust NZ J Ophthalmol 1998;26:195–202.

42. Kolff WJ. The beginning of the artificial eye program. ASAIO J 2000;46:1–2.

43. Bartholow R. Experimental investigations into the functions of the human brain. Am J Med Sci 1874;67:305.

44. Foerster J, Breslau O. Beitrage zur Pathophysiologie der Sehbahn und der Sehsphare. J Psychol Neurol 1929;29:463–485.

45. Krause F, Schum H. Die epiliptischen Erkankungen. In: Kunter H, ed. Neue Deutsche Shirurgie. Stuttgart: Enke, 1931:482–486.

46. Penfield W, Jasper H. Epilepsy and the Functional Anatomy of the Human Brain. London: Churchill, 1954.

47. Penfield W, Rasmussen T. The Cerebral Cortex of Man. New York: Macmillan, 1952.

48. Brindley GS, Lewin WS. The sensations produced by electrical stimulation of the visual cortex. J Physiol 1968;196:479–493.

49. Dobelle WH, Mladejovsky MG. Phosphenes produced by electrical stimulation of human occipital cortex and their application to the development of a prosthesis for the blind. J Physiol 1974;243:553–576.

50. Bak M, Girvin JP, Hambrecht FT, Kufta CV, Loeb GE, Schmidt EM. Visual sensations produced by intracortical microstimulation of the human occipital cortex. Med Biol Eng Comput 1990;28:257–259.

51. Button J, Putnam T. Visual responses to cortical stimulation in the blind. J Iowa State Med Soc 1962;52:17–21.

52. Brindley GS, Lewin W. The visual sensations produced by electrical stimulation of the medial occipital cortex. J Physiol 1968;194:54–55P.

53. Brindley GS, Gautier-Smith PC, Lewin W. Cortical blindness and the functions of the non-geniculate fibres of the optic tracts. J Neurol Neurosurg Psychiatry 1969; 32:259–264.

54. Brindley GS, Rushton DN. Implanted stimulators of the visual cortex as visual prosthetic devices. Trans Am Acad Ophthalmol Otolaryngol 1974;78:OP741–OP745.

55. Klomp GF, Womack MV., Dobelle WH. Fabrication of large arrays of cortical electrodes for use in man. J Biomed Mater Res 1977;11:347–364.

56. Dobelle WH. Cortical stimulation: artificial vision by visual cortex stimulation. Retina 2000: management of posterior segment disease. Am Acad Ophthalmol 2000:125–126.

57. Monroe R. Pigmentosa patients get retina on a chip. EyeNet 2000;4:14.

58. Humayun MS. Retinal stimulation: restoration of vision in blind individuals using a Multiple-Unit Artificial Retina Chipset (MARC) System. Retina 2000: management of posterior segment disease. Am Acad Ophthalmol 2000:121–123.

59. Humayun MS, Prince M, de Juan E, Barron Y, Moskowitz M, Klock IB, Milam AH. Morphometric analysis of the extramacular retina from postmortem eyes with retinitis pigmentosa. Invest Ophthalmol Vis Sci 1999;40:143–148.

60. Brummer SB, Turner MJ. Electrochemical considerations for safe electrical stimulation of the nervous system with platinum electrodes. IEEE Trans Biomed Eng 1977;24:59–63.

61. Majji AB, Humayun MS, Weiland JD, Suzuki S, D'Anna SA, de Juan E. Long-term histological and electrophysiological results of an inactive epiretinal electrode array implantation in dogs. Invest Ophthalmol Vis Sci 1999;40:2073–2081.

62. Margalit E, Fujii GY, Lai JC, Gupta P, Chen SJ, Shyu JS, Piyathaisere DV, Weiland JD, De Juan E, Humayun MS. Bioadhesives for intraocular use. Retina 2000;20:469–477.

63. Humayun MS, Sato Y, Propst R, de Juan E. Can potentials from the visual cortex be elicited electrically despite severe retinal degeneration and a markedly reduced electroretinogram? Ger J Ophthalmol 1995;4:57–64.

64. Clark GM, Tong YC, Patrick JF. Introduction. In: Clark GM, Tong YC, Patrick JF, eds. Cochlear Prostheses. Melbourne, Australia: Churchill Livingstone, 1990:1–14.

65. Thompson R, Barnett D, Humayun MS, Dagnelie G. Reading speed and facial recognition using simulated prosthetic vision. ARVO abstracts. Invest Ophthalmol Vis Sci 2000;41(Suppl):S860.

66. Cha K, Horch KW, Normann RA. Mobility performance with a pixelized vision system. Vision Res 1992;32:1367–1372.

67. Cha K, Horch K, Normann RA. Simulation of a phosphene-based visual field: visual acuity in a pixelized vision system. Ann Biomed Eng 1992;20:439–449.

68. Ross RD. Is perception of light useful to the blind patient? Arch Ophthalmol 1998; 116:236–238.

69. Humayun MS, Propst R, de Juan E, McCormick K, Hickingbotham D. Bipolar surface electrical stimulation of the vertebrate retina. Arch Ophthalmol 1994; 112:110–116.

24

Genetics of Age-Related Macular Degeneration

Philip J. Rosenfeld

Bascom Palmer Eye Institute, University of Miami School of Medicine, Miami, Florida

I. INTRODUCTION

Age-related macular degeneration (AMD) is not the typical kind of disease that usually comes to mind when we think of an inherited disorder. Rather, it is a disease that can present with a variety of phenotypes within two broad categories known as nonneovascular (dry) and neovascular (wet) AMD. In the elusive search for the cause of this disease, investigators have always been in a quandary whether to consider AMD as a continuum of disease severity or as distinct clinical entities within the two broad categories. Are there some subtypes that are destined to remain nonneovascular while others are destined to progress to the neovascular form? Within the dry AMD subtype, are there some individuals with early disease who are predestined to progress to central geographic atrophy while others will retain some central macular function? Are there others who progress to wet AMD and have occult choroidal neovascularization (CNV) and will not progress to classic CNV? Are there still others who will always progress directly to classic CNV without initial evidence of occult CNV? If such subgroups of individuals exist, how can they be identified before the disease progresses and can anything be done to prevent this progression? These are some of the issues that have been tackled by investigators over the years, and some progress has been made in identifying phenotypic characteristics and environmental factors that are predictors of disease progression and severity. However, little success has been realized in altering the overall natural history of the disease.

Until recently, most of the focus has been on the study of environmental factors and how they influence the progression of disease and on the study of the early macular phenotype and how it can predict disease severity. Now the evidence is mounting that heredity plays a more important role than initially suspected in determining the cause and progression of disease. The challenge for the geneticists is to apply their rigorous analytical discipline to a disease with such a variable phenotype and prognosis. For example, should geneticists study everyone with AMD as a homogeneous group or should they subdivide AMD patients into subtypes within subtypes? Initially, being able to define their

457

population is crucial for the geneticist, but once a gene is identified, it then becomes fairly straightforward to broaden one's definition to include oher populations with AMD and determine whether the genetic findings extend across phenotypic categories. By defining the genes one at a time, the geneticist and the clinician will be able to understand how individual genes influence phenotype, either by acting alone or as part of a complex web of gene-gene interactions, and how environmental factors influence the genes. With this knowledge, we will be able to identify those at risk of developing the disease, to predict disease progression, and to develop treatments to prevent vision loss. This review will cover our present understanding of AMD as a complex inherited disorder and the likely directions for research in the near future.

II. AMD AS A GENETIC DISEASE

The genetic basis of AMD was relatively ignored for many years as environmental and dietary issues were the primary focus of epidemiological investigations during the 1970s and 1980s. These epidemiological studies indicated an increased risk for smokers and some associations with dietary factors, resulting in an interest in dietary supplements such as antioxidants and micronutrients such as lutein in the treatment of AMD. Various hypotheses were tested in these epidemiological studies such as the role of diet, cardiovascular disease, hypertension, and sunlight exposure in AMD, but no conclusive causal relationship was established. Yet there is a suggestion that these environmental factors could influence the severity of disease. Overall, these studies have shown that these increased risks are relatively small compared to the increased risk associated with heredity. What is truly advantageous about the genetic approach to the study of AMD is that there is no need for a biological hypothesis or model, and there should be no investigator bias in identifying the cause of disease. Moreover, the genetic approach allows for the discovery of novel causes for disease that might not be suspected from biochemical or cell biological studies.

Several recent advances in human genetics have changed the way we approach AMD and other age-related disorders. First, we now appreciate that aging and many diseases associated with aging can be thought of as genetically complex, meaning that the disease is caused by numerous predisposing genes, and multifactorial, meaning that both genetic and environmental factors contribute to the disease (1–5). Second, our ability to analyze complex genetic traits has greatly improved over the last several years. Diseases once thought unapproachable by genetic analysis because of their complexity can now be dissected using new statistical methodologies. Several complex diseases previously associated with aging and environmental exposure risks have now been found to have a strong genetic component. Examples of such diseases include Alzheimer's disease, diabetes mellitus, hypertension, and obesity (6–16) Third, the inheritance of AMD has become increasingly evident from studies demonstrating a strong familial prevalence for the disease.

A familial tendency to develop AMD was first identified in 1876 by Hutchinson (17) and later confirmed by a few additional reports throughout most of the twentieth century. However, the reports of familial AMD were largely ignored until recently, in part because the pattern of inheritance was not immediately obvious to the clinician largely because of its late age of onset. Family members were unreliable when it came to reporting a family history of AMD even when a positive family history was obvious from the typical symptoms often displayed by parents and relatives in their later years. A positive family history was rarely documented because vision loss from AMD usually occurs during an individual's late 60s or early 70s, and the parents of patients with AMD are usually deceased by the time the diagnosis was obvious. Usually, AMD was not recognized in the parents of patients even if they had the disease but they died before they had experienced significant vision loss. Often, the subtle signs of the disease would have been missed in past decades. Historical accounts of whether a parent was affected by AMD are often confounded by other causes of vision loss, such as cataracts or glaucoma, or the vision loss was inaccurately attributed to these other diagnoses. Sometimes, the use of a different diagnostic term such as "central chorioretinitis" rather than AMD led to confusion among family members. It is even possible that family members were unaware of vision loss in their elderly relatives because decreased vision may have been better tolerated and not thought noteworthy since many people expected decreased vision to be a natural consequence of aging. Even if vision loss did occur, its severity could have been concealed by a decreased dependence on reading or driving owing to the tendency of previous generations to live in close proximity to one another and provide support for one another.

Even if one were not confronted with the unreliability and ambiguities surrounding the diagnosis of AMD in previous generations, the late onset of the condition itself, natural death rates, and small families would create a situation in which many people with an inherited form of AMD would appear to have sporadic disease. Additionally, the heredity of a late-onset disease like AMD has been difficult to appreciate because of the uncertainties in the diagnosis among the children of an affected individual since they are often too young to reliably manifest the disease. A simulation study examining a late-onset dominant disorder with family sizes compatible with those in the United States and with a disease having the frequency and age of onset comparable to AMD revealed that only 15–20% of patients with the disease would report a positive family history even if all of the cases were actually genetic and the reporting was completely accurate (18). With such a low percentage of patients capable of reporting a positive family history of AMD, it is not surprising that clinicians failed to perceive AMD as an inherited disease.

One obvious way to appreciate the inheritance of a disease is to observe the transmission of disease from one generation to another. Owing to the late onset of AMD, this approach is not usually practical or feasible. Another way to appreciate inheritance is to consider the increased prevalence of disease among siblings. However, obtaining reliable prevalence data among siblings is not so easily accomplished. The trend in American society for increasing mobility within families often results in siblings living far apart and unaware of one another's visual status. Even if siblings are affected with AMD, they might not be aware of their disease until they have experienced significant vision loss. Eye care providers are often reluctant to label a patient with the diagnosis of "early" AMD because of the emotional stigma associated with this condition, the absence of effective treatment in most cases, and the unpredictable progression of vision loss. Personal and emotional factors may make family members reluctant to tell others of their diagnosis or their vision difficulties. Often, owing to family conflicts, siblings may not communicate with one another as they get older, so reliable family histories are impossible to obtain.

When siblings do share the diagnosis of AMD, it does not exclude the possibility that the disease is due to environmental influences since siblings usually share similar environmental exposures as children and adolescents. In addition, as adults, family members often choose similar lifestyles. However, twin studies have long been recognized as a means of separating environmental and genetic influences. During early life, dizygotic twins and monozygotic twins are thought to have identical environmental exposures. The extent to which pairs of twins will share the same ocular findings is referred to as disease concordance. Thus, any differences in the degree of concordance among monozygotic twins compared to dizygotic twins would largely be due to heredity. As summarized below, the combination of epidemiological studies, population studies, family studies, and twin studies have provided compelling evidence that inheritance, far more than environmental factors, is responsible for the majority of an individual's risk of developing AMD.

III. AMD GENETIC STUDIES

To determine whether is a strong genetic component to a disease, investigators must first agree upon the definition of the disease and then demonstrate an increased prevalence of the disease among related individuals. Defining AMD is complicated by its clinical heterogeneity. Different clinical criteria for AMD based on fundus appearance, visual acuity, bilaterality, and age have been proposed for study purposes (19–28). While grading systems are similar, subtle and not so subtle differences make it difficult to compare studies. While the term age-related maculopathy (ARM) includes all forms of the disease, from the earliest manifestation with only few discrete drusen, focal pigmentation of the retinal pigment epithelium (RPE), or focal atrophy of the RPE, the term "age-related macular degeneration" is usually reserved for the more advanced fundus changes associated with visual impairment. Moreover, there is some controversy as to what actually constitutes the definition of ARM. Since the definition of ARM is imprecise, most studies have focused on the later stages of the disease where identifying affected individuals with AMD is less ambiguous. Another way to more accurately define your study population is to include a minimal age of onset as part of the definition of the disease. The age restriction attempts to avoid the diagnostic dilemma surrounding younger family members who may have a separate hereditary macular dystrophy or may present with equivocal evidence of early ARM. In contrast to this approach, some clinicians have proposed that AMD is part of a continuum that includes the "juvenile" or early-onset macular dystrophies and that such age distinctions may be misleading. To some extent, the diagnosis of AMD is made once other known causes for macular degeneration have been excluded. Although most analyses are performed on individuals with unambiguous disease, studies often collect information on all individuals regardless of the extent of fundus findings and vision loss so that informative family members are not excluded. This family information, initially excluded from the analyses, can then be included once an association has been identified between a genetic locus and the disease. By adding in these excluded family members, the investigator can determine whether the association between the locus and the disease is strengthened or weakened. This type of approach can help identify the early, more ambiguous stages of the disease. For example, it is still not established whether if clinical distinctions of ARM or AMD phenotypes (i.e., large versus small drusen, number of drusen, soft versus hard drusen, or geographic atrophy versus choroidal neovascular membranes) are meaningful with regard to the genes that confer susceptibility. Only after some of the genetic loci that contribute to AMD are identified will investigators be able to broaden their diagnostic criteria and approach the issue of phenotype-genotype correlations. Thus, the initial burden on clinicians in genetic studies of AMD is to be confident of the diagnosis by identifying criteria (i.e., age, fundus appearance, visual acuity) that can unambiguously constitute the disease.

A. Population Prevalence Studies

AMD as an inherited disease can only be appreciated through population-based screening and exhaustive family studies. Population based studies have examined the prevalence of AMD among racially or ethnically diverse groups and among groups that are geographically or ethnically restricted with limited outbreeding. Large diverse populations will reflect the overall complexity of AMD, while more restricted populations can provide a powerful means of decreasing the complexity of the disease and focusing the search for AMD-related genes. One of the limitations of studying large populations is that the interplay of genetic and environmental influences cannot be easily teased apart. Despite this limitation, these studies can be helpful in directing our attention to certain populations where the disease is more prevalent. Once the prevalence is established, we can look for additional evidence to suggest either a genetic or environmental basis for the disease. Such population studies have suggested an increased prevalence of severe vision loss from AMD among certain racial and ethnic groups, and a decreased prevalence among other groups (29–47).

In the United States, Europe, Africa, and Asia, the prevalence of AMD has been examined among "whites," "blacks," "Hispanics," Greenlanders, in particular Inuits, Chinese, and Japanese. While some investigators have found little difference among races in the prevalence of drusen, the so-called early stage of the disease, this diagnostic category is often ambiguous and there is little agreement on what qualifies as a precursor to AMD. This is why most racial comparisons rely on the prevalence of the more advanced form of the disease associated with vision loss. Severe vision loss from AMD appears to be more common among "whites," Chinese, Japanese, and Inuits as compared to "blacks" and "non-white Hispanics."

Another way of assessing genetic risk is to look at the incidence of disease in two populations of the same race but separated geographically from one another. Cruickshanks et al. (38) studied the prevalence of AMD within two geographically separated non-Hispanic "white" groups. When comparing the two groups, Cruickshanks et al. controlled for known environmental influences and confounding factors such as ancestry, education, income, marital status, menopausal status, diabetes, smoking, exercise, alcohol consumption, body mass, blood pressure, cardiovascular disease history, pulse rate, hypertension, cholesterol, and hematocrit. They found a 33% difference in the prevalence of AMD between the groups from the Beaver Dam study and from the San Luis Valley in Colorado. The authors concluded that genetic differences between these two populations, rather than environmental differences, might play an important role in explaining the difference in prevalence of AMD in these populations. In another study, a low incidence of late AMD, 0.5% in those over age 70, was found in a "white" population in southern Italy (35). These investigators conclude that a genetic difference in this "white" Italian population probably accounts for the low incidence of disease. However, it is entirely possible that some undocumented environmental influences, such as light exposure and diet, could account for the difference between "white" populations.

Investigators not only examine the prevalence of AMD within populations, they also examine how the prevalence has changed over time. If there has been a change, investigators often point to changes in environmental factors as the cause and assume the genetics of a population has remained relatively constant. Risk factors such as cardiovascular disease, decreased dietary antioxidants, or chronic light damage combined with increased longevity are often cited as being responsible for the increasing age-specific incidence of

AMD within a population (48,49). However, if one takes into account improved awareness of the disease, increased longevity, better diagnostic acumen among eye specialists, and improved diagnostic terminology, it is unclear whether the age-specific incidence is increasing or the disease was simply underdiagnosed in previous generations. This type of uncertainty surrounds the dramatic increasing incidence of AMD within the Japanese population over the past 30 years. Is this increasing incidence due to better diagnostic capability or the introduction of new environmental factors? The answer is not known, but even if the disease incidence has been influenced by a newly introduced environmental factor among the Japanese, this does not exclude heredity as playing a major role in AMD. This increased incidence within the population over time may reflect a genetic susceptibility to new environmental factors. This is what is meant by the term "multifactorial" (i.e., influenced by both genetic and environmental factors) when used to describe the inheritance of AMD. It is interesting that there is no difference in the prevalence of AMD found among European and Asians living in the same city. This finding suggests that if a genetic basis for disease exists in the "white" European population, then a genetic basis may exist for the Asian population as well.

B. Family Aggregation Studies

Both qualitative and quantitative evidence for the role of heredity in AMD has been provided by familial aggregation and segregation studies. Like large population studies, family studies examine the predilection for disease among individuals who share similar DNA. However, unlike population studies, there is less genetic heterogeneity within families and everyone in the family is assumed to have been exposed to similar environmental influences.

Familial cases of AMD have been reported from Europe, North America, and Asia (17,24,50–61). The first report of a familial tendency to inherit drusen at an older age was by Hutchinson in 1876 (17). In this report, Hutchinson described three sisters ranging from 40 to 60 years old with characteristic fundus findings "in which the choroid becomes speckled with minute dots of yellowish white deposit." He proceeds to describe the later stages of the disease characterized by "atrophy of choroidal tissue and production of some pigment." The disease is described as progressing in stages from minute yellow-white spots to a coalescence of these spots followed by hemorrhage at the yellow spot and resulting in atrophy.

Nearly 100 years passed before the familial tendency to inherit AMD was revisited. Francois (50) reported that senile macular dystrophy was common in brothers and sisters. He subsequently reported one pedigree with all three siblings affected with AMD and five pedigrees depicting multigenerational inheritance (51). Bradley (52) described the inheritance of senile macular dystrophy in two brothers and wrote, "Nearly every patient I have seen has had other members of the family similarly affected." Gass (53) performed a four-year study of 200 patients with macular drusen and reported that 38 patients (19%) had a positive family history of similar macular disease. Gass studied only 10 of the 38 families, and the diagnosis of AMD was confirmed in all 10 families either by examination or by review of their medical records.

These previous studies documented the tendency of AMD to occur among first-degree relatives within families. However, when a disease as common as AMD has prevalence in the general population of up to 20%, the tendency of the disease to occur within families may be due to coincidence rather than heredity. For this reason, this familial tendency must be compared to a control population to appreciate the contribution of heredity. Hyman et al. (54) were the first to document the increased prevalence of AMD among relatives of affected patients compared to relatives of unaffected controls. A total of 228 affected subjected were identified and 237 unaffected controls were matched by age and sex. A positive family history of AMD was reported in 21.6% of affected subjects compared to 8.6% of unaffected controls. A statistically significant odds ratio of 2.9 was calculated for an association between AMD and a positive family history involving parents and siblings. In an attempt to validate the history of AMD among siblings, the authors submitted questionnaires to eye examiners and a similar response rate was obtained for the siblings from the affected and unaffected cases. Interestingly, 11.3% of affected siblings reported AMD by history and 19.9% of eye examiners reported AMD by examination. Thus, relying on history alone would result in an underreporting of AMD prevalence within families. In contrast, both history and examination confirmed the decreased prevalence of AMD among siblings of unaffected controls. AMD was not validated among parents of either the affected or unaffected cases. Based primarily on the sibling data, Hyman et al. concluded that familial, genetic, and personal characteristics rather than environmental factors such as chemical work exposure and cigarette smoking mainly influenced AMD. In contrast to the study by Hyman et al., another study from the 1980s by Gibson et al. (62) did not identify an increased prevalence of AMD within families. Gibson's failure to detect a familial prevalence was likely due to measurement errors from the diagnostic criteria used, the reliance on family history alone without examination, and the small number of families and the low statistical power of the study.

In the 1990s, Silvestri et al. (56) reported another case-controlled study comparing the prevalence of AMD among first-degree relatives of patients with AMD with first-degree relatives of age- and sex-matched controls. All patients and controls underwent an ophthalmoscopic examination, and the authors either examined all siblings or reviewed their medical records. Examination or review of medical records could not always confirm the diagnosis of AMD in parents. The study consisted of 36 patients and 36 controls. Twelve parents (33.3%) of affected patients were believed to have AMD. In contrast, none of the control parents where thought to have AMD. While 20 of the 81 siblings of affected subjects were affected with AMD, only 1 of the 78 control siblings was diagnosed with AMD. The relative risk of developing AMD was 19.3 times greater for a sibling of an affected individual than for a sibling of an unaffected control. The authors concluded that hereditary factors are important in the etiology of AMD. This study stands apart from other familial studies because of the low prevalence of AMD among siblings of control cases (1/78).

Heiba et al. (57) explored the familial aggregation of AMD by evaluating the large population of male and female adults in the Beaver Dam Eye Study for evidence of a major gene segregation effect. Sibling correlations were evaluated and segregation analysis was performed on the right and left eyes of individuals from 564 families. Siblings were examined for fundus changes associated with AMD and a statistically significant sibling correlation for these findings was reported. The sister-brother correlation was highest followed by the sister-sister correlation. No statistically significant correlation was found between brothers. These authors conclude that a single major gene effect, inherited in a Mendelian fashion, could account for the high sibling correlation between eyes.

Seddon et al. (58) performed a detailed familial aggregation study of AMD by studying 119 affected individuals and 72 unaffected individuals and their first-degree relatives. First-degree relatives included parents, siblings, and offspring 40 years of age and older.

Medical records were reviewed for 177 case relatives and 146 control relatives. A significantly higher prevalence of AMD was found among first-degree relatives of affected probands (23%) compared to control probands (11.6%) with an age-and-sex-adjusted odds ratio of 2.4 ($p = 0.013$). By separately analyzing the 78 probands with neovascular AMD, the authors demonstrated an even higher prevalence of AMD among first-degree relatives (26%) with an odds ratio of 3.1 ($p = 0.003$). In contrast, the prevalence of AMD among first-degree relatives of the 41 probands with dry ARM was 19.2% with an odds ratio of 1.5 ($p = 0.36$). The authors conclude that the higher prevalence of AMD among first-degree relatives of subjects with AMD, particularly neovascular AMD, suggests a strong familial contribution to the disease. This familial component may be genetic, environmental, or multifactorial, the result of interactions between genes and the environment.

In the Blue Mountains Eye Study, Smith and Mitchell (59) assessed the associations between early and late stages of AMD with reported family histories. This involved a cross-sectional study of 3654 subjects from a defined geographic area west of Sydney (NSW, Australia). Subjects with early and late stages of AMD were identified from masked detailed grading of retinal photographs. Interviewer-administered questionnaires provided data on the family history of AMD. It was found that a first-degree family history of AMD was significantly associated with both late AMD (odds ratio 3.92; 95% confidence interval [CI] 1.34–11.46) and early ARM (odds ratio 2.17; 95% CI 1.04–4.55). The association was highest for the late neovascular form of AMD. In this study, the detection of the association between AMD and a positive family history depended upon a questionnaire rather than the examination of the first-degree relatives. Therefore, it is likely there were affected family members who were underreported. If true, then it seems likely that this report underestimated the true association between AMD and a positive family history. These findings provide persuasive evidence that AMD is an inherited disorder and a stated family history of AMD is an important risk factor for AMD.

Klaver et al. (60) reported on the familial aggregation of AMD as part of the Rotterdam Eye Study. In this study, they examined fundus photographs of first-degree relatives of 87 index cases with AMD and 135 controls. Independent of other risk factors, the prevalence of early (odds ratio = 4.8, 95% CI = 1.8–12.2) and late (odds ratio = 19.8, 95% CI = 3.1–126.0) AMD was significantly higher in relatives of patients with late AMD. The lifetime risk estimate of late AMD was 50% (95% CI = 26–73%) for relatives of patients versus 12% (95% CI = 2–16%) for relatives of controls ($p < 0.001$), yielding a risk ratio of 4.2 (95% CI 2.6–6.8). This means that siblings of late-AMD patients are four times more likely to develop AMD than persons who have no first-degree relative with AMD. Moreover, relatives of patients with AMD expressed the various features of AMD at a younger age. Therefore, it would appear that first-degree relatives of patients with late AMD have an increased risk of developing AMD and this occurs at a relatively young age. This result suggests that genetic susceptibility has an important role in determining the onset and severity of disease.

In addition to studying the prevalence of AMD within families, investigators have attempted to support the genetic basis for AMD by comparing and contrasting the fundus appearances of family members with the disease. Piguet et al. (55) compared the density, size, and confluence of drusen in the central macula as early markers of AMD among affected AMD patients, their siblings, and their spouses. The eyes of 53 sibling pairs were compared to the eyes of 50 spouses as part of a prospective study of AMD. They found marked concordance between siblings in the number and density of drusen (52/53 sibling pairs), but not between spouses (24/50). More recently, de La Paz et al. (24) studied the fundus appearance of AMD in eight families with three or more affected members. In contrast to the study by Piguet et al., de La Paz et al. studied families with advanced AMD and found variable expressivity of the disease within families with the full range of fundus characteristics present. These fundus findings ranged from extensive drusen formation to geographic atrophy and neovascular maculopathy. In this study, the authors provided only a cross-sectional analysis of their cohort and provided no longitudinal analysis describing the progression of disease. They conclude that the variable, expressivity of advanced AMD between family members may represent the effect of modifying genes (complex gene-gene interactions) or the influence of environmental factors on a genetically susceptible group (multifactorial etiology). However, it is difficult to determine whether the reported variable expressivity of AMD within families is any different from the variable expressivity observed when comparing the eyes from the same individual. For this reason, it is important to follow the age-dependent progression of macular findings among family members to determine whether the variability persists or whether family members all tend to develop the same macular features.

Different familial aggregation and segregation studies have resulted in identifying a genetic component to AMD, but these studies differ in the magnitude of this effect. We might expect the magnitude of this genetic component to vary depending upon the population and the prevalence of environmental factors that may influence the disease. Another reason why the magnitude of the effect varies from report to report is that the investigators attempt to appropriately phenotype their populations using different classification schemes. While their attempts are appropriate and commendable, the varying results could be explained, in part, by the differences between these classification schemes.

C. Twin Studies

Studies examining the concordance of AMD among monozygotic and dizygotic twins strongly support the role of heredity in AMD. Monozygotic twins share the same chromosomal DNA while dizygotic twins should be no different than any other nontwin sibling pair. A major advantage of twin studies for age-dependent conditions such as AMD is the elimination of age-adjusted comparisons between siblings within a family. If a disease is influenced solely by genetics, then the disease should have a much higher concordance among monozygotic twins than dizygotic twins. If a trait is 100% penetrant, monozygotic twins should have 100% concordance. If the disease has variable penetrance because of either genetic or environmental influences, then the concordance among identical twins may be less than 100%. If there is no genetic influence on the disease, then there should be little difference in the concordance rates between monozygotic and dizygotic twins. The importance of twin research in the study of inherited ophthalmological diseases was first acknowledged by Waardenburg in 1950 (63). In this paper, he reported a personal communication from Roobol, who described a pair of 63-year-old identical twins who may have been concordant for AMD based on his description of their "senile cystic maculopathy" accompanied by "scattered glistening spots."

In 1958, Waardenburg reported on two sets of aged female twins who were believed to be identical, although no genetic testing was performed (64). These twin pairs were found to be concordant for senile macular dystrophy. Additional isolated case reports have subsequently appeared. Melrose et al. (65) reported on the concordance of AMD in a pair of female "identical looking" twins. The first twin developed choroidal neovascularization in the right eye at the age of 72, and within 16 months, the other twin developed a neovascular membrane in the right eye as well. Meyers and Zachary (66) performed genetic testing to confirm monozygosity of a female twin pair who were concordant for severe AMD. These 85-year-old monozygotic twins progressed to bilateral legal blindness within 3 years of each other. Interestingly, four of their 13 siblings were also reported to have severe AMD. Dosso and Bovet (67) reported on 85-year-old male twins who developed neovascular AMD the same year they both developed hypertension and non-insulin-dependent diabetes. The twins were confirmed to be monozygotic by genetic testing, and both progressed to severe vision loss within 1 year. Klein et al. (68) found high concordance rates in a study of nine monozygotic twins with advanced AMD. One member of the pair was originally diagnosed with the disease. Eight pairs were female and monozygosity of all nine pairs was confirmed through analysis of genetic markers. Each twin pair was concordant for the disease and eight of the nine twin pairs showed similar expressivity. Six of the nine twin pairs had advanced AMD, two twin pairs had extensive drusen of the same type, and one twin pair was discordant. The discordant twin pair had one member with neovascular maculopathy and vision loss in one eye, while the fellow twin had large confluent drusen in both eyes. Based on other studies that suggest that large confluent drusen often precede the development of neovascular maculopathy, this isolated, seemingly discordant set of twins may simply represent a difference in the onset of progression toward the development of choroidal neovascularization and not a true case of discordance.

The high concordance of disease among monozygotic twin pairs with regard to age of onset, symmetry of fundus appearance, and vision loss suggests a significant genetic component to the disease. However, owing to the nonrandom selection process of twin sets in these previous reports, there remains considerable concern about selection bias. A more convincing twin study would involve the random examination of twin pairs for concordance of AMD.

Meyers et al. (69,70) prospectively examined 134 consecutive twin pairs and two triplet sets. They compared the concordance of AMD among these siblings. Genetic laboratory testing confirmed the zygosity of all participants. The concordance rate was 100% (25/25) for the monozygotic twin pairs and 42% (5/12) for the dizygotic twin pairs. The remaining twins and triplets showed no evidence of AMD. While the concordance of disease was 100% among the monozygotic twins, there was variability in the expression of disease between the monozygotic twins. This variability was probably no different from the variability observed between the eyes of the same individual. Clinical appearances among monozygotic twins included neovascular maculopathy in both eyes of both twins in four pairs, neovascular maculopathy in one twin and nonneovascular maculopathy in the other twin among six pairs, and nonneovascular changes in both twins of 15 pairs.

From a study in Iceland, Gottfredsdottir et al. (71) examined the concordance of AMD in monozygotic twin pairs and their spouses. They prospectively studied 50 twin pairs and 47 spouses, and macular findings were graded using an accepted international grading system. Monozygosity was confirmed by genetic laboratory testing. The concordance of AMD was 90% in monozygotic twin pairs, which significantly exceeded the concordance of twin/spouse pairs (70.2%; $p = 0.0279$). In the nine pairs that were concordant, fundus appearance and visual impairment were similar. Environmental factors and medical history were essentially the same in the twin pairs. By comparing the monozygotic twins with their spouses rather than siblings or dizygotic twin pairs, these researchers were more interested in examining the effect of the shared environmental influences later in life (twin-spouse concordance) rather than the influences early in life (twin-sibling concordance).

In a study by Hammond et al. (72), 506 unselected twin pairs (226 monozygotic twin pairs and 280 dizygotic twin pairs) with a mean age of 62 years were examined to determine the influence of genetics on AMD. The AMD was graded using stereoscopic fundus photographs from 501 of the twin pairs. While the overall prevalence of AMD was 14.6% (95% CI = 12.4–16.8%), the concordance between monozygotic twins was only 0.37, compared to 0.19 between dizygotic twins, and the heritability of AMD was estimated as 45% (95% CI = 35–53%). The most heritable phenotypes were soft drusen > 125 μm (57%) and hard drusen ≥ 20 μm (81%), with the latter being dominantly inherited. Although this study confirms an important role for heredity in AMD, the concordance among the identical twins and dizygotic twins appeared low compared to the previous studies

In summary, when all these studies are reviewed, concordance rates for AMD among monozygotic twin pairs suggest a strong genetic component for this disease. While the role of environmental influences can never be excluded, these monozygotic twin studies effectively demonstrate the importance of heredity in AMD. Further support for the role of heredity would come from studies investigating the prevalence of AMD among random monozygotic twins who have been raised apart. Knobloch et al. (73) reported on 18 monozygotic and eight dizygotic twin pairs reared apart. Macular drusen were found in only one monozygotic twin pair and they were concordant for this finding. The absence of drusen among the other twin pairs may also reflect concordance for the absence of AMD though the twins in this study were young, ranging in age from only 11 to 54 years. Therefore, the true prevalence of AMD was not known and the future risk of developing AMD among this cohort is uncertain. A larger twin separation study with older twins is needed to confirm the limited results of this paper.

In summary, when these family studies, particularly the twin studies, are examined in their totality, the conclusions overwhelmingly support a major role for heredity in AMD.

IV. MOLECULAR GENETIC ANALYSIS OF AMD

Two molecular genetic approaches can be used to study AMD. In one approach, nothing is known about the chromosomal loci or genes that are involved in the disease. This approach, known as linkage analysis, establishes the location of one or more susceptibility loci within the genome, and once a locus is identified, the gene within the locus responsible for the disease can be identified. This approach is also known as positional cloning. The

Table 1 Chromosomal Loci and Genes Implicated in Causing or Modulating AMD

Chromosomal locus	Symbol	Gene	Protein	Eye diseases associated with locus/gene	References
1p21–p13	STG1	ABCA4(ABCR)	Retina-specific ATP-binding cassette transporter	Stargardt disease Fundus flavimaculatus AMD	96,98–108
1q25–q31	ARMD1	Unknown	Unknown	AMD	74,82
17q25	Unknown	Unknown	Unknown	AMD	82
19q13.2	APOE	APOE	Apolipoproten E	AMD	132–137

Table 2 Prominent Candidate Genes Excluded as Major Causes of AMD

Chromosomal locus	Gene/protein	Eye disease	Method of exclusion	References
2p16–p21	EFEMP1/EGF-containing fibrillin-like extracellular matrix protein	Mallattia Leventinese Dominant radial drusen Doyne honeycomb retinal degeneration	Candidate linkage analysis Candidate gene analysis	12,80,82,84
6p21.2-cen	RDS peripherin	Dominant retinitis pigmentosa (RP) Digenic RP Dominant adult vitelliform macular degeneration	Candidate linkage analysis	80,129,130
6q12	ELOVL4/elongation of very long fatty acids protein	Dominant Stargardt-like macular degeneration	Candidate gene analysis	80,82,131
6q14–q16.2	MCDR1, PBCRA	Dominant North Carolina macular dystrophy Dominant progressive bifocal chorioretinal atrophy	Candidate linkage analysis	80,82
6q25–q26	RCD1/unknown	Dominant retinal cone dystrophy 1	Candidate linkage analysis	80,82
11q13	VMD2/bestrophin	Best disease Dominant vitelliform	Candidate linkage analysis Candidate linkage analysis	80,82,121
22q12.1–q13.2	TIMP3/tissue inhibitor of metalloproteinase-3	Macular dystrophy Dominant Sorsby fundus dystrophy	Candidate gene analysis Candidate linkage analysis Candidate gene analysis	12,80,82,83

second approach, known as association analysis, includes techniques known as candidate linkage analysis and candidate gene analysis. Association analysis specifically tests whether a known specific chromosomal locus or gene contributes to a disease. These approaches complement one another in the search for genes responsible for AMD. Both techniques require a group of affected subjects who have been reliably diagnosed with the disease. A reliable diagnosis of AMD is essential so that an appropriate correlation can be made between an abnormal chromosomal locus or gene and the disease. For this reason, strict diagnostic criteria are required before analysis can proceed. The linkage approach requires a control population so that the frequencies of allele polymorphisms can be accurately determined. This control population for linkage analysis must be representative of the genetic heterogeneity found within the population with disease; however, no assumptions are made about the disease status of this control group. The association approach, in particular candidate gene analysis, also requires a reliable control group without the disease so that one can distinguish between polymorphisms and true mutations related to the disease. In practice, it is nearly impossible to have a perfect disease-free control group because individuals included in the control group may carry the genetic predisposition for disease but, for some unknown reason, have not manifested obvious signs of disease.

A. Linkage Approach: Parametric Linkage Analysis

Conventional linkage analysis for a trait or disease inherited in an autosomal-dominant or X-linked fashion ideally requires large pedigrees with multiple generations affected. Linkage analysis of an autosomal recessive trait ideally requires an inbred or genetically isolated population. Linkage analysis for any monogenic inherited disorder can also succeed with small families provided the disorder is genetically homogeneous (arising from mutations in a single gene). Linkage analysis establishes the location of a disease locus on the genome (i.e., a particular region of a chromosome) by establishing that the pattern of inheritance of the disease within one or more families is similar to the pattern of inheritance of one or more known polymorphic genetic markers. Genome-wide polymorphic markers are analyzed for each individual within a family or pedigree and a correlation is established between the transmission of particular marker alleles among family members and the pattern of inheritance for the disease. The likelihood that the inheritance of marker alleles and the inheritance of the disease are actually linked compared to the likelihood of this association occurring by random chance is referred to as the logarithm of the odds ratio for linkage (LOD Score). When a conventional linkage model calculates a LOD score of 3, that LOD value indicates that there is a 1000 times greater chance that the marker and the disease are linked and in close proximity compared to the random chance for such an association. Similarly, if one calculates a negative LOD score, then the linkage model for the marker and the disease shows a poor correlation, worse than one would expect by random chance alone.

Conventional linkage analysis has successfully identified the first genetic locus for AMD (74) (Fig. 1). Klein et al. described a large multigenerational family with 10 living individuals diagnosed with bilateral extensive, large, confluent drusen and/or geographic atrophy. This large family with AMD appeared to transmit the disease with an autosomal-dominant inheritance pattern. Conventional linkage analysis of this family has identified a potential AMD locus mapping to chromosome 1q25–q31 with a LOD score of 3.00. The gene symbol for this locus is designated as ARMD1. At the time this paper was published, it was not known whether this family with a predominantly dry AMD phenotype was a rare isolated pedigree or whether this locus represented a major gene responsible for AMD.

B. Linkage Approach: Nonparametric Linkage Analysis

Traditional single-family-based linkage analysis identified the first AMD locus, but this approach is difficult to implement routinely for the study of AMD because these large-AMD families are difficult to find. The rarity of these large pedigrees is due to the late onset of the disease, the usual availability of only one generation that can be reliably diagnosed with the disease, and the uncertainty regarding the diagnosis in mildly affected individuals. Modified genome linkage techniques have been developed to analyze late-onset complex

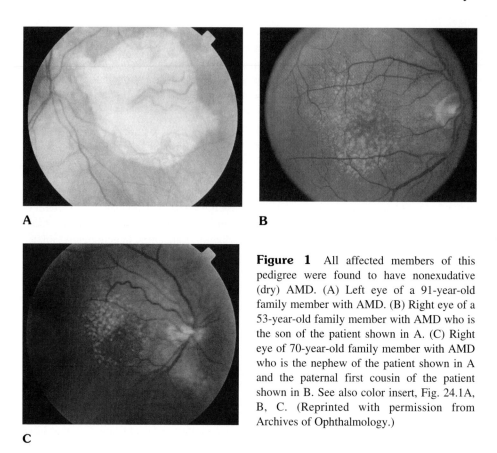

A

B

C

Figure 1 All affected members of this pedigree were found to have nonexudative (dry) AMD. (A) Left eye of a 91-year-old family member with AMD. (B) Right eye of a 53-year-old family member with AMD who is the son of the patient shown in A. (C) Right eye of 70-year-old family member with AMD who is the nephew of the patient shown in A and the paternal first cousin of the patient shown in B. See also color insert, Fig. 24.1A, B, C. (Reprinted with permission from Archives of Ophthalmology.)

inherited traits such as AMD. These approaches have evolved over the past decade and are known as allele-sharing methods (75–80). These newer methods attempt to demonstrate an increased sharing of certain chromosomal regions among affected relatives. Unlike earlier linkage methods, which are termed parametric tests of linkage because one must provide a model for the mode of inheritance (e.g., dominant, recessive, or X-linked), these more recent allele-sharing algorithms are designated nonparametric tests because no assumptions are made about the mode of inheritance or the number of genes involved in the disease. Affected sib-pair analysis was an early form of this method, and newer versions of this approach, such as the affected pedigree member method and SimIBD, have incorporated additional information such as allele frequencies and genetic data from other family members to enhance the ability to detect linkage. The affected pedigree method uses affected siblings and does not require parental testing or the involvement of any other family members, whereas SimIBD incorporates the genetic testing of additional family members whose disease status is uncertain or unaffected. Some programs allow for the analysis of two or more markers that may be linked to the disease, while other programs can incorporate a variety of assumptions and models into the statistical analysis. Using these analytical tools, investigators identify family members with or without AMD (usually siblings) and perform a complete genomewide screen using highly polymorphic markers in an attempt to correlate the coinheritance of a particular chromosomal region with the disease trait.

Several important details need to be addressed to ensure the success of genetic studies that employ the affected sibling pairs. The most important details include (1) sample size and structure (the number of sets of siblings or other affected members within the family), (2) the distances between the polymorphic markers and the disease gene, and (3) the knowledge of the marker allele frequency within the population. The first requirement for this type of linkage analysis, sample size, is highly dependent on the complexity and genetic heterogeneity of the disorder. Until there is an estimate of the number of genes responsible for AMD, it is difficult to estimate the necessary study population. For other complex genetic conditions such as Alzheimer's disease and non-insulin-dependent diabetes, linkage has been reported with as few as 300 subjects (150 sib-pairs). The second issue, the distribution of polymorphic markers that are well-distributed across the genome, is now easily satisfied by the availability of highly polymorphic microsatellite markers and single nucleotide polymorphisms (SNPs) that can be readily amplified by PCR technology and require relatively small amounts of patient DNA. The remaining issue is the availability of a control group, genetically similar to the study group, in which the marker allele frequencies have been determined. As increasing numbers of individuals are genotyped for a wide range of disorders, investigators now have a growing source of information of allele frequencies for these markers within different populations. The allele frequencies are used in the analyses to determine the likelihood that two alleles that are shared between family members represent a portion of the DNA that was inherited from a common ancestor as opposed to the chance that the alleles were inherited from different ancestors. Linkage probability scores are calculated for the different polymorphic loci and the likelihood that a particular locus is associated with the disease is determined. If a positive linkage is established to a particular genomic locus, that locus is narrowed until a mapped candidate gene is identified or the gene is cloned (81)

Using nonparametric linkage analysis, Weeks et al. (80) carried out a genomewide screen for AMD susceptibility loci on a panel of 225 AMD families with up to 212 sib-pairs and then expanded this screen, in a more directed linkage analysis, to include 364 AMD families with 329 affected sib-pairs. These families contained individuals with both atrophic and neovascular forms of AMD, since both forms of AMD are just as likely to have more than one family member with AMD (26). The analyses conducted on these families suggested a positive signal on chromosome 10 that was maintained using three different diagnostic models. This is the first demonstration of a positive result using nonparametric linkage analysis for the study of AMD. Following this initial report, an expanded genomewide linkage analysis of 390 families and 452 sib-pairs revealed the identification of two additional loci with a high likelihood that the loci on chromosomes 1 and 17 represent true AMD susceptibility loci (82) (M.B. Gorin, personal communication, 2001). This second report represented an ongoing effort to expand their first genetic study with additional families and increase their power to detect linkage. This follow-up analysis also identified additional potential loci of lower statistical importance and these sites were located on chromosomes 9, 10, 2, and 12. It is important to appreciate that the locus on chromosome 1 identified using sib-pairs and the nonparametric linkage approach is the same chromosomal region (ARMD1) identified by Klein et al. (74). Thus, using two different approaches, investigators have identified the locus designated ARMD1 as a region that appears to contain a gene responsible for AMD. The nonparametric approach provided independent confirmation of the ARMD1 locus and this confirmation is the first evidence that the nonparametric approach to linkage analysis using sib-pair analysis is capable of identifying a locus responsible for AMD. This confirmation also implies that a significant portion of AMD cases is likely due to mutations in the ARMD1. Moreover, if all the loci identified by Weeks et al. using sibling pairs and the nonparametric approach contain genes responsible for AMD, then these loci probably represent most of the AMD genes. Thus, in the search for genes, sibling pairs with AMD may prove just as useful and more obtainable than the rare large, multigenerational pedigree with AMD.

C. Association Approach: Candidate Linkage Analysis

Association studies utilizing candidate loci or candidate genes may be far better than linkage analyses in identifying genes for complex genetic disorders (14). Association studies, whether they are candidate linkage analysis or candidate gene analysis, require an "educated guess" and focus the search to include specific genes and/or genetic loci that may be involved in the disease. Candidate linkage analysis is accomplished by performing linkage analysis with polymorphic markers in close proximity to a gene or chromosomal locus that is thought to be involved with a particular disease. This approach differs from the candidate-gene-screening methods in which one seeks to identify specific mutations within the coding regions of a gene. By testing for the association of a disease with highly polymorphic markers near a known gene or chromosomal locus, investigators can screen a much larger region and develop a "composite" association of the locus or gene with the disease (i.e., a linkage study examines the impact of all potential mutations without having to identify each individual mutation within the gene). The advantage of pursing polymorphic markers in close proximity to the locus or gene is that it essentially collapses all the disease-causing mutations into a single type of analysis and increases the likelihood that linkage will be detected. This is different than candidate gene analysis (see next section) where the investigator searches through the DNA sequence of the entire gene hoping to find a change that can be associated with the disease. While candidate linkage analysis may be useful in detecting loci and genes that play a major role in a particular disease, it becomes less useful when a particular gene is an infrequent cause of disease. This technique may also fail to demonstrate a gene's role in the disease if an insufficient number of families have been recruited. This could be problematic in the search for AMD genes if many genes cause the disease and each gene contributes only a small percentage of cases.

Potential candidate loci include regions linked to early-onset macular degenerations that share many phenotypic features with AMD such as autosomal-dominant and -recessive Stargardt disease, autosomal-dominant familial drusen, Sorsby fundus dystrophy, Best disease, Malattia Leventinese (ML) (also known as radial drusen and Doyne honeycomb retinal degeneration), pattern dystrophy, North Carolina macula dystrophy (also known as progressive bifocal chorioretinal atrophy), central areolar choroidal dystrophy, and blue cone monochromacy. Additional potential candidate loci can also be chosen based on the hypothesis that a specific chromosomal region may contain a gene that could theoretically affect photoreceptor function, RPE function, retinal/retinol metabolism, fatty acid metabolism, metabolism of extracellular matrix proteins, or any other biological function that may be important to normal functioning of the outer retina and choroid within the macula.

Candidate gene linkage analysis has been performed for the *TIMP-3* gene (83), the cause of Sorsby fundus dystrophy, and for the ML locus (84). de La Paz et al. have excluded the *TIMP-3* gene as a cause for AMD in their affected population, but the ML locus has not been completely excluded as a potential AMD locus. Weeks et al. (80) performed candidate linkage analysis on 364 AMD families and up to 329 affected sib-pairs using markers from 16 plausible candidate regions. These regions included loci for the genes that encode Stargardt disease, Stargardt-like macular dystrophy, ML, North Carolina macular dystrophy, Cohen syndrome, Best macular dystrophy, Sorsby fundus dystrophy *TIMP-3*, cone-rod dystrophy, and seven different types of retinitis pigmentosa. Nine of these candidate regions were excluded, including the region for Stargardt disease, suggesting that the contribution of the Stargardt disease gene *(ABCA4/ABCR)* to AMD must be small and below the detection limits of this analysis. In a follow-up study using additional sib-pairs and chromosomal markers, Gorin et al. (82) once again demonstrated that there was no evidence of any other known candidate gene region playing a major role in the genetics of AMD.

D. Association Studies: Candidate Gene Analysis

The analysis of candidate genes also involves an "educated" guess about the gene that may be involved in a disease. However, unlike candidate linkage analysis described previously, which uses polymorphisms within a specific chromosomal region, candidate gene analysis requires knowing the sequence of a specific candidate gene. Once the gene is chosen, the nucleotide sequence of the gene (usually those portions of the gene that are responsible for the coding of the protein) is compared between patients with the disease and unaffected controls.

How does one know when a change in the gene sequence is the actual cause of the disease rather than a silent polymorphism? As noted previously, the selection of the control population is critical for these studies. Since AMD has a late onset, one must select a control population that is of comparable age and does not have the disease. A younger control population is likely to contain individuals who have not yet developed manifestations of AMD, and this control group would be predicted to contain the mutations that cause the disease at a frequency similar to the prevalence of the disease in the population. Consequently, an older control population in which AMD has been excluded is best. Because one cannot completely exclude the diagnosis of AMD in any control population due to incomplete and age-dependent penetrance and variable expressivity, one must anticipate finding disease-associated nucleotide changes in both the "normal" and the affected populations. Thus, it becomes extremely challenging to distinguish between disease-causing mutations and silent polymorphisms. Without additional evidence that a specific DNA sequence change results in a change in protein structure and function (e.g., null mutation), evidence of disequilibrium (i.e., a nucleotide alteration is present in a higher frequency within the affected population as compared to the frequency within the control population) is a statistical argument, rather than proof of causality. Cosegregation of the DNA change with the disease among family members is another important way to demonstrate that a nucleotide change is a disease-related mutation. In addition, each sequence change must also be analyzed to determine whether the alteration will affect the expression of the gene and/or the structure and function of the corresponding protein. Often, the importance of a sequence alteration is inferred by demonstrating a change within an evolutionarily conserved region of the gene or protein. Finally, proof may require in vitro analysis of the altered gene product (protein) or the creation of a transgenic, knockout, or conditional knockin animal as a model for disease and treatment.

Candidate genes for the study of AMD could include any gene that is known to cause an early-onset form of macular degeneration. This phenomenon, known as "gene sharing," occurs when different or the same mutations in the same gene cause two clinically related, but different, inherited eye diseases. Gene sharing has been shown to occur in a number of inherited ocular traits including retinitis pigmentosa and Leber congenital amaurosis *(RPE65* gene) (85,86); Leber congenital amaurosis and cone-rod dystrophy (87,88); retinitis pigmentosa, pattern dystrophy, and adult vitelliform dystrophy *(RDS/peripherin gene)* (89,90); retinitis pigmentosa and congenital nightblindness (rhodopsin gene) (91); retinitis pigmentosa, cone-rod degeneration, and Stargardt disease *(ABCA4/ABCR* gene) (92,93); autosomal-dominant familial drusen and Stargardt-like macular degeneration (94); juvenile and adult-onset glaucoma (*TIGR* gene) (95).

Although candidate gene analysis seems like a straightforward and noncontroversial approach to demonstrate a causal relationship between a gene and a disease, it can sometimes be quite confusing and controversial. An example of such confusion and controversy surrounds the relationship between the Stargardt gene known as *ABCA4(ABCR)* and AMD. Allikmets et al. (96) reported that mutations in the Stargardt disease gene caused AMD. Stargardt disease (also known as fundus flavimaculatus) is an early-onset, autosomal-recessive macular degeneration characterized by decreased central vision, atrophic changes in the macula, and the appearance of small yellowish flecks at the level of the RPE within the posterior pole, similar to the appearance of some drusen in AMD. The gene encodes a protein that is a member of a well-characterized superfamily of proteins known as ATP-binding cassette (ABC) transporters. The gene is believed to encode a protein that is important for the transport of all-trans retinal from the photoreceptor to the RPE. Disease causing mutations are proposed to cause the accumulation of a condensation product between all-trans-retinal and phosphatidylethanolamine, which subsequently accumulates in RPE cells and is referred to as lipofuscin. This substance is believed to be toxic to the RPE and subsequently causes the macular degeneration (97).

Using the candidate gene approach, Allikmets et al. (96) analyzed a set of 167 unrelated patients with AMD. Subjects with AMD were identified from ophthalmic clinic populations in Boston and Salt Lake City, and screened to exclude other causes of disciform or neovascular maculopathy similar to AMD. The coding regions ofthe *ABCA4(ABCR)* gene that determine the sequence of the protein product were screened exon by exon for sequence variations in the AMD group. If a sequence variation was found to have an affect on the encoded protein sequence within a particular exon, that same region was screened in the control group. The control group was composed of 220 unaffected individuals who were Caucasians from the general population collected for other studies in the United States. No age restriction was placed on the control group. These researchers found that 13 sequence alterations in 26 patients were present at greater frequency in the AMD group than in the control group. Most of the sequence variants were missense changes and rare alleles occurring in one or two individuals. Two exceptions were the sequence changes G1961E and D2177N found in six and seven subjects, respectively. Most of the sequence variations were not known to cause Stargardt disease, although three of the 13 sequence changes were also found in Stargardt patients. The 13 sequence changes that were found more frequently in the AMD group were associated with "dry" AMD characterized by soft and calcific macular and extramacular drusen, drusenoid pigment epithelial detachments, and geographic atrophy. Analyses of the AMD-associated alterations within the gene found some clustering toward the 3' prime end, but most were scattered throughout the coding sequence. The authors conclude that heterozygous mutations in the Stargardt gene may be responsible for up to 16% of AMD cases in their population.

The significance of the *ABCA4(ABCR)* gene sequence changes in AMD was initially challenged by Dryja et al. (98) and Klaver et al. (99), who identified methodological deficiencies in the design of the study. The control group may have been inappropriate as it was recruited from a different regional population than the AMD group, and no objective evidence was provided that the groups were genetically matched. This is important in regard to one sequence variation, R943Q (a nucleotide change that altered the sequence so that arginine is replaced with a glutamine), which was found at a much higher frequency in the control group than the AMD group, 16.25% versus 4.7%, respectively. Three other sequence changes were found more commonly in the control group. Moreover, if all the sequence variants identified by Allikmets et al. account for 16% of AMD cases, then the asymptomatic carrier frequency in the control population would be expected to be 4.8%. However, only 0.45% of the controls were found to have the changes, much lower than the calculated frequency, again suggesting that the control group was not appropriately matched to the AMD group, or the vast majority of sequence changes identified in the *ABCA4 (ABCR)* gene do not cause AMD. Moreover, Dryja et al. and Klaver et al. argue that analysis of the data reveals that there is no statistically significant difference in the frequency of these rare DNA sequence alterations between the AMD and control groups. Consequently, they conclude that no causative connection between the sequence change and the disease is possible. Moreover, they argue that cosegregation of a sequence variation with the disease within families should have been demonstrated to support the conclusion that the Stargardt *ABCA4(ABCR)* gene alterations cause AMD. Finally, Klaver et al. have questioned the diagnosis of AMD in the affected group as the diagnosis was not based on an internationally accepted grading system. In particular, early-stage AMD characterized by a few drusen might not be AMD at all. Moreover, their population of AMD patients may contain some patients with Stargardt disease because end-stage Stargardt disease can be indistinguishable from advanced AMD. In response to these criticisms. Dean et al. (100) attempted to defend their work and offered two possible conclusions regarding their study; either they have an interesting "hypothesis-generating finding" that *ABCA4(ABCR)* mutations may confer an increased risk to AMD or that the *ABCA4(ABCR)* mutations are a cause of AMD.

Since the initial report by Allikmets et al., additional reports have refuted the conclusion that mutations in the *ABCA4(ABCR)* gene are associated with AMD (101–106). Stone et al. (101) showed no role for the *ABCA4(ABCR)* gene in AMD. These investigators screened 182 AMD cases and 96 controls. The control group was specifically chosen to be ethnically matched to the AMD population. This is different than the nonethnically matched control group originally screened by Allikmets et al. (96). Moreover, 60% of the AMD group was shown to have choroidal neovascularization (CNV) in at least one eye. The proportion of patients with CNV in the study published by Allikmets et al. was not documented; however, subsequent studies have found that the dry form of AMD is associated with heterozygous *ABCA4(ABCR)* mutation carriers (107). There are two possible explanations for the discrepancy between reports. First, Stone et al. may not have screened a sufficient number of dry AMD patients to reach clinical significance, and second, Allikmets et al. were really looking at a population of late-onset Stargardt disease patients who were mistakenly diagnosed as having dry AMD. A subsequent paper by Guymer et al. (106) reported on the role of two specific alleles of the *ABCA4(ABCR)* gene in the pathogenesis of AMD. This time, 544 patients with AMD and 689 controls were screened from three continents. The incidences of the G1961E and D2177N variants were compared between the AMD and control groups. Once again, there was no significant difference ($p > 0.1$) between the AMD and control groups. Furthermore, there was no evidence of cosegregation of these alleles with the AMD phenotype among all siblings with AMD in families where at least one individual with AMD had one of the presumed pathogenic alleles. Their conclusion was that mutations in the *ABCA4(ABCR)* gene are not involved in a statistically significant fraction of AMD cases. This paper also emphasized the importance of having ethnically matched controls as there can be wide variations in the frequency of certain alleles that are thought to be pathogenic but are actually found quite frequently in certain control populations.

Kuroiwa et al. (102) also failed to find a relationship between *ABCA4(ABCR)* mutations and AMD. Kuroiwa and colleagues screened 80 unrelated Japanese patients with AMD (67 males and 13 females; mean age, 67.2 years) diagnosed by examination and indocyanine green angiography and compared these patients with 100 age-matched control subjects. The coding sequences were analyzed by the single-strand conformation polymorphism (SSCP) method followed by nucleotide sequencing when necessary. Their results did not support the association between the *ABCA4(ABCR)* gene mutations and neovascular AMD in Japanese patients. A similar type of investigation was performed by De La Paz et al. (103). They screened for *ABCA4(ABCR)* variants among 159 familial cases of AMD from 112 multiplex families and 53 sporadic cases of AMD and compared these patients with 56 racially matched individuals with no known history of AMD from the same clinic population. Analysis for variants was performed by polymerase chain reaction amplification of individual exons of the *ABCA4(ABCR)* gene with flanking primers and a combination of SSCP, heteroduplex analysis, and high-performance liquid chromatography followed by direct sequencing of all abnormal conformers detected using these techniques. Based on these initial findings, De La Paz et al. suggest that *ABCR* is not a major genetic risk factor for AMD in their study population.

In a similar type of study, Rivera et al. (105) assessed the proposed role for *ABCA4(ABCR)* in AMD by studying 200 affected individuals with late-stage disease. In the AMD group, 18 patients were found to harbor possible disease-associated alterations compared to 12 individuals in the control group ($n = 220$). The group with AMD and the control group were analyzed with the same methodology. This difference between groups was not statistically significant; however, their cohort was small compared to the larger cohorts needed to detect rare alleles in complex diseases. Another small study, by Fuse et al. (104) explored whether mutations in the *ABCR(ABCA4)* gene were associated with dry AMD in unrelated Japanese patients. Twenty-five Japanese patients with dry AMD and 40 Japanese controls underwent sequence analysis. A possible pathogenic point mutation in exon 29 was found in one of the 25 dry AMD patients. Other nonpathogenic allelic variations were also detected. The prevalence of the exon 29 sequence variant among AMD patients was 4% while the prevalence in the control group was 5%. In this small study there was no association between the exon 29 allelic variant in the *ABCA4(ABCR)* gene and the diagnosis of dry AMD among these unrelated Japanese patients.

Allikmets (107,108) has continued investigations into the role of *ABCA4(ABCR)* mutations in AMD and continues to report that mutations in the *ABCA4(ABCR)* gene cause AMD. His latest results attempt to refute those studies that fail to find an association between the *ABCA4(ABCR)* gene and AMD. He argues that the *ABCA4(ABCR)* mutations are responsible for nonneovascular forms of AMD and this population should be specifically examined. He also argues that these other laboratories have failed to employ a mutation scanning methodology that detects a majority of all sequence changes. Finally, he emphasizes that about 500 individuals need to be screened to detect the presence of a causative sequence variant having a small effect (109). Thus, the power of a study is increased by increasing the sample size, and he argues that the studies that failed to identify an association between the *ABCA4(ABCR)* gene and AMD failed to study enough patients with nonneo-vascular AMD. To test this hypothesis, Allikmets (107,110) established an expanded collaborative study including 15 centers in North America and Europe. A total of 1385 un-related AMD patients and 1478 comparison individuals were screened for the two most fre-quent AMD-associated variants found in *ABCA4(ABCR)*. These two nonconservative amino acid sequence changes, G1961E and D2177N, were found in one allele of the *ABCA4(ABCR)* gene in 53 patients (approximately 4%), and in 13 control subjects (ap-proximately 0.95%), a statistically significant difference ($p < 0.0001$). The risk of AMD is elevated approximately threefold in D2177N carriers and approximately sevenfold in G1961E carriers. Overall, these two variants are detected in about 4% of nonneovascular AMD cases. With millions of people affected worldwide with AMD, this 4% value repre-sents a substantial number of individuals in whom the mutation that causes their disease may be identified. Whether these sequence changes actually cause disease remains unre-solved, but the controversy regarding the role of the *ABCA4(ABCR)* gene in the pathogen-esis of AMD highlights some of the challenges every investigator must confront when studying a complex genetic disease using candidate gene analysis.

The notion that a heterozygous carrier of a mutation can have a disease that is differ-ent from a disease that occurs when the same mutation is in the homozygous state or in a compound heterozygous state is not unique to Stargardt disease among human diseases. For instance, carriers of an *ATM* mutation can have an increased risk of breast cancer whereas this mutation in the homozygous or compound heterozygous state causes ataxia-telangiec-tasia. Another example involves carriers of a *LDLR* mutation who can have moderately elevated LDL and are prone to coronary artery disease in midlife, but when this same mu-tation is in the homozygous or compound heterozygous state, these individuals have ex-tremely high LDL cholesterol levels and are at risk for myocardial infarction during young adulthood. Yet another example is carriers of a *CFTR* mutation who can have chronic pan-creatitis, but when the mutation is in the homozygous or compound heterozygous state, these individuals develop cystic fibrosis. In a similar fashion, carriers of *ABCR(ABC4)* mu-tations may account for some cases of AMD.

One prediction of this model, that *ABCR(ABCA4)* is a dominant susceptibility locus for AMD, is that parents and grandparents of patients with Stargardt disease are heterozy-gous carriers and at higher risk of developing AMD. Evidence to support this proposal has now been reported (111–116). Lewis et al. (111) examined the *ABCA4(ABCR)* gene in 150 families segregating recessive Stargardt disease. Clinical evaluation of these 150 families with Stargardt disease revealed a high frequency of AMD in first- and second-degree rela-tives. These findings support the hypothesis that some heterozygous *ABCA4(ABCR)* muta-tions may enhance susceptibility to AMD. Shroyer et al. (112) described a pedigree that manifests both Stargardt disease and AMD in which an *ABCA4(ABCR)* mutation cosegre-gates with both disease phenotypes. This pedigree supports the hypothesis that heterozy-gous *ABCA4(ABCR)* mutations may be responsible for AMD. Simonelli et al. (113) as-sessed the clinical phenotypes in 11 Italian families with autosomal-recessive Stargardt disease and fundus flavimaculatus and screened for mutations within the *ABCA4(ABCR)* gene in these families. Clinical evaluation of these families affected with Stargardt disease revealed an unusually high frequency of early AMD in parents of patients with Stargardt disease (6 of 11 families [55%] and 8 of 22 parents [36%], consistent with the hypothesis that some heterozygous *ABCA4(ABCR)* mutations enhance susceptibility to AMD. Souied et al. (114) reported three unrelated families in which AMD was observed in grandparents of patients with Stargardt disease. Compound heterozygous missense mutations were observed in patients with Stargardt disease (arg212cys, arg1107cys, gly1977ser, arg2107his, and le2113met), and heterozygous missense mutations were observed in the grandparents with AMD (arg212cys and arg1107cys). By demonstrating phenotype and genotype findings in three unrelated families segregating patients with Stargardt disease and AMD, the authors propose that the carriers of these *ABCA4(ABCR)* gene mutations may have a higher risk of developing AMD.

Additional studies by Souied et al. (115) examined the familial segregation of *ABCA4(ABCR)* gene mutations in 52 unrelated multiplex cases of exudative AMD. Overall, six heterozygous missense changes were identified. A lack of familial segregation was observed in four of six codon changes (arg943gln, val1433ile, pro1948leu, and ser2255ile). However, two codon changes cosegregated with the disease in two small families: pro940arg and Leu1970phe. Once again, this type of analysis suggests that some mutations in the *ABCA4(ABCR)* gene may be rarely involved in neovascular AMD, with at best two of 52 familial cases (4%) related to this susceptibility factor. Finally, Zhang et al. (116) reported a patient who inherited a mutation in an autosomal-dominant gene for early-onset macular degeneration (ELOVL4) and a likely pathogenic mutation in the *ABCA4(ABCR)* gene resulting in a more severe macular degeneration phenotype. Interestingly, the patient's grandparent with the same heterozygous *ABCA4(ABCR)* mutation developed AMD. These studies suggest that the *ABCA4(ABCR)* gene may be involved in AMD; however, none of these cosegregation studies examining grandparents and/or siblings within families of Stargardt disease patients were conducted in a masked fashion in which the clinician making the phenotypic judgments was masked to the genotypic information. Moreover, all the relatives of the proband were not equally ascertained, so it was impossible to determine whether any family members had AMD without inheriting the sequence variant and how many inherited the sequence variant without having AMD. In these studies, the overall numbers are small and none of these family studies demonstrated a statistically significant association of the presumed pathogenic *ABCA4(ABCR)* mutations with the AMD phenotype. Whether or not *ABCA4(ABCR)* mutations are associated with a disease as complex as AMD will await additional larger, well-designed genetic studies that are duplicated by different groups. The consortiums put together by Guymer et al. and Allikmets et al. are the first examples of these larger multicenter studies, but additional association studies will be necessary to help resolve this ongoing debate.

It is intriguing to speculate that the *ABCA4(ABCR)* gene is in part responsible for AMD. If true, then studies into the biochemistry of the ABCA4(ABCR) protein may help in developing pharmacological therapies for both Stargardt disease and AMD. For example, the biochemical activity of the ABCA4(ABCR) protein has been studied in vitro and biochemical defects have been associated with disease-causing mutations in the *ABCA4(ABCR)* gene (117–119). In addition, these in vitro studies have examined ways to stimulate the biochemical activity of the ABCA4(ABCR) protein. The ATPase activity of the ABCA4(ABCR) protein has been synergistically stimulated by several compounds, including the antiarrhythmic drug known as amiodarone. It is intriguing to speculate that if a drug such as amiodorone could stimulate the protein in vitro, then perhaps drugs could be used to help stimulate the residual activity of the mutant proteins in Stargardt disease and help preserve vision. The goal would be to find a drug that would enhance the normal activity of the protein while suppressing the abnormal activity caused by the mutation. Similarly, in patients who may be at increased risk of developing AMD because they are heterozygous carriers of mutations in the *ABCA4(ABCR)* gene, it may be possible to administer a drug that would stimulate the activity of the wild-type protein rather than the mutant protein. As a result, the detrimental effects of the mutant protein would be minimized and the progression of disease could be slowed.

In the search for other genes that may cause AMD, one attractive candidate is designated *EFEMP1*, the gene responsible for Doyne honeycomb retinal dystophy (DHRD), also known as ML or autosomal-dominant radial drusen. EGF-containing fibrillin-like extracellular matrix protein 1 (EFEMP1) is an example of an extracellular matrix protein that might play an important role in the evolution of AMD. The fundus appearance of the early-onset autosomal-dominant macular disorder caused by mutations in the *EFEMP1* gene is characterized by the appearance of drusen in young adulthood and closely resembles early AMD. However, CNV is not a common feature of this disorder. Of interest, in all 39 families studied with DHRD (ML or autosomal-dominant radial drusen), all affected subjects have the same mutation (arg345trp) in the *EFEMP1* gene (120). While preliminary linkage analysis suggested this locus could be responsible for some families with AMD (84), subsequent analysis by Stone et al. (120) revealed no such association. Stone et al. found no additional pathogenic sequence variants within the coding region of the *EFEMP1* gene in 477 control individuals or in 494 patients with AMD. Souied et al. also examined the role of *EFEMP1* sequence alterations in AMD and found no association with AMD among 52 unrelated French families with multiplex cases of AMD compared to 90 unrelated and unaffected French controls (121). Although there may be mutations within the gene responsible for some sporadic cases of AMD, it seems unlikely that mutations in the *EFEMP1* gene will play a major role in causing AMD.

Another potential candidate includes the gene responsible for Best macular dystrophy, also known as vitelliform macular dystrophy type 2 (VMD2), an autosomal-dominant, early-onset macular degeneration. The gene responsible for Best macular dystrophy is designated *VMD2* (122,123). *VMD2* encodes a transmembrane protein and is expressed in RPE cells. Although the function of the *VMP2* gene product is unknown, it may play a role in the transport or the metabolism of polyunsaturated fatty acids in the retina. Allikmets et al. (124) screened the *VMD2* gene for sequence changes in a collection of 259 AMD patients. Only about 1% of patients with AMD were found to have sequence changes in their *VMD2* genes that would cause changes in the amino acid sequence of the gene product. The authors concluded that there is no statistically significant evidence that this gene plays a significant role in the predisposition of individuals to AMD. A similar conclusion was reached by Kramer et al. (125). In their study, 200 patients with AMD were screened for mutations in *VMD2*. No mutations were found in the AMD group. In contrast to these results, Lotery et al. (126) performed a similar type of sequence analysis in 321 AMD patients, and 192 ethnically similar control subjects, 39 unrelated probands with familial Best disease, and 57 unrelated probands with the ophthalmoscopic findings of Best disease but no family history. These authors found five different probable or possible disease-causing mutations in the 321 AMD patients (1.5%), a fraction that was not significantly greater than in control individuals (0/192, 0%). They felt that these findings, although not statistically significant, suggested that a small fraction of patients with the clinical diagnosis of AMD might have a late-onset variant of Best disease. However, Souied et al. (121) examined the role of *VMD2* sequence alterations in AMD and found no association with AMD among 52 unrelated French families with multiplex cases of AMD compared to 90 unrelated and unaffected French controls. Although the possibility exists that the rare sporadic cases of AMD might be caused by mutations in the *VMD2* gene, these studies strongly suggest that mutations in the Best macular dystrophy gene are not a major cause of AMD.

Another candidate gene includes *TIMP3*, the gene responsible for Sorsby fundus dystrophy, an early-onset, autosomal-dominant disorder characterized by macular degeneration and choroidal neovascularization. The *TIMP3* gene product, an inhibitor of a metalloproteinase known as a Zn-binding endopeptidase, is involved in the degradation of the extracellular matrix. It is attractive to consider the hypothesis that a gene product involved in the metabolism of the extracellular matrix has an important role in the evolution of AMD and choroidal neovascularization. However, as mentioned previously, candidate gene linkage analysis has excluded this locus in AMD (127) and a more detailed screening of the gene has failed to identify any sequence changes *TIMP3* associated with AMD (128). In this study, Felbor et al. (128) screened *TIMP3* for disease-causing mutations in 143 patients with AMD. They identified one sequence alteration (a G-to-C base change) in the 5' prime-untranslated region in a patient with AMD. However, the functional consequences of this mutation are uncertain, and no other disease-causing mutations were found. They did identify a frequent intragenic polymorphism in exon 3 of the *TIMP3* gene (heterozygosity = 0.57) that will be useful for genetic linkage or allele-sharing analyses or both. However, the results suggest that *TIMP3* is not a major factor in the cause of AMD.

Other candidate genes include the *peripherin/RDS* gene, the gene responsible for a variety of retinal disorders such as retinitis pigmentosa, pattern dystrophy, and adult vitelliform dystrophy. However, studies have shown no association between this gene and AMD (129,130). Another potential gene *ELOVL4*, the gene responsible for autosomal dominant drusen and a Stargardt-like dystrophy. A preliminary report suggests that mutations in this gene are not associated with AMD (131).

In most of the studies designed to look for associations between sequence changes within a candidate gene and AMD, most if not all of the genetic analysis is performed on coding regions or exon/intron boundaries within the gene. These regions are examined because it is understood how changes in these sequences could affect gene expression and function. It is entirely possible that mutations reside outside these regions. One might postulate that the types of mutations that would cause a late-onset disease like AMD might be found within regulatory regions of the gene that would have a subtler affect on expression or function. These regulatory regions, which are not routinely screened, would include sequences that constitute the promoter, terminator, or introns of the gene. Such detailed sequence analysis within these regions for each participant in a study is currently just not feasible. However, as mentioned previously, it is feasible to perform association studies using candidate linkage analysis since all the mutations within a gene are screened by looking for linkage with known polymorphic markers either within or near the genes. Therefore, candidate linkage analysis is probably a more useful approach to identify the major genes and loci responsible for AMD. The major drawback of this approach is that candidate linkage analysis will identify only the more common genes and loci. Most likely, a gene would have to be responsible for at least 15–20% of AMD cases before the candidate linkage approach would demonstrate a positive association. A current list of potential candidate genes and loci that could be used for candidate gene screening and linkage analyses can be found at the following website: www.sph.uth.tmc.edu/retnet/home.htm. In conclusion, it would appear that the genes responsible for early-onset Mendelian-type macular degenerations are not major contributors to AMD. However, mutations in these genes may account for a small percent of AMD cases. This may well be the case for the Stargardt gene (*ABCA4/ABCR*).

A candidate gene for AMD does not necessarily have to be a gene that causes an early-onset retinal degeneration. Moreover, a candidate gene for AMD does not even have to be a gene that is expressed only in the retina. We already know that genes that are important for retinal function but are expressed in other tissues as well can cause retina-specific diseases. Examples of such retina-specific diseases caused by non-retina-specific genes include retinoblastoma, gyrate atrophy, choroideremia, and Sorsby fundus dystrophy.

One such candidate gene is the apolipoprotein E(*APOE*)gene. This is an example of how a non-retina-specific gene may play an important role in AMD (132–137). ApoE, the major apolipoprotein of the central nervous system and an important regulator of cholesterol and lipid transport, appears to be associated with neurodegenerative diseases. Polymorphisms within the *APOE* gene are associated with a high risk of developing certain neurodegenerative conditions such as Alzheimer's disease, and the ApoE protein has been demonstrated in disease-associated lesions of these disorders. Souied et al. (132) evaluatedl *APOE* alleles among 116 unrelated patients with neo vascular AMD in one eye and hard drusen or soft drusen in the other eye and compared the frequency of these alleles with 168 age-matched and sex-matched controls subjects. A lower frequency of epsilon-4 allele carriers was found in the neovascular AMD group versus the control group (12.1% vs 28.6%; $p < 0.0009$), and the epsilon-4 allele was less frequent among the AMD group compared to the control group (0.073 vs. 0. 149; $p < 0.006$). This lower frequency was mainly observed in the soft-drusen subgroup. The authors postulated that apoE alleles might affect cholesterol metabolism, which may be related to lipid deposition in Bruch's membrane, drusen formation, and subsequent neovascular changes

Klaver et al. (138) performed an association study with 88 AMD cases and 901 controls derived from the population-based Rotterdam Study in the Netherlands. The *APOE* epsilon-4 allele was associated with a decreased risk (odds ratio 0.43; 95% CI 0.21–0.88), and the epsilon-2 allele was associated with a slightly increased risk of AMD (odds ratio 1.5; 95% CI 0.8–2.82). They also studied apoE immunoreactivity in 15 AMD and 10 control maculae and found that apoE staining was consistently present in the disease-associated deposits in maculae from AMD patients (i.e., drusen and basal laminar deposit). These results suggested that *APOE* may be directly involved in the pathogenesis of AMD and may be a susceptibility gene for AMD. The results reported by Schmidt et al. (135) suggested a protective effect of the *APOE* episilon-4 allele on the risk of developing AMD, but their conclusions were less significant than those of the previous studies. In their report, 230 AMD cases were compared to 230 controls with respect to *APOE* genotypes. Separate analyses were also performed for 129 familial AMD cases and 101 sporadic AMD cases-as these groups might have a different disease etiology. No evidence was found for the risk-increasing effect attributed to the epsilon-2 allele in either familial or sporadic AMD. In addition, there was no evidence for a protective effect of the epsilon-4 allele in the sporadic AMD cases. These authors did find an age- and sex-adjusted odds ratio of 0.66 (95% CI 0.38–1.12, $p = 0.13$) for epsilon-4 carriers among familial AMD cases compared to controls. For the subgroup of individuals younger than 70 years of age, an odds ratio of 0.24 (95% CI 0.08–0.72, $p = 0.004$) was obtained. Interestingly, this modest protective effect was seen only in the familial cases, particularly those younger than 70 years of age. The authors suggested that a more thorough investigation was required to determine whether the effect was restricted to cases with a family history of AMD and whether the effect varied according to age and sex.

In contrast to these studies, Pang et al. (134) examined the frequency of the *APOE* epsilon-4 allele among 98 Hong Kong Chinese with AMD compared to 133 control subjects. In this population, the frequency of epsilon-4 carriers showed a trend toward a decreased prevalence of disease compared to controls, but it was not significant (11.2 vs. 15.0%, $p < 0.52$). Among the 39 patients with neovascular AMD, there was also no significant difference in the epsilon-4 allele frequency (12.8%, $p < 0.93$). In the previous reports, the reduced risk of AMD associated with the epsilon-4 allele was seen most notably in this neovascular AMD subgroup. The lack of a statistically significant effect of epsilon-4 allele may be due to the lower frequency of the epsilon-4 allele in Chinese compared to Europeans. In addition, AMD in the Chinese population may be phenotypically and genetically distinct from the AMD observed in patients with European ancestry. The authors conclude that the epsilon-4 allele of *APOE* is most likely not a major factor influencing AMD risk in the Chinese. However, in patients with European ancestry, it would appear that the *APOE* epsilon-4 allele might be protective against AMD, in particular neovascular AMD.

The risk of neovascular AMD has also been associated with polymorphisms in the gene encoding manganese superoxide dismutase (139, 140). In this study, Kimura et al. chose to study the manganese superoxide dismutase gene because of their hypothesis that xenobiotic-metabolizing enzymes and antioxidant enzymes may contribute to the development of AMD. This is an example of how a biological model for disease causation can direct genetic research. In their hospital-based case-controlled study of 102 consecutive Japanese patients with the neovascular AMD, sequence variation analysis was performed to detect polymorphisms in the cytochrome P-450 1A1, glutathione S-transferases, microsomal epoxide hydrolase, and manganese superoxide dismutase genes. Similar analysis was performed on 200 controls. They found a significant association of the manganese superoxide dismutase gene polymorphism (valine/alanine polymorphism at the targeting sequence of the enzyme) with AMD. Patients with AMD had an increased frequency of the alanine allele and the alanine/alanine genotype (odds ratio = 10.14, 95% CI 4.84–2.13; $p = 0.0005$ after Bonferroni correction). There was also a weak association of a microsomal epoxide hydrolase exon-3 polymorphism with AMD (odds ratio = 2.20, 95% CI 4.02–1.20; $p = 0.020$ after Bonferroni correction). No additional associations were found for the genes that encode cytochrome P-450 1A1, glutathione S-transferases, and microsomal epoxide hydrolase. The authors conclude that this manganese superoxide dismutase gene polymorphism may be associated with neovascular AMD, and an association may also exist for the microsomal epoxide hydrolase gene. These results may be the first genetic clue that genes for xenobiotic-metabolizing enzymes and oxidative enzymes may be involved in the environmental-genetic interactions that influence AMD. Moreover, these genetic findings may prove useful markers for predicting disease severity. Another preliminary positive association between AMD and an antioxidant enzyme was found by Weeks et al. (80). They initially found a potential association of AMD with glutathione peroxidase, but the significance of this association was lost when they performed an expanded genomewide candidate linkage analysis (82).

Another example of how a non-retina-specific process might influence AMD is suggested not by genetic studies but by histopathological studies. Blumenkranz et al. (141) demonstrated an association between dermal elastotic degeneration in sun-exposed skin and choroidal neovascularization in a patient with AMD. This association by Blumenkranz et al. could be explained by the presence of abnormal basement membrane proteins in both the skin and Bruch's membrane. These abnormal proteins could make the skin more susceptible to sun damage and the eye more susceptible to choroidal neovascularization.

V. THE FUTURE OF AMD GENETICS

AMD is most likely a complex genetic disease based on the overwhelming evidence from family and twin studies. To date, there have been no published reports to refute this genetic influence. Whether candidate gene analysis has successfully identified the Stargardt gene *ABCA4(ABCR)* as the first AMD gene remains unresolved. This raises the question of whether a gene can actually be shown to cause a complex disorder or whether a gene can only be shown to infer susceptibility to AMD based on the coinheritance of other susceptibility genes. In a disease with very high penetrance such as digenic retinitis pigmentosa, it was convincingly shown that two different genes needed to be coinherited to cause this retinal degeneration (142). This is an example of polygenic inheritance. What if the penetrance is lower at around 50%? Would it be possible to show causality of a particular gene if a patient inherits the disease-causing allele and does not develop disease? Using the linkage or association approaches to find a gene for a complex genetic disorder, we may never be able to provide conclusive evidence of causality from a single gene and be reduced to arguing relative risks or percentage likelihood of developing the disease. Owing to the complexity of AMD, the unknown number of AMD genes, and the unknown variability of disease penetrance combined with the wide spectrum of disease phenotypes, future discussions may focus on calculating a statistical risk of developing AMD based on the analysis of several genes and environmental conditions, thus establishing a genetic risk assessment. By identifying as many genes as possible, we hope to define a common biological pathway and understand how these genes and their proteins contribute to the disease in a collective fashion.

While AMD is a complex genetic disease, it is also a multifactorial disease in which environmental factors can influence disease penetrance and severity. By understanding all the genes involved in AMD and elucidating their common biological pathway, we will also appreciate how environmental factors influence the disease. Examples of how environmental factors can influence the progression of an inherited retinal degeneration include the roles of vitamin A in slowing the progression of autosomal dominant retinitis pigmentosa (143,144) and in alleviating nightblindness in Sorsby fundus dystrophy (145), the role of a low-protein, low-arginine diet in gyrate atrophy (146), and the role of a low-fat diet with vitamin supplementation in Bassen-Kornzweig disease (147).

In the future, genetic studies will identify at least several of the genes that cause AMD. Patients should be encouraged to participate in these genetic studies. The immediate benefit of gene identification will be genetic screening of individuals at risk for AMD before signs and symptoms develop. Once genes are identified, additional genes encoding proteins that interact with disease-causing genes will also be candidates to explore as potential causes of disease. For example, the gene that causes recessive Stargardt disease *(ABCA4/ABCR)* is thought to interact with the gene that causes a dominant Stargardt-like condition (116). This second gene may also interact with other genes along a common pathway and these other genes may cause macular degeneration as well.

Eventually, once the genes for AMD are identified, clinicians will be able to genotype AMD patients and correlations will be developed between genetic mutations, clinical phenotype, and disease progression. Identification of susceptibility genes will also allow the identification of a high-risk cohort of at-risk individuals for AMD intervention studies that could result in shorter and less costly clinical trials of new therapies. Gene identification will provide the first insight into the mechanism of disease at the cellular level. Elucidation of pathological mechanisms will direct the development of pharmacological therapies. As mentioned previously, Sun et al. (118) reported that the ATPase activity of the

ABCA4(ABCR) protein can be stimulated by the drug amiodarone. Perhaps other commonly available drugs could be shown to be useful for the treatment of AMD once the genes are identified. Another approach would be to develop designer drugs to specifically interact with these AMD genes or their corresponding proteins. By modifying the expression of these genes or altering the activity of the protein, these drugs could minimize the accumulative deleterious effect of the mutant gene over the lifetime of the individual. Of course, these therapies would be tested initially on transgenic animals engineered to contain the abnormal genes that cause AMD. In addition, these animals would be used to test theories about the role of environmental influences on AMD. For example, studies of knockout mice lacking the *ABCA4(abcr)* gene that causes Stargardt disease have been shown to undergo a slow retinal degeneration. If bright light is avoided by these mice, the retinal degeneration may be slowed (148). This observation could be translated to humans and used as a potential treatment to delay the onset of symptoms in patients with Stargardt disease. Hopefully, as we begin to identify the genes that cause AMD and understand the pathogenesis of this disease, we will develop novel therapies and recommend lifestyle modifications that will delay the progression of disease and preserve useful vision for the life of the patient.

VI. SUMMARY

AMD is likely to be a complex genetic disease as shown by population, family, and twin segregation and aggregation studies. The first genetic locus for AMD was designated ARMD1 and identified by conventional linkage analysis using a large multigenerational family with AMD. Another genetic study using sibling pairs and a nonparametric linkage approach confirmed this locus as a potential site for a gene that causes AMD. This second study identified additional chromosomal loci that are likely to contain genes for AMD.

Candidate gene analysis has implicated the Stargardt disease gene designated *ABCA4(ABCR)* as a cause of AMD; however, this finding remains controversial. Contradictory reports have been published that refute the association between AMD and the Stargardt disease gene. Extensive analyses of genes that cause early-onset macular degenerations have not yet identified any other association between these diseases and AMD. There have been several reports that the apolipoprotein E gene may play an important role in determining the risk of developing AMD.

REFERENCES

1. Rose MR, Archer MA. Genetic analysis of mechanisms of aging. Curr Opin Genet Dev 1996;6(3):366–370.
2. Johnson TE. Genetic influences on aging. Exp Gerontol 1997;32(1-2):11–22.
3. Martin GM. Genetic modulation of the senescent phenotype of *Homo sapiens*. Exp Gerontol 1996;31(1–2):49–59.
4. Martin GM, Austad SN, Johnson TE. Genetic analysis of aging: role of oxidative damage and environmental stresses. Nat Genet 1996;13(1):25–34.
5. Osiewacz HD. Genetic regulation of aging. J Mol Med 1997;75(10):715–727.
6. Hanis CL, Boerwinkle E, Chakraborty R, Ellsworth DL, Concannon P, Stirling B, Morrison VA., Wapelhorst B, Spielman RS, Gogolin-Ewens KJ, Shepard JM, Williams SR, Risch N, Hinds, Iwasaki N, Ogata M, Omori Y, Petzold C, Rietzch H, Schroder HE, Schulze J, Cox NJ,

Menzel S, Boriraj VV, Chen X, et al. A genome-wide search for human non-insulin-dependent (type 2) diabetes genes reveals a major susceptibility locus on chromosome 2 [see comments]. Nat Genet 1996;13(2):161–166.

7. Luo DF, Bui MM, Muir A, Maclaren NK, Thomson G, She JX. Affected-sib-pair mapping of a novel susceptibility gene to insulin-dependent diabetes mellitus (IDDM8) on chromosome 6q25–q27. Am J Hum Genet 1995; 57(4):911-919.

8. Bailey-Wilson JE, Bamba V. Sib-pair linkage analyses of Alzheimer's disease. Genet Epidemiol 1993;10(6):371–376.

9. Pericak-Vance MA, Haines, JL. Genetic susceptibility to Alzhiemer disease. Trends Genet 1995;11(12):504–508.

10. Bouchard C. Genetics of human obesity: recent results from linkage studies. J Nutr 1997;127(9):1887S–1890S.

11. Chagnon YC, Perusse L, Bouchard C. Familial aggregation of obesity, candidate genes and quantitative trait loci. Curr Opin Lipidol 1997;8(4):205–211.

12. Williams GH, Fisher ND. Genetic approach to diagnostic and therapeutic decisions in human hypertension [see comments]. Curr Opin Nephrol Hypertens 1997;6(2);199–204.

13. Lifton RP. Genetic determinants of human hypertension. Proc Natl Acad Sci USA 1995;92(19):8545–8551.

14. Risch P, Merikangas K. The future of genetic studies of complex human disease. Science 1996;273:1516–1517.

15. Becker KG. Comparative Genetics of type 1 diabetes and autoimmune disease: common loci, common pathways? Diabetes 1999;48(7):1353–1358.

16. Myers AJ, Goate AM. The genetics of late-onset Alzheimer's disease. Curr Opin Neurol 2001;14(4):433–440.

17. Hutchinson J. Symmetrical central choroido-retinal disease occuring in senile persons. R Lond Ophthalmic Hosp Rep 1876;8:231–244.

18. Sibert A, Goldgar D. Relationship between family history, family size, and penetrace: a population simulation. Am J Hum Genet 1997;61(4):A212.

19. Bressler SB, Maguire MG, Bressler NM, Fine SL. Relationship of drusen and abnormalities of the retinal pigment epithelium to the prognosis of neovascular macular degeneration. The Macular Photocoagulation Study Group. Arch Ophthalmol 1990;108(10):1442–1447.

20. Kelin R, Davis MD, Magli YL, Segal P, Klein BE, and Hubbard L. The Wisconsin age-related maculopathy grading system. Ophthalmology 1991;98(7):1128–1134.

21. Klein R, Klein BEK, Linton KLP. Prevalence of age-related maculopathy. Ophthalmology 1992; 99(6):933-943.

22. Bird AC, Bressler NM, Bressler SB, Chisholm IH, Coscas G, Davis MD, PT de Jong, Klaver CC, Klein BE, Klein R, et al. An international classification and grading system for age-related maculopathy and age-related macular degeneration. The International ARM Epidemiological Study Group. Surv Ophthalmol 1995; 39(5):367–374.

23. Age-Related Eye Disease Study Manual of Procedures. Bethesda, MD: National Eye Institute, 1992.

24. De La Paz MA, Pericak-Vance, MA JL, Hanies Seddon JM. Phenotypic heterogeneity in families with age-related macular degeneration. Am J Ophthalmol 1997;124(3):331–343.

25. Preferred Practice Pattern: Age-Related Macular Degeneration. San Francisco: American Academy of Ophthalmology, 1994.

26. Keverline MR, Mah TS, Keverline PO, and Gorin MB. A practice-based survey of familial age-related maculopathy. Ophthalmic Genet 1998;19(1):19–26.

27. Curcio CA, Medeiros NE, and Millican, CL. The Alabama Age-Related Macular Degeneration Grading System for donor eyes. Invest Ophthalmol Vis Sci 1998;39(7):1085–1096.

28. The Age-Related Eye Disease Study (AREDS): design implications AREDS report no. 1. The Age-Related Eye Disease Study Research Group. Control Clin Trials 1999;20(6):573–600.

29. Chumbley LC. Impressions of eye diseases among Rhodesian blacks in Mashonaland. S Afr Med J 1977;52:316–318.

30. Gregor Z, Joffe L. Senile macular changes in the black African. Br J Ophthalmol 1978;62:547–550.
31. Klein BE, Klein R. Cataracts and macular degeneration in older Americans. Arch Ophthalmol 1982;100:571–573.
32. Sommer A, Tielsch JM, Katz J, Quigley HA, Gottsch JD, Javitt JC, Martone JF, Royall RM, Witt KA, Ezrine S. Racial differences in the cause-specific prevalence of blindness in East Baltimore. N Engl J Med 1991;325:1412–1417.
33. Pieramici DJ, Bressler NM, Bressler SB, Schachat AP. Choroidal neovascularization in black patients. Arch Ophthalmol 1994;112(8):1043–1046.
34. Capone AJ Wallace RT, Meredith TA. Symptomatic choroidal neovascularization in blacks. Arch Ophthalmol 1994;112(8):1091–1097.
35. Ponte F, Giuffre G, Giammanco R. Prevalence and causes of blindness and low vision in the Casteldaccia Eye Study. Graefes Arch Clin Exp Ophthalmol 1994;232(8):469–472.
36. Schachat AP, Hyman L, Leske MC, Connell AMS, Wu SY, Group BES. Features of age-related macular degeneration in a black population. Arch Ophthalmol 1995;113:728–735.
37. Klein R, Rowland ML, Harris MI. Racial/ethnic differences in age-related maculopathy. Third National Health and Nutrition Examination Survey. Ophthalmology 1995;102(3):371–381.
38. Cruickshanks KJ, Hamman RF, Klein R, Nondahl DM, Shetterly, SM. The prevalence of age-related maculopathy by geographic region and ethnicity. The Colorado-Wisconsin Study of Age-Related Maculopathy. Arch Ophthalmol 1997;115(2):242–250.
39. Das BN, Thompson JR, Patel R, Rosenthal AR. The prevalence of eye disease in Leicester: a comparison of adults of Asian and European descent. J R Soc Med 1994; 87(4):219–222.
40. Ho T, Law NM, Goh LG, Yoong T. Eye diseases in the elderly in Singapore [see comments]. Singapore Med J 1997;38(4):149–155.
41. Jampol LM, Tielsch, J. Race, macular degeneration, and the Macular Photocoagulation Study [editorial]. Arch Ophthalmol 1992; 110(12):1699–700.
42. Chang TS, Hay D, Courtright P. Age-related macular degeneration in Chinese-Canadians. Can J Ophthalmol 1999;34(5):266–271.
43. Lim JI, Kwok A, Wilson DK. Symptomatic age-related macular degeneration in Asian patients. Retina 1998;18(5):435–438.
44. Friedman DS, Katz J, Bressler NM, Rahmani B, Tielsch JM. Racial differences in the prevalence of age-related macular degeneration: the Baltimore Eye Survey. Ophthalmology 1999;106(6):1049–1055.
45. Rosenberg T. Prevalence of blindness caused by senile macular degeneration in Greenland. Arctic Med Res 1987;46(2):64–70.
46. Rosenberg T. Prevalence and causes of blindness in Greenland. Arctic Med Res 1987;46(1):13–7.
47. Yuzawa M, Tamakoshi A, Kawamura T, Ohno Y, Uyama M, Honda T. Report on the nationwide epidemiological survey of exudative age-related macular degeneration in Japan. Int Ophthalmol 1997;21(1):1–3.
48. Evans K, Bird AC. The genetics of complex ophthalmic disorders. Br J Ophthalmol 1996;80(8):763–768.
49. Evans J, Wormald R. Is the incidence of registrable age-related macular degeneration increasing? Br J Ophthalmol 1996;80:9–14.
50. Francois J. The differential diagnosis of tapetoretinal degenerations. Arch Ophthalmol 1958;59:88–120.
51. Francosis J. L'heredite des degenerescences macularies siniles. Arch Ophthalmol 1969;29:899–902.
52. Bradley AE. Dystrophy of the macula. Am J Ophthalmol 1966;61(1):1–24.
53. Gass JDM. Drusen and disciform macular detachment and degeneration. Arch Ophthalmol 1973;90:206–217.
54. Hyman LG, Lilienfeld AM, FD Ferris Fine SL. Senile macular degeneration: a case-control study. Am J Epidemiol 1983;118(2):213–227.

55. Piguet B, Wells JA, Palmvang IB, Wormald R, Chisholm IH., Bird AC. Age-related Bruch's membrane change: a clinical study of the relative role of heredity and environment. Br J Ophthalmol 1993;77(7):400–403.

56. Silvestri G, Johnston PB, Hughes AE. Is genetic predisposition an important risk factor in age-related macular degeneration? Eye 1994;8(Pt 5):564–568.

57. Heiba IM, Elston RC, Klein BE, Klein, R. Sibling correlations and segregation analysis of age-related maculopathy: the Beaver Dam Eye Study. Genet Epidemiol 1994;11(1): 51–67.

58. Seddon JM, Ajani UA, Mitchell BD. Familial aggregation of age-related maculopathy. Am J Ophthalmol 1997;123(2):199–206.

59. Smith W, Mitchell P. Family history and age-related maculopathy: the Blue Mountains Eye Study. Aust NZ J Ophthalmol 1998;26(3):203–206.

60. Klaver CC, Wolfs RC, Assink JJ, van Duijn CM, Hofman A, de Jong PT. Genetic risk of age-related maculopathy. Population-based familial aggregation study. Arch Ophthalmol 1998;116(12):1645–1651.

61. Yoshida A, Yoshida M, Yoshida S, Shiose S, Hiroishi G, Ishibashi T. Familial cases with age-related macular degeneration. Jpn J Ophthalmol 2000;44(3):290–295.

62. Gibson JM., Shaw DE, Rosenthal AR. Senile cataract and senile macular degeneration: an investigation into possible risk factors. Trans Ophthalmol Soc UK 1986;105(Pt 4): 463–468.

63. Waardenburg PJ. Twin research in ophthalmology. Doc Ophthalmol 1950;4:154–199.

64. Waardenburg PJ. Two sets of aged female monozygotic twins who both suffered from senile macular dystrophy. Eighteenth International Congress of Ophthalmology: abstracts of reports, symposia, discussions, and free communications. Vol. International Congress Series #20. Amsterdam: Excerpta Medica Foundation, 1958, c27.

65. Melrose MA, Magargal LE, Lucier AC. Identical twins with subretinal neovascularization complicating senile macular degeneration. Ophthalmic Surg 1985;16(10):648–651.

66. Meyers SM, Zachary AA. Monozygotic twins with age-related macular degeneration. Arch Ophthalmol 1988;106:651–653.

67. Dosso AA, Bovet J. Monozygotic twin brothers with age-related macular degeneration. Ophthalmologica 1992;205(1):24–28.

68. Klein ML, Mauldin WM, Stoumbos VD. Heredity and age-related macular degeneration. Observations in monozygotic twins. Arch Ophthalmol 1994;112(7):932-937.

69. Meyers SM. A twin study on age-related macular degeneration. Trans Am Ophthalmol Soc 1994;92:775–843.

70. Meyers SM, Greene T, Gutman FA. A twin study of age-related macular degeneration. Arch Ophthalmol 1995;120:757–766.

71. Gottfredsdottir MS, Sverrisson T, Musch DC, Stefansson E. Age-related macular degeneration in monozygotic twins and their spouses in Iceland. Acta Ophthalmol Scand 1999;77(4):442–425.

72. Hammond CJ, Webster AR, Snieder H, Bird AC, Gilbert CE, Spector TD. Genetic influence on early age-related macular degeneration: a population–based twin study. Ophthalmology 2002;109:730–736.

73. Knobloch WH, Leavenworth NM, Bouchard TJ, Eckert ED. Eye findings in twins reared apart. Ophthalmic Paediatr Genet 1985;5(1):59–66.

74. Klein ML, Schultz DW, Edwards A, Matise TC, Rust K, Berselli CB, Trzupek K, Weleber RG, Ott J, Wirtz MK, Acott, TS. Age-related macular degeneration. Clinical features in a large family and linkage to chromosome 1q. Arch Ophthalmol 1998;116(8):1082–1088.

75. Weeks DE, Lange K. The affected-pedigree-member method of linkage analysis. Am J Hum Genet 1988;42(2):315–326.

76. Lander ES, Schork NJ. Genetic dissection of complex traits. Science 1994;265:2037–2048.

77. Weeks DE, Harby, LD. The affected-pedigree-member method: power to detect linkage. Hum Hered 1995;45(1):13–24.

78. Davis S, Goldin LR, Weeks DE. imIBD: A powerful robust nonparametric method for detecting linkage in general pedigrees. In: Pawlowitzki I-H, Edwards JH, Thompson EA, eds. Genetic Mapping of Disease Genes. Academic Press: San Diego, 1997:193–203.

79. Davis S, Weeks DE. Comparison of nonparametric statistics for detection of linkage in nuclear families: single-marker evaluation. Am J Hum Genet 1997;61(6):1431–1444.

80. Weeks DE, Conley YP, Mah TS, Paul TO, Morse L, Ngo-Chang J, Dailey JP, Ferrell RE, Gorin MB. A full genome scan for age-related maculopathy. Hum Mol Genet 2000;9(9):1329–1349.

81. Brown DL., Gorin MB, Weeks DE. Efficient strategies for genomic searching using the affected-pedigree-member method of linkage analysis. Am J Hum Genet 1994;54(3):544–552.

82. Weeks DE, Conley P, Tsai HJ, Mah TS, Rosenfeld PJ, Paul TO, Eller AW, Morse LS, Dailey JP, Ferrell RE, Gorin MB. Age-related maculopathy: an expanded genome-wide scan with evidence of susceptibility loci within the 1q31 and 17q25 regions. Am J Ophthalmol 2001;132(S):682–692.

83. de La Paz MA, Pericak-Vance MA, Lennon F, Haines JL, Seddon JM. Exclusion of TIMP3 as a candidate locus in age-related macular degeneration. Invest Ophthalmol Vis Sci 1997;38(6):1060-1065.

84. de La Paz MA, Haines JL, Heinis R, Agarwal R, Lennon F, Pericak-Vance MA. Linkage studies of the Mallatia Leventinese (ML) locus to age-related macular degeneration. Am J Hum Genet 1997; 61(4):A273.

85. Gu. SM, Thompson DA, Srikumari CR, Lorenz B, Finckh U, Nicoletti A, Murthy KR, Rathmann M, Kumaramanickavel G, Denton MJ, Gal A. Mutations in RPE65 cause autosomal recessive childhood-onset severe retinal dystrophy. Nat Genet 1997;17(2)194-197.

86. Marlhens F, Bareil C, Griffoin JM, Zrenner E, Amalric P, Eliaou C, Liu SY, Harris E, Redmond TM, Arnaud B, Claustres M, Hamel CP. Mutations in RPE65 cause Leber's congenital amaurosis [letter]. Nat Genet 1997;17(2):139–141.

87. Freund CL, Gregory-Evans CY, Furukawa T, Papaioannu M, Looser J, Ploder L, Bellingham J, Ng D, Herbrick JA, Duncan A, Scherer SW, Tsui LC, Loutradis-Anagnostou A, Jacobson SG, Cepko CL, Bhattacharya SS, McInnes RR, Cone-rod dystrophy due to mutations in a novel photoreceptor-specific homeobox gene (CRX) essential for maintenance of the photoreceptor. Cell 1997;91(4):543–553.

88. Freund CL Wang QL, Chen S, Muskat BL, Wiles CD, Sheffield VC, Jacobson SG, McInnes RR, Zack DJ, Stone EM. De novo mutations in the CRX homeobox gene associated with Leber congenital amaurosis [letter]. Nat Genet 1998;18(4):311–312.

89. Nichols BE, Drack AV, Vandenburgh K, Kimura AE, Sheffield VC, Stone EM. A 2 base pair deletion in the RDS gene associated with butterfly-shaped pigment dystrophy of the fovea [published erratum appears in Hum Mol Genet 1993;2(8):1347]. Hum Mol Genet 1993;2(5):601–603.

90. Felbor U, Schilling H, Weber BHF. Adult vitelliform macular dystrophy is frequently associated with mutations in the peripherin/RDS gene. Hum Mutat 1997;10:301–309.

91. Dryja TP, Berson EL, Rao V Oprian DD. Heterozygous missense mutation in the rhodopsin gene as a cause of congenital stationary nightblindness. Nat Genet 1993;4:280–283.

92. Cremers FP, van de Pol DJ, van Driel M, den Hollander AI, van Haren FJ, Knoers NV, Tijmes N, Bergen AA, Rohrschneider K, Blankenagel A, Pinckers AJ, Deutman AF, Hoyng CB, Autosomal recessive retinitis pigmentosa and cone-rod dystrophy caused by splice site mutations in the Stargardt's disease gene ABCR. Hum Mol Genet 1998;7(3):355–362.

93. Martinez-Mir A, Paloma E, Allikmets R, Ayuso C, del Rio T, Dean M, Vilageliu L, Gonzalez-Duarte R, Balcells S. Retinitis pigmentosa caused by a homozygous mutation in the Stargardt disease gene ABCR. Nat Genet 1998;18(1)11–12.

94. Zhang K, Kniazeva M, Han M, Li W, Yu Z, Yang Z, Li Y, Metzker ML, Allikmets R, Zack DJ, Kakuk LE, Lagali PS, Wong PW, MacDonald IM, Sieving PA, Figueroa DJ, Austin CP, Gould RJ, Ayyagari R, Petrukhin K. A 5-bp deletion in ELOVL4 is associated with two related forms of autosomal dominant macular dystrophy. Nat Genet 2001;27(1):89–93.

95. Stone EM, Fingert JH, Alward WLM, Nguyen TD, Polansky JR, Sunden SLF, Nishimura D, Clark AF, Nystuen A, Nichols BE, Mackey DA, Ritch R, Kalenak JW, Craven ER, Sheffield VC. Identification of a gene that causes primary open angle glaucoma [see comments]. Science 1997;275(5300):668–670.

96. Allikmets R, Shroyer NF, Singh N, Seddon JM, Lewis RA, Bernstein PS, Peiffer A, Zabriskie NA, Li Y, Hutchinson A, Dean M, Lupski JR, Leppert M. Mutation of the Stargardt disease gene (ABCR) in age-related macular degeneration [see comments]. Science 1997;277 (5333):1805-1807.

97. Lewis RA, Lupski JR. Macular degeneration: the emerging genetics. Hosp Pract (Off Ed) 2000; 35(6):41-50,56–58.

98. Dryja TP, Briggs CE, Berson EL, Rosenfeld PJ, Abitbol M. ABCR gene and age-related macular degeneration (Technical Comment). Science 1998;279:p1107.

99. Klaver CCW, Assink JJM, Bergen AAB, van Duijn CM. ABCR gene and macular degeneration (Technical Comment). Science 1998;279:1107.

100. Dean M, Allikmets R, Shroyer NF, Lupski JR, Lewis RA, Leppert M, Bernstein PS, Seddon JM. ABCR gene and age-related macular degeneration (Technical Comment). Science 1998;279:1107.

101. Stone EM, Webster AR, Vandenburgh K, LM Streb, Hockey RR, Lotery AJ, Sheffield VC. Allelic variation in ABCR associated with Stargardt disease but not age-related macular degeneration [letter]. Nat Genet 1998;20(4):328–329.

102. Kuroiwa S, Kojima H, Kikuchi T, Yoshimura N. ATP binding cassette transporter retina genotypes and age related macular degeneration: an analysis on exudative non-familial Japanese patients. Br J Ophthalmol 1999;83(5):613–615.

103. De La Paz MA, Guy VK, Abou-Donias, Heinis R, Brachen B, Vance JM, Gilbert JR, Gass JD. Haines JL, Pericak-Vance MA. Analysis of the Stargardt disease gene (ABCR) in age-related macular degeneration. Ophthalmology 1999;106(8):1531–1536.

104. Fuse N, Suzuki T, Wada Y, Yoshida M, Shimura M, Abe T, Nakazawa M, Tamai M. Molecular genetic analysis of ABCR gene in Japanese dry form age-related macular degeneration. Jpn J Ophthalmol 2000;44(3):245–249.

105. Rivera A, White K, Stohr H, Steiner K, Hemmrich N, Grimm T, Jurklies B, Lorenz B, Scholl HP, Apfelstedt-Sylla E, Weber BH. A comprehensive survey of sequence variation in the ABCA4 (ABCR) gene in Stargardt disease and age-related macular degeneration. Am J Hum Genet 2000;67(4):800–813.

106. Guymer RH, Heon E, Lotery AJ, Munier FL, Schorderet DF, Baird PN, McNeil RJ, Haines H, Sheffield VC, Stone EM. Variation of codons 1961 and 2177 of the Stargardt disease gene is not associated with age-related macular degeneration. Arch Ophthalmol 2001;119(5):745–751.

107. Allikmets R. Further evidence for an association of ABCR alleles with age-related macular degeneration. The International ABCR Screening Consortium. Am J Hum Genet 2000;67(2):487–491.

108. Allikmets R. Simple and complex ABCR: genetic predisposition to retinal disease. Am J Hum Genet 2000;67(4):793–799.

109. Long AD, Langley CH. The power of association studies to detect the contribution of candidate genetic loci to variation in complex traits. Genome Res 1999; 9(8):720–731.

110. Allikmets R. Molecular genetics of age-related macular degeneration: current status. Eur J Ophthalmol 1999;9(4):255–265.

111. Lewis RA, Shroyer, Singh N, Allikmets R, Hutchinson A, Li Y, Jupski JR, Leppert M, Dean M. Genotype/phenotype analysis of a photoreceptor-specific ATP-binding cassette transporter gene, ABCR, in Stargardt disease. Am J Hum Genet 1999;64(2):422–434.

112. Shroyer NF, Lewis RA, Allikmets R, Singh N, Dean M, Leppert M, Lupski JR. The rod photoreceptor ATP-binding cassette transporter gene, ABCR, and retinal disease: from monogenic to multifactorial. Vision Res 1999;39(15):2537–2544.

113. Simonelli F, Testa F, de Crechio GE, Rinaldi E, Hutchinson A, Atkinson A, Dean M, D'Urso, Allikmets R. New ABCR mutations and clinical phenotype in Italian patients with Stargardt diseas. Invest Ophthalmol Vis Sci 2000;41(3):892–897.

114. Souied EH, Ducroq D, Gerber S, Gherber I, Rozet JM, Perrault I, Munnich A, Dufier JL, Coscas G, Soubrane G, Kaplan J, Age-related macular degeneration in grandparents of patients with Stargardt disease: genetic study. Am J Ophthalmol 1999;128(2):173–178.

115. Souied EH, Ducroq D, Rozet JM, Gerber S, Perrault I, Munnich A, Coscas G, Soubrane G, Kaplan J, ABCR gene analysis in familial exudative age–related macular degeneration. Invest Ophthalmol Vis Sci 2000;41(1):244–247.

116. Zhang K, Kniazeva M, Hutchinson A, Han M, Dean M, Allikmets R. The ABCR gene in recessive and dominant Stargardt diseases: a genetic pathway in macular degeneration [In Process Citation]. Genomics 1999;60(2):234–237.

117. Sun H, Nathans J. ABCR: rod photoreceptor-specific ABC transporter responsible for Stargardt disease. Methods Enzymol 2000;315(4):879–897.

118. Sun H, Molday RS, Nathans J. Retinal stimulates ATP hydrolysis by purified and reconstituted ABCR, the photoreceptor-specific ATP-binding cassette transporter responsible for Stargardt disease. J Biol Chem 1999;274(12):8269–8281.

119. Sun H, Smallwood PM, Nathans J. Biochemical defects in ABCR protein variants associated with human retinopathies. Nat Genet 2000;26(2):242–246.

120. Stone EM, Lotery AJ, Munier FL, Heon E, Piguet B, Guymer RH, Vandenburgh K, Cousin P, Nishimura O, Swiderski RE, Silvestri G, Mackey DA, Hageman GS, Bird AC, Sheffield VC, Schorderet DF. A single EFEMP1 mutation associated with both Malattia Leventinese and Doyne honeycomb retinal dystrophy. Nat Genet 1999;22(2):199–202.

121. Souied EH. Ducroq D, Rozet JM, Gerber G, Perrault I, Munnich A, Coscas G, Soubrane G, Kaplan J. Analysis of the VMD2 and the EFEMP1 genes in familial cases of exudative age-related macular degeneration. Invest Ophthalmol Vis Sci 2001;42(4):S448.

122. Petrukhin K Koisti MJ, Bakall B, Li W, Xie G, Marknell T, Sandgren O, Forsman K, Holmgren G, Andreasson S, Vujic M, Bergen AA, McGarty-Dugan V, Figueroa D, Austin CP, Metzker ML, Caskey CT, Wadelius C. Identification of the gene responsible for Best macular dystrophy. Nat Genet 1998;19(3):241–247.

123. Marquardt A, Stohr H, Passmore LA, Kramer F, Rivera A, Weber BH. Mutations in a novel gene, VMD2, encoding a protein of unknown properties cause juvenile-onset vitelliform macular dystrophy (Best's disease). Hum Mol Genet 1998;7(9):1517–1525.

124. Allikmets R, Seddon JM, Bernstein PS, Hutchinson A, Atkinson A, Sharma S, Gerrard B, W Li, Metzker ML, Wadelius C, Caskey CT, Dean M, Petrukhin K. Evaluation of the Best gene in patients with age-related macular degeneration and other maculopathies. Hum Genet 1999;104(6):449–453.

125. Kramer F, White K, Pauleikhoff D, Gehrig A, Passmore L, Rivera A, Rudolph G, Kellner U, Andrassi M, Lorenz B, Rohrschneider K, Blankenagel A, Jurklies B, Schilling H, Schutt F, Holz FG, Weber BH, Mutations in the VMD2 gene are associated with juvenile-onset vitelliform macular dystrophy (Best disease) and adult vitelliform macular dystrophy but not age-related macular degeneration. Eur J Hum Genet 2000. 8(4):286–292.

126. Lotery AJ, Munier FL, Fishman GA, Weleber RG, Jacobson SG, Affatigato LM, Nichols BE, Schorderet DF, Sheffield VC, Stone, EM. Allelic variation in the VMD2 gene in Best disease and age-related macular degeneration. Invest Ophthalmol Vis Sci 2000;41(6):1291–1296.

127. De La Paz MA, Pericak-Vance MA, Lennon F, Hanies JL, Seddon JM. Exclusion of TIMP3 as a candidate locus in age-related macular degeneration. Invest Ophthalmol Vis Sci 1997;38(6):1060–1065.

128. Felbor U, Doepner D, Schneider U, Zrenner E, Weber, BH. Evaluation of the gene encoding the tissue inhibitor of mctalloproteinases-3 in various maculopathies. Invest Ophthalmol Vis Sci 1997;38(6):1054–1059.

129. Shastry BS Trese, MT. Evaluation of the peripherin/RDS gene as a candidate gene in families with age-related macular degeneration. Ophthalmologica 1999;213(3):165–170.

130. Baird PN, Tomlin BM, McNeil RM. Weih LM, McCarty CA, Cain M, Guymer RM. Do single nucleotide polymorphisms (SNPs) in the peripherin/RDS gene play a role in AMD? Invest Ophthalmol Vis Sci 2001:42(4):S638.

131. Kakuk LE, Zhang, K Swaroop A,Yashar BM, Yang Z, Y Li, Petrunkhin K, Sieving PA, Ayyagari R, Allikmets R. Analysis of the ELOVL4 gene in patients with AMD and dominant macular dystrophies. Invest Ophthalmol Vis Sci 2001;42(4):S638.

132. Souied EH Benlian P, Amouyel P, Feingold J, Lagarde JP, Munnich A, Kaplan J, Coscas G, Soubrane, G. The epsilon4 allele of the apolipoprotein E gene as a potential protective factor for exudative age-related macular degeneration. Am J Ophthalmol 1998;125(3):353–359.

133. Klaver CC, Kliffen M, van Duijn CM, Hofman A, Cruts, M Grobbee DE, van Broeckhoven C, de Jong, PT. Genetic association of apolipoprotein E with age-related macular degeneration. Am J Hum Genet 1998;63(1):200–206.

134. Pang CP, Baum L, Chan WM, Lau TC, Poon PM, Lam DS. The apolipoprotein E epsilin4 allele is unlikely to be a major risk factor of age-related macular degeneration in Chinese. Ophthalmologica 2000:214(4):289–291.

135. Schmidt S, Saunders AM, de La Paz MA, Postel EA, Heinis RM, Agarwal A, Scott WK, Gilbert JR, McDowell JG, Bazyk A, Gass JD, Haines JL, Pericak-Vance MA, Association of the Apolipoprotein E gene with age-related macular degeneration: possible effect modification by family history, age, and gender. Mol Vis 2000;6:287–293.

136. Klaver CCW, van Leeuwen R, van Duijn CM, Slooter A, Hofman A, de Jong PT. Apolipoprotein E polymorphism and drusen, pigmentary changes, and late age-related maculopathy. The Rotterdam Study. Invest Ophthalmol Vis Sci 2001;42(4):S310.

137. Pericak-Vance MA, Schmidt S, Gorin MB, Haines JL, Ferrell R, Klaver CC, Postel EA, van Duijn CM, Saunders AM, Weeks DE. Association of the apolipoprotein E (APOE) gene with age-related macular degeneration (AMD). Invest Ophthalmol Vis Sci 2001;42(4):S311.

138. Klaver CC, Kliffen M, van Duijn CM, Hofman A, Cruts M, Grobbee DE, van Broeckhoven C, de Jong PT. Genetic association of apolipoprotein E with age-related macular degeneration [published erratum appears in Am J Hum Genet 1998;63(4):1252]. Am J Hum Genet 1998; 63(1):200–206.

139. Kimura K, Isashiki Y, Sonoda S, Kakiuchi-Matsumoto T, Ohba N. Genetic association of manganese superoxide dismutase with exudative age-related macular degeneration. Am J Ophthalmol 2000;130(6):769–773.

140. Ohba N. Introduction to genetics in ophthalmology, value of family studies. Jpn J Ophthalmol 2000:44(3):320–321.

141. Blumenkranz MS, Russell SR, Robey MG, Kott-Blumenkranz R, Penneys N. Risk factors in age-related maculopathy complicated by choroidal neovascularization. Ophthalmology 1986;93(5):552–558.

142. Kajiwara K, Berson EL, Dryja TP. Digenic retinitis pigmentosa due to mutations at the unlinked peripherin/RDS and ROM1 loci. Science 1994;264(5165):1604–1608.

143. Berson EL, Rosner B, Sandberg MA, Hayes KC, Nicholson BW, Weigel-DiFranco, Willett W. A randomized trial of vitamin A and vitamin E supplementation for retinitis pigmentosa. Arch Ophthalmol 1993;111.

144. Sandberg MA, Weigel-DiFranco C, Rosner B, Berson, EL. The relationship between visual field size and electroretinogram amplitude in retinitis pigmentosa. Invest Ophthalmol Vis Sci 1996;37(8):1693–1698.

145. Jacobson SG, Cideciyan AV, Regunath G, Rodriguez FJ, Vandenburgh K, Sheffield VC, Stone EM. Night blindness is Sorsby's fundus dystrophy reversed by vitamin A. Nat Genet 1995:11(1):27–32.

146. Kaiser-Kupfer MI, Caruso RC, Valle D. Gyrate atrophy of the choroid and retina. Long-term reduction of ornithine slows retinal degeneration. Arch Ophthalmol 1991;109(11):1539–1548.

147. Runge P, Muller DP, McAllister J, Calver D, Lloyd JK, Taylor D. Oral vitamin E supplements can prevent the retinopathy of abetalipoproteinaemia. Br J Ophthalmol 1986;70(3):166–173.

148. Mata NL, Tzekov RT, Liu X, Weng J, Birch DG, Travis GH. Delayed dark adaptation and lipofusein accumulation in aber $+/-$ mica: implications for involvement of *ABCR* in age-related macular degeneration. Invest Ophthalmol 2001;42(8):1685–1690.

25

Retinal Pigment Epithelial Cell Transplantation in Age-Related Macular Degeneration

Lucian V. Del Priore and Tongalp H. Tezel
Columbia University, New York, New York

Henry J. Kaplan
University of Louisville, Louisville, Kentucky

I. INTRODUCTION

Age-related macular degeneration (AMD) is the leading cause of blindness in the United States and Western Europe (1). The natural history of subfoveal neovascularization in AMD is poor, as loss of six lines or more of best-corrected visual acuity will occur in 30–50% of patients with ill-defined or well-defined subfoveal neovascularization within 2 years (2–4). The poor visual outcome for patients with subfoveal neovascularization in AMD has led to the exploration of several therapeutic modalities for the treatment of this condition. Subfoveal laser photocoagulation was the first treatment shown to be better than natural history in a randomized clinical trial for a select subgroup of eyes with AMD (5,6), but many ophthalmologists did not adopt this treatment strategy because subfoveal thermal laser results in a significant postoperative reduction in visual acuity and the recurrence rate is high (5). Photodynamic therapy (PDT) can halt or reverse visual loss in patients who have subfoveal choroidal neovascularization that is >50% classic, but most patients with wet AMD have lesions that are not PDT-eligible (7,8). Other alternatives have been explored including radiation therapy (9,11), retinal translocation (12–15), pharmacological therapy with interferon, thalidomide, or other drugs (16–18), and subfoveal surgery (19–26).

The role of subfoveal surgery alone in the management of exudative AMD is being investigated in the Subfoveal Surgery Trial sponsored by the National Eye Institute (27,28). A definitive determination of whether subfoveal surgery is better than observation awaits the results of this trial. However, careful examination of nonrandomized series suggests that the results of subfoveal surgery alone for wet AMD are less than ideal. Subfoveal surgery does not lead to significant visual improvement in most patients with AMD and recovery of vision to better than 20/100 is uncommon (19–22). It is likely that several factors are responsible for the lack of visual improvement seen after submacular surgery for wet AMD, including removal of the native retinal pigment epithelium (RPE) with the subfoveal choroidal neovascular complex (29). Removal of the native RPE may lead to the development or progression of subfoveal choriocapillaris atrophy (29), and successful RPE transplantation may prevent or reverse choriocapillaris atrophy. Transplantation of the RPE has been attempted in small numbers of patients undergoing surgical excision of subfoveal neovascularization and in a few patients with nonexudative AMD (30–40). We herein review the current status of RPE transplantation for the management of AMD, including the clinical results that have been obtained in small numbers of patients who have undergone this procedure. We will also discuss companion laboratory studies that give us insight into the hurdles that must be overcome before significant visual recovery can occur after RPE transplantation.

II. RATIONALE FOR RPE TRANSPLANTATION IN AMD

In 1991, Thomas and Kaplan reported two patients who experienced significant visual improvement after surgical excision of subfoveal choroidal neovascularization from presumed ocular histoplasmosis syndrom (POHS) (24). One patient improved from 20/200 preoperatively to 20/40, whereas the other patient improved from 20/200 to 20/25. de Juan and Machemer (35) had previously performed diskiform scar excision in four patients with end-stage AMD, but the report by Thomas and Kaplan was the first to demonstrate that excellent visual acuity was possible after submacular surgery. Since these initial publications, several authors have reported small, uncontrolled series of patients undergoing submacular surgery for AMD (19–26, 36–39). At the current time, the exact role of submacular surgery in the management of choroidal neovascularization is being evaluated as part of the Subfoveal Surgery Trial, and determining whether subfoveal surgery is better than the natural history awaits the results of this trial (27,28). However, examination of the results of nonrandomized studies of submacular surgery suggests that significant visual improvement is limited after submacular surgery for AMD, and that RPE removal may be an important factor in limiting postoperative visual recovery.

Thomas and co-workers reported that the visual acuity improved in 5/41 AMD eyes (12%) after submacular surgery but a final acuity of 20/40 or better was achieved in only 5% of the eyes (22). We previously reported 40 patients with subfoveal choroidal neovascularization secondary to AMD (29). All patients except one had a postoperative Snellen visual acuity of 20/100 or worse. Roth et al. also reported 38 patients with AMD and well-demarcated membranes on fluorescein angiography that underwent submacular surgery (36). Three months after surgery, 7/38 eyes improved (18%), 8/38 were worse (21%), and 23/38 were unchanged (60%). The authors concluded that submacular surgery should not be routinely offered to patients with AMD using the current technology. Merrill et al. reported 64 AMD patients undergoing submacular surgery assisted by the injection of tissue plasminogen activator (37). The final visual acuity was improved in 19/64 eyes (30%), stable in 27 eyes (42%), and worse by three or more lines in 18 eyes (28%). Again, less than 10% of eyes achieved a final vision of 20/100 or better. Lewis and co-workers performed a randomized, double-blind clinical trial to determine whether injection of tissue plasminogen activator at the time of subfoveal membrane removal was helpful (38). Eighty eyes of 80 patients with subfoveal choroidal neovascularization secondary to AMD were randomized to subretinal injection of tissue plasminogen activator or balanced salt solution before membrane excision. Since best-corrected postoperative visual acuity was 20/320 in both groups, the authors concluded that use of this drug before subfoveal surgery is of no visual anatomical benefit in AMD patients. Thus, nonrandomized case series of patients undergoing submacular surgery for AMD demonstrate that recovery of central visual acuity to better than 20/100 is unusual in AMD eyes. Early results from the Submacular Surgery Trial for recurrent subfoveal neovascularization reinforce this observation (27,28).

The visual results after surgery for POHS are clearly better than the results after submacular surgery for AMD. Holekamp et al. reported 117 patients who underwent surgical removal of subfoveal neovascularization in POHS with follow-up of 18 months (26). In this study, 35% of patients achieved a postoperative visual acuity of 20/40 or better and 40% had improvement of three or more Snellen lines after surgery with a recurrence rate of 44%. Berger et al. reported 63 eyes of 62 patients undergoing surgery for subfoveal choroidal neovascularization in POHS (25). The median patient age was 42 years (range 16–68) and the median follow-up time was 24 months (range 6–48). Visual acuity improved by two or more lines in 24/63 (38%), was unchanged in 21/63 (33%), and was worse in 18/63 (29%); 11/63 eyes (17%) achieved a final vision of 20/50 or better. Recurrence of the choroidal neovascular membrane occurred in 24/63 eyes (38%) but was less common in patients who had not undergone previous laser photocoagulation (29%) than in patients receiving prior laser treatment (47%). Postoperative complications included macular striae in 4/63 (6%), rhegmatogenous retinal detachment in 2/63 (3%), peripheral retinal tear in 1/63 (1.6%), and progression of cataract in 19/63 (30%). No patients required cataract extraction for visually significant cataract during the follow-up period.

Thus, evidence from nonrandomized case series demonstrates that there is a significant difference in the visual prognosis after submacular surgery for patients with AMD versus POHS. Many factors could be responsible for this observed difference, including advanced patient age in AMD, disease within Bruch's membrane in AMD, the size of the choroidal neovascular complex (larger in AMD eyes compared to POHS), the location of the ingrowth site, and the relationship of the choroidal neovascular membrane to the native RPE (39). Patients with POHS and other disorders may have a better prognosis because the choroidal neovascular membrane lies anterior to the RPE and can thus be removed while leaving the native RPE intact (39). However, in AMD eyes the choroidal neovascular complex is frequently deep to the native RPE, so surgical membrane excision denudes Bruch's membrane of native RPE.

The consequences of RPE removal during submacular surgery are significant because removal of the native RPE leads to progressive choriocapillaris atrophy and limits visual recovery after submacular surgery (40–43). The subfoveal choriocapillaris can be perfused 1–2 weeks after submacular surgery in AMD eyes but become nonperfused without further surgery or laser photocoagulation (40). Thach et al. examined the choroidal perfusion after surgical removal subfoveal membranes in 12 eyes of 11 AMD patients (44). Stereoscopic fluorescein and indocyanine green angiograms of the excision bed revealed hypofluorescence with visible perfusion in the underlying median and large choroidal vessels in all eyes. On the basis of these observations the authors concluded that the choriocapillaris and small choroidal vessels were frequently abnormal or absent in the bed of the removed neovascular membrane. We cannot exclude the possibility that some nonperfusion of the subfoveal choriocapillaris is present in patients before submacular surgery. However, patients who develop subfoveal choroidal neovascularization experience sudden and severe visual loss, demonstrating that the perfusion of the choriocapillaris is sufficient to support good visual function even if it is not normal.

Experimental evidence suggests that the native RPE is removed with the choroidal neovascularization in AMD. Grossniklaus and Green examined specimens removed from the subretinal space as part of the Submacular Surgery Trial (45). Most of these patients (61 of 78) had AMD and the balance had POHS or idiopathic neovascularization. The specimens contained fibrovascular tissue, fibrocellular tissue, and hemorrhage. Vascular endothelium and RPE were the most common cellular constituents. As expected, the membranes from AMD patients were more likely to be beneath the RPE and the size of the RPE defect was larger in AMD eyes. Histopathological examination of an eye from a patient who had undergone surgical excision of a choroidal neovascular membrane in AMD revealed an RPE defect in the center of the dissection bed with incomplete resurfacing of the RPE defect after surgery (46,47). Thus, AMD patients are more likely to have a bare area of Bruch's membrane after surgery and the RPE defect is more likely to persist after surgery in these eyes.

Extensive experimental evidence suggests that RPE removal at the time of submacular surgery would lead to progressive atrophy of the subfoveal choriocapillaris. Destruction of the RPE with sodium iodate leads to changes in the RPE and choriocapillaris within 1 week and marked choriocapillaris atrophy within 1 month (48). In contrast, the choriocapillaris has a normal appearance in areas where the RPE still appears healthy. Similar changes are seen after intravitreal ornithine injection and in an experimental model of thioridizine retinopathy (49–52). Repopulation of Bruch's membrane occurs after RPE removal in the cat with choriocapillaris preservation under areas of healed RPE and choriocapillaris atrophy in nonhealed areas (53). RPE removal in the nontapetal porcine eye yields similar results (54–56). Bruch's membrane becomes repopulated with a monolayer or multilayer of variably pigmented cells 1 month after surgical debridement of the RPE. In these regions, the outer nuclear layer and outer limiting membrane remained intact and the choriocapillaris appeared patent. In regions of poor RPE healing, the lumen of the choriocapillaris was collapsed and the choriocapillaris endothelium was separated from its basement membrane (55,56).

Thus, a combination of experimental and clinical studies suggests that the following sequence of events occurs after choroidal neovascular membrane excision (Fig. 1). Subfoveal surgery can be performed without disturbing the native RPE in some eyes, but choroidal neovascular membrane excision results in a focal RPE defect in AMD eyes and in some younger eyes with other diseases. If the native RPE is not disturbed, the underlying choriocapillaris will not undergo secondary atrophy. If the native RPE is removed, the defect will heal by migration and proliferation of new RPE from the edge of the epithelial defect if the native basal lamina is intact. The proliferating RPE are hypopigmented, making it difficult to visualize these cells in vivo. There are no changes in the choriocapillaris if the area of the RPE defect is completely and rapidly repopulated by hypopigmented RPE. Incomplete or delayed healing of the RPE defect will lead rapidly to atrophy of the choriocapillaris although the medium and large vessels of the choroid can remain patent.

The functional consequences of subfoveal choriocapillaris atrophy are significant because atrophy of the subfoveal choriocapillaris is correlated with poor visual recovery after surgery. Over 90% of AMD eyes and 37% of POHS eyes have atrophy of the subfoveal choriocapillaris after submacular surgery (41,42), and the rate of visual improvement to

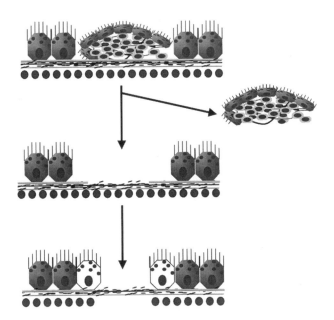

Figure 1 (Top) Sub-RPE choroidal neovascular membrane typical in age-related macular degeneration. (Middle) Membrane removal denudes the native RPE from Bruch's membrane and excises fragment of the inner aspects of Bruch's membrane. Native RPE cannot heal the epithelial defect completely in the absence of native basal lamina. (Bottom) Nonpigmented RPE may heal the defect partially in the presence of residual basal lamina, but will not heal the epithelial defect in the absence of basal lamina. An RPE defect leads to atrophy of the subfoveal choriocapillaris.

better than 20/50 was worse for AMD eyes than for POHS (41,42). Within the POHS subgroup, the subfoveal choriocapillaris was perfused in 24/38 (63%) eyes and nonperfused in 14/38 (37%) eyes. Best-corrected visual acuity improved by at least two lines in 17/24 (71%) perfused eyes and 2/14 (14%) nonperfused eyes ($p = 0.0089$). Additionally, a best-corrected vision of 20/100 or better was achieved in 18 (75%) of the perfused eyes and only four (29%) nonperfused eyes ($p < 0.05$). Thus, both the final visual acuity and improvement in visual acuity were correlated with postoperative perfusion of the subfoveal choriocapillaris (42).

III. RPE HARVESTING TECHNIQUE

We have previously described a method for harvesting and storage of intact adult human RPE sheets prior to transplantation (57). Briefly, human cadaver eyes are cleaned of extraocular tissue and the suprachoroidal space of the posterior pole is sealed with cyanoacrylate glue (58). A small scleral incision is made 3 mm posterior to the limbus until the choroidal vessels are exposed. Tenotomy scissors are introduced through this incision into the suprachoroidal space and the incision is extended circumferentially. Four radial relaxing incisions are made in the sclera and the sclera is peeled away from the periphery to the optic nerve with care not to tear the choroid. The eye cup is then incubated with 25 U/mL of Dispase (Gibco) for 30 min, rinsed with carbon dioxide–free medium, and a circumferential incision is made into the subretinal space along the ora serrata. The loosened RPE sheets are separated from the rest of the ocular tissue and placed on a slice of 50% gelatin on a 25 mm $\times$ 75 mm $\times$ 1 mm glass slide (Fisher Scientific, Pittsburgh, PA) with the apical RPE surface facing upward. Contamination with choroidal cells is avoided by directly visualizing the RPE sheets under a dissecting microscope while they are being harvested. The glass slide containing the gelatin film with the RPE sheet is then placed in a 100 mm $\times$ 15 mm polystyrene dish and incubated in a humidified atmosphere of 5% CO_2 and 95% air at 37°C for 5 min to allow the gelatin to melt and encase the RPE sheet. The specimen is kept at 4°C for 5 min to solidify the liquid gelatin and then stored in carbon dioxide–free medium (pH = 7.4) at 4°C. Harvested sheets are stained with cytokeratin to ensure purity of the cell population.

Transmission electron microscopy shows intact RPE cells with well-developed microvilli, basal infoldings, and intercellular connections. The initial viability of intact RPE sheets is 86% with a progressive decline in viability with increased storage time. Cells harvested within 24 h after death maintain greater viability than those harvested after 24 h ($p < 0.05$) and maintain 82% viability for as long as 48 h if stored at 4°C.

IV. CLINICAL RESULTS OF RPE TRANSPLANTATION

The goal of RPE transplantation is to repopulate Bruch's membrane with donor RPE prior to the development of widespread atrophy of the choriocapillaris. Some preliminary experimental evidence suggests that RPE transplanted into a debrided bed will support the native choriocapillaris, and healthy RPE may reverse choriocapillaris atrophy after it develops (48). To date all human studies of RPE transplantation in exudative AMD have been performed at the same time as submacular surgery, rather than after subfoveal choriocapillaris atrophy has progressed. The following studies have been reported to date:

Peyman et al. performed submacular scar excision with translocation of an autologous RPE pedicle flap or transplantation of an allogeneic RPE-Bruch's membrane explant in two patients (59). The final visual acuity was 20/400 in the first patient and count fingers at 2 ft in the second patient. Neither of these patients was immune suppressed.

Algvere et al. initially reported subretinal membrane removal with transplantation of fetal human RPE patches in five AMD patients, and subsequently reported on a larger series of 17 eyes (30–32). Cystoid macular edema developed and the grafts became encapsulated by white fibrous tissue within several months after surgery but none of these patients received systemic immune suppression. Scanning laser ophthalmoscopic microperimetry demonstrated that patients were able to fixate over the area of the RPE graft immediately after surgery, but an absolute scotoma developed in this region several months after surgery. These results are not surprising because the patients were not immune suppressed, and RPE transplanted into the subretinal space will be rejected (60,61).

Subfoveal membranectomy with transplantation of adult human RPE sheets has been performed in 11 AMD patients who were immune suppressed postoperatively with prednisone, cyclosporine, and immuran (33). Eligibility criteria included the presence of drusen, patient age > 60, best-correct acuity ≤ 20/63 (Bailey-Lovie chart), and subfoveal neovascularization ≤ 9 disk areas on preoperative fluorescein angiography. The mean visual acuity, contrast sensitivity, and reading speed did not change significantly for 6 months postoperatively. Transplants showed no signs of rejection in patients able to

Table 1 Summary of Clinical Results on RPE Transplantation

	No. of eyes	RPE source	Immune suppress	Best VA	Encapsulation
Peyman (57)	2 Diskiform	1 Homologous	No	20/400	Yes
		1 Autologous			No
Algvere (30–32)	5 RPE Patch/wet	Fetal	No	20/400	Yes
	4 RPE Patch/dry				
	5 RPE Suspensions/ dry				
	2 RPE Suspensions/ RPE Tear				
Kaplan (33)	11 Wet AMD	Adult	Yes	20/200 (20/100 in 1 eye)	No[a]
Weisz (34)	1 Dry AMD	Fetal	No	20/500	Yes[b]

[a] Grafts did not encapsulate unless immune suppression was discounted.
[b] Post-op subretinal fibrosis developed. Patient had serum antibodies to rhodopsin and phosducin after surgery but preoperative levels were not recorded.

continue immune suppression for the first 6 months after surgery, but patients who discontinued immune suppression developed signs of graft rejection 2 weeks later. Histopathology is available on an 85-year-old woman who died 4 months after RPE sheet transplantation (62). A complete autopsy demonstrated the cause of death to be congestive heart failure. A patch of hyperpigmentation was visible at the transplant site under the foveola after surgery. Mound-like clusters of individual round, large densely pigmented cells were present in the subretinal space and outer retina in this area and the transplant site did not contain a uniform monolayer in most areas. There was loss of the photoreceptor outer segments and native RPE in the center of the transplant bed, with disruption of the outer nuclear layer predominantly over regions of multilayered pigmented cells. Cystic spaces were present in the inner and outer retina. A residual intra-Bruch's membrane component of the original choroidal neovascular complex was present under the transplant site. The poor morphology at the transplant site was consistent with the lack of visual improvement seen after surgery in this patient.

Weisz et al. (34) delivered a patch of fetal RPE under the retina in one patient with geographic atrophy. Visual acuity remained stable at 20/80 1 month after surgery but deteriorated to 20/500 by 5 months postoperatively. Mild subretinal fibrosis developed after surgery. The patient demonstrated a systemic immune response to phosducin and rhodopsin postoperatively in the absence of systemic immune suppression. Table 1 summarizes the clinical results that have been obtained to date.

V. LABORATORY INSIGHTS INTO CLINICAL RESULTS

Several investigators have previously characterized the molecular constituents that may play an important role in the reattachment of human RPE to human Bruch's membrane. The basal surface of RPE cells contains a β_1-subunit of integrin (63,64) and the inner aspect of Bruch's membrane contains laminin, fibronectin, heparan sulfate, and collagen (65). Several studies suggest that the attachment of RPE to coated artificial surfaces can be mediated by an interaction between the β_1-subunit of integrin and known extracellular matrix molecules. For example, RPE cells bind to petri dishes coated with laminin or fibronectin but do not attach to untreated petri dishes (64). The synthetic tetrapeptide RGDS (arginine-glycine-aspartate-serine), which is derived from the cell-binding domain of fibronectin, decreases RPE binding to laminin-coated or fibronectin-coated dishes (66). When added simultaneously with the cells, binding of RPE to fibronectin-coated dishes and laminin-coated dishes can be blocked by an antibody to the β_1-subunit of integrin but RPE cell binding to charged tissue culture plastic is not affected by the antibody (66). When RPE are initially allowed to attach and spread on fibronectin- or laminin-coated petri dishes, addition of antibodies to fibronectin or laminin causes the attached cells to detach from the surface and round up (66). Thus, in vitro binding studies suggest that RPE attachment to plastic surfaces coated with laminin or fibronectin is mediated by an interaction between the β_1-integrin subunit and laminin and fibronectin coating the surface.

Molecular binding studies demonstrate a role for integrins and extracellular matrix ligands in mediating RPE attachment to Bruch's membrane in a more direct fashion (67). In these studies passaged human RPE are seeded onto RPE-derived extracellular matrix or human Bruch's membrane explants denuded of cells by treatment with 0.02 N ammonium hydroxide. Coating the surface of either RPE-derived extracellular matrix in petri dishes or Bruch's membrane explants with the fibronectin, laminin, vitronectin, or type IV collagen increased the RPE attachment rate. Exposing RPE to anti-β_1 integrin antibodies or RGDS, or precoating the surface with antibodies to fibronectin, laminin, vitronectin, or type IV collagen, decreased the RPE attachment rate to both surfaces. These experiments demonstrate that the attachment of human RPE cells to human Bruch's membrane or to RPE-derived extracellular matrix proteins is mediated by an interaction between the β_1-subunit of integrin on the RPE surface and ligands in the extracellular matrix that include laminin, fibronectin, vitronectin, and type IV collagen (67).

Understanding the mechanism of attachment of RPE cells to Bruch's membrane is important because this interaction is necessary to prevent RPE apoptosis (68). In vitro experiments demonstrate the importance of this effect. Second-passage human RPE were plated onto tissue culture plastic precoated with extracellular matrix, fibronectin, laminin, uncoated tissue culture plastic, untreated plastic, and untreated plastic coated with 4% agarose. Reattachment rates were determined for each substrate 24 h after plating. The TUNEL (terminal deoxynucleotidyl transferase-mediated dUTP nick end labeling) technique was used to determine apoptosis rates in attached cells, unattached cells, and the entire cell population. Attachment rates were as follows: ECM-coated tissue culture plastic > fibronectin-coated tissue culture plastic > laminin-coated tissue culture plastic > uncoated tissue culture plastic > untreated plastic > agarose-coated untreated plastic. Apoptosis rates for the entire cell population were increased as the RPE cell attachment rate decreased, and the proportion of apoptotic cells in the entire population was inversely related to the percent attached cells ($r = -0.95$). These results imply that RPE cells that are removed from their substrate prior to transplantation must reattach rapidly to a substrate to prevent apoptosis (Fig. 2).

These results have clinical relevance because all layers of Bruch's membrane are not intact after submacular surgery and in vitro studies of human RPE attachment to human Bruch's membrane demonstrate that the layer of Bruch's membrane available for cell

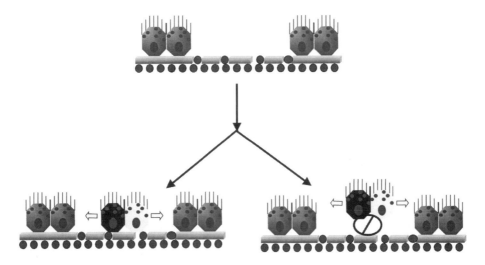

Figure 2 (Top) Sub-RPE choroidal neovascular membrane typical in age-related macular degeneration. (Bottom, left) Goal of RPE transplantation is to repopulate an area of bare Bruch's membrane with healthy donor RPE and thus avoid secondary choriocapillaris atrophy. (Bottom, right) Transplanted RPE must reattach to host Bruch's membrane in order to survive after transplantation. Unattached cells will not survive.

attachment can have a profound effect on cell behavior (69–71). In these studies 6-mm punches of peripheral Bruch's membrane were stabilized on 4% agarose and placed in 96-well plates with Bruch's membrane facing upward. Removing each apical layer sequentially exposed the RPE basal lamina, inner collagen layer, elastin layer, and outer collagen layer. First-passage human RPE harvested from a single donor (age = 52 years) were plated onto the surface (15,000 viable cells/explant) and the RPE reattachment rate to each layer of Bruch's membrane was determined. The RPE reattachment rate was highest to the inner aspects of Bruch's membrane and decreased as deeper layers of Bruch's membrane were exposed (i.e., basal lamina > inner collagen layer > elastin layer > outer collagen layer). The reattachment rate to the inner collagen layer, elastin layer, and outer collagen layer harvested from elderly donors (age > 60) was less than the reattachment rate to the corresponding layers harvested from younger donors (age < 50). Thus, the ability of harvested RPE to reattach to human Bruch's membrane depends on the anatomical layer of Bruch's membrane present in the host tissue. Similarly, the fate of transplanted RPE depends on the layer of Bruch's membrane available for cell attachment (70,71). The RPE apoptosis rate of attached cells increased as deeper layers of Bruch's membrane were exposed. Both the proliferation rate and mitotic index of the grafted cells were higher on the basal lamina layer than on deeper layers. Adult human RPE cells plated onto basal lamina repopulated the explant surface within 14 ± 3 days whereas cells plated onto inner collagen layer and elastin eventually died and never reached confluence. This suggests that age-related structural and functional changes that occur in the inner collagen layer, elastin layer, and outer collagen layer limit the ability of adult human RPE to repopulate these layers in elderly individuals (Fig. 3).

In contrast, cultured fetal human RPE seeded at a higher density may be able to repopulate human cadaver Bruch's membrane in vitro (72). One hour after seeding onto the

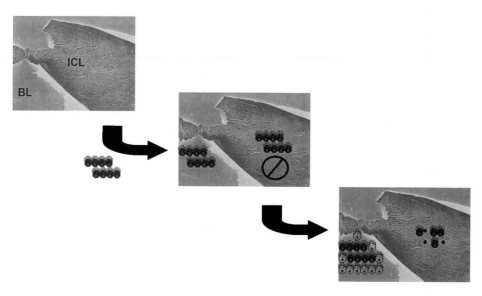

Figure 3   (Top, left) Transmission electron micrograph of human Bruch's membrane in which a tear through the basal lamina (BL) exposes the inner collagen layer (ICL). (Middle) Transplanted RPE attach to older basal lamina but not to older ICL. (Bottom, right) Transplanted RPE proliferate on the basal lamina layer but not the ICL.

surface plated RPE start to attach and flatten, and the cells cover the entire debrided surface in a monolayer within 4–6 h after seeding. Cells attached to the inner collagen layer tended to be flatter than cells attached to residual native basal lamina. At 12 and 24 h, expression of hexagonal shape, tight junctions, and apical microvilli were observed more frequently in cells attached to native basal lamina. No newly formed basement membrane was observed at these time points. Thus it appears that the presence of native RPE basement membrane promoted the early attachment of the cells and more rapid expression of normal morphology.

These results have several implications for the management of subfoveal choroidal neovascularization in exudative AMD. Many technical problems associated with RPE transplantation have been resolved, since instrumentation currently exists to harvest and then deliver dissociated RPE suspensions or RPE harvested as a patch or a sheet into the subretinal space. Transplanted RPE may survive when transplanted onto normal Bruch's membrane, yet Bruch's membrane is unlikely to be normal in AMD patients who will undergo cell transplantation. First, structural changes are present in all layers in Bruch's membrane in AMD patients including the accumulation of basal laminar and basal linear deposits, cross-linking of collagen within the inner and outer collagen layer, and calcification and fragmentation of the elastin layer (73–76). These changes may preclude successful repopulation of Bruch's membrane by transplanted RPE. Second, the inner aspects of Bruch's membrane are removed during submacular surgery. Thus, RPE transplanted after submacular surgery will have to reattach to an abnormal substrate to prevent death of the transplant by apoptosis. Bare areas of Bruch's membrane will have to be repopulated with RPE within 1 week or choriocapillaris atrophy will develop under these bare areas.

VI. FUTURE DIRECTIONS

At the current time many unresolved issues may influence the ability of transplanted cells to repopulate Bruch's membrane and numerous questions need to be addressed before successful cell transplantation can occur. In the absence of an animal model for AMD the approach to this problem must rely on a mixture of in vivo studies of cell transplantation in healthy animals, in vitro studies of cell reattachment to human Bruch's membrane diseased with AMD, and a small number of clinical trials on AMD patients. Several important variables need to be investigated.

A. Source of Cells

The ideal source for human transplantation studies is not known. Adult human RPE are readily available from donor Eye Bank eyes but it is not known whether these cells are the best source or whether the age of the donor RPE makes any difference. Fetal human RPE may be able to repopulate Bruch's membrane better than adult RPE but there are ethical and legal issues involved with the use of human fetal cells, and fetal cells cannot be autologous. Use of immortalized human RPE cells lines has been proposed, but the effects of immortalization or passaging in tissue culture on the distribution of cell surface receptors necessary for cell attachment to Bruch's membrane have not been considered in prior studies. There is some concern about tumorigenic potential if immortalized cells are used. Several authors have already used iris pigment epithelial cells because these cells are related embryological to the RPE, are readily available, and will not be rejected inmunologically (77,78). However, iris pigment epithelial transplantation combined with subfoveal surgery has not led to a dramatic improvement in vision to better than 20/200.

    Several other cell sources that may be useful for RPE transplantation have not been investigated fully. First, the recent isolation of retinal progenitor cells (stem cells) raises the interesting possibility of using these cells to repopulate denuded areas of Bruch's membrane (79). This is an attractive possibility because a small population of such retinal progenitor cells could yield a large population of cells for transplantation, and isolation of progenitors from adults could avoid problems of immune rejection. Second, xenotransplantation of porcine cells has already been performed in the management of central nervous system disease including stroke and Parkinson's disease (80,81). These cells have been well tolerated after transplantation into the central nervous system in patients and the possibility of using fetal xenografts could provide an attractive alternative to the use of human tissue.

B. Immune Suppression

A second issue that needs to resolved is related to the immune suppression necessary to ensure graft survival. In the original paper by Algvere et al. (30), the fundus photograph strongly suggests that immune rejection developed in these nonsuppressed individuals since the grafts became encapsulated and cystoid macular edema developed within 3 months. Similar changes were not seen in the study of adult RPE transplantation in which patients received systemic immune suppression with cyclosporin, immuran, and prednisone (30). Thus, systemic immune suppression appears to be sufficient to prevent ophthalmic signs of graft rejection but local suppression with slow-release devices (intravitreal cyclosporin implants, for example) would be preferable.

C.   Status of Bruch's Membrane After Submacular Surgery

The status of Bruch's membrane is important for the ultimate success of cell transplantation. Disease within Bruch's membrane and iatrogenic removal of the inner layers of Bruch's membrane during submacular surgery affect the ability of transplanted RPE to repopulate this structure. Several approaches could be used to rectify this problem including cleaning of Bruch's membrane surface deposits, deposition of soluble extracellular matrix ligands, or placement of an artificial substrate, such as lens capsule, extracellular matrix, or healthy Bruch's membrane, into the subretinal space. Successful application of these techniques in vivo has yet to be demonstrated.

D.   Timing of Surgery/Identification of Surgical Candidates

The issue regarding the timing of surgery is still to be resolved. Patients with diskiform scars have evidence of significant atrophy of the outer retina over the neovascular tissue. Thus, prompt intervention may be necessary to improve the visual prognosis. Also choriocapillaris atrophy may develop under the fovea in patients with chronic subfoveal neovascularization, so prompt surgery may improve preservation of this vascular supply as well.

VII.   SUMMARY

The development of techniques to surgically excise choroidal neovascular membranes has introduced the possibility of surgically reconstructing the subretinal space in patients who have subfoveal choroidal neovascularization in AMD, POHS, and other disorders. Early attempts at reconstructing the anatomy of the subretinal space were focused on simple surgical excision of choroidal neovascularization. Subfoveal membrane excision can lead to good visual results if the subfoveal RPE is not removed at the time of surgery, or if the RPE is removed and adjacent RPE then repopulates the subfoveal area of Bruch's membrane within 1 week after surgery. The presence of native or regenerated RPE is required to prevent postoperative atrophy of the subfoveal choriocapillaris, because the subfoveal choriocapillaris will undergo atrophy if Bruch's membrane remains devoid of RPE for ≥ 1 week after subfoveal surgery. Persistent bare areas of Bruch's membrane will be present in patients who have large defects in the RPE monolayer, or in whom advanced patient age or disease to the inner aspects of Bruch's membrane prevents complete RPE resurfacing by migration and proliferation of adjacent RPE. Initial studies on RPE cell transplantation have not led to dramatic visual improvements, but the presence of disease within Bruch's membrane, iatrogenic removal of the inner layers of Bruch's membrane, and immune rejection of the transplant have limited visual recovery after surgery. The next challenges in submacular surgery are to deliver RPE into the subretinal space as an organized monolayer, ensure the rapid attachment of these cells to Bruch's membrane, and prevent immunological rejection of these cells. Cell survival immediately after transplantation is important to prevent atrophy of the subfoveal choriocapillaris. Development of an elusive animal model would facilitate progress in this field, because in the absence of an animal model conclusions must be drawn from a combination of in vitro studies studying cell attachment to normal and diseased Bruch's membrane, in vivo studies of cell transplantation in normal animals, and a limited number of in vivo studies of RPE transplantation in individuals with AMD. At the dawn of the new millennium, the challenge is great but the potential benefit of success is even greater because of the sheer number of patients who are affected by this devastating disease.

ACKNOWLEDGMENT

This work was supported in part by an unrestricted grant from Research to Prevent Blindness, Inc., New York.

REFERENCES

1. Bressler NM, Bressler SB, Fine SL. Age-related macular degeneration. Surv Ophthalmol 1988;32:375–413.
2. Bressler NM, Frost LA, Bressler SB, Murphy RP, Fine SL. Natural course of poorly defined choroidal neovascularization associated with macular degeneration. Arch Ophthalmol 1988;106:1537–1542.
3. Stevens TS, Bressler NM, Maguire MG, Bressler SB, Fine SL, Alexander J, Phillips DA, Margherio RR, Murphy PL, Schachat AP. Occult choroidal neovascularization in age-related macular degeneration: a natural history study. Arch Ophthalmol 1997;115:345–350.
4. Bressler SB, Bressler NM, Fine SL, Hillis A, Murphy RP, Olk RJ, Patz A. Natural course of choroidal neovascular membranes within the foveal avascular zone in senile macular degeneration. Am J Ophthalmol 1982;93:157–163.
5. Macular Photocoagulation Study Group. Laser photocoagulation of subfoveal neovascular lesions in age-related macular degeneration. Results of a randomized clinical trial. Arch Ophthalmol 1991;109:1220–1231.
6. Macular Photocoagulation Study Group. Laser photocoagulation of subfoveal recurrent neovascular lesions in age-related macular degeneration results of a randomized clinical trial. Arch Ophthalmol 1991;109:1232–1241.
7. TAP Study Group. Photodynamic therapy of subfoveal choroidal neovascularization in age-related macular degeneration with verteporfin: one-year results of 2 randomized clinical trials— TAP report. Treatment of age-related macular degeneration with photodynamic therapy. Arch Ophthalmol 1999;117:1329–1345.
8. Miller JW, Schmidt-Erfurth U, Sickenberg M, Pournaras CJ, Laqua H, Barbazetto I, Zorafos L, Piguet B, Donati G, Lane AM, Birngruber R, van den Berg H, Strong A, Manjuris U, Gray T, Fsadni M, Bressler NM, Gragoudas ES. Photodynamic therapy with verteporfin for choroidal neovascularization caused by age-related macular degeneration: results of a single treatment in a phase 1 and 2 study. Arch Ophthalmol 1999;117:1161–1173.
9. Finger PT, Chakravarthy U, Augsburger JJ. Radiotherapy and the treatment of age-related macular degeneration. External beam radiation therapy is effective in the treatment of age-related macular degeneration. Arch Ophthalmol 1998;116:1507–1511.
10. Bergink GJ, Hoyng CB, van der Maazen RW, Vingerling JR, van Daal WA, Deutman AF. A randomized controlled clinical trial on the efficacy of radiation therapy in the control of subfoveal choroidal neovascularization in age-related macular degeneration: radiation versus observation. Graefe's Arch Clin Exp Ophthalmol 1998;236:321–325.
11. Spaide RF, Guyer DR, McCormick B, Yanuzzi LA, Burke K, Mendelsohn M, Haas A, Slakter JS, Sorenson JA, Fisher YL, Abramson D. External beam radiation therapy for choroidal neovascularization. Ophthalmology 1998;105:24–30.
12. Machemer R, Steinhorst UH. Retinal separation, retinotomy, and macular relocation: II. A surgical approach for age-related macular degeneration? Graefe's Arch Clin Exp Ophthalmol 1993;231:635–641.

13. Ninomiya Y, Lewis JM, Hasegawa T, Tano Y. Retinotomy and foveal translocation for surgical management of subfoveal choroidal neovascular membranes. Am J Ophthalmol 1996;122:613–621.
14. de Juan E Jr, Lowenstein A, Bressler NM, Alexander J. Translocation of the retina for management of subfoveal choroidal neovascularization. II: A preliminary report in humans. Am J Ophthalmol 1998;125:635–646.
15. Pieramici DJ, De Juan E, Fujii GY, Reynolds SM, Melia M, Humayun M, Schachat AP, Hartranft CD. Limited inferior macular translocation for the treatment of subfoveal choroidal neovascularization secondary to age-related macular degeneration. Am J Ophthalmol 2000;130:419–428.
16. Donahue SP, Wall M, Weingeist TA. Interferon treatment of SRNV. Ophthalmology 1994;101:624–625.
17. Fung WE. Interferon alpha 2a for treatment of age-related macular degeneration. Am J Ophthalmol 1991;112:349–350.
18. Engler CB, Sander B, Koefoed P, Larsen M, Vinding T, Lund-Andersen H. Interferon alpha-2a treatment of patients with subfoveal neovascular macular degeneration: a pilot investigation. Acta Ophthalmol 1993;71:27–31.
19. Berger AS, Kaplan HJ. Clinical experience with the surgical removal of subfoveal neovascular membranes short-term postoperative results. Ophthalmology 1992;99:969–975.
20. Lambert HM, Capone A, Aaberg TM, Sternberg P, Mandell BA, Lopez PF. Surgical excision of subfoveal neovascular membranes in age-related macular degeneration. Am J Ophthalmol 1992;113:257–262.
21. Coscas G, Meunier I, Chirurgie des membranes neovasculaires sous-rétiniennes macularies. Ophtalmol 1993;16:633–641.
22. Thomas MA, Grand MG, Williams DF, Lee CM, Pesin SR, Lowe MA. Surgical management of subfoveal choroidal neovascularization. Ophthalmology 1992;99:952–968.
23. Lambert HM, Capone A, Aaberg TM, Sternberg P, Mandell BA, Lopez PF. Surgical excision of subfoveal neovascular membranes in age-related macular degeneration. Am J Ophthalmol 1992;113:257–262.
24. Thomas MA, Kaplan HJ. Surgical removal of subfoveal neovascularization in the presumed ocular histoplasmosis syndrome. Am J Ophthalmol 1991;111:1–7.
25. Berger AS, Conway M, Del Priore LV, Walker RS, Pollack JS, Kaplan HJ. Submacular surgery for subfoveal choroidal neovascular membranes in patients with presumed ocular histoplasmosis. Arc Ophthalmol 1997;115:991–996.
26. Holekamp NM, Thomas MA, Dickinson JD, Valluri S. Surgical removal of subfoveal choroidal neovascularization in presumed ocular histoplasmosis: stability of early visual results. Ophthalmology 1997;104:22–26.
27. Submacular Surgery Trials Pilot Study Investigators. Submacular surgery trials randomized pilot trial of laser photocoagulation versus surgery for recurrent choroidal neovascularization secondary to age-related macular degeneration: I. Ophthalmic outcomes submacular surgery trials pilot study report number 1. Am J Ophthalmol 2000;130:387–407.
28. Submacular Surgery Trials Pilot Study Investigators. Submacular surgery trials randomized pilot trial of laser photocoagulation versus submacular surgery for recurrent choroidal neovascularization secondary to age-related macular degeneration: II. Quality of life outcomes submacular surgery trials pilot study report number 2. Am J Ophthalmol 2000;130:408–418.
29. Del Priore LV, Kaplan HJ, Berger AS. Retinal pigment epithelial transplantation in the management of subfoveal choroidal neovascularization. Semin Ophthalmol 1997;12:45–55.
30. Algvere PV, Berglin L, Gouras P, Sheng Y. Transplantation of fetal retinal pigment epithelium in age-related macular degeneration with subfoveal neovascularization. Graefe's Arch Clin Exp Ophthalmol 1994;232:707–716.
31. Gouras P, Algvere P. Retinal cell transplantation in the macula: new techniques. Vis Res 1996;36:4121–4125.

32. Algvere PV, Berglin L, Gouras P, Sheng Y, Kopp ED. Transplantation of RPE in age-related macular degeneration: observations in disciform lesions and dry RPE atrophy. Graefe's Arch Clin Exp Ophthalmol 1997;235:149–158.

33. Kaplan HJ, Del Priore LV, Tezel TH, Berger AS. Retinal pigment epithelial transplantation for subfoveal neovascularization in age-related macular degeneration: a clinical trial. The Retina Society, Washington, DC, September 1998.

34. Weisz JM, Humayun MS, De Juan E, Del Cerro M, Sunness JS, Dagnelie G, Soylu M, Rizzo L, Nussenblatt RB. Allogenic fetal retinal pigment epithelial cell transplant in a patient with geographic atrophy. Retina 1999;19:540–545.

35. de Juan E, Machemer R. Vitreous surgery for hemorrhagic and fibrous complications of age-related macular degeneration. Am J Ophthalmol 1988;105:25–9.

36. Roth DB, Downie AA, Charles ST. Visual results after submacular surgery for neovascularization in age-related macular degeneration. Opthalm Surg Lasers 1997;28:920–925.

37. Merrill PT, LoRusso FJ, Lomeo MD, Saxe SJ, Khan MM, Lambert HM. Surgical removal of subfoveal choroidal neovascularization in age-related macular degeneration. Ophthalmology 1999;106:782–789.

38. Lewis H, VanderBrug Medendorp S. Tissue plasminogen activator-assisted surgical excision of subfoveal choroidal neovascularization in age-related macular degeneration: a randomized, double-masked trial. Ophthalmology 1997;104:1847–1851.

39. Gass JD. Biomicroscopic and histopathologic considerations regarding the feasibility of surgical excision of subfoveal neovascular membranes. Am J Ophthalmol 1994;118:285–298.

40. Nasir M, Sugino I, Zarbin MA. Decreased choriocapillaris perfusion following surgical excision of choroidal neovascular membranes in age-related macular degeneration. Br J Ophthalmol 1997;81:481–489.

41. Pollack JS, Del Priore LV, Smith ME, Feiner MA, Kaplan HJ. Postoperative abnormalities of the choriocapillaris in exudative age-related macular degeneration. Br J Ophthalmol 1996;80:314–8.

42. Akduman L, Desai V, Del Priore LV, Olk PJ, Kaplan HJ. Perfusion of the subfoveal choriocapillaris affects visual recovery after submacular surgery in presumed ocular histoplasmosis syndrome. Am J Ophthalmol 1997;123:90–96.

43. Desai VN, Del Priore LV, Kaplan HJ. Choriocapillaris atrophy after submacular surgery in the presumed ocular histoplasmosis syndrome. Arch Ophthalmol 1995;113:408–409.

44. Thach AB, Marx JL, Frambach DA, LaBree LD, Lopez PF. Choroidal hypoperfusion after surgical excision of subfoveal neovascular membranes in age-related macular degeneration. Int Ophthalmol 1996-97;20:205–213.

45. Grossniklaus HE, Green WR. Histopathologic and ultrastructural findings of surgically excised choroidal neovascularization. Submacular Surgery Trials Research Group. Arch Ophthalmol 1998;116:745–749.

46. Rosa RH, Thomas MA, Green WR. Clinicopathologic correlation of submacular membranectomy with retention of good vision in a patient with age-related macular degeneration. Arch Ophthalmol 1996;114:480–487.

47. Hsu JK, Thomas MA, Ibanez H, Green WR. Clinicopathologic studies of an eye after submacular membranectomy for choroidal neovascularization. Retina 1995;15:43–52.

48. Korte GE, Reppucci V, Henkind P. RPE destruction causes choriocapillaris atrophy. Invest Ophthalmol Vis Sci 1984;25:1135–1145.

49. Miller FS III, Bunt-Milam AH, Kalina RE. Clinical-ultrastructural study of thioridazine retinopathy. Ophthalmology 1982;89:1478–1488.

50. Henkind P, Gartner S. The relationship between retinal pigment epithelium and the choriocapillaris. Trans Ophthalmol Soc UK 1983;103:444–447.

51. Kuwabara T, Ishikawa Y, Kaiser-Kupfer MI. Experimental model of gyrate atrophy in animals. Ophthalmology 1981;88:331–335.

52. Takeuchi M, Itagaki T, Takahashi K, Ohkuma H, Uyama M. Changes in the intermediate stage of retinal degeneration after intravitreal injection of ornithine. Nippon Ganka Gakkai Zasshi 1993;97:17–28.
53. Leonard DS, Zhang XG, Panozzo G, Sugino IK, Zarbin MA. Clinicopathologic correlation of localized retinal pigment epithelium debridement. Invest Ophthalmol Vis Sci 1997;38:1094–1109.
54. Del Priore LV, Kaplan HJ, Valentino TL, Hornbeck R, Jones Z, Mosinger-Ogilvie J, Swinn M. Debridement of the pig retinal pigment epithelium in vivo. Arch Ophthalmol 1995;113:939–944.
55. Valentino TL, Kaplan HJ, Del Priore LV, Fang R, Berger A, Silverman MS. Retinal pigment epithelial repopulation in monkeys after submacular surgery. Arch Ophthalmol 1995;113:932–938.
56. Del Priore LV, Kaplan HJ, Silverman MS, Hornbeck R, Jones J, Swinn M. Debridement of the pig retinal pigment epithelium in vivo. Arch Ophthalmol 1995;113:939–944.
57. Tezel TH, Del Priore LV, Kaplan HJ. Harvest and storage of adult human retinal pigment epithelial sheets. Curr Eye Res 1997;16:802–809.
58. Pfeffer B. Improved methodology for cell culture of human and monkey retinal pigment epithelium. Prog Retin Res 1991;10,251–291.
59. Peyman GA, Blinder KJ, Paris CL, Alturki W, Nelson NC, Desai U. A technique for retinal pigment epithelial transplantation for age-related macular degeneration secondary to extensive subfoveal scarring. Ophthalm Surg 1991;22:102–108.
60. Jiang LQ, Jorquera M, Streilein JW. Immunologic consequences of intraocular implantation of retinal pigment epithelial allografts. Exp Eye Res 1994;58:719–728.
61. Ye J, Wang HM, Ogden TE, Ryan SJ. Allotransplantation of rabbit retinal pigment epithelial cells double-labelled with 5-bromodeoxyuridine (BrdU) and natural pigment. Curr Eye Res 1993;12:629–639.
62. Del Priore LV, Kaplan HJ, Tezel TH, Hayashi N, Green WR. Retinal pigment epithelial cell transplantation after subfoveal membranectomy in age-related macular degeneration: clinicopathologic correlation. Am J Ophthalmol 2001;131:472–480.
63. Chu P, Grunwald GB. Identification of the 2A10 antigen of retinal pigment epithelium as a beta 1 subunit of integrin. Invest Ophthalmol Vis Sci 1991;32:1757–1762.
64. Chu P, Grunwald GB. Functional inhibition of retinal pigment epithelial cell-substrate adhesion with a monoclonal antibody against the beta 1 subunit of integrin. Invest Ophthalmol Vis Sci 1991;32:1763–1769.
65. Das A, Frank RN, Zhang NL, Turczyn TJ. Ultrastructural localization of extracellular matrix components in human retinal vessels and Bruch's membrane. Arch Ophthalmol 1990;108:421–429.
66. Avery RL, Glaser BM. Inhibition of retinal pigment epithelial cell attachment by a synthetic peptide derived from the cell-binding domain of fibronectin. Arch Ophthalmol 1986;104:1220–1222.
67. Ho TC, Del Priore LV. Reattachment of cultured human retinal pigment epithelium to extracellular matrix and human Bruch's membrane. Invest Ophthalmol Vis Sci 1997;38:1110–1118.
68. Tezel TH, Del Priore LV. Reattachment to a substrate prevents apoptosis of human retinal pigment epithelium. Graefe's Arch Clin Exp Ophthalmol 1997;235:41–47.
69. Del Priore LV, Tezel TH. Reattachment rate of human retinal pigment epithelium to layers of human Bruch's membrane. Arch Ophthalmol 1998;116:335–341.
70. Tezel TH, Del Priore LV, Kaplan HJ. Fate of human retinal pigment epithelial cells seeded onto layers of human Bruch's membrane. Invest Ophthalmol Vis Sci 1999;40:467–476.
71. Tezel TH, Del Priore LV. Repopulation of different layers of host human Bruch's membrane by retinal pigment epithelial cell grafts. Invest Ophthalmol Vis Sci 1999;40:767–774.
72. Castellarin AA, Sugino IK, Vargas JA, Parolini B, Lui GM, Zarbin MA. In vitro transplantation of fetal human retinal pigment epithelial cells onto human cadaver Bruch's membrane. Exp Eye Res 1998;66:49–67.

73. Burns RP, Feeney-Burns L. Clinico-pathologic correlations of drusen of Bruch's membrane. Trans Am Ophthalmol Soc 1980;78:206–225.
74. Sarks SH, Sarks JP. Age-related macular degeneration: atrophic form. In: Ryan S, Schachat AP, Murphy RM, Patz A, eds. Retina, Vol. 2. St. Louis: CV Mosby Co, 1989:149–173.
75. Sarks SH, Van Driel D, Maxwell L, Killingsworth M. Softening of drusen and subretinal neovascularization. Trans Ophthalmol Soc UK 1980;100:414–22.
76. Green WR, Key SN. Senile macular degeneration: a histopathologic study. Trans Am Ophthalmol Soc 1977;75:180–254.
77. Rezai KA, Kohen L, Weidemann P, Heimann K. Iris pigment epithelium transplantation. Graefe's Arch Clin Exp Ophthalmol 1997;65:23–29.
78. Thumann G, Aisenbrey S, Schraermeyer U, Lafaut B, Esser P, Walter P, Bartz-Schmidt KU. Transplantation of autologous iris pigment epithelium after removal of choroidal neovascular membranes. Arch Ophthalmol 2000;118:1350–1355.
79. Tropepe V, Coles BL, Chiasson BJ, Horsford DJ, Elia AJ, McInnes R, van der Kooy D. Retinal stem cells in the adult mammalian eye. Science 2000;287:2032–2036.
80. Edge AS, Gosse ME, Dinsmore J. Xenogeneic cell therapy: current progress and future developments in porcine cell transplantation. Cell Transplant 1998;7:525–539.
81. Deacon T, Schumacher J, Dinsmore J, Thomas C, Palmer P, Kott S, Edge A, Penney D, Kassissieh S, Dempsey P, Isacson O. Histological evidence of fetal pig neural cell survival after transplantation into a patient with Parkinson's disease. Nat Med 1997;3:350–353.

26

Assessment of Visual Function and Quality of Life in Patients with Age-Related Macular Degeneration

Paul J. Mackenzie
University of British Columbia, Vancouver, British Columbia, Canada

Thomas S. Chang
Doheny Retina Institute of the Doheny Eye Institute, University of Southern California Keck School of Medicine, Los Angeles, California

I. INTRODUCTION

Age-related macular degeneration (AMD) remains the leading cause of severe irreversible visual loss in North Americans over the age of 50 (1–5). The prevalence of AMD is known to increase with age with approximately 10% of individuals in their seventh decade of life having signs of the disease and over 30% involvement for individuals over 75 years of age. The disease is broadly divided into exudative and atrophic forms with over 90% of those sustaining visual loss being attributed to the exudative form. Precursor lesions have been identified for both mechanisms of visual loss. In patients who develop choroidal neovascularization, the presence of large, soft confluent drusen typically precedes the exudative phase. Similarly, the presence of crystalline drusen is often predictive for those who go on to develop geographic atrophy. In the majority of circumstances, patients will often volunteer a subjective progressive change in their visual perception prior to the development of these vision-threatening processes. This is often not appreciated with Snellen acuity measurement. This inherent limitation of Snellen acuity to reflect visual function is one of the principal reasons for the development of functional outcome/quality-of-life (QOL) assessments. Snellen acuity is a monocular measure of the ability to discern a stationary, high-contrast single object presented to the very center of the visual field at a standardized distance. Visual function is a binocular process of perception in nonideal everyday conditions and one that has no single measure. In addition, visual function involves perception in more than just the very central few degrees of visual angle. One final difference between the two measures is that central acuity is measured as a categorical variable (i.e., stepwise levels) while visual function is typically described in terms of a continuous variable.

To better describe this continuous measure of binocular visual function, we look to the concepts of health-related quality-of-life studies (HRQOL). Functional assessment and quality of life analysis is a field of growing importance in medicine as it offers a method of

511

incorporating patients' perceptions into the clinical setting to assist in providing optimum patient care. In AMD, clinicians have been shown to underestimate the extent to which the disease negatively impacts upon their patients (6). The concept involves utilization of standardized questionnaires supplied to patients in a uniform format and scored in a systematic manner. Two broad categories of functional outcome assessments are currently in use:

1. Generic QOL assessments
2. Functional outcome assessments

Examples of common instruments used in both of these categories will be given. One general caveat should be mentioned regarding all QOL instruments in that the specific questionnaire must be tested for validation for each specific use or disease state.

II. GENERIC QUALITY-OF-LIFE ASSESSMENTS

HRQOL is a multidimensional concept that encompasses physical, emotional, and social aspects associated with a given disease or its treatment. Measurement of HRQOL can potentially help clinicians and researchers identify predictors of patient outcome and provide information on the recovery process. The Short Form-36 (SF-36) is one of the most widely used health status evaluation tools. The instrument consists of 36 items and provides a comprehensive evaluation of eight health concepts: physical functioning, bodily pain, role limitations due to physical health problems, role limitations due to personal or emotional problems, general mental health, social functioning, energy/fatigue, and general health perceptions (7–9). Table 1 provides a description of the subscales of the SF-36.

As a comprehensive QOL instrument, the SF-36 has often been used to complement vision-specific instruments, as discussed below (10–12). In these studies, correlations between the vision-specific instruments and the SF-36 subscales have usually been fairly low

Table 1 Description of the Subscales of the Short-Form 36 (SF-36)

SF-36 subscale	Description
Physical health scales	
Physical functioning	Limitations in performing a range of physical activities, from basic activities of daily living to extremely vigorous physical activities
Role-physical	Problems with work or daily activities as a function of physical health
Bodily pain	The degree to which bodily pain exists and causes limitations
General health	How subjects view their current personal health and whether it is likely to get worse
The Physical Composite Scale (PCS) is a composite of the above 4 subscales.	
Mental health scales	
Vitality	The reported level of tiredness and energy
Social functioning	Limitations in social interactions due to either physical or emotional problems
Role-emotional	Problems at work or in everyday activities due to emotional problems
Mental health	The degree of depression, nervousness, peace, and calm experienced by subjects
The Mental Composite Scale (MCS) is a composite of the four mental health subscales.	

Source: Adapted from SF-36 Health Survey Manual and Interpretation Guide. Boston: The Health Institute, New England Medical Center, 1993.

Table 2 Correlations Between SF-36 Subscales and VF-14, Weighted Visual Acuity, and Clinical AMD Severity and Weighted Comorbidity Scale in Patients with AMD (*n* = 159)

SF-36 subscale	VF-14 score	AMD severity	WCS score	Weighted visual acuity
Physical functioning	0.39**	−0.22*	−0.39**	−0.26**
Role-physical	0.30**	−0.19*	−0.40**	−0.22**
Bodily pain	0.18*	0.06	−0.42**	−0.08
General health	0.18*	0.02	−0.41**	−0.14
Vitality	0.30**	−0.04	−0.32**	−0.19*
Social functioning	0.25**	−0.13	−0.32**	−0.20*
Role-emotional	0.15	−0.09	−0.26**	−0.06
Mental health	0.08	0.00	−0.26**	−0.12
PCS (composite)	0.39**	−0.17	−0.49**	−0.26**
MCS (composite)	0.06	−0.03	−0.23*	−0.06

*$p < 0.05$.
**$p < 0.01$.
Source: Reprinted with permission from Assessment of vision-related function in patients with age-related macular degeneration. Ophthalmology. In press.

as would be expected for the application of a generic instrument to a specific function. A recent study looked at visual functioning in retinal patients using the Visual Function-14 (VF-14), the SF-36, and a third instrument, the Weighted Comorbidity Scale (WCS) (12). The latter provides information about nonocular medical comorbidities that may impact on either visual function or physical/mental well-being (13). Correlations between the SF-36 subscales and measures of visual functioning such as the VF-14 score and visual acuity were low, ranging from 0.12 to 0.25. Once again, this would be expected as the generic methodology of the SF-36 is not designed to differentiate levels of visual function. In a second study conducted by our research group (14), the findings were duplicated when a specific subset of retinal patients with AMD were assessed, as shown in Table 2. These and other studies (10,11) have suggested that the SF-36 does not provide specific information about vision-related QOL in patients with AMD but rather provides a broader view of the health of patients with AMD. Because the SF-36 has been so broadly and extensively used, it allows comparison of different disease populations to each other and to normal populations in the United States, Australia, United Kingdom, and more recently in Canada (15–19). For example, our study (14) provides the following picture of the overall physical and mental well-being of patients with AMD as compared to the general population.

Table 3 illustrates a comparison of SF-36 scores in patients with AMD with population norms for the United States (15) and Canadian (19) general populations. This type of data is helpful in assessing the relative overall physical and mental well-being of patients with AMD as compared to the general population. Of the eight SF-36 scales, four are used to assess physical health; these are Physical Functioning, Role-Physical, Bodily Pain, and General Health. A difference of five points between populations represents a difference that is likely clinically relevant (15). AMD patients report similar values to population norms on the Bodily Pain Scale, which captures the degree to which bodily pain exists and causes limitations. The General Health scale provides an assessment of how subjects view their current personal health and whether it is likely to get worse. Patients with AMD have scores that are five points lower than U.S. population norms and 10 points lower than Canadian population norms, a difference likely to be clinically relevant. AMD patients' responses

Table 3 Mean SF-36 Scores in Patients with AMD in Comparison to Norms for General U.S. Population and General Canadian Population Patients

SF-36 subscale	AMD	U.S. general population	Canadian general population
Physical functioning	72 (29)	84 (23)	86 (20)
Role-physical	63 (42)	81 (34)	82 (33)
Bodily pain	72 (27)	75 (23)	76 (23)
General health	67 (23)	72 (20)	77 (18)
Vitality	57 (22)	61 (21)	66 (18)
Social functioning	81 (26)	83 (23)	86 (20)
Role-emotional	85 (39)	81 (33)	84 (32)
Mental health	74 (20)	74 (18)	78 (15)
PCS (composite)	45 (11)	50 (9.9)	51 (9.0)
MCS (composite)	50 (11)	50 (10)	52 (9.1)

Source: Reprinted with permission from Assessment of vision-related function in patients with age-related macular degeneration. Ophthalmology. In press.

were 12–16 points lower than population norms on the Physical Functioning Scale. This scale assesses how limited subjects believe themselves to be in performing a range of physical activities, from basic activities of daily living to extremely vigorous physical activities. Finally, the largest difference of nearly 20 points was seen on the Role-Physical Scale, which assesses problems with work or daily activities as a function of physical health. The SF-36 data suggest that patients with AMD believe they are in poorer physical health than does the general population. In addition to the four physical health scales, a single Physical Composite Scale (PCS) can be generated from the four scales to provide a single composite score of physical health. Consistent with the above data, PCS scores were lower in AMD patients than in general population norms in the United States and Canada. These data therefore suggest that patients with AMD may fare worse than individuals without AMD in issues involving physical well-being and activity.

In contrast, when we look at the mental health of patients with AMD in comparison to population norms without AMD, the scores appear to be at or near population norms. Again, four of the SF-36 scales attempt to assess different facets of mental health (Table 1). The Vitality Scale assesses the reported level of subjects' tiredness and energy. The Social Functioning Scale measures the degree to which social interactions are interfered with due to either physical or emotional problems. The Role-Emotional Scale refers to problems at work or in everyday activities due to emotional problems. The Mental Health Scale assesses the degree of depression, nervousness, peace, and calm experienced by subjects. Of these four scales, only the Role-Emotional Scale showed clinically relevant differences between AMD patients and population norms (Table 3). These data suggest that, despite significant visual disability, general emotional health as assessed by the SF-36 is only minimally affected in patients with AMD. This conclusion is supported by the SF-36 Mental Composite Scale (MCS), generated from the four mental health scales. In a recent study of AMD patients, the correlations between the MCS and visual acuity in the better eye, visual acuity in the worse eye, and the clinical severity of AMD were near zero (11). In our study of AMD patients, the correlation between the MCS and weighted visual acuity was −0.06; the correlation between MCS and the clinical severity of AMD was 0.03 (Table 2). No differences were seen in MCS scores between individuals with AMD and general population norms. Additionally, patients with AMD scored no different from the general population on the Mental Health Scale, an indicator of depression. These results support the conclusion that the mental health of patients with AMD is at population levels and does not vary with the extent of their AMD. Other factors, such as the rate of progression of visual loss, the degree of disparity in visual functioning between the eyes, and the use of low-vision services, may play significant roles in how patients approach their visual disability. In addition, vision-specific mental health issues such as perceptions about prognosis may also have a significant impact, as discussed below.

Generic QOL instruments enhance the information gathered from vision-specific instruments by providing important contextual information on the general state of health and by allowing comparison to other populations of individuals. Although very useful for a variety of health outcome evaluation purposes, the SF-36 short-form health survey takes 10–12 min to complete and is too long for inclusion in large-scale measurement and monitoring efforts. An abbreviated version of the SF-36, the SF-12, has been developed recently (20). The average time to complete SF-12 questionnaire is less than 2 min. By using a shorter, simpler battery of tests, significant study efficiency improvements and cost savings may be realized by achieving higher instrument completion rates and reducing time spent by the respondent and interviewer during the survey.

While imposing less encumbrance on the respondents and interviewers administering the survey, the SF-12 was shown to produce the physical and mental component summary scores (PCS and MCS) of the SF-36 with considerable accuracy. A cohort of 836 patients with retinal diseases were evaluated by our research group comparing both the 36-item short-form scales and summary measures were replicated for the 12-item Physical and Mental Component Summaries by Ware, et al. (20). Evaluation of a subset of 12 items from the SF-36 Health Survey explained at least 90% of the variance in SF-36 physical and mental health summary measures in patients with AMD. Results of this study suggest that the shorter, more user-friendly SF-12 may play an increasing role in the measurement of generic QOL assessments in ophthalmic studies in the future.

III. FUNCTIONAL OUTCOME ASSESSMENT

Functional outcome assessments are standardized vision-related QOL instruments designed to measure the vision-specific limitations of patients. This approach recognizes a middle ground between visual acuity and generic QOL instruments. On one hand, a generic QOL instrument provides context about the mental and physical state of a group of patients, but may not be sensitive enough to measure the impact of a specific visual disability. On the other hand, visual acuity, although objective and easily understood and communicated, provides only limited information about patients' functional limitations. The example of reading ability illustrates the limited information provided by Snellen visual acuity. While high-contrast visual acuity is certainly an important factor that influences reading ability, there is more to reading than resolving monochrome targets of stationary single letters under conditions of maximum contrast at distance. Reading usually occurs under less ideal conditions with smaller letters within a distracting background. These letters are presented at near distance, in uneven lighting, and with less than 100% contrast. In addition to central visual acuity, effective reading may involve a motion-dependent, low-contrast visual channel involved in coordinating visual input with saccades (21). Reading ability has been shown to be predicted better by low-contrast visual acuity and by contrast sensitivity than by high-contrast visual acuity (22,23). Therefore, in reading tasks, while central vision tests under ideal conditions are important, other aspects of visual function are stronger predictors of function. Understanding these factors may improve our understanding of how patients view their limitations, not only in reading but in other visual functions.

Several instruments of visual functioning have been developed. Three of these tools, the National Eye Institute Visual Function Questionnaire (NEI-VFQ), the Activities of Daily Vision Scale (ADVS), and the Visual Function 14 (VF-14), have gained increasing acceptance in the recent literature.

A. National Eye Institute Visual Function Questionnaire

The NEI-VFQ was designed as a comprehensive functional assessment tool, applicable to a variety of sight-limiting diseases (24). It has been used in a number of patient groups including individuals with glaucoma, cataract, diabetic retinopathy, cytomegalovirus retinitis, and AMD (10). The scale reports an overall score of visual functioning and separate scores for 12 subscales, including near vision, distance vision, color, ocular pain, driving, peripheral vision, and some broader measures such as general health and vision-specific expectations. The strength of the NEI-VFQ is that it was developed using focus groups of patients from a variety of ophthalmic diseases, therefore providing a theoretical basis for using the tool to compare across a variety of ocular conditions (24). A study of 108 patients with AMD reported that the NEI-VFQ adequately represents visual functioning and can discriminate visual disability from nonvisual disability. Additional evidence supporting the validity of the NEI-VFQ was provided by the high correlations between the NEI-VFQ and other scales of visual functioning including the VF-14 and the ADVS (10). Although the NEI-VFQ shows promise as a valid measure of visual functioning in AMD patients, the 51-item questionnaire may be too unwieldy for many outcome studies. Furthermore, the study described above (10) involved patients with moderate or severe AMD and therefore cannot attest to reliability or validity in patients with mild AMD. A more recently developed 25-item version of the NEI-VFQ may prove to be a more useful outcomes research tool; however, reliability and validity analysis in a large sample of patients with a broad spectrum of AMD severity has yet to be reported.

B. Activities of Daily Vision Scale

The ADVS consists of 21 multiple-choice items designed to assess visual functioning along five subscales: night driving, daytime driving, distance vision activities that do not require driving, near vision activities, and activities subject to glare (25). Although originally developed to assess visual functioning following cataract surgery (26), the instrument has been validated for other visual diseases including glaucoma (27) and diabetic retinopathy (28). The ADVS has been recently applied to the study of visual functioning in patients with AMD (11). AMD severity was found to be associated with lower levels of reported visual functioning, particularly for near vision and driving activities. However, the correlation between AMD severity and the ADVS disappeared after adjusting for visual acuity. This may suggest that central acuity adequately captured patients' reported level of visual functioning. Alternatively, this lack of independent correlation between ADVS and AMD severity may have been a result of the small number of patients with severe AMD or unique features of the ADVS questionnaire or the AMD severity grading scale used in the study.

C.   The Visual Function 14

The VF-14 was developed by Steinberg et al. (29). It is an index of visual function that was designed to assess patients undergoing cataract surgery (30–32). The focus of the VF-14 on common activities of daily living has made it applicable to a range of ophthalmological patients, including corneal disease (33) and glaucoma patients (34). It has also been translated for use in other languages (35). The succinct format of the VF-14 has made it a popular choice owing to its ease of administration and high rate of patient compliance. Its use of a single domain of vision as a "composite measure of functional disability attributable to visual impairment" (29) allows for a useful measure of a patient's functional status and comparison among eye diseases. The VF-14 contains 14 questions about the degree of difficulty that is experienced by patients because of their vision in performing vision-related daily activities such as reading, seeing steps, and watching television.

In a previous article, the VF-14 was demonstrated to be a reliable, valid, and sensitive measure of visual function in retinal patients (12). Individuals living with retinal disease were found to perceive significant functional limitations in their daily activities because of their visual function. As AMD is the leading cause of blindness in North American patients over 50 (1–5), we investigated the potential utility of the VF-14 in assessing visual function in 159 patients with this condition (14). In this study we sought to compare VF-14 scores with visual acuity, with the severity of macular pathology, and three patient global self-assessment instruments. The global self-assessment questions required patients to rate the degree of satisfaction with their vision, trouble with vision, and an overall rating of their vision. The use of patient global self-assessment questions for this purpose has been reported previously (29,35–37).

Table 4 illustrates the aspects of visual functioning that are assessed by the VF-14, ranked in order of most difficulty reported by patients with AMD. Patients reported having

Table 4   VF-14 Question Responses Ranked by Percentage Reporting Some Difficulty

Question (# applicable)	Extent of difficulty (%)				
	None	Little	Moderate amount	Great deal	Unable to do
Reading small print (157)	20	23	17	23	17
Doing fine handiwork (145)	30	26	15	15	15
Driving during the night (109)	30	25	15	7	23
Reading a newspaper or book (158)	30	19	16	22	13
Reading signs (158)	44	29	12	10	6
Writing checks/completing forms (153)	49	20	11	12	9
Watching television (156)	50	23	14	12	1
Seeing steps, stairs, curbs (156)	56	26	8	9	0
Reading large-print material (158)	60	15	12	8	6
Playing table games (131)	60	18	9	7	6
Driving during the day (119)	62	13	3	3	18
Cooking (145)	64	16	13	6	1
Sports involvement (96)	65	15	9	2	9
Recognizing people at close distances (156)	72	12	7	8	1

Source: Reprinted with permission from Assessment of vision-related function in patients with age-related macular degeneration. Ophthalmology. In press.

Table 5 Correlations Between VF-14, Weighted Visual Acuity, Clinical Disease Severity, Trouble with Vision, Satisfaction with Vision, and Overall Quality of Vision in Patients with AMD ($n = 159$)

	VF-14 score	Trouble with vision	Satisfaction	Overall vision	AMD severity	WCS score	Weighted visual acuity
VF-14/score							
Trouble with vision	−0.67**						
Satisfaction with vision	0.62**	−0.72**					
Overall quality of vision	0.67**	−0.74**	0.69**				
AMD severity	−0.49**	0.40**	−0.44**	−0.54**			
WCS score	−0.08	0.19*	−0.17	−0.15	0.00		
Weighted visual acuity	−0.69**	0.51**	−0.50**	−0.56**	0.66**	0.03	

WCS, Weighted comorbidity scale.
* $p < 0.05$.
** $p < 0.01$.
Source: Reprinted with permission from Assessment of vision-related function in patients with age-related macular degeneration. Ophthalmology. In press.

the most difficulty with reading small print, doing fine handiwork, and night driving. Patients reported the least impairment with recognizing people at close distances, sports involvement, and cooking. We assessed the validity of the VF-14 in patients with AMD by using the patient global self-assessment questions. Since these scales most directly evaluate subjective degree of impairment, they provide a useful tool in validation studies. In our study we used three global self-assessment questions: patients' reports of trouble with vision, satisfaction with their vision, and overall assessment of their vision on an analog scale (see Table 5). The VF-14 was more highly related than visual acuity to the global self-assessment questions in patients with AMD, and therefore more representative of the amount of trouble and satisfaction patients have with their vision. These data contribute to the validity of the VF-14 as a valid measure of visual function in patients with AMD.

A second method of testing the usefulness of a questionnaire involves the determination of discriminant validity; that is, a construct should not correlate with dissimilar, unrelated variables. Therefore, it was hypothesized that the SF-36, a general QOL instrument that includes functional status questions, would show a weaker correlation to the global self-assessment scales and to visual acuity than would the VF-14 (a vision-specific instrument). Second, it was hypothesized that the SF-36 would show a stronger correlation with nonocular medical comorbidity (measured by the WCS) than would the VF-14. As shown in Table 2, AMD patients demonstrated significant, but weak, correlations between the SF-36 Physical Component Summary (PCS) and the global scales. Correlations between VF-14 score and global scales, by contrast, were considerably stronger (Table 5). Conversely, the correlation between the SF-36 PCS and the Weighted Comorbidity Scale was stronger than the VF-14 correlation with the WCS. Therefore, the discriminant validity of the VF-14 is supported by this study group, providing further strength for the utility of this instrument in patients with AMD.

Table 6   Scoring System for Rating AMD Severity

Exudative changes		Nonexudative changes	
E 0	Nonexudative changes	NE 0	No dry changes
E 1	Drusen (small hard or large soft)	NE 1	Crystalline drusen
E 2	RPE detachment	NE 2	Early geographic atrophy (extra or juxtafoveal)
E 3	Occult CNVM	NE 3	Late geographic atrophy (subfoveal)
E 4	CNVM (type I or II)		
E 5	Diskiform scar		
E 6	SRH (>3 disk diameters)		
Unilateral rating for each eye			
Mild	E 0, E 1, NE 0, NE 1		
Moderate	E 2, E 3, or NE 2		
Moderately severe	E 4		
Very severe	E 5, E 6, or NE 3		
AMD severity (bilateral: better eye/worse eye)			
Grade 1	Mild/mild		
Grade 2	Mild/moderate		
Grade 3	Mild/moderately severe		
Grade 4	Mild/very severe or moderate/moderate		
Grade 5	Moderate/moderately severe		
Grade 6	Moderately severe/moderately severe or moderate/very severe		
Grade 7	Moderately severe/very severe or very severe/very severe		

Source: Reprinted with permission from Assessment of vision-related function in patients with age-related macular degeneration. Ophthalmology. In press.

The VF-14 was correlated with the SF-36 physical composite scale (PCS) but not with the mental composite scale (MCS). This may indicate that one limitation of the VF-14 is that it does not assess the mental aspects of health-related QOL in patients with AMD. Indeed, focus groups used to develop the NEI-VFQ reported mood and mental health problems as the fourth most common type of problem associated with their condition, after reading, driving in daytime, and seeing clearly (24). Furthermore, patients with AMD scored significantly lower than controls on the NEI-VFQ vision-specific mental health subscale (10). However, our data indicated no relationship between SF-36 mental health scores and visual acuity or AMD severity. Furthermore, overall the MCS score distribution had a mean of 50 and a standard deviation of 11, similar to general population norms. These data suggest that the overall mental health of patients with AMD is at or near normal levels; however, these patients may experience vision-specific mental health problems, including issues such as worry about future vision, embarrassment, and loss of control due to visual loss. A comparison of VF-14 with the more detailed NEI-VFQ on the same population of patients with AMD would be informative as to whether the NEI-VFQ is able to account for a greater amount of variance in reported visual functioning. Other factors, for example, rate of progression of visual loss, the degree of disparity in visual functioning between the eyes, and the use of low-vision services, may also play significant roles in how patients approach their visual disability.

The clinical severity of AMD was graded from patient charts on a seven-point scale as shown in Table 6. A severity of one indicated mild AMD in one or both eyes, and a severity of seven indicated severe AMD in both eyes. As with visual acuity, VF-14 scores were significantly negatively correlated with the severity of AMD, indicating that reported visual functioning on the VF-14 decreased as clinical AMD severity increased. However, clinical AMD severity was not a significant predictor of VF-14 score independently of visual acuity. These results were therefore similar to the study by Mangione et al. using the ADVS (11) despite several differences in study methodology as follows. First, the patient database in our group included a greater number of patients with moderate and severe AMD. Second, Mangione et al. used the 21-item activities of daily vision scale (ADVS) whereas our study employed the VF-14. Third, AMD severity was rated according to different criteria in the two studies. In the study by Mangione et al. the classification system placed emphasis on differentiation between stages of nonexudative AMD. All changes of exudative AMD were grouped into one category. In contrast, our classification system was developed to highlight changes that occur in patients with exudative disease. These studies together suggest that visual acuity captures a large proportion of the deficits in visual functioning associated with AMD. However, as 54% of the variance in VF-14 scores was accounted for in the linear regression, other factors not included in the current study account for a significant proportion of reported visual functioning deficits.

In our study, AMD severity predicted VF-14 scores independently of visual acuity in the worse eye in 51 patients with 20/20 vision in one eye. Thus, in patients with 20/20 vision in the better eye, the unilateral presence of AMD significantly impairs reported visual functioning beyond what is accounted for by worse-eye vision. This impairment could be related to the effect of the loss of binocularity, contrast sensitivity, or another component of vision beyond acuity. A further possible explanation for the effect of unilateral AMD on reported visual functioning may involve the experience of having AMD unilaterally. Worry about the loss of vision in the better eye may play a role in how patients perceive their current visual functioning. Another possible explanation of these data is that the difference in vision between the two eyes, which is larger in patients with unilateral AMD, may be an important factor in patients' perceptions of their functioning. A recent study from Hart et al. (38) lends support to the latter interpretation. They reported on a 22-item visual-functioning questionnaire that was developed in Britain specifically for patients with AMD, termed the Daily Living Tasks Dependent on Vision (DLTV). In their study, although visual acuity predicted a large proportion of visual functioning, the difference in vision between the two eyes significantly contributed to the total variation in DLTV scores. Interestingly, the DLTV does not include questions about driving ability or sports participation, but does probe other activities, including enjoyment of scenery if out for a drive, pouring a drink, and the ability to cut food on a plate. A comparison of the DLTV with the VF-14 would identify whether such questions would further increase the validity of the VF-14.

IV. SUMMARY

The validation of VRQOL instruments serves several purposes. First, comparisons can be made between the level of functioning in patients with different eye diseases. For example, patients with AMD have been recently reported to experience greater trouble with their vision-related activities than patients with cataract for a given level of visual acuity (38). With better understanding of the utility of VRQOL instruments in patients with AMD it is hoped that more will be learned about the subjective changes in visual perception not accounted for by Snellen acuity. As VRQOL instruments gain greater familiarity and acceptance they will likely play a larger role as outcome measures for randomized clinical trials.

In particular with clinical trials that report "stabilization of visual acuity" as a primary outcome measure, secondary measures such as VRQOL outcomes may help to determine optimal treatment for patients with AMD.

REFERENCES

1. Ferris FL. Senile macular degeneration: review of epidemiologic features. Am J Epidemiol 1983;118:132–151.
2. Ferris FL, Fine SL, Hyman LG. Age-related macular degeneration and blindness due to neovascular maculopathy. Arch Ophthalmol 1984;102:1640–1642
3. Leibowitz HM, Krueger DE, Maunder LR, Mi Hon RC, Kini MM, Kahn HA, Nickerson RJ, Pool J, Colton TL, Ganley JP, Loewenstein JI, Dawber TK. The Framingham Eye Study Monograph. Surv Ophthalmol 1980;24(Suppl):335–610.
4. Klein R, Klein BEK, Linton KLP. Prevalence of age-related maculopathy: the Beaver Dam eye study. Ophthalmology 1992;99:933–943.
5. Tielsch JM, Javitt JC, Coleman A, Katz J, Sommer A. The prevalence of blindness and visual impairment among nursing home residents in Baltimore. N Engl J Med 1995; 332:1205–1209.
6. Brown GC, Brown MM, Sharma S. Difference between ophthalmologists' and patients' perceptions of quality of life associated with age-related macular degeneration. Can J Ophthalmol 2000;35:127–133.
7. Ware JE Jr, Sherbourne CD. The MOS 36-item short-form health survey (SF-36), I. Conceptual framework and item selection. Med Care 1992;30:473–483.
8. McHorney CA, Ware JE Jr, Raczek AE. The MOS 36-item short-form health survey (SF-36), II: psychometric and clinical tests of validity in measuring physical and mental health constructs. Med Care 1993;31:247–263.
9. McHorney CA, Ware JE Jr, Lu JFR, Sherbourne CD. The MOS 36-item short-form health survey (SF-36), III: tests of data quality, scaling assumptions, and reliability across diverse patient groups. Med Care 1994;32:40–66.
10. Mangione CM. Lee PP. Pitts J. Gutierrez P. Berry S. Hays RD. Psychometric properties of the National Eye Institute Visual Function Questionnaire (NEI-VFQ). NEI-VFQ Field Test Investigators. Arch Ophthalmol 1998;116(11):1496–1504.
11. Mangione CM, Gutierrez, MA, Lowe G, Orav EJ, Seddon JM. Influence of age-related maculopathy on visual functioning and health-related quality of life. Am J Ophthalmol 1999;128:45–53.
12. Linder M, Chang TS, Scott IU, et al. Validity of the visual function index (VF-14) in patients with retinal disease. Arch Ophthalmol 1999;117:1611–1616.
13. Scott IU, Schein OD, West S, Bandeen-Roche K, Enger C, Folstein MF. Functional status and quality of life measurement among ophthalmic patients. Arch Ophthalmol 1994;112:329–335.
14. Mackenzie PJ, Chang TS, Scott IU, Linder M, Hay D, Feuer WJ, Chambers K. Assessment of vision-related function in patients with age-related macular degeneration. Ophthalmology. In press.
15. Ware JE, Snow KK, Kosinski M, Gandek V. SF-36 Health Survey Manual and Interpretation Guide. Boston: The Health Institute, New England Medical Center, 1993.
16. Nilsson UL. Visual rehabilitation of patients with advanced diabetic retinopathy: a follow-up study at the Low Vision Clinic, Department of Ophthalmology, University of Linkoping. Doc Ophthalmol 1986;62:369–382.
17. Wetzler HP, Radosevich DM. Health status questionnaire (SF-36) technical report. Interstudy 1992.
18. Thalji L, Haggerty CC, Rubin R. 1990 national survey of functional health status: final report. Chicago: National Opinion Research Center, 1991.
19. Hopman WM, Towheed T, Anastassiades T, et al. Canadian normative data for the SF-36 health survey. Can Med Assoc J 2000;163:265–271.

20. Ware JE Jr, Kosinski M, Keller SD. SF-12: how to score the SF-12 physical and mental health summary scales. The Health Institute, New England Medical Center, Boston, 1995.
21. Livingstone MS, Rosen GD, Drislane FW, Galaburda AM. Physiological and anatomical evidence for a magnocellular defect in developmental dyslexia. Proc Natl Acad Sci USA 1991;88:7943–7947.
22. Alexander MF, Maguire MG, Lietman TM, et al. Assessment of visual function in patients with age-related macular degeneration and low visual acuity. Arch Ophthalmol 1988;106:1543–1547.
23. Hazel CA, Petre KL, Armstrong RA, et al. Visual function and subjective quality of life compared in subjects with acquired macular disease. IOVS 2000;41:1309–1315.
24. Mangione CM, Berry S, Spritzer K, Janz NK, Klein R, Owsley C, Lee PP. Identifying the content area for the 51-item National Eye Institute Visual Function Questionnaire. Arch Ophthalmol 1998;116:227–233.
25. Mangione CM. Phillips RS. Seddon JM. Lawrence MG. Cook EF. Dailey R. Goldman L. Development of the "Activities of Daily Vision Scale." A measure of visual functional status. Med Care 1992;30:1111–1126.
26. Mangione CM. Phillips RS. Lawrence MG. Seddon JM. Orav EJ. Goldman L. Improved visual function and attenuation of declines in health-related quality of life after cataract extraction. Arch Ophthalmol 1994;112:1419–1425.
27. Sherwood MB, Garcia-Siekavizza A, Meltzer MI, Hebert A, Burns AF, McGorray S. Glaucoma's impact on quality of life and its relation to clinical indicators: a pilot study. Ophthalmology 1998;105:561–566.
28. Lee PP, Whitcup WM, Hays RD, Spritzer K, Javitt J. The relationship between visual acuity and functioning and well-being among diabetics. Qual Life Res 1995;4:319–323.
29. Steinberg EP, Tielsch JM, Schein OD, Javitt JC, Sharkey P, Cassard SD, Legro MW, Diener-West M, Bass ED, Damiano AM. The VF-14: an index of functional impairment in cataract patients. Arch Ophthalmol 1994;112:630–638.
30. Steinberg P, Tielsch JM, Schein OD, Javitt JC, Sharkey P, Cassard SD, Legro MW, Diener-West M, Bass EB, Damiano AM. National study of cataract surgery outcomes. Variation in 4-month postoperative outcomes as reflected in multiple outcome measures. Ophthalmology 1994;101:1131–1140.
31. Cassard SD, Patrick DL, Damiano AM, Legro MW, Tielsch JM, Diener-West M, Schein OD, Javitt JC, Bass EB, Steinberg EP. Reproducibility and responsiveness of the VF-14: an index of functional impairment in cataract patients. Arch Ophthalmol 1994;112:630–638.
32. Desai P, Reidy A, Minassian DC, Vafidis G Bolger J. Gains from cataract surgery: visual function and quality of life. Br J Ophthalmol 1996;80:868–873.
33. Courtright P, Poon CI, Richards JSF, Chow DL. Visual function amoung corneal disease patients waiting for penetrating keratoplasty in British Columbia. Ophthalmol Epidemiol 1998;5:13–20.
34. Lee BL, Gutierrez P, Gordon M, Wilson MR, Cioffi GA, Ritch R, Sherwood M, Mangione CM. The Glaucoma Symptom Scale. A brief index of glaucoma-specific symptoms. Arch Ophthalmol. 1998;116;861–866.
35. Gresset J, Boisjoly H, Nguyen TQ, Boutin J, Charest M. Validation of French-language versions of the Visual Functioning Index (VF-14) and the Cataract Symptom Score. Can J Ophthalmol 1997;32:31–37.
36. Scott IU, Smiddy WE, Feuer W, Merikansky A. Vitreoretinal surgery outcomes: results of patient satisfaction/functional status survey. Ophthalmology 1998;105:795–803.
37. Damiano AM, Steinberg, EP, Cassard SD, Bass EB, Diener-West M, Tielsch J, Schein OD, Javitt J, Kolb M. Comparison of generic versus disease-specific measures of functional impairment in patients with cataract. Med Care 1995;33 (Suppl 4):AS120–AS130.
38. Hart PM, Chakravarthy U, Stevenson MR, Javison JQ. A vision specific functional index for use in patients with age related macular degeneration. Br J Ophthalmol 1999;83:1115–1120.

27
Clinical Research Trials

A. Frances Walonker and Rohit Varma

Doheny Eye Institute, University of Southern California Keck School of Medicine, Los Angeles, California

I. INTRODUCTION

A. Historical Review

Of the estimated 34.8 million people in the United States who were 65 years of age or older in 2000, approximately 1.2 million had some form of visual impairment associated with age-related macular degeneration (AMD). Approximately 200,000 of these will have experienced a rapid, devastating loss of vision due to choroidal neovascularization (CNV), whereas the remaining 1.0 million may experience a slow, progressive retinal atrophy and possibly a severe visual handicap (1). Most may have difficulty performing routine visual tasks, such as driving, reading printed material, or recognizing the faces of their friends.

As the U.S. population continues to age, more and more persons will become visually impaired from AMD—more, in fact, than from any other eye disease. In AMD with CNV, decreased vision results from scarring in the macular region. The scarring is caused by the ingrowth of abnormal blood vessels from the choriocapillaris through breaks in Bruch's membrane. Clinical research shows that laser treatment can reduce the risk of extensive scarring in selected cases of "classic" or well-defined AMD. However, these effects last for only 1–2 years in at least half of the patients treated because neovascularization recurs on the foveal edge of the laser scar, with subsequent foveal scarring and severe visual loss (2).

Laser photocoagulation has not been shown to be effective in more than 75% of those patients who are at risk of going blind from CNV. Many of these patients may develop scarring caused by "occult" or "poorly defined" choroidal neovascularization that often progresses to severe visual loss.

Because a large number of individuals have AMD complicated by CNV, effective treatment of even 25% of all cases (2) can lead to significant savings to society and can decrease the number of people requiring Social Security and other disability payments (not to mention the effects on patients' dignity and independence), with savings far outweighing the costs of clinical research, management, and treatment.

In the past, the National Eye Institute has funded investigator-initiated grants that looked at such topics as the aging retina, cone photopigments, and the effect of light or chemical factors on the integrity of the photoreceptor/retinal pigment epithelial complex. The first randomized clinical research study that looked at the treatment of macular degeneration was the Macular Photocoagulation Study (MPS).

1. The Macular Photocoagulation Study (MPS)

The MPS Group published its first reports in 1982. The studies evaluated the usefulness of laser photocoagulation in the treatment of macular degeneration. These studies showed that laser treatment reduced the risk of severe visual loss in eyes with extrafoveal choroidal neovascular membranes secondary to macular degeneration [confluent laser treatment for well-defined, classic, choroidal neovascularization in which the posterior edge of the neovascularization was at least 1 mm from the foveal center (2)]. Subsequent studies evaluating photocoagulation for presumed ocular histoplasmosis (3) and idiopathic neovascularization (4) came to the same conclusion: the photocoagulation effectively treated extrafoveal membranes.

However, long-term follow-up revealed that extrafoveal choroidal neovascularization recurred in a high proportion of the patients. These findings were corroborated by investigators in other countries. It appeared that nearly 75% of these recurrences occurred within the first year. This led investigators to hope that if no recurrence occurred in the first year, the possibility of new neovascularization was low (5).

In the past 18 years, the search for a more long-lasting cure for macular degeneration with choroidal neovascularization has led to many different approaches. Treatments studied have included photodynamic therapy, submacular surgery, external-beam radiation, medications such as interferon and thalidomide, and various oral supplements that are believed to be preventive. At present, a number of randomized clinical research trials are looking at various therapies for macular degeneration. Basic scientists are working hand in hand with clinicians to find a cure for this blinding disease.

B. Clinical Relevance

Prior to the (MPS) Macular Photocoagulation Study, there was no proven treatment for AMD with CNV. The use of low-vision aids and mobility training were recommended but little could be done other than observe the natural history of AMD with CNV. The MPS showed that laser photocoagulation of AMD with CNV prevented the most severe types of vision loss, compared to no treatment. The study was also important as a natural-history study of macular degeneration (2). Since the 1980s this randomized controlled clinical trial has served as a benchmark for AMD research, against which other treatment trials can be measured.

II. CLINICAL RESEARCH METHODOLOGY

The path a new idea takes from the patient's problem to the basic research laboratory to the clinical research center and ultimately back to the treatment of the patient in the clinical setting is extensive and expensive. The final research question can be answered and practice guidelines established, but the cost in time commitment and dollars is great.

The pathway from the patient and back again to the patient starts when the ophthalmologist sees a patient with a disease that either has no cure or would benefit from an improved treatment. Case-series studies, in which an investigator has noted some interesting or intriguing observation, frequently lead to the generation of a hypothesis that will subsequently be investigated. The ophthalmologist then teams up with the basic scientist to address this problem. Together, they design appropriate laboratory research to address the question. Results from these basic science studies lead to preliminary clinical investigations of a possible new diagnostic technique, a treatment, or a drug. A small group of carefully selected patients participate in a pilot study to study the safety of these new treatments. If successful, such a pilot study generates a single-center clinical trial to further evaluate the safety and efficacy of the treatments.

Subsequently a full-scale, multicenter, randomized clinical research trial is initiated to recruit enough patients to prove the safety and the efficacy of the new procedure, operation, test, or drug. These new approaches are tested for their effects on the quality of life of patients with the initial disease.

The randomized clinical research trial is the gold standard, or reference, in medicine as it provides the greatest justification for concluding causality and is subject to the least number of problems or biases. Clinical trials are the best type of study to use when the objective is to establish efficacy of a treatment or a procedure. Clinical trials in which patients are randomly assigned to different treatments are the strongest design of all.

These innovative approaches to clinical practice are then taught to other ophthalmologists through continuing medical education courses, publications in peer review journals, and presentations at national and international scientific meetings. Finally, the new techniques, medications, or test materials are available to all patients under standard practice guidelines for diagnosis and treatment for disease.

This path from clinical problem to clinical cure, from an idea in the clinic to the research laboratory, and finally back to the patient in the clinic is difficult, challenging, and expensive. Yet the future of maintaining healthy eyes and vision for all of us depends on the success of this vision research process.

A. Design of a Clinical Research Trial

The initial step in determining whether a research proposal would fulfill all the ethical and investigational guidelines necessary to protect human subjects involved in a clinical research trial is to go through a formal decision-making process. After all the data from previous observational, basic laboratory (in vitro and animal studies), case report studies, Phase I, and Phase II studies have been analyzed, a protocol is established under which the trial will be conducted. A manual of procedures is developed outlining every detail of the research study so that every participant in the study is aware of the protocol detail and is able to follow this protocol without deviation, maintaining the standardization of testing and of any other procedure. These steps are as follows.

1. The Rationale

The ophthalmologist will team up with a basic science researcher or will work in his/her own laboratory to design a series of experiments that may address a specific problem. The results of these experiments, done again and again and replicated in other laboratories, may suggest an intervention or therapy that would be tested on some laboratory animal under the strict guidelines of a research laboratory. The results would be the basis for a limited trial on a small group of carefully selected patients. If these patients reacted well to the therapy, the next phase would be a single-clinical-center study, a pilot study, of patients with a specific disease.

This is the initial stage of the research trial. All the data from prior studies are then analyzed along with any new information, and the rationale for conducting this particular study is outlined. The objectives of the study, the safety and efficacy of the treatment, and the experimental plan, including the design, are then detailed.

2. The Protocol

The protocol for the study will include:

> Background of the disease to be studied and the results of all previous related research, both basic science and clinical; all information to support the justification of this research project and the impact it will have on the population in general and the population with this specific disease entity; the expected benefits to be obtained from the study.
>
> Subject selection criteria with the inclusion and exclusion criteria with justification for both. Justification for or against inclusion/exclusion of vulnerable subjects.
>
> Discussion of the appropriateness of the research methods and statistical justification for the chosen sample size with the statistical method of analysis explained.
>
> Provisions for managing any adverse reaction.
>
> Detailed description of the procedures to be performed with the frequency of these procedures outlined and the time commitment of the patient explained.

3. The Informed Consent

Before any research trial that includes human subjects can be instituted, an Institutional Review Board (IRB) must approve all the components of the trial. The responsibility of an IRB is to establish the requirements and procedures for requests for the performance of human research, development, demonstration, or other activities involving patients or patient products, outside the scope of established and accepted methods. The IRB monitors approved research in accordance with the requirements of the Office of Protection from Research Risks (OPRR) and the regulations of the Food and Drug Administration (FDA), National Institutes of Health (NIH) and Department of Health and Human Services (DHHS). The IRB uses a group process to review research protocols and related material, e.g., informed consent documents and investigator brochures, to ensure the following:

> Risks to human subjects are minimized by using procedures that are consistent with sound research design and that do not unnecessarily expose subjects to risk. Whenever appropriate, such procedures already will have been performed on subjects for diagnostic or therapeutic purposes.
>
> Risks to subjects are reasonable in relation to the anticipated benefits (if any) to the subjects and the importance of the knowledge that may be expected from the result.
>
> The selection of the subjects is equitable; i.e., the study subjects are of both genders and from different racial/ethnic groups, and no age limitations exist other than those associated with a disease entity.
>
> Informed consent will be sought from each prospective subject or the subject's legally authorized representative and will be documented in accordance with and to the extent required by informed consent regulations.

Where appropriate, the research plan makes adequate provision for monitoring the data collected to ensure the safety of subjects.

Adequate provisions are in place to protect the privacy of the subjects and to maintain confidentiality of the data.

Appropriate additional safeguards have been included in the study to protect the rights and welfare of subjects who are members of a vulnerable group.

The IRB has the authority to disapprove, modify, or approve studies based on consideration of human subject protection aspects. It also has the authority to suspend or terminate a study, to place restrictions on a study, and to require progress reports and oversee, the conduct of the study.

The informed consent the patient will sign before entering into a clinical research trial will also include the length of the patient's participation, the alternatives to this treatment modality, the risks involved in this trial, and a statement allowing the patients to withdraw from the trial at any time without consequence.

4. The Manual of Procedures

The manual of procedures for the clinical research study is divided into several sections. Each section covers in detail a different component of the study.

The background of the research design.
Directory of personnel/committees
The research plan

1. Objectives
2. Treatment groups: control versus treatment
3. Outcome variables
4. Eligibility and exclusion criteria
5. Randomization
6. Statistical consideration

Examination descriptions and schedules

1. Screening evaluation
2. Baseline visits
3. Follow-up visits
4. Study visit windows
5. Missed visit and inactive patient considerations

Examination procedures

1. List of examination procedures
2. Equipment and facilities
3. Refraction protocol
4. Visual acuity protocol
5. Intraocular pressure protocol
6. Ophthalmic examination protocol
7. Other testing protocols as appropriate for a particular trial

Ancillary testing protocols

1. Performance
2. Labeling/processing

Surgical protocols

1. Description of the surgical procedures/laser procedures
2. Description of the postoperative medications to be used

Certification of personnel

1. Detailed description of the performance required for each role in the trial
2. Performance evaluation methods
3. Certification procedures
4. Importance of standardization

Data collection

1. Patient identification/name codes
2. Case report forms
3. Mailing instructions
4. Procedures for tracing patients
5. Reports on adverse events
6. Edit queries
7. Monitoring visits/data collection corroboration

Data safety and monitoring

1. Functions of the committee
2. Frequency of meeting
3. Endpoints

Statistics

1. Detail of the statistical methods used
2. Justification of the patient sample size chosen
3. Randomization process and justification

B. Settings for Research Trials

Advancing medical knowledge—through screening, surgery, and pharmaceutical intervention—has prolonged the life of many people with disabling chronic disease conditions and increased the number of survivors of traumatic injury. At the present, 13% of the population is over the age of 65; by the year 2040, this number will have grown to 23% of the population (7). By 2040, 70 million people will have some form of activity limitation, whether mental, physical, or visual, that will require intervention from the health care systems in some form. Research into the most effective care for persons with chronic disease, including eye disorders in particular, and efforts at prevention will be at the forefront of future clinical research. The projected cost of health care in the year 2040 is $906 billion, a huge percentage of the GNP of the United States and the highest of the entire world's developed countries (7).

With such huge expenditures anticipated for health care, and in response to continued pressure by government regulatory agencies to drive down costs, evaluation of cost in conducting research is suggested. Researchers must include cost research objectives, such as costs associated with screening programs, alternative treatments and procedures, use of new technology, and implementation of new regulatory measures associated with programs and trials. The results obtained from including cost analysis in research help health care decision makers weigh the costs and consequences of competing treatment alternatives. Cost information provides additional data that can supplement clinical judgment when making therapeutic choices. Therefore, clinicians and researchers at major academic institutions need to focus on advancing the care and prevention of eye disease. Efforts should be based on rigorous clinical methods, i.e., randomized controlled clinical trials and analysis of economic and humanistic outcomes. With research of this nature, the results can be applied directly to the patient, where they will accomplish the greatest good. This is especially true when these outcomes may mean the difference between sight and blindness, and when they impact on the outcome measures of quality of life and, ultimately, life expectancy.

C. Limitation of Randomized Clinical Trials

The cost of developing the necessary infrastructure to support the scientific and clinical activities involved in conducting major national and international clinical research makes it prohibitive except for large academic ophthalmology centers.

Most major academic ophthalmology centers involved in clinical and basic science research are referral centers for patients with complicated disease who have not responded to standard therapy or who have a disease with no known cure. This population would comprise the carefully selected patients who could be enrolled in a clinical research trial to address the safety and efficacy of a new treatment approach. However, because of the nature of this population, i.e., those with severe disease as well as those with rare and complicated disease, the numbers of patients who would be eligible to enter a clinical research trial would be limited, making recruitment difficult. This places a potential for selection bias on these clinical research studies, such that when the studies are completed, they may not translate to the population in general.

On the other hand, a more common disease entity, such as macular degeneration, with its potential for marked vision loss if untreated, offers access to more subjects for inclusion in a clinical trial. These patients are seen routinely in the private-practice ophthalmologist's office and may now be involved in limited clinical research. The disadvantage to academic institutions that have invested in the development of an infrastructure to rigorously support all basic and clinical research is that they no longer have access to this large patient population. The disadvantage to the patient may be that the strict protocol that is the hallmark of academic institutional research may not be adhered to so rigorously in a community where that infrastructure is not present.

Another limitation is access to the underserved—those people who have no access to health care providers, because of either lack of insurance or distance from those same providers. These patients are likely to postpone needed care until their conditions have escalated in severity. This group would have no representation in the clinical research arena; the subsequent lack of diversity in the research population may result in possible bias.

The tremendous increases in new technology have not been accompanied by changes in the evaluation of new approaches. As a result, new approaches become established that may harm many patients, and researchers may have difficulty obtaining approval to perform properly designed clinical trials from the human subjects committees that oversee the ethics of research because of the presumed standard of practice that is present in the field.

III. RESEARCH STAFF AND DOCUMENTATION

The goal of all clinical research is to provide information that will help the practitioner treat his or her patients more effectively. The clinical trial provides the best means to quantify and compare objectively the benefits and risks of new or alternative treatments for disease, especially when the difference between a new or old treatment is not clear or when a large number of factors may influence the course of the disease or the outcomes of the treatment (6). To ensure that the treatment groups are compared objectively, standardized methods of gathering data, training and certifying the personnel who collect the data, and treating patients either surgically or pharmaceutically are imperative. Continuous monitoring of adherence to protocol, accumulating data in a uniform way, and recertifying personnel on a frequent basis will eliminate any concerns of bias or ambiguity when the data are presented. All data accumulated on a case report form, the form that is submitted to a central data collection agency, must be documented in the patient file and these two documents must be reconciled at all times. All clinical research studies are monitored at regular intervals to ensure that all information is recorded on all the legal documents and that no data are missing or unsubstantiated. The success of all clinical research is totally dependent on this accurate and standardized collection of data and strict adherence to the protocols (8).

IV. SUMMARY

MPS was the first clinical study to look at macular degeneration The aging population numbers 34.8 million with 1.2 million having some form of visual impairment.

Clinical research is the best means to quantify and objectively compare the benefits and risks of new or alternative treatments for disease or injury especially when:

1. The difference between a new or old treatment is not clear.
2. The disease naturally follows a chronic, variable, and erratic course.
3. A large number of factors, known or unknown, may influence both the course of the disease and the outcome of the treatment.

A well-designed and well-conducted randomized clinical trial incorporates the following:

1. High ethical standards—of paramount importance are patient welfare, informed consent, adherence to protocol, and careful data monitoring.
2. Control groups that match treatment groups.
3. Random assignment of patients to both study and control groups when comparability of results among groups is essential.
4. Masking to minimize bias of both the examiner and the patient, if possible.
5. Enrollment of an adequate number of patients enrolled in the trial for the results to be statistically significant.
6. Completeness of patient follow-up.
7. Use of statistical methods for data analysis.
8. Continuous monitoring of adherence to protocol and accumulation of data by the Data Safety Monitoring Committee (DSMC), the study Advisory Committee, the Executive Committee, and the Steering Committee to ensure the safety of the subjects involved in the trial (8).

REFERENCES

1. A profile of older Americans. Administration on Aging (AoA), U.S. Department of Health and Human Services, 2000.
2. Macular Photocoagulation Study Group. Argon laser photocoagulation for senile macular degeneration. Results of a randomized clinical trial. Arch Ophthalmol 1982;100:912–918.
3. Macular Photocoagulation Study Group. Argon laser photocoagulation for ocular histoplasmosis. Results of a randomized clinical trial. Arch Ophthalmol 1983;101:1347–1357.
4. Macular Photocoagulation Study Group. Argon laser photocoagulation for idiopathic neovascularization. Results of a randomized clinical trial. Arch Ophthalmol 1983;101:1358–1361.
5. Macular Photocoagulation Study Group. Recurrent choroidal neovascularization after argon laser treatment for neovascular maculopathy: Arch Ophthalmol 1986;104:503–512.
6. Walonker A F, Sturrock D. The Ryan Leopold Beckman Center for Clinical Research, Masters thesis, School of Public Health, UCLA, 1999.
7. Chronic Care in America. A 21st Century Challenge. Prepared by the Institute for Health and Aging, University of California, San Francisco for the Robert Wood Johnson Foundation, Princeton, NJ, August 1996.
8. Clinical trials supported by the National Eye Institute, U.S. Department of Health and Human Services, 1987.

Index